Anatomy and Physiology for
MIDWIVES

Anatomy and Physiology for
MIDWIVES

Fourth Edition

Jane Coad BSc PhD PGCEA
Professor in Nutrition, Massey University,
Palmerston North, New Zealand

and

Kevin Pedley BSc DPhil
Associate Professor in Physiology, Massey University,
Palmerston North, New Zealand

with

Melvyn Dunstall BSc MSc PGCEA RM RGN
Formerly Deputy Research & Development Manager, Lead Midwife for
Research, Frimley Health NHS Foundation Trust, Surrey, UK

ELSEVIER   Edinburgh   London   New York   Oxford   Philadelphia   St Louis   Sydney 2020

First edition 2001
Second edition 2005
Third edition 2011
Fourth edition 2020

The right of Jane Coad, Kevin Pedley and Melvyn Dunstall to be identified as authors of this work has been asserted by them in accordance with the Copyright, Designs and Patents Act 1988.

Notices

Practitioners and researchers must always rely on their own experience and knowledge in evaluating and using any information, methods, compounds or experiments described herein. Because of rapid advances in the medical sciences, in particular, independent verification of diagnoses and drug dosages should be made. To the fullest extent of the law, no responsibility is assumed by Elsevier, authors, editors or contributors for any injury and/or damage to persons or property as a matter of products liability, negligence or otherwise, or from any use or operation of any methods, products, instructions, or ideas contained in the material herein.

ISBN: 978-0-7020-6668-9

Content Strategist: Alison Taylor
Senior Content Development Specialist: Helen Leng
Project Manager: Joanna Souch
Design: Margaret Reid
Illustration Manager: Muthukumaran Thangaraj
Illustrator: Robert Britton
Marketing Manager: Kristen Oyirifi

Printed in India

Last digit is the print number: 9 8 7 6 5

Working together
to grow libraries in
developing countries

www.elsevier.com • www.bookaid.org

CONTENTS

PREFACE

Many of the most magical and fascinating aspects of physiology are associated with reproduction, from before conception, through fetal development and the maternal responses to the growing fetus, to the signalling and progression of labour, continued development of the neonate, optimized by maternal behaviour and lactation and the mother's subsequent return to fertility. Reproductive physiology continues to be a fast-moving field, as recent advances in fertility treatment, postnatal care of premature infants, and the impact of the gestational environment and early nutrition on later health, make evident.

Midwives are expected to understand in depth, the science underpinning midwifery practice but have often had little background in this exciting field. Midwives also often find themselves to be bombarded with questions from interested, fascinated and increasingly well-informed prospective parents due to information (and misinformation) readily available via the Internet. This book aims to support midwifery and physiology students and practising midwives wanting more detailed scientific knowledge that can be applied within the practice setting.

The book provides a thorough review of anatomy and physiology applicable to midwifery and reproductive physiology from first principles through to current research. It acknowledges the importance of the research base and aims to integrate theory and practice.

The chapters are organized such that learning objectives lead into the body of the chapter. Case studies illustrate some of the theoretical aspects and provide the reader with the opportunity to reflect on the implications for practice. Wherever possible, information is supported by illustrations. At the end of each chapter, key points are provided and the applications of the scientific content to clinical practice are summarized. Each chapter is comprehensively referenced and has a list of annotated recommendations for further reading.

Chapter 1 begins by introducing the reader to the basic unit of structure, the cell, and describes the relationship between cellular structure and function. It provides an introduction to the major tissue types and physiological systems found within the body and reviews the principles of regulation and maintenance of homeostatic systems.

Chapter 2 focuses on the reproductive and urinary systems of the human. The basic anatomy and physiology of the urinary system are explored in the first part of this chapter. The female reproductive tract and the organs associated with it are then described, relating both their structure and function specifically to childbirth. The last part of this chapter focuses on the male reproductive organs and the process of spermatogenesis.

Chapter 3 introduces the principles of endocrinology, laying the foundation for understanding the changes that occur in pregnancy. It describes the different types of hormones, how and where they are produced, and their modes of action.

Chapter 4 covers the endocrine control and regulation of reproductive cycles. Ovarian function and follicular development lead on to gamete formation in the female and consideration is given as to why this is so dramatically different to spermatogenesis in the male. One of the essential roles of reproductive cycles is the coordination of oogenesis and the cyclical changes within the endometrium that are necessary to optimize fertilization and implantation. Thus, the menstrual cycle is described in depth in this chapter. Some of the hormonal causes of infertility are discussed, as is the use of endocrine manipulation to achieve or prevent contraception. The chapter concludes with brief descriptions of the physiological changes at puberty and menopause.

Chapter 5 integrates the concepts introduced in the first four chapters by focusing on how sexual differentiation is achieved and examines the biological basis for the differences in reproductive physiology and behaviour in women and men.

Chapter 6 describes fertilization, very early development and implantation of the zygote and the maternal physiological responses that allow successful fertilization and implantation. The principles and techniques used in assisted reproductive technologies (ART) are briefly described.

Chapter 7 introduces the basic concepts of genetics, highlighting an essential component of the human reproductive strategy in how genetic mixing and thus variation within the species are achieved. An introduction to the aetiology and types of genetic disease and approaches used in genetic testing and screening are also included.

Chapter 8 presents the development and function of the placenta and its interaction with maternal physiology. It also discusses some of the causes and effects of placental pathology.

Chapter 9 provides a comprehensive overview of the development of the embryo and its physiological systems.

The factors that promote and influence fetal growth are also discussed in this chapter.

Chapter 10 brings the reader back to maternal physiology, by introducing and giving an overview of immunological issues and principles related to pregnancy. The maternal acceptance of the fetus and its implications are discussed, as are the effects of pregnancy upon the maternal immune system. A section is included on the interaction of the maternal and fetal immune systems, using some clinical conditions as examples of these interactions. The neonate's vulnerability to infection is described in relation to midwifery care, together with the principles of immunization. Finally, the specific effects of the human immunodeficiency virus (HIV) and the influenza virus in pregnancy are considered.

Chapter 11 explores one of the most striking aspects of reproductive physiology; the extent and speed of the physiological changes that occur within the pregnant female and why these changes occur and how they are orchestrated in order to facilitate an optimal outcome of pregnancy. These changes are related to how the woman experiences pregnancy and the signs, symptoms and discomforts she might encounter.

Chapter 12 provides a brief overview of nutrition and the nutritional requirements in pregnancy. This lays the basis for exploring how maternal nutrition and health can influence pregnancy outcomes not only for the mother but also for the fetus, both *in utero* and throughout life.

Chapter 13 specifically explores the physiology of parturition and how maternal physiology is altered to facilitate this. Current theories and evidence relating to the timing and initiation of labour in humans are discussed. An overview is provided of pain physiology related to labour and how this is affected by pain-relieving interventions. This chapter includes a section that explores the effects of labour upon fetal physiology.

Chapter 14 discusses how, following birth, the physiological changes that occur during pregnancy are dramatically and efficiently reversed in the puerperium. This period of maternal recovery is often overlooked but is a vulnerable time for maternal morbidity and mortality.

Chapter 15 focuses on the transition to neonatal life, including how these changes are assessed.

Chapter 16 highlights the physiology of lactation and how this meets the unique requirements of the neonate, not only from a nutritional perspective but also from an immunological and developmental basis. It is essential that midwives understand the physiological aspects of lactation in order to promote breastfeeding, as the evidence is overwhelming that successful breastfeeding positively influences the health and well-being, both physically and mentally, of the infant for the rest of its life.

The demand for this book came primarily from our midwifery students, including preregistration students, midwives returning to practice and those undertaking post-registration study, and our physiology students, especially those studying human lifecycle physiology and nutrition, at Massey University. Enthusiastic questions, demands for explanations, the evident relish for understanding the theory related to practice and excitement about physiology stimulated the birth and continued development of the book, resulting in this extensively updated fourth edition. We hope that readers will continue to enquire about and enjoy this exciting field so that they can successfully utilize scientific knowledge in the ongoing development and promotion of effective midwifery practice and physiology research.

Jane Coad
Melvyn Dunstall
Kevin Pedley

ACKNOWLEDGEMENTS

It is almost 20 years since we began working on the first edition of this book and, as in the previous editions, we would like, once again, to thank our patient families and friends who again provided us with the encouragement and support to complete the fourth edition of this book. The fourth edition has been enriched by the inclusion of Kevin Pedley as an author; his expertise and background in cell physiology teaching and research, particularly its clinical application to fertility and parturition, are most valuable. In addition, all the case studies have been reviewed and updated by Melvyn Dunstall, who has drawn yet again on his extensive experience in clinical practice.

We would like to thank all our colleagues and students at Massey University in New Zealand and Frimley Health NHS Foundation Trust for their continued help, support and guidance in the development of this latest edition. Of particular note are Dr Louise Brough and Dr Janet Weber who generously shared their knowledge about nutrition in pregnancy and infancy; and Katie Schraders who critically reviewed Chapter 12.

Our midwifery and physiology students and other readers of the book have continued to ask questions and demand answers and their views and opinions have, once again, shaped the development of this latest edition and we continue to be indebted to them all. Within the clinical situation, there is now an even greater need for evidence-based practice and students and practitioners demand a knowledge base that will support this. Finally, we continue to owe much to the production team at Elsevier, especially Helen Leng, Alison Taylor and Joanna Souch. We would like to thank them all for their help, guidance and perseverance in supporting us in completing the fourth edition.

After 39 years of working in the NHS, with over 35 years in midwifery practice, it is time for me to retire, so this will be the last edition of the book that I will be fully associated with. There are many people I would like to thank personally, who have so positively contributed to my professional development; too many to mention individually.

Over the years there have been many changes within the clinical practice setting and it is a full-time commitment to keep up with and assimilate new evidence into practice. However, this is what makes midwifery so exciting and challenging. This constant requirement to learn will feed that innate midwifery desire to provide and facilitate the safest and best care for mothers, babies, fathers and their families.

I wish all up-and-coming midwives will enjoy their careers as much as I have. My final message to you is that the gathering and integrating of evidence-based knowledge into practice is the 'Science' underpinning midwifery, but the 'Art' is to apply it humanly, non-judgmentally and most importantly with compassion and grace in combination with the understanding, consideration and support for women to help them make their own decisions and choices. Remember, midwives do not deliver babies – they are birthed by their mother – and each birth is a unique and defining situation for all those privileged to be present.

MD

LIST OF ABBREVIATIONS

AII	angiotensin II	BSSL	bile salt stimulated lipase (also called bile salt dependent lipase, BSDL)
AA	arachidonic acid (or ARA)	BV	bacterial vaginosis
aCGH	array comparative genomic hybridization	BWPW	birthweight: placental weight
ABP	androgen-binding protein	CAG	cytosine-adenine-guanine trinucleotide
ACTH	adrenocorticotrophic hormone (corticotrophin)	CAH	congenital adrenal hyperplasia
AD	Alzheimer's disease	CAIS	complete androgen insensitivity syndrome
ADAM	a disintegrin and metalloprotease	CaM	calcium-binding protein (calmodulin)
ADH	antidiuretic hormone (vasopressin)	cAMP	cyclic adenosine monophosphate
AFP	alpha-fetoprotein	CAP	contraction-associated protein
AGE	advanced glycation end-products	CBG	corticosteroid-binding globulin
AIDS	acquired immune deficiency (immunodeficiency) syndrome	CCK	cholecystokinin
		CCT	controlled cord traction
AMH	anti-Müllerian hormone, also known as Müllerian-inhibiting substance, MIS or Müllerian-inhibiting hormone, MIH	CD	cluster of differentiation (cell surface glycoprotein, e.g. CD4 and CD8)
		CDH/CHD	congenital dislocation of the hips also known as congenital hip dysplasia
ANP	atrial natriuretic peptide	CEU	contrast enhanced ultrasound
ANS	autonomic nervous system	CfDNA/	
AOA	assisted oocyte activation	cffDNA	cell-free DNA/cell-free fetal DNA
APC	antigen-presenting cell	cGMP	cyclic guanosine monophosphate
APP	amyloid precursor protein	CKD	chronic kidney disease
AR	androgen receptor	CMV	cytomegalovirus
ARBD	alcohol-related birth defects	CNS	central nervous system
ARND	alcohol-related neurodevelopmental disorder	CoA	coenzyme A
		COC	combined oral contraceptive
ART	assisted reproductive technology or antiretroviral therapy	COX	cyclooxygenase
		CP	cerebral palsy
AS	Angelman syndrome	CpG	Cytosine-phosphate-guanine dinucleotide
ASB	artificially sweetened beverages	CRH	corticotrophin-releasing hormone
ASD	atrial septal defect	CRH-BP	corticotrophin-releasing hormone-binding protein
ASPM	abnormal spindle-like microcephaly-associated protein		
		CRISPR	clustered randomly interspaced palindromic repeats
ATP	adenosine triphosphate	CRL	crown–rump length
AV	arteriovenous	CSF	cerebrospinal fluid or cytostatic factor
AVN	atrioventricular node	CT	computed tomography (scan)
BAT	brown adipose tissue (brown fat)	CVS	chorionic villus sampling
BAV	bicuspid aortic valve	CYP	cytochrome P450 family of enzymes
BMI	body mass index	DA	ductus arteriosus
BMR	basal metabolic rate	D&C	dilatation and curettage
BPA	bisphenol A	DCT	distal convoluted tubule
BPD	biparietal diameter or bronchopulmonary dysplasia	DDT	dichlorodiphenyltrichloroethane (pesticide)
2,3-BPG	2,3-bisphosphoglycerate (also called 2,3-DPG, 2,3-diphosphoglycerate)	DES	diethylstilboestrol
BFHI	Baby Friendly Hospital Initiative		

DHA	docosahexaenoic acid (an Omega 3 fatty acid)	FISH	fluorescent in situ hybridization
DHEAS	dehydroepiandrosterone sulphate	FMc	fetal microchimerism
5α-DHT	5α-dihydrotestosterone	FPU	fetal–placental unit
DI	donor insemination	FRT	female reproductive tract
DIC	disseminated intravascular coagulation	FSH	follicle-stimulating hormone
DIT	diet-induced thermogenesis	GALT	gut-associated lymphoid tissue
DSD	disorder of sex development	GBS	group B Streptococcus
D-MER	dysphoric milk ejection reflex	GC	glucocorticoid
DMT1	divalent metal transporter 1	GDM	gestational diabetes mellitus
DNA	deoxyribonucleic acid	GERD	gastroesophageal reflux disease
DOHaD	Developmental Origins of Health and Disease	GFR	glomerular filtration rate
		GH	growth hormone
DSM	Diagnostic and Statistical Manual of Mental Disorders (of the American Psychiatric Association)	GH-V	growth hormone variant (also called GH2)
		GI	glycaemic index
DVT	deep vein thrombosis	GIFT	gamete intrafallopian transfer
E1	oestrone	GIP	gastric inhibitory poly peptide
E2	oestradiol-17β	GL	greatest length or gastric lipase
E3	oestriol	GLUT	glucose transporter family
ECG	electrocardiogram	GM-CSF	granulocyte–macrophage colony-stimulating factor
ECMO	extracorporeal membrane oxygenation		
ECP	emergency contraceptive pill	GnRH	gonadotrophin-releasing hormone
ED	erectile dysfunction	GOR/GORD	gastro-oesophageal reflux/ gastro-oesophageal reflux disease
EDC	endocrine disrupting chemical		
EDD	estimated date of delivery	GP	general practitioner
ED-PAF	embryo-derived platelet-activating factor	GPCR	G-protein coupled receptor
EDRF	endothelium-derived relaxing factor	GPX	glutathione peroxidase
EGF	epidermal growth factor	gRNA	guide RNA
ENaC	epithelial sodium channel	GSC	germline stem cell
EPA	eicosapentaenoic acid (an omega-3 fatty acid)	GTD	gestational trophoblastic disease
		GWG	gestational weight gain
EPO/rEPO	erythropoietin/recombinant erythropoietin	HAMLET	Human Alpha-lactalbumin Made LEthal to Tumour cells
		Hb/HbF/	
EPOR	excitement-plateau-orgasmic-resolution (model)	HbA	haemoglobin fetal-type Hb/adult type Hb
		HbS	sickle haemoglobin (also called HbC)
ER	endoplasmic reticulum	hCG	human chorionic gonadotrophin
ERM	Ets-related molecule (a transcription factor)	hCG-H	hyperglycosylated human chorionic gonadotrophin
ERPC	evacuation of retained products of conception	hCG-S	sulphated human chorionic gonadotrophin
ESC	embryonic stem cell	HDL	high-density lipoprotein
ET	embryo transfer	HDL-c	cholesterol associated with high-density lipoproteins
FAS	fetal alcohol syndrome		
FASD	fetal alcohol spectrum disorders	HDNB	haemorrhagic disease of the newborn (old term for VKDB)
FBM	fetal breathing movements		
FGM	female genital mutilation	HELLP	haemolysis, elevated liver enzymes and low platelet counts
FGF	fibroblast growth factor		
FGR	fetal growth restriction	HFCS	high fructose corn syrup
FHR	fetal heart rate	HFEA	Human Fertilisation and Embryology Authority, UK
FHV	fetal heart variability		
FIL	feedback inhibitor of lactation	HG	hyperemesis gravidarum

HGP	human genome project	LC-PUFA	long-chain polyunsaturated fatty acid
HH	hypogonadotrophic hypogonadism	LDL	low-density lipoprotein
Hib	Haemophilus influenzae type b	LDL-c	cholesterol associated with low-density lipoproteins
HIE	hypoxic-ischaemic encephalopathy		
HIV	human immunodeficiency virus	LH	luteinizing hormone
HLA	human leukocyte antigen (major histocompatibility complex, MHC)	LHRH	luteinizing hormone releasing hormone
		LIF	leukaemia-inhibitory factor
hMG	human menopausal gonadotrophin	LGA	large for gestational age
HMO	human milk oligosaccharide	LMP	last menstrual period
HPA	hypothalamic–pituitary–adrenal (axis)	LPL	lipoprotein lipase
HPG	hypothalamic–pituitary–gonadal (axis)	LSCS	lower-segment caesarean section
hPL	human placental lactogen	LUS	lower uterine segment
HPV	human papillomavirus	LV	left ventricle
HRT	hormone replacement therapy	MAC	membrane attack complex
11β-HSD2	11β-hydroxysteroid dehydrogenase 2	M-cell	microfold cell
		MCV	mean (blood) cell volume
HSC	haemopoietic stem cells	MDG	Millennium Development Goals (United Nations)
5HT	5-hydroxytryptamine (serotonin)		
HSV	herpes simplex virus	MECs	mammary epithelial cells (lactocytes)
HZFO	hamster zona-free ovum	MenSC	menstrual blood stem cells
IAAO	indicator amino acid oxidation method of determining protein	MESA	microepidermal sperm aspiration
		MFG/	
IAP	intrapartum antibiotic prophylaxis	MFGM	milk fat globule/milk fat globule membrane
IBD	inflammatory bowel disease		
ICSI	intracytoplasmic sperm injection	MHC	major histocompatibility complex proteins (human leukocyte antigen, HLA)
IDA	iron deficiency anaemia		
IDD	iodine deficiency disorders		
IDDM	insulin-dependent diabetes mellitus	MI	myocardial infarction
IDO	indoleamine 2,3-dioxygenase	MIS	Müllerian-inhibiting substance (also known as Müllerian-inhibiting hormone, MIH)
Ig	immunoglobulin		
IGF	insulin-like growth factor		
IGF-BP	insulin-like growth factor binding protein	MLCK	myosin light-chain kinase
IGFR	IGF receptor	MMN	multiple micronutrient
IL	interleukin family of cytokines (e.g. IL-12)	MMP	matrix metalloproteinases
		MMR	measles, mumps and rubella (vaccines)
IMSI	intracytoplasmic morphologically-selected sperm injection	MRI	magnetic resonance imaging
		mRNA	messenger ribonucleic acid
IOM	Institute of Medicine (USA)	MRSA	methicillin-resistant Staphylococcus aureus
IOP	intraocular pressure		
IP3	inositol trisphosphate	MSAF	meconium-stained amniotic fluid
IPI	interpregnancy interval	MSAFP	maternal serum alpha(α) fetoprotein
IU/i.u.	international units	MSH	melanocyte-stimulating hormone
IUD	intrauterine device	MSU	midstream specimen of urine
IUGR	intrauterine growth retardation (also called fetal growth retardation, FGR)	mtDNA	mitochondrial DNA
		NEC	necrotizing enterocolitis
IUI	intrauterine insemination	NEFA	non-esterified (or free) fatty acids
IVF	in vitro fertilization	NET	neutrophil extracellular trap
kDa	kilodaltons	NICE	National Institute for Health and Care Excellence, UK (formerly National Institute for Clinical Excellence 1999-2005)
KS	Klinefelter syndrome		
LA	left atrium		
LARC	long acting reversible contraception		
LBW	low birthweight	NGS	next generation sequencing (of DNA)

NK cell	natural killer cell	PID	pelvic inflammatory disease
NO	nitric oxide	PIP2	phosphatidylinositol 4,5-bisphosphate (PtdIns(4,5)P2)
NPN	non-protein nitrogen		
NPU	net protein utilization	PKU	phenylketonuria
NPY	neuropeptide Y	PLA2	phospholipase A2
NREM	nonrapid eye movement (deep) sleep	PLC	phospholipase C or pregnancy-lactation cycle
nRNA	nuclear (pre-messenger) ribonucleic acid		
NSAID	nonsteroidal anti-inflammatory drug	PLRP2	pancreatic lipase-related protein 2
NSP	nonstarch polysaccharide	PMCS	perimortem caesarean section (or resuscitative hysterotomy)
NST	nonshivering thermogenesis		
NT	nuchal translucency	PMDD	premenstrual dysphoric disorder
NTD	neural tube defect	PMS	premenstrual syndrome
NVP	nausea and vomiting in pregnancy	PNMT	phenylethanolamine-n-methyltransferase
OAT	oligoasthenoteratozoospermia (oligospermia); low sperm count with decreased sperm motility and increased abnormal morphology	POA	preoptic area (of hypothalamus)
		POMC	proopiomelanocortin
		POP	progesterone only pill (preparation)
		PPD	postpartum depression (and anxiety)
17α-OHP	17α-hydroxyprogesterone	PPH	postpartum haemorrhage
OHSS	ovarian hyperstimulation syndrome	PPHN	persistent pulmonary hypertension of the newborn
OS	oxidative stress		
OTA	ochratoxin A	PPROM	preterm premature rupture of (fetal) membranes
OTR	oxytocin receptor		
OXY	oxytocin	PPI	proton-pump inhibitors
PAE	prenatal alcohol exposure	PPT	postpartum thyroiditis
PAF	platelet activating factor	PRL	prolactin
PAMP	pathogen-associated molecular patterns	PROM	premature rupture of the membranes
PAPP-A	pregnancy-associated plasma protein A	PRR	pattern recognition receptors
PCB	polychlorinated biphenyl	PSA	prostate specific antigen
PCD	primary ciliary dyskinesia	PTH	parathyroid hormone
PCR	polymerase chain reaction	PUFA	polyunsaturated fatty acid
PCT	proximal convoluted tubule	PUL	pregnancy of unknown location
PCV	pneumococcal vaccine	PVR	pulmonary vascular resistance
PCOS	polycystic ovary syndrome	PWS	Präder–Willi syndrome
PDA	patent ductus arteriosus	PZD	partial zona dissection
PDCAAS	protein digestibility corrected amino acid score	qPCR	quantitative polymerase chain reaction
		RA	retinoic acid or right atrium
PDE	phosphodiesterase	RAAS	renin–angiotensin aldosterone system
PE	pulmonary embolism	RAR	retinoic acid receptor
PESA	percutaneous epididymal sperm aspiration	RCOG	Royal College of Obstetrics and Gynaecology, UK
		RCT	randomized control trial
pFAS	partial fetal alcohol syndrome	RDI	recommended dietary intake
PFO	patent forum ovale	RDS	respiratory distress syndrome
PG	prostaglandin	RE	retrograde ejaculation
PGC	primordial germ cell	REM	rapid eye movement (sleep)
PGD	preimplantation genetic diagnosis	RER	rough endoplasmic reticulum
PGDH	prostaglandin dehydrogenase	Rh	Rhesus
PGH	placental growth hormone	RIF	repeated implantation failure
PGI2	prostacyclin	RLS	restless legs syndrome
PGS	preimplantation genetic screening	RNA	ribonucleic acid
PHV	peak height velocity	rRNA	ribosomal ribonucleic acid
Pi	inorganic phosphate	ROS	reactive oxygen species
PIBF	progesterone-induced blocking factor		

RPOC	retained products of conception
RSA	recurrent spontaneous abortion
RSV	respiratory syncytial virus
RV	right ventricle
RXR	retinoid X receptor
SAN	sinoatrial node (pacemaker)
SaO2	oxygen saturation of arterial blood
SCD	sickle cell disease
SCN	suprachiasmatic nuclei
SDG	Sustainable Development Goals (United Nations)
SePP	selenoprotein P
SER	smooth endoplasmic reticulum
SGA	small for gestational age
SHBG	sex hormone binding globulin
SIDS	sudden infant death syndrome ('cot death')
sIg	secretory immunoglobulin
SLE	systemic lupus erythematosus
SNP	single nucleotide polymorphism
SPA	surfactant protein A
SPD	symphysis pubis diastasis (or dysfunction)
SPTL	spontaneous (or idiopathic) preterm labour
SRE	steroid response element
SRY	sex determining region of Y chromosome (note *SRY* refers to the human gene for SRY)
SSB	sugar-sweetened beverage
SSC (or S2S)	skin-to-skin contact
SSRI	selective serotonin reuptake inhibitor
STD	sexually transmitted disease
STI	sexually transmitted infection
STRA8	gene Stimulated by Retinoic Acid 8
SUA	single umbilical artery
SUN	'Scaling Up Nutrition' (UN)
SUZI	subzonal sperm injection
SVR	systemic vascular resistance
T1DM	Type-1 diabetes mellitus
T2DM	Type-2 diabetes mellitus
T3	triiodothyronine
T4	thyroxine
TAG (TG)	triacylglycerides (or triglycerides)
TB	tuberculosis
TBG	thyroxin-binding globulin
TBP	thyroid-binding protein
TCA	tricarboxylic acid
Tc cells	cytotoxic T-cells
tDC	tolerogenic dendritic cells
TEF	thermic effect of food

TENS	transcutaneous electrical nerve stimulation
TESE	testicular sperm extraction
TGF	transforming growth factor
THC	tetrahydrocannabinol
Th cells	T helper cells
TLR	Toll-like receptors
TNF	tumour necrosis factor
Treg cells	regulatory T-cells (formerly called suppressor T-cells)
tRNA	transfer ribonucleic acid
TS	Turner syndrome
TSH	thyroid-stimulating hormone
TSI	thyroid-stimulating immunoglobulin
TTN	transient tachypnoea of the newborn
TTTS	twin-to-twin transfusion syndrome
TxA2	thromboxane A2
UCP	uncoupling protein
UI	urinary incontinence
uLGL	uterine large granular leukocytes
uNK	uterine natural killer (cells)
UVR	ultraviolet radiation
UTI	urinary tract infection
VDBP	vitamin D binding protein
VDJ	variable, diverse and joining (gene segment)
VDR	vitamin D receptor
VEGF	vascular endothelial growth factor
VIP	vasoactive intestinal peptide
VKDB	vitamin K deficiency bleeding (formerly HDNB)
VLDL	very-low-density lipoprotein
V/Q	ventilation perfusion ratio
VTE	venous thromboembolism
WAT	white adipose tissue
WBW	World Breastfeeding Week
WHI	Women's Health Initiative (studies on HRT)
WHO	World Health Organization
ZIFT	zygote intrafallopian transfer
ZP	zona pellucida

Introduction to Physiology

- To describe the structure of a typical cell and the role of its organelles.
- To discuss how cell differentiation and organization permit physiological function.
- To recognize the features and characteristics of different tissue types that facilitate their function.
- To describe the provision of oxygen and nutrients to cells and how the waste products of metabolism are excreted.

- To identify key features of physiological control mechanisms.
- To describe the principles and components of a homeostatic system.
- To discuss examples of physiological homeostasis.
- To be able to explain basic physiology to women so that they are able to understand how pregnancy alters the way a woman's body functions, in order to support her pregnancy and prepare her physiologically for nurturing her newborn infant.

INTRODUCTION

Physiology is the biological science that explores how living organisms are able to function in order to survive and reproduce successfully. Physiology investigates the relationship between the structure and function of body systems. Physiological systems are complex structures, which serve a particular function such as blood circulation or respiration. Organs are made up of cells organized into different tissue types such as nerve tissue or muscle tissue. The physiological systems communicate and interact with each other. A key concept of physiology is that life is only possible within some tightly regulated conditions such as temperature and ion concentration. Homeostasis describes an organism's ability to control its internal environment and maintain a stable condition; this allows the organisms to adjust to, and survive in, a broad range of environments. This book focuses on human reproductive function. This chapter aims to provide an illustrated introduction to, and an overview of, some of the basic physiological concepts referred to and developed in subsequent chapters, with specific reference to reproduction. (For more details, readers are recommended to look at the list of Annotated Further Reading at the end of the chapter.)

CHAPTER CASE STUDY

Zara is a 29-year-old primipara who presents herself at the midwife's clinic, which is held at her GP's surgery, giving a history of a positive pregnancy test.
- If Zara had accessed preconceptual care what advice do you think she should have been given in her preparation for pregnancy?
- What information would be available in Zara's medical records that would be useful to the midwife in her initial assessment of Zara's pregnancy?
- How could this information be used by the midwife to inform Zara of the physiological changes that have started to occur in her body?
- What assessments would enable the midwife to judge whether Zara's pregnancy is progressing normally even at this early stage.

THE CELL

The cell is the fundamental unit of structure and function of all living organisms. The evolution of multicellular organisms has led to the differentiation of cells, which means that different cells have evolved to perform specific functions and processes that contribute to the wellbeing of the organism as a whole. Differentiated cells form tissues that combine with other tissues to form organs, which are linked together in physiological systems (Fig. 1.1). However, although cells can be highly specialized, they all share common features of the single cellular organisms from which higher life-forms evolved. A typical human cell is about 10 μm in diameter. The largest human cell is the oocyte (see Chapter 6); it is about 100 μm in diameter so it can just be seen with the naked eye. The follicular cells surrounding the oocyte have a more typical human cell size. The sperm cell is one of the smallest human cells. Smaller cells and organelles can be visualized by light and electron microscopy.

Cell Structure

Most cells contain cytoplasm and are enclosed within a plasma membrane. Within a typical cell are various structures, called organelles (Table 1.1), and a specialized part of the cell, called the nucleus (Fig. 1.2). The fluid surrounding the organelles is called cytosol.

CELLS AND TISSUES

Although about 200 types of cells with different structures can be identified within the body, cells can be grouped together in functional categories (Table 1.2). The study of the physical characteristics of cells is called histology (Box 1.1). There are four types of tissue: epithelial tissue, muscle tissue, connective tissue and nervous tissue.

Epithelial Tissue

Epithelial cells line or cover the internal and external surfaces of body organs (Fig. 1.3), forming the outer layer of the skin, the mucous membranes, the lining of the blood vessels, lungs, gut, reproductive and urinary tracts. Endocrine and exocrine glands are also formed from epithelial tissue. Epithelial cells are tightly packed, often into epithelial sheets in which the cells are 'polarized' and have different characteristics on their apical (top) surface and their basal surface (which is in contact with the basement membrane). The basement membrane forms scaffolding to epithelial tissue and allows diffusion of nutrients from the underlying blood vessels. Epithelial cells are relatively undifferentiated and tend to undergo frequent mitotic divisions (see Chapter 7). This is because they are often exposed to wear and tear and so replacement epithelial cells are generated from a basal layer where cell division takes place. Specialized functions of differentiated epithelial cells include absorption, secretion, excretion, transport, protection and sensation (e.g. mechanosensory, chemosensory, thermosensory attributes).

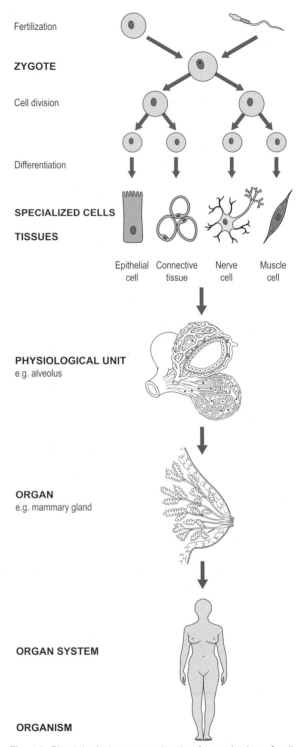

Fig. 1.1 Physiological systems: levels of organization of cells, tissues, organs and physiological systems, using breast tissue as an example.

TABLE 1.1 Cell Components

Cell Component	Structure	Function
Cell membrane	The cell membrane is composed of a phospholipid bilayer embedded with various protein structures such as hormone receptors, ion channels and antigen markers	The membrane acts as a differentially permeable barrier between the cell and its immediate environment
The nucleus	The nucleus is bound by a membrane, similar to the plasma membrane of the cell; this contains openings referred to as nuclear pores, which allow the movement of substances into and out of the nucleus	The nucleus contains deoxyribonucleic acid (DNA), the genetic instructions for the organism. Most of the time, the DNA is organized as chromatin threads; these condense into chromosomes prior to cell division. The nucleus stores and replicates DNA, which is expressed to synthesize proteins (gene expression) via a second type of nucleic acid, ribonucleic acid (RNA). These proteins determine the structure and function of the cell
Endoplasmic reticulum	This is a system of membranes, enclosing a space (lumen), which is continuous with the nuclear membrane. Endoplasmic reticulum (ER) exists as rough (granular) endoplasmic reticulum (RER) and smooth (agranular) endoplasmic reticulum (SER)	RER appears rough because of the attached ribosomes. RER is involved in protein packaging. SER is involved in lipid and steroid synthesis and the regulation of intracellular calcium levels
Mitochondria	Spherical or elongated rod-like structures surrounded by a folded inner membrane and a smooth outer membrane. There are more mitochondria in cells that are metabolically active and have a high energy requirement	Chemical processes involved in the formation of adenosine triphosphate (ATP). The cristae (inner membrane folds) are the site of oxidative phosphorylation and the electron transport chain of aerobic respiration. Krebs (tricarboxylic acid or TCA) cycle and the oxidation of fatty acids take place within the matrix. Mitochondria contain mitochondrial DNA, which is maternally inherited and contains the genes for only 13 of >600 mitochondrial proteins
Golgi apparatus (complex)	A series of flattened curved membranous sacs	Modifies proteins from the RER and sorts them into secretory vesicles
Lysosomes	Spherical or oval organelles enclosed by a single membrane	Enclose acidic fluid containing digestive enzymes, which act as a 'cellular stomach' breaking down cellular debris
Peroxisomes	Similar structure to lysosomes	Destroy reactive oxygen species and protect cell
Cytoskeleton	Filamentous network	Involved in maintaining cell shape and motility

Epithelial cells often form a barrier, which allows secretion and absorption of substances from one compartment to another. The skin is a specialized epithelial layer. The basal layer produces cells that have lost their nuclei and have become enriched with the protein keratin. The outer layers of skin cells are dead and so lack cytoplasm; it is these keratinized dead cells that provide the barrier (waterproof) function of the skin. Epithelial cells are classified by shape (cuboidal, columnar or squamous) and the number of layers. If there is a single layer of cells and all cells are in contact with the basement membrane, the epithelium is described as simple; if there is more than one layer of cells (such as skin), it is stratified. Squamous epithelium consists of flattened cells allowing efficient diffusion of substances such as oxygen and carbon dioxide in the alveoli of the lungs. Epithelia can create a low-friction surface by secreting a layer of mucus onto their surface and allow directional transport and fluid absorption, for example in the gut, by having different transporters on their apical and basal membranes. Pseudostratified cells are a single layer of cells that appear to consist of more than one layer and may have cilia (fine hair-like extensions that can waft

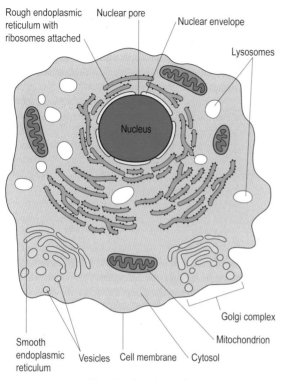

Rough endoplasmic reticulum with ribosomes attached

Nuclear pore

Nuclear envelope

Lysosomes

Nucleus

Smooth endoplasmic reticulum

Vesicles   Cell membrane   Cytosol

Golgi complex

Mitochondrion

Fig. 1.2 A typical cell.

fluid). The respiratory epithelium secretes mucus to trap pathogens then moves this mucus to the nose (and handkerchief) using millions of cilia.

Cell Junctions

Cells in epithelia are held together by cell junctions, which can be classified into three groups. Tight junctions seal cells together in an epithelial sheet so that the movement of solutes through the space between cells (intercellular space) is restricted. This supports the unidirectional transcellular transport of solutes and water across an epithelial sheet, for example nutrient absorption in the gut or water reabsorption in the kidney tubule. The second group, anchoring junctions, connect the cytoskeleton of a cell to either the cytoskeleton of an adjacent cell or to the extracellular matrix, allowing the intrinsically flimsy structure of the cell to be incorporated into a strong epithelial sheet, able to withstand the forces of, for example digesta movement through the intestine. Finally, communicating junctions allow small molecules to pass directly from cell to cell, to allow coordination of cellular responses via shared signalling mechanisms. A good example of this is seen in uterine smooth muscle, where the number of gap junctions increases dramatically as parturition approaches so that

uterine contractions are more powerful and coordinated to propel the fetus towards the birth canal (see Chapter 13).

Muscle Tissue

Muscle cells (myocytes) contain contractile elements, so the cells can generate the mechanical force required for movement of the body or substances within the body (Fig. 1.4) or change shape and size. Muscle tissue is formed from the mesodermal layer of the embryo (see Chapter 9). There are three types of muscle tissue: skeletal, cardiac and smooth muscle. Skeletal muscle may be attached to bones and controls movement and position (posture) of the skeleton. Skeletal muscle can also be attached to the skin, for instance the muscles of the face involved with expression. Contraction of skeletal muscle is usually under voluntary or conscious control (movements are initiated by the central nervous system [CNS]). Skeletal muscle is often described as 'striated' because of the striped appearance of the sarcomeres of the muscle observed under the light microscope. Skeletal muscle fibres can be subdivided into slow (type I) and fast (type II) twitch fibres. Slow twitch fibres appear red because they have a lot of capillaries to support oxidative metabolism. They are rich in myoglobin and mitochondria and rely upon aerobic metabolism. Fast twitch muscles, particularly type IIx fibres, use anaerobic metabolism. Fast twitch fibres contract more strongly and generate a lot of force but they tire easily, whereas slow twitch fibres can contract for prolonged periods. Skeletal muscle is usually anchored to bone by tendons.

Cardiac muscle is only found in the heart; it has some structural similarity with skeletal muscle (appears striated) but rather than the muscle fibres being organized in regular parallel bundles characteristic of skeletal muscle, cardiac muscle fibres branch. Smooth muscle and cardiac muscle are usually under involuntary control (meaning there is no conscious awareness of the control).

Smooth muscle surrounds many of the 'tubes' in the body (such as those in the vascular system, gut, airways and urinary system), maintaining the function of several body systems. Smooth muscle cells are linked by gap junctions, and muscle contraction is relatively slow but can be sustained for long periods. Blood pressure is maintained by the contraction of a smooth muscle layer in the walls of the blood vessels. If the smooth muscle constricts, described as 'vasoconstriction', the internal lumen of the vessel will decrease in diameter and blood pressure will increase. 'Vasodilation' (or vasodilatation) is the opposite condition: the smooth muscle relaxes and the lumen diameter increases, so blood pressure falls. Coordinated synchronized waves of smooth muscle contraction and relaxation, for instance in the gut, renal system and uterine tubes, generate peristaltic waves; these produce unidirectional

TABLE 1.2 Functional Classification of Cells

Cell Group	Epithelial Cells	Support Cells	Contractile Cells	Nerve Cells	Germ Cells	Blood Cells	Immune Cells	Hormone-secreting Cells
Example	Lining gut and blood vessels; covering skin	Fibrous support tissue, cartilage, bone	Muscle	Brain	Spermatozoa Ova	Circulating 1. Red cells 2. White cells 3. Platelets	Lymphoid tissues, nodes and spleen	Islets, thyroid adrenal
Function	Barrier; absorption; secretion	Organize and maintain body structure	Movement	Direct cell communication	Reproduction	1. Oxygen transport 2. Defence	Defence	Indirect cell communication
Special features	Tightly bound together by cell junctions	Produce and interact with extracellular matrix material	Contractile proteins	Release chemical messengers directly on to other cells	Haploid (i.e. half-normal chromosome number)	1. Proteins bind oxygen 2. Proteins destroy bacteria 3. Blood clotting	Recognize and destroy foreign material	Secrete chemical messengers into blood

BOX 1.1   Histology

The study of tissue structure is described as histology. The functions of tissues are reflected in the microscopic structure of the cells of which the tissue is composed. For example, cells that are metabolically active contain many mitochondria, whereas cells that produce hormones or enzymes, for instance, will contain a large proportion of ER. Specific tissues and cellular structures are often identified by the application of various chemicals that stain particular tissues. Histology is important in diagnosing cancer, as the cancerous tissue often has histological characteristics different from those of the normal tissue in which the cancer has developed. Malignant cancerous tumours have highly differentiated cells, which means they often appear different from the normal tissue cells from which they arose; they often have a simpler structure and usually a very fast rate of cell division. These cells are less likely to adhere to neighbouring cells as normal cells do, so they are shed into the circulatory system and are carried to other parts of the body where they seed more tumours (secondary tumours or metastases). Benign tumours usually have undifferentiated cells, which may closely resemble the cells of the tissue from which they arose and tend only to grow in the one position. Although cancers in pregnancy are rare, many cancerous cells may respond to oestrogen (sometimes referred to as oestrogen dependent); therefore, cancer growth during pregnancy can be quite rapid and unpredictable.

movement of the contents within the lumen of the tube (Fig. 1.5). Whilst a peristaltic pattern of contraction occurs following food consumption to propel the lumen contents progressively through the gut, a different nonpropulsive pattern of alternate contraction and relaxation by the longitudinal and circular smooth muscle layers is also demonstrated; this 'segmentation' facilitates mixing of the food, combining it with secretions from the gut and thus promoting digestion and maximizing contact of the absorptive epithelium with the products of digestion.

Connective Tissue

Connective tissue functions to connect (or separate), anchor and support body structures (Fig. 1.6). It is often classified as connective tissue proper (and subdivided into loose connective tissue, dense regular connective tissue or dense irregular connective tissue) and special connective tissue (e.g. bone and cartilage, adipose tissue, blood and lymphatic fluid). Connective tissue cells, such as fibroblasts, are spread in an extracellular fluid, which may have a liquid or gel-like composition. Connective tissue proper usually has fibres (collagen and/or elastic fibres), ground substance and cells. Connective tissue cells (such as fibroblasts) often produce an extracellular matrix composed of proteins in a ground substance of sugars (e.g. glycosaminoglycans), proteins (e.g. proteoglycans) and minerals. The ground substance is important in limiting the spread of pathogens in the body. Other functions of connective tissue include facilitating the diffusion of nutrients and oxygen from capillaries to cells and waste products back to capillaries, providing elasticity and strength and resisting stretching.

Connective tissue is found in all body tissues so that connective tissue disorders, some of which are inherited such as Marfan syndrome and Ehlers-Danlos syndrome, can also affect many parts of the body. Pathology in a variety of these disorders is often seen in the heart and blood vessels, in bones and joints and in skin but can also have implications for women in pregnancy and labour and/or their offspring, who could inherit the disorder.

Bone is a type of connective tissue, whereas collagen is an example of an extracellular matrix. Adipose tissue is composed of specialized cells that store fat for future energy requirements and have an endocrine role. Adipose tissue also acts as an insulating layer to conserve body heat loss and so contributes to the maintenance of the homeothermic status of the organism. Fibrous tissue is an example of dense connective tissue. It is a tough tissue that forms ligaments, tendons and protective membranes. The meninges that cover the brain and spinal cord are another type of connective tissue. Blood and lymphatic fluid are also often considered to be connective tissue.

Nervous Tissue

Nervous tissue includes the cells of the CNS (brain and spinal cord) and the peripheral nervous system (nerves). Neurons or nerve cells are specialized to initiate and conduct electrical signals; they have a cell body, axons (long projections that carry the action potential to the next neuron or target tissue) and dendrites that receive the electrochemical stimulation from neurotransmitters (Fig. 1.7). Neurons require the presence of glial cells (neuroglia) for nourishment and support; glial cells are also involved in the propagation of the electrical impulses in the neurons. As neurons are so highly specialized, they do not usually undergo further mitotic divisions once developed. Therefore, in the fetal and early neonatal period, the number of neurons produced far exceeds the level required for normal neurological function. To survive and function, neurons need regular stimulation. Throughout life, millions of neurons become dysfunctional and die, a process which increases markedly in later life and can lead to

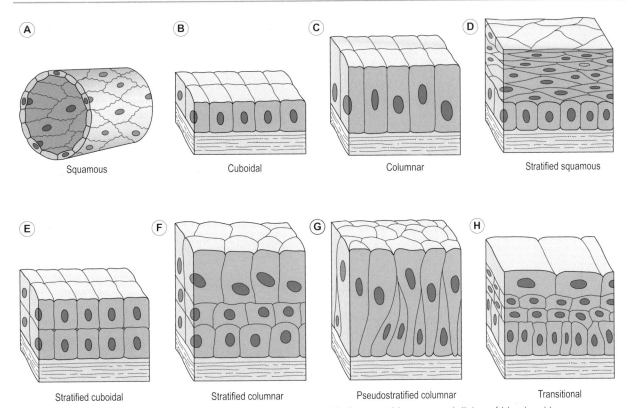

Fig. 1.3 Types of epithelial cell: (A) simple squamous epithelium provides a smooth lining of blood and lymphatic vessels (endothelium), alveoli of lung and glomeruli of kidney; (B) simple cuboidal epithelium is often found on absorptive or secretory surfaces such as in kidney tubules; (C) simple columnar epithelium is often associated with secretory and absorptive tissues and may have microvilli, as in the gut; it may also be ciliated, as in the upper airways; (D) stratified squamous epithelium protects the mouth and oesophagus and vagina from abrasion; (E) stratified cuboidal epithelium protects glands such as mammary glands, salivary and sweat glands; (F) stratified columnar epithelium also protects and may be involved in secretion such as glands and the male urethra; (G) pseudostratified columnar epithelium can appear stratified but all cells are in contact with the basement membrane and cells are often ciliated as in the upper part of the respiratory tract; (H) transitional epithelium lines the bladder and other organs of the urinary system allowing the tissue to stretch and expand.

neurological decline and a range disorders, predominantly in the elderly, which are referred to as dementia.

THE STRUCTURAL ORGANIZATION OF THE BODY

The body's organization can be understood by considering each component organ system separately. However, these systems all work together, as a whole. Together the systems provide nutrients and oxygen for the cells and the excretion of waste products (Fig. 1.8). Movement is controlled and the temperature is maintained. Survival until reproductive function is completed has allowed the species to multiply. Cells are bathed in extracellular fluid, comprised of the interstitial fluid surrounding the tissue cells, the plasma within the blood vessels and other body fluids such as cerebrospinal fluid (CSF) in the CNS.

Homeostasis

Homeostasis is the term used to describe the processes of the various physiological systems that maintain relative constancy of the internal environment. Multicellular animals are able to maintain an internal stability that is essential for the optimal functioning of all body systems, whereas simple unicellular organisms tend to inhabit stable environments or have adapted to overcome fluctuations in the environment, for instance by forming spores during dry periods. Unicellular organisms rely on basic nutrients

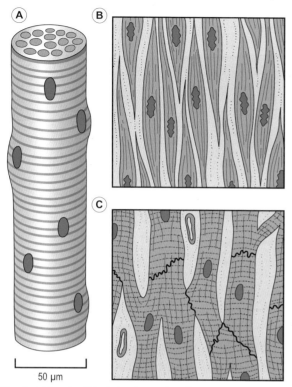

50 μm

Fig. 1.4 Muscle: (A) skeletal muscle; (B) smooth muscle; (C) cardiac muscle. (Adapted with permission from Brooker, 1998.)

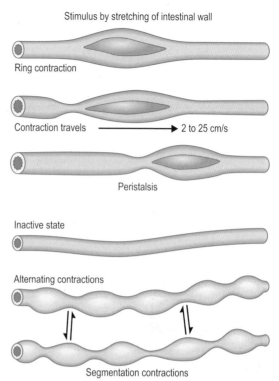

Fig. 1.5 Peristaltic waves and segmentation. Peristalsis is achieved through the interaction of both longitudinal and circular smooth muscle fibres found in vessels with patent lumen. The peristaltic waves are responsible for (usually) unidirectional movement of the contents within the lumen. Segmentation results in the mixing of the lumen contents with digestive enzymes and other secretions and increasing exposure of the absorptive surface of the gut with products of digestion.

being present in the environment to allow cell growth and reproduction.

The evolution of multicellular organisms and the development of motility meant that these animals were able to move within the environment to seek out the conditions that suited them best and so optimize their ability to reproduce. Mammals have developed homeostatic mechanisms to a high degree. Motility, together with the homeostatic challenge of counteracting fluctuations in the external environment, places a huge energy burden upon these individuals. This increased energy requirement is above the basal metabolic rate, which is the rate of energy required to maintain essential functioning only.

Examples of homeostasis include the maintenance of glucose (see Chapter 3) and electrolyte concentrations within a tight range, regulating pH and water balance, regulating blood pressure, haemostasis (maintenance of an adequate circulatory system facilitating the passage of nutrients and oxygen into and waste products out of the organism) and thermoregulation (maintenance of a constant internal temperature). Homeostasis is regulated by the nervous system, the endocrine system and behavioural factors that are dependent on conscious or subconscious

action by the organism. A homeostatic control system can be considered to have three main components: a sensing component or regulator, which monitors (or senses) the variable and detects changes; a control centre, which sets the upper and lower limits of the physiological range to be maintained; and an effector system, which generates responses to correct any deviation from the physiological range thus restoring the composition of the internal environment (Fig. 1.9). (This type of system, involving a process called negative feedback, is dealt with in more detail in Chapter 3, p. 75). Failure of appropriate homeostasis, including natural processes of ageing, results in disease.

Thermoregulation

Temperature regulation is a well-characterized example of homeostasis (Fig. 1.10). Enzymes regulating biochemical changes, and physiological and metabolic functions, have optimal activity within a narrow temperature range.

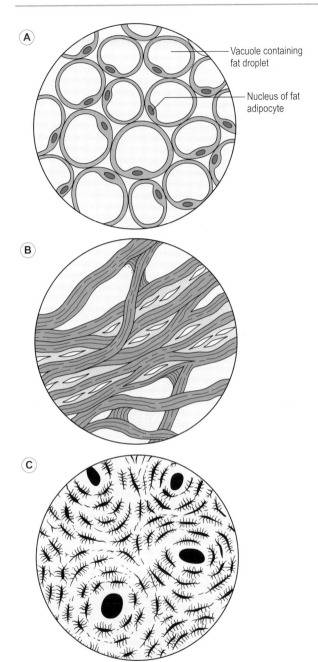

Fig. 1.6 Connective tissue: (A) loose connective tissue, e.g. adipose tissue; (B) dense regular connective tissue, e.g. tendons; (C) dense irregular connective tissue, e.g. dermis.

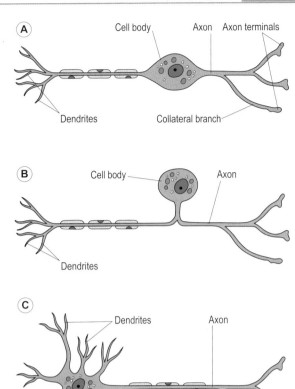

Fig. 1.7 Types of neuron: (A) bipolar; (B) unipolar; (C) multipolar.

animal, which generates heat from metabolism, is well prepared to react quickly and efficiently to changes in the environment, unlike a cold-blooded (poikilothermic) animal, in which body temperature largely reflects the ambient temperature of the environment.

The Nervous System

The nervous system coordinates body functions, both voluntary and involuntary. It monitors physiological processes by processing input from the senses, integrating them and initiating responses or motor output. The nervous system in humans is an organization of billions of neurons, or nerve cells, and these are supported by >10 times as many glial cells, which maintain the structural integrity of the nervous system and are essential for the function of neurons. The nervous system is comprised of the CNS (brain and spinal) and the peripheral nervous system comprised of the remaining neurons throughout the body (Fig. 1.11). The skull and the vertebral column protect the brain and the spinal cord. Neurons usually consist of a cell body and dendrites (long extensions) and an axon, which carries

Outside this physiological temperature range, the protein structure of the enzyme begins to denature, so the configuration (shape) of the enzyme distorts, which affects its functional activity. A warm-blooded (homeothermic)

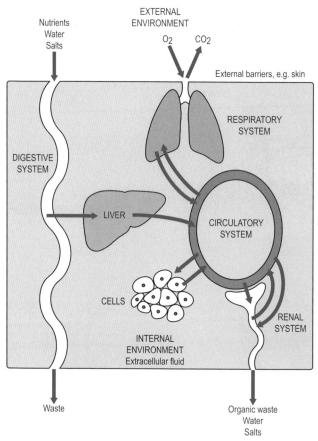

Fig. 1.8 Organization of the body.

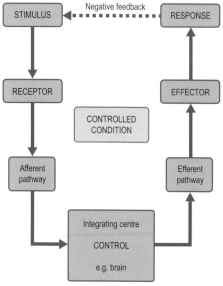

Fig. 1.9 The principles of homeostasis.

information from the cell body to, or from, the CNS. Axons can have very different lengths to conduct signals over a range of distances with neurons in the sciatic nerve, for example stretching from the base of the spine to the big toe, approximately 1 m in length. A nerve is a collection of axons running alongside each other over the same distance. A ganglion is a collection of cell bodies of neurons within the peripheral nervous system. Ganglions are located in dorsal (back) or ventral (front) branches of the spinal cord. The spinal cord and spinal nerves are organized on a segmental basis; this corresponds to the embryonic origin of the dermatomes (see Chapter 9). Cranial nerves carry information between the brain and regions of the head. Neurons that carry information from the peripheral NS towards the brain, entering the dorsal roots of the spinal cord, are sensory or afferent neurons. Neurons carrying information from the CNS to the effectors such as skeletal muscles or endocrine glands, and leaving the spinal cord at the ventral roots, are motor or efferent neurons (Fig. 1.12). Neurons that carry information between a sensory neuron

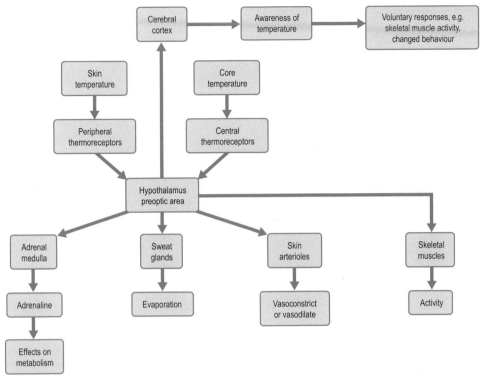

Fig. 1.10 Temperature regulation: a homeostatic system in operation.

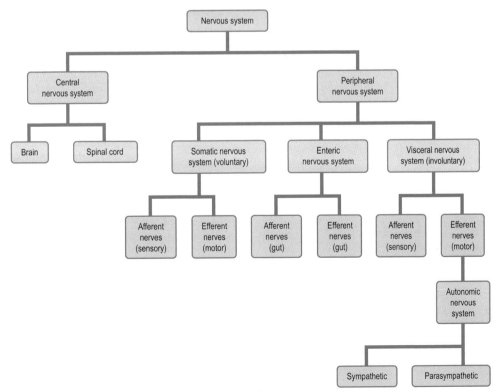

Fig. 1.11 Organization of the nervous system.

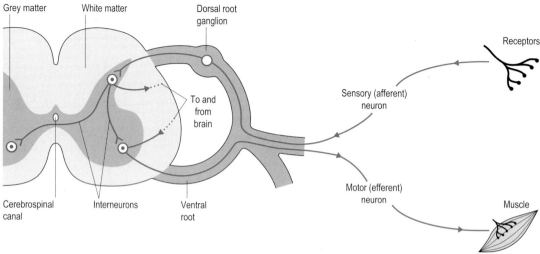

Fig. 1.12 Afferent and efferent neurons.

and the CNS (or between the CNS and a motor neuron) are known as interneurons.

The Action Potential

Neurons carry information or nerve impulses by changing the electrical charge along their axon length so the transmembrane polarity changes rapidly from negative to positive and back. This change in electrical charge is termed an 'action potential'. Electrical impulses are summated in the axon hillock of the cell body and when these reach the axon, sodium channels open, allowing the movement of extracellular sodium ions (Na^+) down their electrochemical gradient into the axon. As the sodium ions carry a positive charge, the immediate local area around the sodium channels inside of the axon becomes electrically positive compared with the immediate area outside and so the membrane becomes temporarily depolarized. At the height of the action potential (about 1 ms) the sodium channels close and potassium channels open so that potassium ions (K^+) move out of the axon down their electrochemical gradient. The result is the restoration of the resting membrane potential, described as 'repolarization'. That segment of the axon then enters a refractory period when no further action potential can be produced. However, depolarization in one small segment of the neuron leads to depolarization in the next segment; the rapid movement of the altered electrical activity is therefore propagated along the length of the neuron.

The action potential moves along the axon to the synapse, a junction with another neuron or the target tissue such as muscle or a secretory gland. There is a gap between two neurons at the synapse. Information transmission across this gap is by chemicals called neurotransmitters. These are released from the first neuron, travel across the synapse and trigger an action potential in the second neuron. The connection between a stimulating neuron and a muscle is called a neuromuscular junction. Action potentials move faster in axons of greater diameter, and if the axon is insulated by a myelin sheath. Myelin sheaths surround the neuron for short lengths, punctuated by the nodes of Ranvier. Action potentials in myelinated nerves are not propagated as waves but move by saltatory conduction, whereby they 'hop' along the nerve between the nodes of Ranvier in a fast and efficient manner. Action potentials are conducted along myelinated axons at up to 50× faster than nonmyelinated axons and this is essential to normal neuronal function. Multiple sclerosis is a neurological autoimmune disease in which immune cells attack and damage the myelin sheath causing dysfunction of the CNS.

The Somatic and Autonomic Nervous Systems

The somatic nervous system controls muscles that change position. These muscles are called skeletal or voluntary muscles as they are controlled voluntarily, whereas smooth muscle and cardiac muscle are controlled involuntarily by the autonomic nervous system (ANS). The ANS controls the internal functions of the body such as circulation, respiration, digestion and metabolism.

Traditionally, the ANS has been divided into the sympathetic and parasympathetic systems (Table 1.3); these two branches of the ANS are described as working in tandem, either synergistically or antagonistically. The sympathetic nervous system controls the responses

TABLE 1.3	**The Autonomic Nervous System**	
	Sympathetic Division	**Parasympathetic Division**
Characteristics	Preganglionic outflow originates in thoracolumbar portion of spinal cord Chain of ganglia Postganglionic fibres distributed throughout body Divergence of pathways, so system as a whole is usually stimulated. 'Fear, fight and flight'	Preganglionic outflow originates in midbrain, hindbrain and sacral portions of spinal cord Terminal ganglia near or in effector organs Postganglionic fibres mainly associated with head and viscera Little divergence, so limited parts of the system are stimulated 'Resting and digesting'
Examples of effect	Eye: dilation of pupil Cardiovascular system: increased heart rate and increased strength of myocardial contraction, vasoconstriction of peripheral vessels and increased blood pressure Lungs: dilation of bronchioles Bladder: increased muscle tone Uterus: contraction in pregnant woman; relaxation in nonpregnant woman Penis: ejaculation	Eye: constriction of pupil Cardiovascular system: decreased heart rate and vasodilation of peripheral vessels and decreased blood pressure Lungs: constriction of bronchioles Bladder: increased contraction Penis: vasodilation and erection

and provision of energy required for stressful situations; it is often known as the fear–fight–flight system. Effects of the sympathetic system include increased heart rate and blood pressure, pupillary and bronchial dilation, increased skeletal muscle blood flow (at the expense of blood flow to other tissues), increased glycogenolysis and lipolysis to increase energy provision and other responses that facilitate fight or escape and heightened awareness to threatening situations. The sympathetic system operates in conjunction with the endocrine system, facilitating the release of adrenaline, which augments the manifesting of fear–fight–flight reflexes. Conversely, the parasympathetic branch of the ANS is more influential in periods of rest and inactivity and favours rest, increased digestive activity and restoration. Effects of parasympathetic nervous activity include increased blood flow to the gut and skin, stimulated salivary gland secretion and peristalsis, and slowing of the heart rate. In the ANS, two neurons carry information from the CNS to the target organ; these travel via autonomic ganglia and are termed 'preganglionic' and 'postganglionic' neurons. There is a third subdivision of the ANS called the enteric nervous system, which regulates smooth muscle and secretion in the gut.

The Brain

The brain is the centre of the nervous system; it is the most complex organ, which, in humans, contains 100 billion neurons with one quadrillion (10^{15}) connections and, not surprisingly with this complexity, its function is not fully understood. The vertebrate brain develops from three anterior bulges of the neural tube (see Chapter 9), which are the brain stem, the cerebellum and the cerebrum. The brain stem is formed of the medulla oblongata (which controls autonomic functions), the pons (which relays information to and from the higher centres of the brain) and the midbrain (which integrates sensory information). The brain stem is an evolutionarily older structure, which regulates essential automatic and integrative functions; it is often called the 'lower brain' and is particularly important in maintaining homeostasis and in coordinating movement. The cerebellum coordinates and error-checks motor activities and perceptual and cognitive factors.

The most highly evolved structure of the brain is the cerebrum. The outer layer of the brain is the grey matter of the cerebral cortex, which is divided into the left and right hemispheres (Fig. 1.13). The left and right hemispheres of the cerebrum have different functions, for example the ability to form words is associated with the left hemisphere whereas abstract reasoning skills is the right hemisphere. This separation is called lateralization. Different regions of the cortex are associated with different functions; they are illustrated in the 'sensory homunculus' (Fig. 1.14). Communication between the left and right cerebral cortices is via the corpus callosum, the largest bundle of nerve fibres in the entire nervous system, with >200 million axons. This structure has been shown to be very well developed when left–right coordination is high, for example in pianists, with other

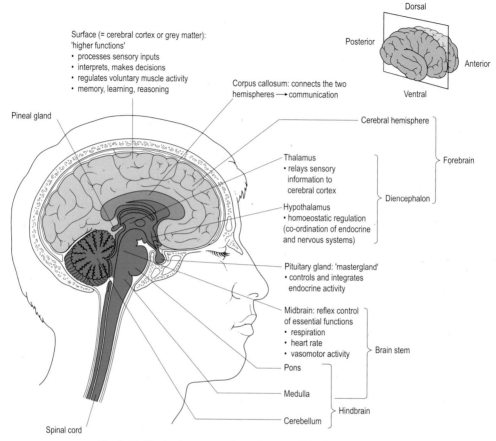

Fig. 1.13 The brain: an overview of some of the functional areas.

brain regions also changing significantly with the demands of musical practice (Gärtner et al., 2013). The reticular formation acts as a sensory filter and is concerned with states of waking and alertness. The hypothalamus is involved in motivation and regulation and integration of many metabolic and autonomic processes. The hypothalamus controls body temperature, hunger and thirst and circadian cycles, and links the nervous and endocrine systems. The cerebellum is mainly concerned with coordination of movement and repetitive performance of previously learned tasks.

The Digestive System

As animals grew larger, they could not rely upon obtaining nutrients through diffusion and random contact with the environment. As mammals evolved, they became able to feed intermittently. They could do this because they had developed the ability to digest (break down) large organic macromolecules into smaller molecules through the action of digestive enzymes. Mechanisms for food storage, such as the deposition of fat within adipose tissue, enabled periods of food shortage to be overcome. The ability to synthesize

new tissue with energy expenditure is termed 'anabolism'. When tissue is broken down there is a reverse process termed 'catabolism'; this usually results in the production of energy and waste products, which require excretion.

The gastrointestinal tract, or gut, is a long tube that runs from mouth to anus (Table 1.4) in which food is digested and absorbed, to extract energy and nutrients; the remaining waste is expelled. Food enters the mouth; here it is tasted, masticated (mechanically broken down, thus increasing its surface area) and lubricated, and enzymes are added before it is passed through the oesophagus to the stomach. The stomach is a bag-like swollen structure where the first major digestive processes occur. Hydrochloric acid secreted into the stomach maintains a pH of about 2–2.5 after food intake; this has an important role in destroying microorganisms and denaturing proteins, which allows enzymes to access them. There is some protein breakdown in the stomach through the action of pepsin and the food is mixed well. The semifluid mix of partially digested food, or chyme (pronounced 'kime'), then moves into the duodenum where most of the digestion and absorption take place. Digestive enzymes and

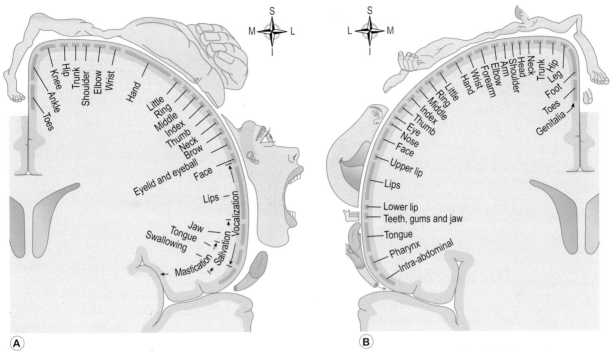

Fig. 1.14 The 'homunculus': a representation of the (A) motor and (B) sensory areas of the brain illustrating the proportion of brain tissue dedicated to these areas. (Reproduced from Waugh A, Grant A: *Ross and Wilson anatomy & physiology in health and illness*, 12 ed, Elsevier 2014, Fig. 7.22.)

bicarbonate ions (which neutralize the acidic pH) are produced from the pancreatic exocrine tissue and secreted into the duodenum. Bile salt secretion from the gall bladder is important for the digestion of fats.

The small intestine is a major site of absorption and has a very large surface area provided by a number of structural modifications. Finger-like projections of the intestinal wall called villi (Fig. 1.15) and tiny projections on the surface of the individual epithelial cells called microvilli (or the 'brush border') together increase the surface area of the small intestine by 60- to 120-fold compared with a smooth tube of the same dimensions. Many textbooks have suggested that these and other modifications result in a 260–300 m² surface area of the human gut mucosa, approximately the area of a tennis court. More recent studies, however, report a much smaller (though still impressive) surface area of about 32 m² (Helander and Fändriks, 2014). Villi are absent from the large intestine but microvilli increase its surface area by approximately 6.5-fold. The epithelial cells lining the absorptive surfaces of the gastrointestinal system have membrane-bound enzymes, for further digestion of the food molecules, and specific transporters for absorbing different molecules into the bloodstream. As mentioned above, the tight junctions present between adjacent intestinal epithelial cells ensure

that leakage of these transported molecules back into the lumen is prevented and that specific transporters involved in nutrient absorption cannot swap places between the apical and basolateral membranes, which would undermine the entire process.

Cells of the mucosa (that lines the gut) have a very rapid turnover; the entire cell lining is regenerated every 3–5 days. The stem cells of the intestinal epithelium are located in the crypts that lie between the villi. These stem cells divide and differentiate into the six differentiated cell types present in the small intestinal mucosa: absorptive enterocytes, secretory enteroendocrine, goblet and Paneth cells, and or M-(or microfold-)cells and tuft cells (Fig. 1.15d). Enterocytes comprise >90% of the cells present; enteroendocrine cells produce hormones (such as somatostatin, cholecystokinin, motilin and others), which are vital for gut function and the gut–brain axis; goblet cells produce mucus to lubricate and protect the epithelium; Paneth cells produce antimicrobial proteins to protect the gut. The production of these cell types in the correct numbers at the right time is essential for the maintenance of normal gut function. Agents that inhibit cell division such as radiation and chemotherapy drugs compromise the intestinal epithelium and total surface area so may affect nutrient absorption.

TABLE 1.4   The Digestive System

Region of Gastrointestinal System	Main Digestive Events
Mouth	• Taste • Mechanical digestion (chewing, mastication) • Food moistened and lubricated, to facilitate passage down oesophagus • Starch digestion (amylase)
Oesophagus	• Peristalsis enables transfer of food bolus to stomach • Buccal amylase activity continues

Stomach	• Stores, mixes, dissolves, releases food
	• Hydrochloric acid (HCl)
	  • lowers pH to 2
	  • kills microbes
	  • denatures proteins
	  • converts pepsinogen to pepsin
	• Mucus: protects gastric lining
	• Pepsin: protein digestion

Pancreas	• Enzyme production: digestion • Bicarbonate: neutralizes pH
Liver	• Bile production
Gall bladder	• Bile concentration and coordinated release facilitating emulsification of fats
Small intestine	• Digestion and absorption of most nutrients • Absorption of water
Large intestine	• Passage of undigested matter • Absorption of water and vitamins • Provides environment for commensal symbiotic bacteria (gut microbiota)
Rectum	• Storage of undigested matter • Defecation

The absorbed nutrients pass from the capillaries of the small intestine into the hepatic portal vein and are transported to the liver. The wall of the gut is lined with smooth muscle, which undergoes synchronous contraction, generating waves of peristaltic movement propelling the food along the gut. The control of the smooth muscle is via the enteric nervous system.

The large intestine (or colon) is important in the maintenance of fluid and iron balance and the absorption of vitamins. It is colonized and inhabited by trillions of bacteria known as the gut microbiota (Box 1.2), many of which synthesize vitamins, including vitamin B_{12}, vitamin K, thiamin and riboflavin, which can be absorbed across the gut wall. Mobility of food through the gut is increased if there are more undigested nonstarch polysaccharides (fibre) present. Some breakdown of these polysaccharides occurs by bacterial action, which can produce gas (flatus): nitrogen, carbon dioxide, hydrogen, methane and hydrogen sulphide.

Secretion and motility of the gut are controlled by nervous stimulation (Fig. 1.16). There are three phases or stages of nervous control. The cephalic phase is stimulated by the smell, taste, sight and thought of food, which increase motility and hydrochloric acid secretion. When food reaches the stomach it causes distension, increased acidity and increased protein digestion and peptide formation, which stimulate the gastric phase of control. The hormone gastrin is released, which stimulates secretion of acid and affects motility in the lower regions of the gut. The third phase of control is the intestinal phase, which is stimulated by food within the lumen of the intestine. The intestinal phase causes the reflex inhibition of gastric secretion.

The digestive system interacts with the immune system; effectively, the lining of the digestive system is an exterior surface of the body in contact with potentially pathogenic microorganisms that are ingested from food. Most of the body's immune cells (~70%) are located at the digestive system mucosal interface as individual cells and forming the gut-associated lymphoid tissue (GALT), which surveys and protects the digestive system. In addition, the digestive system provides the habitat for trillions of microorganisms (~10^{14}) about 10 times the total number of human cells, with a biomass of at least 1

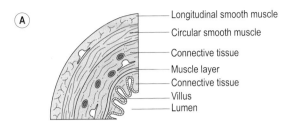

Longitudinal smooth muscle
Circular smooth muscle
Connective tissue
Muscle layer
Connective tissue
Villus
Lumen

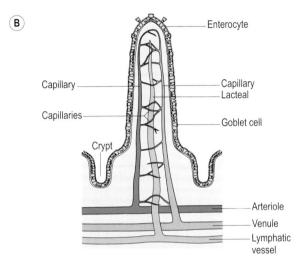

Enterocyte

Capillary

Capillary
Lacteal

Capillaries

Goblet cell

Crypt

Arteriole
Venule
Lymphatic vessel

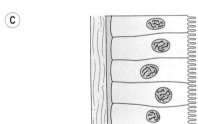

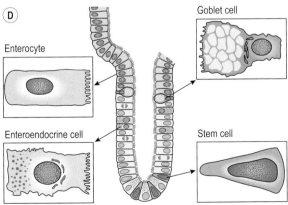

Enterocyte

Goblet cell

Enteroendocrine cell

Stem cell

Fig. 1.15 Structure of the small intestinal villi: (A) transverse section through the intestinal wall; (B) a villus; (C) details of the epithelium; (D) cell types of the villus.

BOX 1.2   Gut Microbiota

Although there are trillions of microbiota in the gut (10 bacteria cells per one human cell!), they are small and probably only contribute about a kilogram of the total body mass. They do, however, contribute >5 million different genes – over 100-fold more than the total number of genes in the human genome. The microbiota have been described as 'the forgotten organ'; it is becoming increasingly evident that it plays an extraordinary role in human health. The human immune system is significantly influenced by the composition of the gut microbiota; dysbiosis or abnormal composition is associated with increased likelihood of autoimmune diseases such as rheumatoid arthritis and type 1 diabetes and metabolic conditions such as type 2 diabetes. The microorganisms that constitute the microbiota are nonpathogenic in the optimal ratio and do not cause disease unless the balance of the microorganisms changes. They are therefore commensal bacteria that live in symbiosis with their human host. The profile of microbiota is different in individuals who are obese; it has less diversity and increased proportions of bacteria which can increase the efficiency of energy extracted from otherwise indigestible carbohydrates. The human skin also offers a niche for microorganisms. Although the optimal composition of microbiota has not yet been definitively established, it is clear that some events during the fetal and postnatal lifecycle have significant and lasting effects on the microbiota and on the infant's developing immune system. These include mode of delivery (vaginal birth results in inoculation of the newborn with maternal microbiota); method of feeding (many components of human breast milk promote 'healthy' microbiota), timing of weaning and foods that are introduced, and use of antibiotics. It is also suggested that maternal diet in pregnancy and lactation may play a role in the establishment of the microbiota of the infant and some microorganisms are introduced in the amniotic fluid and breast milk.

kg). Most of the gut microbiota (microorganisms) reside in the colon and provide a repository of functional genes (known as the 'microbiome') that make a significant contribution to host processes such as protecting against pathogens, interacting with the immune system, promoting gut development and synthesizing essential nutrients such as vitamins.

The Respiratory System

Respiration is essential for the functioning of all living organisms. Physiological respiration is the exchange of gases between the environment and the body. The term 'cellular respiration' refers to the metabolic processes in cells by which substrates (such as glucose, fatty acids and amino acids) are oxidized to water and carbon dioxide, releasing biochemical

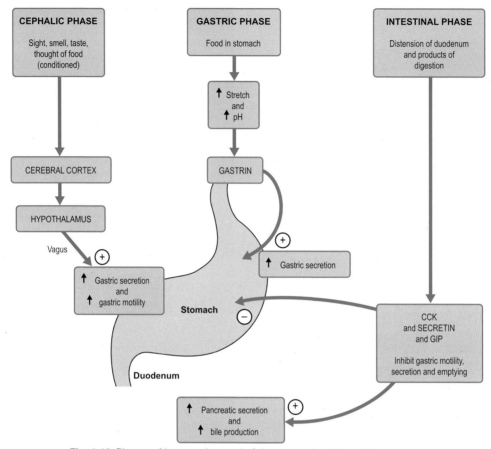

Fig. 1.16 Phases of hormonal control of the stomach and associated organs.

energy in the form of ATP and heat. There are two types: aerobic and anaerobic. In aerobic respiration, organic molecules from ingested food are oxidized to produce energy (Fig. 1.17). Anaerobic respiration is when energy is produced in the absence of oxygen. This form of respiration is relatively inefficient compared with aerobic respiration, for example producing two molecules of ATP per glucose molecule, compared with approximately 30 molecules of ATP from oxidative metabolism of glucose to CO_2 and water.

Anaerobic respiration is common among single-celled organisms. Large animals, such as humans, can produce some energy anaerobically, for instance in times of acute stress and rapid muscle activity when oxygen demand exceeds oxygen supply. However, anaerobic respiration results in the rapid accumulation of toxic metabolites. In simple organisms, these may simply diffuse out of the cell into the environment, but for large animals this rapid excretion cannot be achieved and so anaerobic processes are self-limiting. 'Asphyxia' is the term that describes irreversible damage to cells due to the build-up of these toxins (see Box 15.1 for a description of 'Fetal asphyxia').

Aerobic respiration is an extension of anaerobic respiration. The metabolites such as pyruvate, produced under anaerobic processes such as glycolysis, are further broken down producing carbon dioxide, water and significantly more energy. Aerobic respiration requires the presence of oxygen and mitochondria, the sites of the enzymes involved in these biochemical pathways. Cells require a continuous source of oxygen for metabolism.

The respiratory system consists of the lungs, the branching airways, the gaseous exchange membranes, the rib cage and respiratory muscles. Ventilation is the mechanical activity that moves gases in and out of the lungs; the movements of the intercostal muscles and diaphragm allow filling and emptying of the lungs (Fig. 1.18). An adult at rest will take 10–16 breaths/min and inspire about 250 mL of oxygen and expire about 200 mL of carbon dioxide every minute. The respiratory tract provides a large surface area that, while optimizing gas exchange, is vulnerable, as it is constantly exposed to microorganisms. An important function of the respiratory system is to defend itself and prevent pathogens gaining access to the body (Box 1.3).

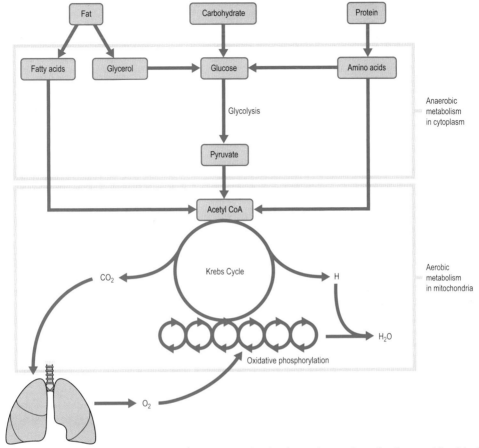

Fig. 1.17 A summary of metabolism: substrate molecules (such as glucose from food) are oxidized (using respiratory oxygen), producing carbon dioxide (expired) and energy in the form of ATP.

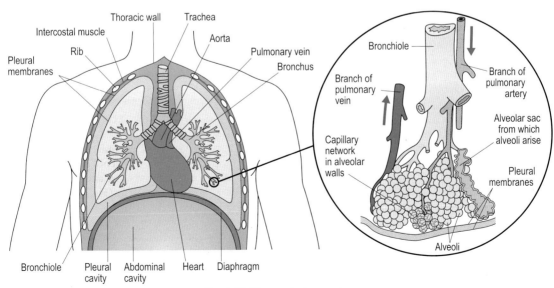

Fig. 1.18 The respiratory system.

BOX 1.3 Defence Mechanisms of the Respiratory System

The vasculature, which warms and moistens the inhaled air

Mucus secretion, which forms a sticky layer (blanket) that traps infective agents, foreign particles and other debris

Ciliated cells: the cilia, which beat >1000 times/min, waft the mucus blanket propelling it upwards away from the gas exchanging region to the pharynx where it is swallowed or coughed out. (This combination of mucus and cilia is known as the 'mucociliary escalator'.)

Branching of the bronchial tree, which increases the chances of an inhaled particle coming into contact with the mucus blanket

Phagocytes (macrophages and neutrophils), which engulf inhaled particles and microorganisms

Immunologically active secretions such as specific antibodies (secretory immunoglobulin A), complement, lysozyme, lactoferrin, interferon and phagocytosis promoters

Irritation responses and protective reflexes such as coughing and sneezing

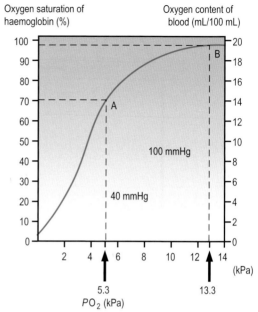

Fig. 1.19 The oxygen–haemoglobin dissociation curve. (Reproduced with permission from Brooker, 1998.)

Gas exchange occurs across the capillary and moist membranes of the alveoli, which are very thin (~0.2 μm), lined with squamous epithelium and therefore have a very low diffusion distance. Oxygen from the inspired air diffuses into the capillaries where it binds temporarily to haemoglobin in the red blood cells. The binding of oxygen to haemoglobin can be graphically described by the oxygen–haemoglobin dissociation curve (Fig. 1.19). Haemoglobin has a high affinity for oxygen at higher concentrations and its binding sites are saturated with oxygen in the alveoli. At low concentrations of oxygen, haemoglobin has a low affinity for oxygen, so it releases oxygen at the tissues. Binding of oxygen to haemoglobin is altered by carbon dioxide, pH, temperature and the glycolytic intermediate 2,3-bisphosphoglycerate (also known as 2,3-diphosphoglycerate). These alter the shape of the haemoglobin molecule, which affects its oxygen-binding sites. Substances that reduce haemoglobin–oxygen affinity increase the release of oxygen (so the curve is shifted towards the right and oxygen is unloaded more readily at the tissues).

Carbon dioxide diffuses from the tissues into the capillaries. It is mostly taken up by the red blood cells where it reacts with water to form carbonic acid. This reaction is catalysed by the enzyme carbonic anhydrase in the red blood cells. Carbonic acid is unstable and dissociates to bicarbonate and hydrogen ions (Fig. 1.20); the bicarbonate diffuses out of the red blood cell into the plasma. This accounts for about 70% of the carbon dioxide in the blood; about 23% is bound to haemoglobin in red blood cells and the remaining 7% is dissolved in the plasma.

The respiratory control centre, in the medulla oblongata of the brain stem, affects the activity of the inspiratory and expiratory neurons that control the respiratory muscles, which contract to allow inspiration and expiration. The respiratory centre receives information from stretch receptors in the lungs and from the peripheral and central chemoreceptors that monitor the pH and oxygen content of the blood (Fig. 1.21).

There is homeostatic regulation of acid–base balance to maintain pH within narrow parameters at around 7.3 (Fig. 1.22). This regulation involves both the respiratory and the renal systems (see Chapter 2).

The Cardiovascular System

The cardiovascular system includes the heart, the blood vessels and the blood. The blood is pumped around a network of blood vessels (Fig. 1.23). Arteries transport blood away from the heart and have thick muscular walls. Veins carry blood towards the heart; they function as a capacitance system. The blood vessels are differentiated by their structure and the direction that blood flows (not by whether the blood is oxygenated or not). Capillaries link the arterial and venous systems and allow exchange of substances between the blood and the tissues.

The heart functions as a double pump, pumping blood to the tissues of the body and the lungs (Fig. 1.24). Blood

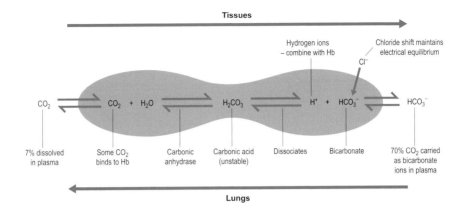

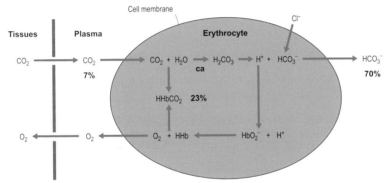

Fig. 1.20 Carbon dioxide transport. (Reproduced with permission from Brooker, 1998.)

from the right ventricle of the heart is pumped via the pulmonary artery to the capillaries surrounding the alveoli of the lungs where the blood is oxygenated. Oxygenated blood returns to the left atrium of the heart in the pulmonary veins. The oxygenated blood is then pumped from the left ventricle via the aorta and the systemic circulation, around the body to the tissues and back to the right atrium of the heart. There are two circulatory routes, which do not fit the general pattern of double circulation. The portal blood blow from the hypothalamus to the anterior pituitary gland (see Chapter 3) is one of these. The other is associated with the gut. The deoxygenated (but nutrient-enriched) blood from the digestive system drains into the hepatic portal vein, which goes to the liver, allowing the liver to take up absorbed nutrients (and neutralize any absorbed toxins). From the liver, blood drains to the hepatic veins then into the inferior vena cava and from there to the heart.

The coronary circulation is the circulation of blood within the vessels of the heart. Blood flow to the brain is via a circular arrangement of vessels (the circle of Willis); this ensures that there will always be sufficient oxygen and nutrients, albeit at the expense of other parts of the body when the circulatory system is under stress. The blood–brain barrier protects the brain against the entry of some harmful substances, such as toxins.

The adult heart beats about 70 times/min at rest, forcing blood from the ventricles into the pulmonary artery and the aorta. The increased volume of blood entering the circulation causes a fluctuating increase in blood pressure. The highest blood pressure occurs after ventricular contraction (or systole), which adds the ejection fraction (the volume of blood pushed out of the ventricle) to the blood in the main arteries; this is systolic blood pressure. Diastolic blood pressure is the lowest blood pressure, which occurs when the ventricles are in diastole (relaxed). Blood pressure can be measured using a sphygmomanometer to record pressure within an artery and a stethoscope to listen to the turbulence of blood within the blood vessels (this is called 'auscultation') (Fig. 1.25). The amount of blood that leaves the heart per minute is described as the cardiac output. This is the volume of blood ejected from the ventricles each time the heart beats multiplied by the number of beats per minute (Fig. 1.26). The amount of oxygen that reaches the cells of the tissue depends on the proportion of the cardiac output the tissue receives.

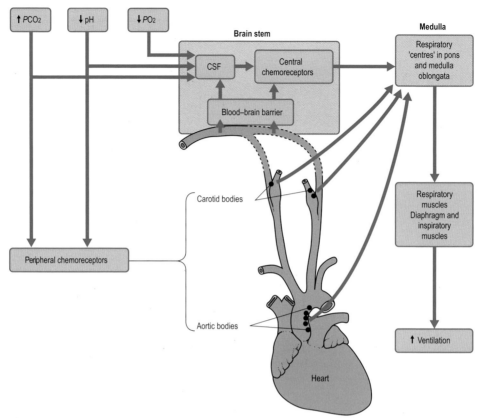

Fig. 1.21 Chemoreceptor control of respiration: the regulation of ventilation is achieved via peripheral and central chemoreceptors, which sample the blood, and then via a neuronal pathway influencing the rate and depth of breathing. CSF, cerebrospinal fluid.

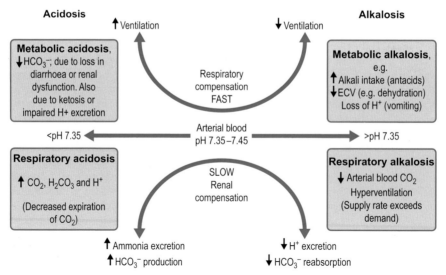

Fig. 1.22 Acid–base balance.

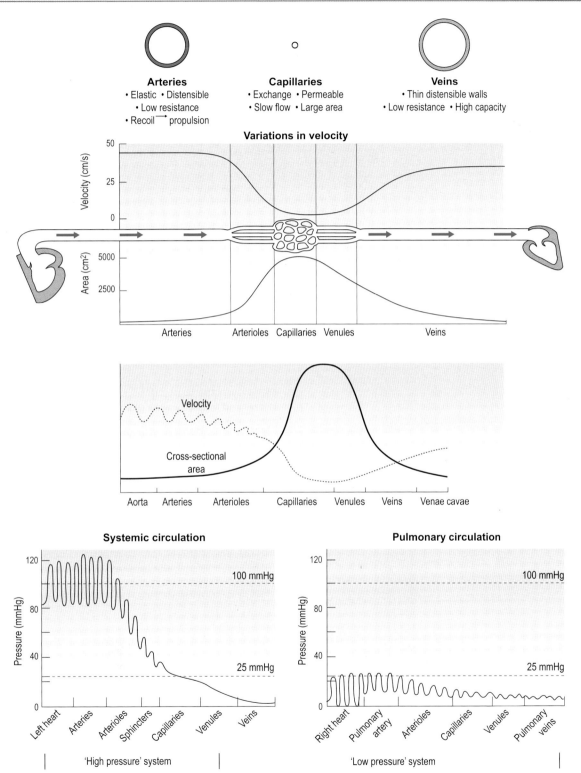

Fig. 1.23 Blood vessels: the major role of arteries is in the generation of elastic recoil, which propels the blood around the body. The capillaries are involved in gas exchange and the veins act as capacitance vessels returning blood to the heart.

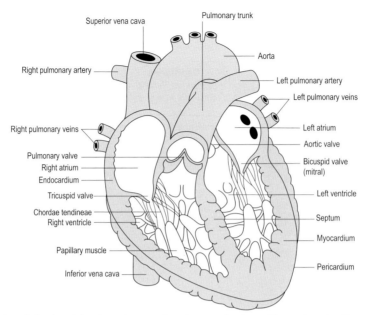

Fig. 1.24 Interior of the heart to show layers, chambers and valves. (Reproduced with permission from Brooker, 1998.)

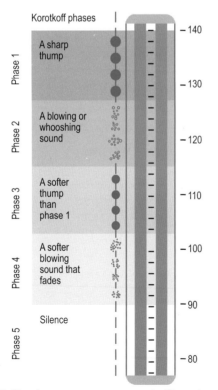

Fig. 1.25 Blood pressure measurement. (Reproduced from Perry AG, Potter PA: *Mosby's pocket guide to nursing skills & procedures*, 9 ed, Elsevier 2019, Fig. 8.1.)

The heart's internal pacemaker, the sinoatrial node (SAN), sets the heart rate. The SAN spontaneously depolarizes and triggers a wave of electrical activity, which stimulates the heart muscle to contract (Fig. 1.27). The SAN is innervated by both parasympathetic and sympathetic nerves. Receptors throughout the body respond to changes in blood pressure and respiratory gas level. These baroreceptors and chemoreceptors, respectively, transmit information to afferent nerves in the medulla of the brain (the brain stem) that control efferent nerves to the heart, lungs and blood vessels (Fig. 1.28).

The total capacity of blood vessels in the body exceeds the volume of the blood. To maintain homeostasis and tissue requirements, the cardiovascular system is carefully regulated to ensure optimal oxygenation of the tissues. The control of blood flow is regulated by an increase (vasodilation) or a decrease (vasoconstriction) of the diameter of the blood vessels, which changes the flow of blood in the vessel as well as peripheral resistance (also called 'systemic vascular resistance'; SVR). The diameter of the blood vessels is altered by the activity of sympathetic nerves that innervate the smooth muscle in the vessel walls. Increased sympathetic activity in the flight or fight response, as mentioned above, can redirect blood flow to the tissues that need more O_2 and nutrients, while triggering vasoconstriction of blood vessels in other tissues. Adrenaline (epinephrine) will trigger vasodilation of the blood vessels in skeletal muscle, which express β-adrenergic receptors, so that

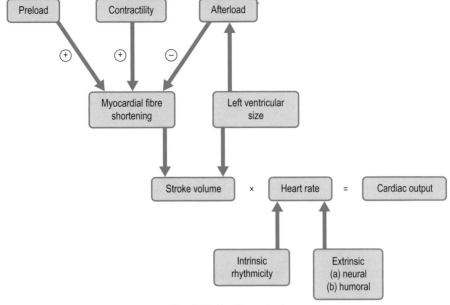

Fig. 1.26 Cardiac output.

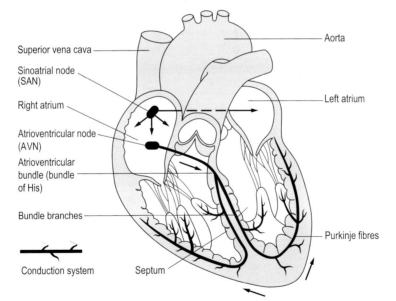

Fig. 1.27 Sinoatrial node (SAN) depolarization: the conduction pathway of the heart enables the organ's co-ordinated and rhythmic beating.

blood supply is increased to support the 'flight-or-fight' response. Conversely, adrenaline will trigger vasoconstriction in intestinal blood vessels via α-adrenergic receptors, thus shifting the supply of blood from the gut to skeletal muscle. In addition, the same β-adrenergic receptor type on liver cells will signal the breakdown of stored glycogen to release glucose into the bloodstream to support muscle contraction. Blood vessel diameter is also controlled locally by tissue metabolites. This autoregulation increases blood flow to metabolically active tissues.

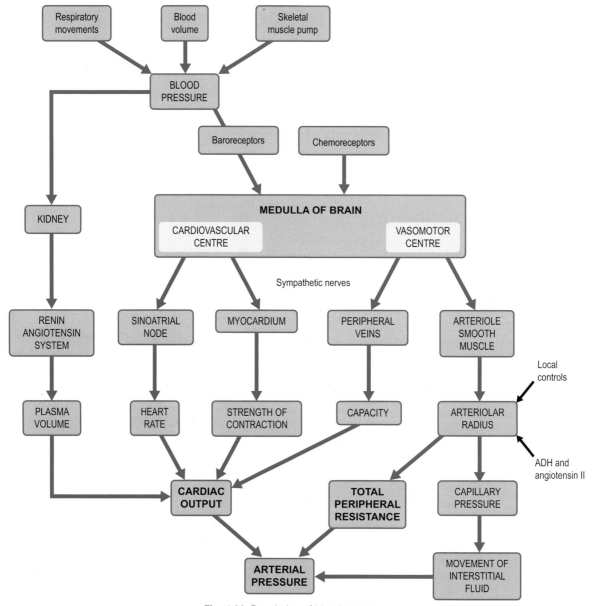

Fig. 1.28 Regulation of blood pressure.

The circulation of blood in the capillaries is called microcirculation; about 7% of total circulating blood volume is in the microcirculation. Capillaries are effectively leaky and allow fluid from the blood, but not red blood cells and large plasma proteins, to leave the blood by diffusion to form interstitial fluid, which delivers oxygen and nutrients to the tissue supplied by the capillaries. Most of the fluid returns to the capillary but some is collected by the lymphatic system (see p. 27).

Blood

Blood is a suspension of cells in plasma (see Table 1.2). Blood cells are all derived from haematopoietic stem cells in the bone marrow. The majority (>99%) of cells are red blood cells (or erythrocytes). Red blood cells contain haemoglobin, a protein containing iron, which binds to oxygen. Iron, folic acid and vitamin B_{12} are required for the production of erythrocytes. The kidneys produce

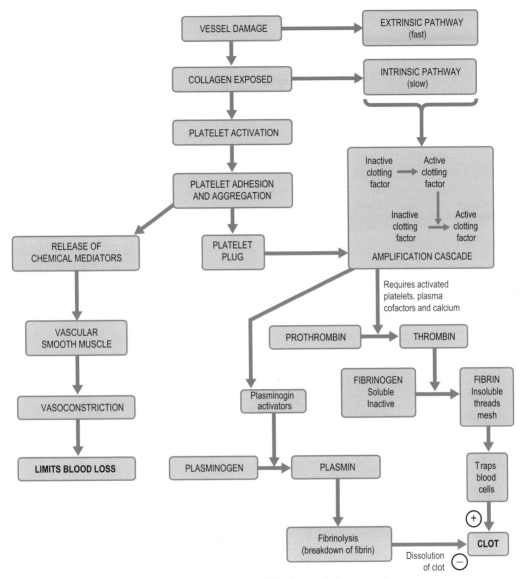

Fig. 1.29 Haemostasis: the blood coagulation cascade.

a hormone, erythropoietin, in response to low oxygen levels, which stimulates an increase in the production of red blood cells (erythropoiesis) from the bone marrow. Leukocytes, or white blood cells, include polymorphonuclear leukocytes (neutrophils, eosinophils and basophils) and the agranular monocytes and lymphocytes; white blood cells and platelets are also produced in the bone marrow (in a process called 'myelopoiesis'). The role of white blood cells is the defence of the body (see Chapter 10). Platelets are cellular fragments of megakaryocytes, which are an essential component

of the blood-clotting mechanism (Fig. 1.29). Plasma is predominantly water and contains proteins (albumin, globulins and some clotting factors, such as fibrinogen), nutrients, hormones, waste products and ions. The normal range of blood pH is 7.35–7.45 (Fig. 1.30); the pH is maintained by buffering, and the renal and respiratory systems.

The Lymphatic System

The lymphatic system is part of the circulatory system and consists of a network of thin branching vessels, lymph nodes, lymphatic organs (thymus and bone marrow, which produce lymphocytes) and the spleen and lymphatic fluid (Fig. 1.31). About 20 L of fluid in total leaves the capillary blood and enters the interstitial tissue, of this about 17 L returns to the venous end of the capillaries (Fig. 1.32). The lymphatic system collects the remaining 3 L of interstitial fluid bathing tissue and returns it to the blood. Lymphatic fluid has a similar composition to plasma; it contains white blood cells such as lymphocytes, proteins, waste products, cellular debris and bacteria. The lymphatic system has no pump and lymph vessels have one-way valves like veins, and depend on the movement of skeletal muscle and intrinsic contractions of the lymphatic vessels to propel the fluid, which moves slowly under low pressure. The lymphatic fluid in the vessels is drained into lymphatic ducts, which then drain into the subclavian veins so lymphatic fluid is returned to the blood circulatory system.

The lymphatic system transports lymphocytes and is important in defending the body against microorganisms (see Chapter 10) and against metastasis of tumours. Lymph nodes in the lymphatic system contain lymphocytes and act as collecting filters for viruses and bacteria, which are then destroyed. Lymphatic vessels (lacteals) are also present in the lining of the digestive tract and transport digested lipids that have been absorbed in the small intestine to the thoracic duct so they enter the venous circulation.

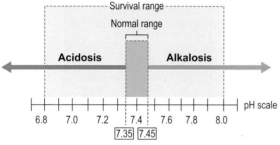

Fig. 1.30 Acid–base balance: the maintenance of blood pH.

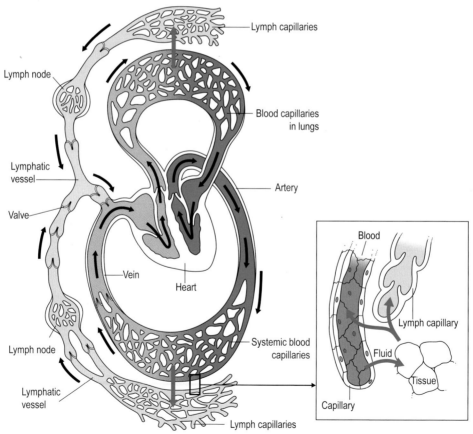

Fig. 1.31 The lymphatic system.

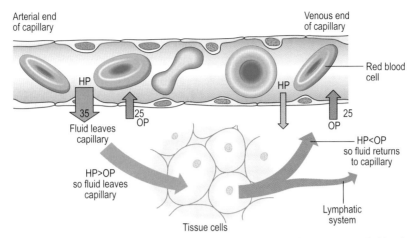

Fig. 1.32 Capillary exchange. At the arterial end of the capillary, the dominant pressure is blood pressure so fluid leaves the blood and bathes over the cells. Most fluid, now depleted in nutrients and oxygen, returns to the venous end of the capillary where the dominant driver is the osmotic pressure of the plasma proteins. About 15% of interstitial fluid is transported back to the blood via the lymphatic system.

METABOLISM

Energy Production and Storage

Cells have a continuous requirement for energy and adenosine triphosphate (ATP). The energy from ATP drives virtually all the body processes but there is very little ATP present at any one time, just enough to provide energy requirements for only a few minutes. Every tissue requires energy but some, such as muscles, have a very variable energy requirement. Meals provide fuel from food components, which are oxidized to provide ATP and heat. However, the intake of food is irregular and does not coordinate with the requirement for energy. The energy substrates from a meal are usually absorbed within 3 h; as the next meal can be hours away, animals have evolved efficient methods of storing energy substrates.

The main storage forms of energy are glycogen in the liver and skeletal muscle and triacylglycerides in adipose tissue. Carbohydrates are the major fuels for the brain and nervous tissue. Oxidation of glucose occurs in several stages (Fig. 1.33). Glycolysis takes place in the cell cytosol and produces a little ATP anaerobically. If oxygen is present, the products of glycolysis can be oxidized through the tricarboxylic acid (TCA) cycle (Krebs cycle) and oxidative phosphorylation (the electron transport chain), both of which occur in mitochondria. This increased efficiency of ATP production takes place only in cells that have mitochondria and adequate provision of oxygen. In tissues lacking mitochondria, such as red blood cells, or those with insufficient oxygen, such as active muscle, there is a build-up of the key intermediate pyruvate. Pyruvate can be converted into lactate and oxidized by the heart and kidneys or converted to glucose by the liver and kidneys.

About 500 g of the glucose polymer, glycogen, is stored: 100 g in the liver, which can release the glucose when required (by glycogenolysis), and 400 g in the skeletal muscles, which is reserved for use by the muscle. Triacylglycerides are stored in virtually unlimited amounts, as observed in obesity. As they do not mix with water, the storage form is very calorie dense and efficient. Triacylglycerides (triglycerides) are composed of three fatty acids bound to a glycerol backbone. The glycerol can be converted into glyceraldehyde-3-phosphate and enter the glycolysis pathway, thereby providing a substrate for the brain to oxidize for energy. Fatty acids are released with free glycerol from the adipose tissue and can be oxidized by the liver, muscles and kidneys. Fatty acids cannot cross the blood–brain barrier and cannot be converted to glucose so they provide little substrate for the brain directly but are used preferentially by other tissues thus sparing available glucose for the brain. Ketone bodies are water-soluble derivatives of fatty acids formed by the liver during starvation or prolonged severe exercise. When sufficient concentrations of ketone bodies accumulate, the brain and kidney use them to generate ATP. Certain amino acids are also ketogenic and can be converted into ketone bodies. Overproduction of ketone bodies, as in uncontrolled diabetes, overwhelms the buffering capacity of the body and can cause life-threatening acidosis (known as ketosis or ketoacidosis).

There is no reserve storage form of protein independent of function. Protein can be metabolized to provide energy but at the expense of the breakdown of structural

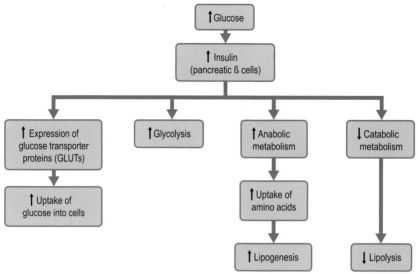

Fig. 1.33 Oxidation of glucose.

and functional components of the body. The use of protein as a fuel potentially damages the body, so it is used only as a 'last resort' when the protein is broken down and the amino acids are converted into components of the glycolytic pathway to produce energy. However, proteins constitute a large proportion of body structure and therefore can provide a substantial source of energy when other supplies have been exhausted. Protein in excess of requirements can be irreversibly converted into glucose or triacylglycerides.

The brain consumes about a quarter of the body's daily energy production when the body is at rest. The brain's requirement for fuel drives energy metabolism. The main fuel storage form of the body is triacylglycerides, but the brain cannot use fatty acids directly. Although the brain can oxidize ketone bodies, derived from fatty acids, for 80% of its energy requirements, 20% must come from glucose. Glucose comes from the diet or from breakdown of liver glycogen (glycogenolysis) or synthesis of glucose from amino acids or glycerol (gluconeogenesis) in the liver. Other cells therefore utilize other substrates in preference to glucose. The hierarchy of fuel use means that the brain utilizes ketone bodies, when they are available, or glucose. Muscle has a major reserve of protein and glycogen. Muscle spares brain fuel by preferentially oxidizing fatty acids, thus sparing ketone bodies and glucose for the brain. Since muscle lacks the glucose-6-phosphatase enzyme needed to produce free glucose from glycogen breakdown, the glycogen stored in muscle is specifically available for muscle use.

The external environment is continually fluctuating and energy requirements are constantly changing. However, the body maintains homeostasis or internal stability by ensuring a constant level of amino acids and glucose in the blood, despite intermittent high loads following a meal. The level of ATP within cells is kept relatively constant although the rate of usage is variable; for instance, activity increases the energy requirement of a muscle by up to 20-fold. Cellular energy requirement is regulated very sensitively; metabolic pathways that predominate after a meal (called the absorptive state) are different from those between meals (the postabsorptive state) (Fig. 1.34). Dominance of the pathways is via substrate concentration, changes in enzyme activity or amount (via gene expression) and altered transport of substrates, often controlled by hormones. Interconversion from one metabolic step to the next is regulated by substrate activation, where the substance stimulates its own use, and product inhibition, where the product prevents the reaction from continuing. Enzymes and transporters can be relocated between different cellular compartments (compartmentation) to regulate metabolic pathways and enzymes catalysing the same reaction may exist as isoenzymes in different types of tissue, having different affinities for their substrates. This means that different concentrations of substrate are required for the biochemical pathway to progress.

Blood Sugar Regulation

When plasma glucose concentration rises after a meal, secretion of insulin from pancreatic β-cells is stimulated and plasma levels of insulin increase. Insulin triggers the translocation of vesicles containing the insulin-sensitive glucose transporter, GLUT4, from intracellular sites to the cell membrane of the insulin-sensitive tissues, skeletal

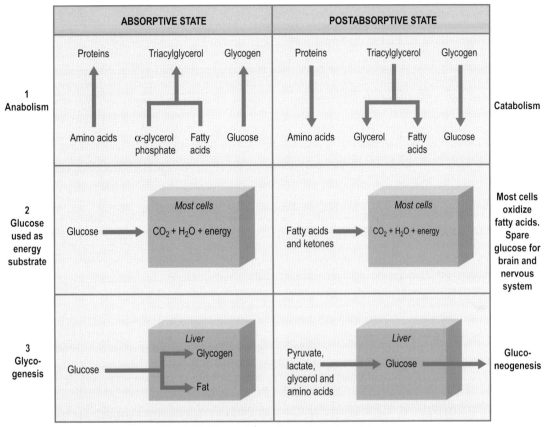

	ABSORPTIVE STATE	POSTABSORPTIVE STATE	
1 **Anabolism**	Proteins Triacylglycerol Glycogen ↑ ↑ ↑ Amino acids α-glycerol phosphate Fatty acids Glucose	Proteins Triacylglycerol Glycogen ↓ ↓ ↓ Amino acids Glycerol Fatty acids Glucose	**Catabolism**
2 **Glucose used as energy substrate**	*Most cells* Glucose → CO₂ + H₂O + energy	*Most cells* Fatty acids and ketones → CO₂ + H₂O + energy	**Most cells oxidize fatty acids. Spare glucose for brain and nervous system**
3 **Glyco-genesis**	*Liver* Glucose → Glycogen / Fat	*Liver* Pyruvate, lactate, glycerol and amino acids → Glucose →	**Gluco-neogenesis**

Fig. 1.34 Absorptive and postabsorptive states.

and cardiac muscle and adipocytes. This increases the uptake of glucose into the cell and promotes the anabolic (storage) biochemical pathways (Fig. 1.35). Tissues that have a constant requirement for glucose, such as brain cells, do not have insulin-sensitive glucose transporters but do express the high-affinity transporter, GLUT3, as well as GLUT1. Under conditions of low plasma glucose concentration, for example during overnight fasting, secretion of glucagon from pancreatic α-cells is increased, which acts to mobilize liver glycogen (glycogenolysis) and switch on glucose production by liver (gluconeogenesis) so that plasma glucose levels are raised. This homeostatic regulation of plasma glucose levels by opposing hormones insulin and glucagon maintains plasma glucose levels within a very narrow range (~4.5–7 mM). Adrenaline, secreted from the adrenal medulla in response to sympathetic innervation, causes a rapid mobilization of fuels for 'fight or flight' (see p. 13). Adrenaline stimulates glycogen breakdown in both muscle and liver but glucose is released only from the liver, and increases lipolysis in adipose tissue so that levels of glucose and fatty acids increase to provide additional metabolic fuel.

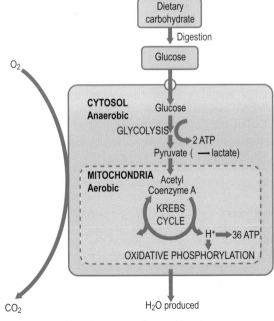

Fig. 1.35 The effects of insulin.

Application to Practice

Physiological observations to assess maternal well-being

To assess wellbeing during pregnancy, practitioners must consider how physiological parameters are altered in pregnant women and when these altered parameters become abnormal in relation to pregnancy, but observations to assess wellbeing cannot be considered in isolation. It is important to monitor respiratory rate as well as blood pressure, pulse and temperature. A rising respiratory rate can be an early indicator of respiratory distress. Ideally, respiratory rate should be counted without informing the woman so that she is not aware that her breathing is being assessed because that is likely to affect the respiratory rate. Tachypnoea (rapid breathing) is a significant clinical feature that should not be dismissed as being caused by anxiety or stress, or related to pain. If tachypnoea is present with a rapid pulse and a fall in blood pressure, then the maternal condition might be deteriorating because of cardiovascular problems, such as haemorrhage or sepsis. It is common for oxygen saturation to be monitored to assess respiratory function; however, oxygen saturation is often maintained in the presence of tachypnoea (98% +) and a fall in oxygen saturation is therefore a late indicator of advanced maternal distress.

A raised temperature is a significant indicator of sepsis; however, if sepsis is severe, body temperature measured orally or in the axilla may be misleadingly low because of peripheral vascular shutdown caused by toxicity. Thus, an abnormally low temperature can also indicate advanced sepsis. In such cases, core temperature should be measured, for example by use of a rectal probe. The greater the difference between core and peripheral temperature, the more likely it is that sepsis is severe.

If the pulse rate is higher (beats/min) than the systolic blood pressure (measured in millimetres of mercury; mmHg), this also indicates serious deterioration in the wellbeing of the woman.

Blood pressure is usually lower and pulse rate is slightly faster in pregnancy, so direct comparisons to nonpregnant values are not valid. Whenever possible, midwives should access prepregnancy observations, for example, from well-women clinic records, family planning clinics, GP notes, etc., thus providing a reference point when assessing normal physiological changes in pregnancy. Women who do not have lower blood pressure in the first trimester than their prepregnant parameter are at greater risk of hypertensive problems in pregnancy and in later life or may have underlying renal problems.

Blood pressure must be measured using a cuff appropriate to the size of the woman's arm. If automated machines are being used to measure blood pressure, it is essential that they are regularly calibrated.

Women should have direct access to midwives or lead maternity carers as soon as pregnancy is confirmed so that pregnancy care can be planned to meet their individual needs. The women will experience the physiological changes described within this book, so the midwife must be able to reassure the women that these are normal and also to be able to recognize when such changes are not occurring normally.

KEY POINTS

- Cells have different anatomical structures, which are related to their physiological functions.
- Cells are organized together to form tissues, which are organized into organs and the physiological systems of the body.
- The role of the physiological systems is to provide internal stability or homeostasis, which will ensure that the cells' variable but essential requirements for energy are met by an adequate supply of oxygen and nutrients.
- As the enzymes and transporters that regulate cellular activity are proteins, they are affected by fluctuations in pH and temperature, so homeostasis has to maintain optimum temperature and acid–base balance.

APPLICATION TO PRACTICE

The basic physiology described in this chapter relates to the nonpregnant state. During pregnancy, there are many physiological changes, explored throughout the rest of this book. A basic knowledge of physiology is essential so that the complexities of the physiological changes in pregnancy can be understood, assessed and explained. This knowledge is also essential for the midwife to be able to monitor the development of pregnancy effectively and make appropriate referrals when deviations from normal are suspected.

ANNOTATED FURTHER READING

Alberts B, Bray D, Lewis J, et al.: *Molecular biology of the cell*, ed 6, New York, 2014, Garland.
A beautifully written and well-illustrated text on molecular and cellular biology, which is accessible, easy to read and up-to-date; the cell biologist's 'Bible'.
Koeppen BM, Stanton BA: *Berne & Levy physiology*, ed 7, St Louis, 2017, Elsevier.
A comprehensive and well-illustrated textbook, which emphasizes physiological concepts and basic principles of organ systems.
Koeppen BM, Stanton B: *Renal physiology*, ed 5, Mosby, 2012.
Provides a useful reference to the core concepts of normal renal physiology including clinical applications and cellular and molecular aspects
Raff H, Widmaier EP, Strang KT: *Vander's human physiology: the mechanisms of body function*, ed 15, New York, 2018, McGraw-Hill.
An updated version of the classical textbook, which provides a useful guide to the principles of human physiology using clear diagrams and flow diagrams; the new edition includes more clinical application and physiological inquiry questions designed to promote critical thinking.
Salway J: *Metabolism at a glance*, ed 4, Oxford, 2016, Blackwell.
A revised and extensively illustrated large-format book, which provides a comprehensive review of basic human metabolism, including inborn errors of metabolism and clinical aspects of metabolism. Metabolic pathways are summarized as segments with a clear diagrammatic pathway map on one page and an outline of the metabolism on the facing page.
Salway J: *Medical biochemistry at a glance*, ed 3, Oxford, 2012, Wiley-Blackwell.
A useful overview of human biochemistry and its application to clinical medicine, which provides a synopsis using detailed flowcharts and explanatory diagrams.
Tortora GJ, Derrickson BH: *Principles of anatomy and physiology*, ed 15, New York, 2017, John Wiley and Sons.
A clear, comprehensive and generously illustrated textbook (supported by an online learning environment) providing an in-depth overview of physiology and anatomy. It is targeted at students in a range of health professions and includes clinical applications and study outlines.
Ward JPT, Linden RWA: *Physiology at a glance*, ed 4, Oxford, 2017, Wiley-Blackwell.
Another of the popular 'at-a-glance' series of books, which provides clear and concise summaries and useful tables related to the core concepts and structure-function relationships of physiological systems. The companion website provides a range of resources such as flashcards, revision notes and interactive test questions.

REFERENCES

Brooker CG: *Human structure and function*, ed 2, St Louis, 1998, Mosby, pp 15, 30, 32, 33, 88, 207, 211, 228, 277, 279, 296, 372, 383.
Gärtner H, Minnerop M, Pieperhoff P, et al.: Brain morphometry shows effects of long-term musical practice in middle-aged keyboard players, *Front Psychol* 4:636, 2013.
Helander HF, Fändriks L: Surface area of the digestive tract – revisited, *Scand J Gastroenterol* 49:681–689, 2014.

The Reproductive and Urinary Systems

INTRODUCTION

This chapter reviews the basic anatomy of human reproductive and urinary systems. The human urinary system differs only slightly between the male and female, mostly in relation to the structure of the external genitalia and length of the urethra. The function of the urinary system is also essentially the same in men and women. However, the renal system can be severely stressed by pregnancy, mostly because of its close proximity to the reproductive organs and the major changes in fluid balance resulting in fluid retention during pregnancy. The midwife needs to understand the basics of normal renal physiology in order to understand the changes that take place in the renal system during pregnancy and how these may affect the general condition of the woman. For example, not only are the regulation and retention of fluid altered in pregnancy but also excretion of glucose and other substances is affected by these changes. Drug excretion via the kidneys may also be modified, so long-term medication may need to be changed as pregnancy progresses. The effectiveness of medication may be reduced and altered drug dosage may also be required. (Specific changes in the renal system in pregnancy are covered in Chapter 11.)

THE URINARY SYSTEM

The urinary system is composed of two kidneys, which produce urine, two ureters which carry this urine from the kidneys to the bladder which collects and stores the urine, and a urethra from which urine is discharged to the exterior (Fig. 2.1). The uroepithelium, which lines the renal pelvis, ureters and bladder, is not just a passive impermeable barrier; it can modulate the composition of urine and also transmit information about the extracellular environment such as the bladder pressure and composition of the urine to the underlying nervous, muscular and connective tissues (Birder and Wyndaele, 2013).

CHAPTER CASE STUDY

Zara, during the booking appointment, is asked by the midwife to provide a mid-stream specimen of urine to screen for infection. The midwife notes that the specimen appears cloudy, although Zara does not have any other signs of a urinary tract infection.

- Are there any reasons apart from infection that could explain the cloudiness of the specimen?
- If the culture of the specimen proves positive, how will this be managed and what advice should the midwife give to Zara?

- If the analysis of the specimen showed a bacteraemia of group B (haemolytic) streptococcus (GBS infection), what would be the significance of this, how should it be managed and what are the possible future consequences for Zara and her baby?
- If protein was detected in Zara's urine, how could this be explained and what should the midwife do about it?
- Are there any other factors not related to infection that may suggest an abnormal situation? How might these be relevant to Zara's health?

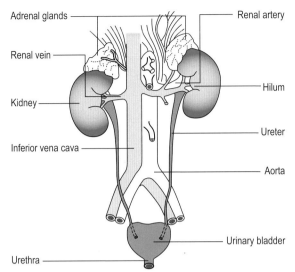

Fig. 2.1 The urinary system. (Reproduced with permission from Brooker, 1998.)

The Kidneys

The kidneys have a broad range of other functions (Box 2.1) as well as producing urine. The kidneys are situated upon the posterior wall of the abdominal cavity, one on either side of the vertebral column at the level of the thoracic and lumbar vertebrae (just below the rib cage). The right kidney is slightly lower than the left owing to its inferior relationship to the liver. Each kidney is about 10 cm long, 6.5 cm wide and about 3 cm thick (about the size of a clenched fist). Each kidney weighs about 100 g (a small proportion of the total body mass), but they receive about 25% of the cardiac output (which per unit of tissue is about eight times higher than the blood flow to muscles undergoing heavy exercise). The renal blood supply arises from the aorta via the renal arteries and returns to the inferior vena cava via the renal veins. Each kidney is enclosed by a thick fibrous capsule and has two distinct layers: the reddish-brown cortex, which has a rich blood supply, and the inner medulla, within which the structural and functional units of the kidney, the nephrons, are found (Fig. 2.2).

The Nephron

Each kidney has approximately one million nephrons (though the number declines with increasing age), each of which is about 3 cm long. The nephron is a tubule that is closed at one end and opens into the collecting duct at the other. The nephron has six distinct regions, each of which is adapted to a specific function (Fig. 2.3). There are two types of nephron. Most (85–90%) are cortical nephrons;

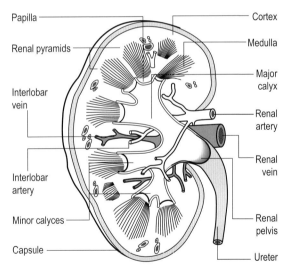

Fig. 2.2 The structure of the kidney (longitudinal section). (Reproduced with permission from Brooker, 1998.)

these have short loops of Henlé and are mainly concerned with the control of plasma volume during normal conditions. The juxtamedullary nephrons, which have longer loops of Henlé extending into the renal medulla, facilitate increased water retention (and thus the production of hyperosmotic or concentrated urine) when the availability of water is restricted.

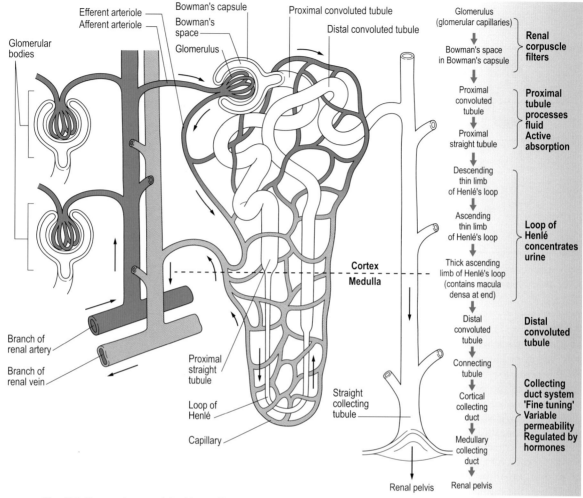

Fig. 2.3 The nephron and double capillary arrangement. The panel on the right shows the functions of the regions of the nephron.

The renal corpuscle comprises the Bowman capsule, a blind-ended tube, and the glomerulus, a coiled arrangement of capillaries around which the Bowman capsule is invaginated forming a cup-like structure around the glomerulus. The glomerulus provides a large area of capillary vessels from which substances can leave, crossing the specialized flattened epithelial cells to enter the capsule of the nephron. There is a double capillary arrangement (see Fig. 2.3) whereby afferent arterioles supply the glomerular capillaries and efferent arterioles lead from the glomerulus to a second capillary bed supplying the rest of the nephron. Differential vasoconstriction of the afferent and efferent arterioles maintains a constant blood pressure within the glomerulus, which results in a constant rate of filtration.

Urine production relies on three steps: simple filtration, selective reabsorption and secretion (Fig. 2.4).

Filtration

Filtration is a nonselective passive process that occurs through the semipermeable walls of the glomerulus and glomerular capsule. All substances with a molecular mass of <68 kilodaltons (kDa) are forced out of the glomerular capillaries into the Bowman capsule. Therefore, water and small molecules such as glucose, amino acids and vitamins enter the nephron, whereas blood cells, plasma proteins and other large molecules are usually retained in the blood. The presence of blood (haematuria; gross haematuria is visible by eye) or protein (proteinuria) in the urine indicates compromised

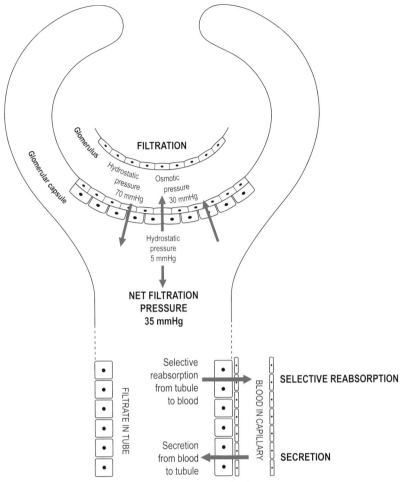

Fig. 2.4 Urine production.

renal function and may be caused by urinary tract infections (UTIs), hypertension or preeclampsia. The content of the Bowman capsule is 'glomerular filtrate' and the rate at which this is formed is referred to as the 'glomerular filtration rate' (GFR). The glomerular filtrate is processed by the nephron to form urine. The kidneys form a total (cumulative) of about 180 L of dilute filtrate each day (a GFR of about 125 mL/min). Most of it is immediately selectively reabsorbed so the final volume of urine produced is about 1–1.5 L/day, dependent on fluid intake and other fluid loss such as sweat.

Box 2.2 describes an example of disrupted renal function in pregnancy that is detected by abnormal urine composition.

Selective Reabsorption

Substances from the glomerular filtrate are reabsorbed by the nephron and transported into the surrounding

---

BOX 2.2 Hypertension in Pregnancy

Hypertensive disorders in pregnancy can disrupt renal function. The detectable presence of protein within the urine (proteinuria) may indicate that larger molecules than normal are being forced into the Bowman capsule. This is caused by the increased blood pressure resulting in abnormal ultrafiltration. Women who have a degree of renal damage prior to pregnancy are unlikely to be able to adapt to the pregnancy-induced physiological changes as effectively as women with normal renal function. These women tend to develop high blood pressure during early pregnancy and so do not normally demonstrate such a marked physiological reduction in blood pressure parameters, putting both the mother and fetus at risk.

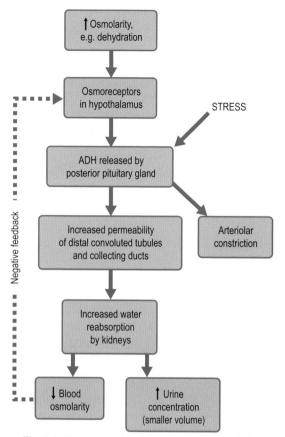

Fig. 2.5 The action of antidiuretic hormone (ADH).

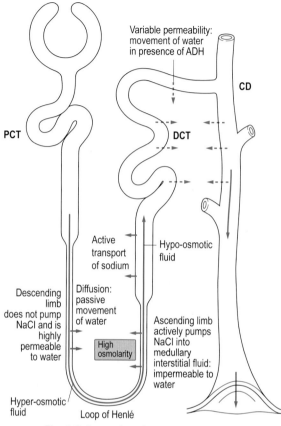

Fig. 2.6 Formation of concentrated urine.

capillaries. The proximal convoluted tubule (see PCT in Fig. 2.6) is the widest and longest part of the whole nephron (approximately 1.4 cm long). The epithelial cells lining the nephron contain a large number of mitochondria to provide energy for facilitating active transport as most of the reabsorption of the glomerular filtrate takes place here. Some substances, such as glucose and amino acids, are completely reabsorbed and are not normally present in urine. Reabsorption of waste products is largely incomplete, so, for instance, a large proportion of urea is excreted. The reabsorption of other substances is under the regulation of several hormones. Antidiuretic hormone (ADH) controls the insertion of aquaporin water channels into the walls of the distal convoluted tubule (see DCT in Fig. 2.6) and collecting ducts (see CD in Fig. 2.6), which allows water to leave the filtrate, thus producing a smaller volume of more concentrated urine (Fig. 2.5). The formation of concentrated urine is facilitated by the physical arrangement of the loop of Henlé and its surrounding capillaries, which create and maintain the conditions for the reabsorption of

BOX 2.3   Hypertonic Urine

The evolution of the mammalian kidney has enabled mammals to become highly adapted to terrestrial living. The kidney aids water conservation by producing urine that is able to be concentrated far more than the internal body fluid environment. The scarcer water is within the environment, the longer the nephron to conserve water.

water by osmosis (Fig. 2.6; Box 2.3). Calcitonin increases calcium excretion and parathyroid hormone (via vitamin D) enhances reabsorption of calcium from renal tubules. Aldosterone affects the reabsorption of sodium (Fig. 2.7). Atrial natriuretic peptide (ANP) inhibits NaCl reabsorption in the DCT and cortical collecting duct of the nephron. ANP also increases the GFR by dilating the afferent glomerular arterioles and constricting the efferent glomerular arteriole, thus increasing NaCl excretion.

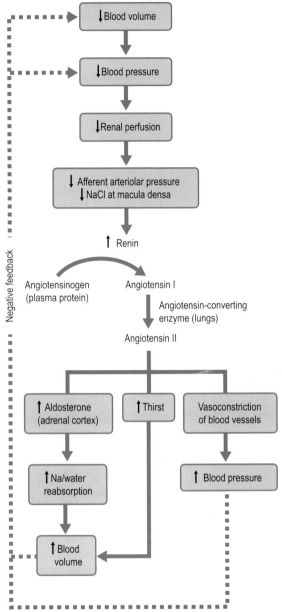

Fig. 2.7 Aldosterone regulation of sodium (Na) excretion.

Secretion

Some waste products, such as creatinine, plant toxins and drug metabolites, may be actively transported directly into the glomerular filtrate from the surrounding blood capillaries. Other components such as hydrogen ions, ammonium and potassium ions are secreted into the filtrate as part of the adjustment of body pH and electrolyte balance. The cells of the renal tubules synthesize some substances, such as ammonium ions and peptides, which can be secreted into the filtrate.

The Ureters

The ureters, which are tubes ~25–30 cm long and 3 mm in diameter, transport the urine from the kidneys to the bladder. From each kidney, the collecting ducts open into the renal pelvis, which leads to the ureter. The walls of the renal pelvis have a smooth muscle layer, which has intrinsic activity (i.e. not controlled by nerves but self-generated within the tissue), generating peristaltic waves of contraction every 10 s. These unidirectional waves of contraction propel urine down through the ureters to the bladder. Each ureter is also lined with smooth muscle and transitional epithelium; the lumen has a star-shaped cross-section.

The ureters lie upon the posterior abdominal wall outside the peritoneal cavity, entering the bladder at an oblique angle, one at each side of the base of the specialized muscle area called the trigone, which has its apex at the urethral opening. As urine accumulates in the bladder, the ureters are compressed, effectively forming a valve (the vesicoureteral valve), which prevents urinary reflux.

The Bladder

The bladder is a distensible hollow organ, also composed of smooth muscle, which acts as a reservoir for urine. It is lined with transitional epithelium, which occurs exclusively in the urinary system, which appears as one or two layers of cells when the bladder is full of urine and distended but appears to be many layers of cells when the lining is relaxed in the empty bladder. The bladder is intermittently emptied under conscious control. Stretch receptors within the muscle and trigone provide the signals that indicate that the bladder is full. The normal capacity of the bladder is ~700–800 mL; however, the natural desire to void urine becomes conscious when the volume of urine in the bladder reaches approximately 300 mL. Inflammation in the trigone region caused by infection and or trauma often results in a frequent and urgent desire to void urine but on voiding only small amounts of urine are passed.

As the bladder lies below the uterus, its capacity is compromised by the growing uterus in early pregnancy. Later on, once the pregnant uterus has become an abdominal organ, the pressure on the bladder is relieved. Finally, at the end of pregnancy, bladder capacity is again compromised as the presenting part of the fetus engages, occupying space within the true pelvic cavity and thus restricting the space available to the bladder.

The Urethra

Urine is voided via the urethra. The female urethra is considerably shorter and straighter than the male urethra:

only 4 cm in length compared with ~20 cm in males. This anatomical difference predisposes women towards an increased incidence of ascending UTIs. Thus, a colony count of more than 100,000 bacterial cells/mL of urine is considered to be pathologically significant and is usually referred to as 'bacteriuria'. There are small mucus-secreting glands in the urethra that help to protect the epithelium from the corrosive urine. The upper internal sphincter, at the exit from the bladder, is composed of smooth muscle and is under autonomic control. The external sphincter is composed of skeletal muscle and is under voluntary control. The urethra in the man has a dual role as the route for urine and the delivery of spermatozoa, via coitus. (Structural differences related to the development of the external genitalia are covered in Chapter 5.) Trauma to the pelvic floor during childbirth may result in neurological damage affecting the function of the internal sphincter resulting in urgency of urination (micturition). Urgency to void is increased by the degree of weakness in the sphincter and the amount of urine held in the bladder. The risk of postpartum urinary incontinence (UI) is increased with older age, higher body weight, smoking, parity and family history; women who experience transient UI in pregnancy or postnatally are more likely to have problems with UI in later life. Pelvic floor muscle training during the antenatal and postnatal periods may prevent UI (Wesnes and Lose, 2013). Treatment options for persistent UI, which has a significant effect on quality of life, range from a variety of surgical procedures to pharmacological treatment and lifestyle and behavioural modification (Castro et al., 2015).

Urine

Urine has a specific gravity of 1.010–1.030 and is usually slightly acidic (pH 6.5–7.0), depending on the diet and time of day. The volume and final concentration of urea and solutes depend on fluid intake. Sleep and muscular activity also inhibit urine production. The amber colour is due to urobilin, the bile pigment. Urine has a characteristic smell, which is not unpleasant when fresh. Unpleasant odour or cloudiness in a fresh urine specimen usually indicates a bacterial infection (Box 2.4).

Control of Micturition

Micturition (urination) is a coordinated response that is due to the contraction of the muscular wall of the bladder, reflex relaxation of the internal sphincter of the urethra and voluntary relaxation of the external sphincter (Fig. 2.8). It is assisted by increased pressure in the pelvic cavity as the diaphragm is lowered and the abdominal muscles contract. Over-distension of the bladder is painful and can cause involuntary relaxation of the external sphincter resulting in urgency of micturition, incontinence and

---

BOX 2.4   Urinary Tract Infections (UTIs)

Pregnancy further increases the risk of UTIs and so a routine culture and sensitivity test to detect bacteriuria is common practice. Some women with bacteriuria may be asymptomatic, for example, for group B haemolytic streptococcus. If group B streptococcus (GBS) is detected in a urine sample, antibiotic therapy is recommended (Hughes et al., 2017), as this represents a high bacterial load, which could put the neonate at risk of infection following birth (see Chapter 10). Of all adults in the UK, 20–40% (including pregnant women) are colonized with GBS and so are carriers of the organism. GBS is the most common cause of severe and early onset infection in newborn infants.

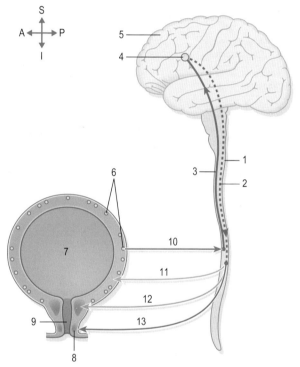

Fig. 2.8 Control of micturition. A, Anterior; I, inferior; P, posterior; S, superior; 1, spinal cord; 2, voluntary inhibition of the micturition reflex; 3, nerve impulse going to the cerebral cortex; 4, cerebral cortex; 5, brain; 6, stretch receptors; 7, full bladder; 8, external urethral sphincter; 9, urethra; 10, nerve impulses going to the spinal cord; 11, nerve impulses stimulate contraction of the detrusor muscle; 12, nerve impulses stimulate relaxation of the internal urethral sphincter; 13, a conscious effort to control the external urethral sphincter thwarts the micturition reflex. (Reproduced from Muller A: *Ross & Wilson pocket reference guide to anatomy and physiology*, 5 ed, Elsevier, 2014, Ch. 13.)

overflow. The tone of this sphincter is also affected by psychological stimuli (such as waking or getting ready to leave the house) and external stimuli (such as the sound of water or the feel of the lavatory seat). Any factor that raises the intra-abdominal and intravesicular pressures (such as laughter, sneezing or coughing) in excess of the urethral closing pressure can result in stress incontinence.

Accumulation of urine increases bladder wall tension, stimulating the stretch receptors of the bladder, which relay parasympathetic sensory impulses to the brain, generating awareness. However, there is conscious descending inhibition of the reflex bladder contraction and relaxation of the external sphincter. Entry of urine into the urethra irritates and stimulates stretch receptors, augmenting the sensory pathways as the bladder fills. Micturition is thus postponed until a socially acceptable time and place. This inhibition of the spinal reflex and contraction of the external sphincter is a learned response. Infants tend to develop bladder control when they are about 2 years old. Irritation of the bladder or urethra, for instance as a result of infection, can also initiate the desire to urinate regardless of the bladder capacity.

Normal physiological control of micturition requires an intact nerve supply to the urinary tract, normal muscle tone (of bladder, urethral sphincters and pelvic floor muscles), absence of any obstruction to flow, normal bladder capacity and, finally, the absence of psychological factors that may inhibit the micturition cycle (such as embarrassment and discomfort).

THE FEMALE REPRODUCTIVE TRACT

The main features of the female reproductive tract (FRT) distinguishing it from the male are that the female reproductive organs are internal and, in the nonpregnant state, are situated within the true pelvic cavity. The FRT consists of two ovaries, two uterine (fallopian) tubes, the uterus and cervix, the vagina and external genitalia. The female reproductive system undergoes considerable changes throughout life from childhood through reproductive life (Box 2.5) to menopause. Superimposed on these changes are the effects of the menstrual cycle (see Chapter 3). Prevention of infection in the FRT is essential; the cervix, endometrium and uterine tubes secrete a broad spectrum of >20 different antimicrobial substances that act as the first line of defence against pathogens entering the lower FRT (Wira et al., 2014). These secretions are under hormonal control, which means that the FRT is protected in different ways throughout the menstrual cycle and particularly during the vulnerable period of fertilization and implantation.

The Ovaries

The ovaries are dull-white almond-shaped bodies, ~4 cm long. They lie posteriorly and laterally relative to the body of

---

BOX 2.5 Changes to the Female Genital Tract at Puberty

- Hair appears on the mons veneris and subcutaneous fat accumulates
- Secretory glands mature and become active
- Labia majora and minora become pigmented with melanin
- Enlargement of the clitoris occurs
- Vaginal epithelium thickens and becomes responsive to oestrogen
- Vaginal pH decreases as lactobacilli metabolize glycogen from cell secretions
- Uterus grows and cervix doubles in length

---

the uterus and below the uterine tubes. They are anchored by the ovarian ligaments and attached to the posterior layer of the broad ligament, a fold within the peritoneum that extends from and around the uterus (Fig. 2.9). The blood supply to the ovary is via the ovarian artery, which runs alongside the ovarian ligament, and the ovarian branch of the uterine artery (see Fig. 2.12). This dual blood supply is important in maintaining reproductive function; if the ovary becomes twisted, for instance because it is displaced by a tumour or cystic growth, the ovarian ligament may occlude the blood supply from the ovarian artery. This torsion of the ovary can cause ischaemia of the tissues and intense pain.

The ovaries are composed of two distinct layers: the outer layer is the cortex and the inner section is referred to as the medulla. The ovary is contained within a sheath of connective tissue, the tunica albuginea. The cortex contains the developing follicles that contain the primary oocytes and is also responsible for the production of the female steroid hormones oestrogen and progesterone (see Chapters 4 and 5). The medulla is composed primarily of connective tissue and blood vessels and provides precursors to facilitate steroid production within the cortex. The ovary has two main functions: to produce fertilizable oocytes, which can undergo full development, and to secrete the steroid hormones, which prepare the reproductive tract for fertilization and to establish and support the pregnancy.

The long-held generally accepted belief that all oocytes (and follicles) in the human ovaries were formed in the fetal period (prenatal 'total endowment' or ovarian reserve) has been challenged. Studies of oogenesis have identified the presence of germline stem cells (GSCs) and the presence of genes characteristically expressed by primordial germ cells in adult human ovaries (Virant-Klun, 2015), which appear to suggest *de novo* oogenesis and ovarian regeneration could occur in postnatal life. However, the evidence that follicular and oocyte renewal continue through female

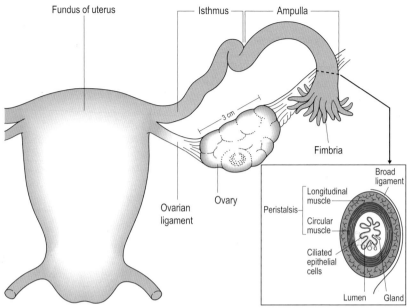

Fig. 2.9 Position of the ovary, and ovarian and broad ligaments. (Reproduced with permission from Sweet, 1996.)

reproductive life in humans remains controversial (see Chapter 6). Postnatal oogenesis would have important clinical significance for the treatment of female infertility.

The Uterine (Fallopian) Tubes

The uterine tubes are ~12 cm long; they have walls of smooth muscle and are lined with ciliated epithelial and secretory cells. The uterine tubes are mobile and not fixed to the ovaries. The distal end of the uterine tube has specialized structures called fimbriae, which surround the opening into the tube. The fimbriae lie in close proximity to the ovary and, at ovulation, assist the entry of the ovum into the uterine tube by a wafting action, which facilitates movement of the interperitoneal fluid. The lining of the uterine tubes lies in many folds (or plicae) and is composed of ciliated columnar epithelial cells interspersed with mucus-secreting goblet cells. The cilia facilitate the movement of the ovum down the uterine tube; this is augmented by coordinated peristaltic contractions of the smooth muscle. The distal end of the uterine tube has a slightly wider area, called the ampulla, where fertilization of the ovum by the sperm usually occurs.

If both uterine tubes are completely blocked, fertilization is prevented as the sperm are unable to access the ovum. If one uterine tube is patent or only partially blocked, then sperm may encounter and fertilize an ovum within the peritoneal cavity. However, if a fertilized ovum enters a partially or totally obstructed uterine tube or one where the cilia are damaged, its passage to

CASE STUDY 2.1

Julie, during her (first) booking appointment, informs the midwife that she had previously suffered an ectopic pregnancy with her last pregnancy, which was treated conservatively with methotrexate.

What does the midwife need to do to ensure that Julie's pregnancy is progressing normally? What are the signs and symptoms of an ectopic pregnancy; and when are they most likely to become apparent?

What information should Julie have received following her ectopic pregnancy and what information should you give her now and would she require any further care and follow-up?

Julie has attended the booking appointment 5 weeks following her last menstrual period (LMP), because of her previous history. The midwife refers Julie for an ultrasound scan, which reports a pregnancy of unknown location (PUL). What is the meaning of this, how should it be managed and what advice should be given to Julie?

the uterus will be impeded and so the pregnancy may develop within the uterine tube or peritoneal cavity (Case study 2.1; Box 2.6).

Infection of the genital tract with *Chlamydia trachomatis* is the most prevalent sexually transmitted bacterial infection worldwide. It can cause urethritis but is usually

BOX 2.6 Ectopic Pregnancy

An ectopic pregnancy is one that implants in the uterine tubes or, more rarely, the cervix, ovaries or abdomen. It is relatively common as it occurs in about 1% of all pregnancies and although the fatality rate is much reduced, ectopic pregnancy still remains a significant cause of maternal morbidity and mortality (NICE, 2012). It is usually confirmed by an ultrasound scan revealing an empty uterine cavity and a positive pregnancy test. Raised human chorionic gonadotrophin (hCG) levels confirm pregnancy but levels are lower in ectopic pregnancy than in uterine pregnancy. The term 'pregnancy of unknown location' (PUL) is used to describe a pregnancy where there is a positive pregnancy (hCG) test but no intra- or extrauterine pregnancy can be visualized on a transvaginal ultrasound scan (Fields and Hathaway, 2016). In these cases, it is recommended that serial hCG measurements be made to monitor whether the PUL is failing (the hCG ratio is used to compare initial or baseline hCG levels with those at various later time points) and also that serum progesterone measurements are made to predict the likely outcome (higher levels are associated with pregnancies subsequently demonstrated to be viable). Women who have a PUL may subsequently be found to have a viable intrauterine pregnancy but some have a spontaneous abortion and up to 20% are diagnosed with an ectopic pregnancy.

Most ectopic pregnancies are due to implantation in the ampulla of the uterine tube but about 5% occur in other sites such as on the scar tissue from a caesarean section (NICE, 2012). The usual first warning sign of an ectopic pregnancy is abdominal pain or bleeding after intercourse at around 8 weeks' gestation, which may present with symptoms mimicking gastrointestinal disease (misdiagnosis of ectopic pregnancy as gastroenteritis is associated with maternal mortality). Ectopic pregnancy should be suspected in all women of childbearing age who present with fainting or sudden unexpected collapse (NICE, 2012); no form of contraception is 100% effective, so pregnancy should not be excluded in women who use contraception. If the uterine tube ruptures, the woman may become clinically shocked owing to excessive bleeding into the peritoneal cavity. The growing fetus can be surgically removed together with the damaged uterine tube if necessary (this is referred to as a salpingectomy). Occasionally, an abdominal pregnancy may ensue if implantation occurs on the peritoneum. The pregnancies rarely go to term; however, delivery of live infants via abdominal surgery has been documented. This phenomenon underpins scientific interest enabling men to have babies through a process of peritoneal implantation. The main causes of tubal blockage are infection (usually due to pelvic inflammatory disease), the formation of scar tissue from surgery or trauma and congenital malformation. High levels of steroid hormones can also affect ciliary movement. If a tubal pregnancy is diagnosed early before trauma occurs, it can be treated by the intramuscular administration of the drug methotrexate. Methotrexate is a chemotherapeutic drug, which inhibits folic acid metabolism (by inhibiting difolate reductase so DNA synthesis ceases) thus targeting rapidly dividing tissue such as the trophoblast; the embryo is eventually reabsorbed. Methotrexate has side-effects on mucosal surfaces as they also have a fast rate of cell division and can cause conjunctivitis, gastrointestinal disturbances and stomatitis (inflammation of the mucous membranes in the mouth). Women may experience some degree of abdominal pain because of tubal miscarriage; it can be difficult to distinguish this from tubal rupture. Although the uterine tube is saved, the risk of another ectopic pregnancy is high. As the rate of sexually transmitted disease is increasing and there are more assisted conceptions and caesarean sections, the rate of ectopic pregnancy is expected to increase (Knight et al., 2017).

---

asymptomatic. It can be transferred by vaginal, anal or oral sex, during childbirth and through direct contact with infected tissue, which may cause conjunctivitis for instance. Infection, by *Chlamydia trachomatis* or *Neisseria gonorrhoeae* for instance, can cause pelvic inflammatory disease (PID), which is associated with a high risk of ectopic pregnancy, tubal infertility and chronic pelvic pain. Although the prime site of chlamydial infection is usually within the columnar epithelial cells of the cervix, the infection can quickly ascend to the upper reproductive tract probably by attaching to sperm or by being transported in the flow of fluids. Extragenital infections, for instance of the oropharynx and rectum, can also occur (Chan et al., 2016). Infection of the female reproductive tract leads to production of proinflammatory cytokines, which interact with the immune system (see Chapter 10) causing inflammation and tissue destruction. The prevalence of *Chlamydia* infection is increasing; increased detection of infection and use of more sensitive tests may contribute to this increase. The risk for infection is associated with young onset of sexual activity, number of sexual partners, irregular use of condoms and history of sexually transmitted infections. Screening and effective antibiotic treatment of affected individuals and their partners are essential components of

Chlamydia prevention programmes. *Chlamydia* infection is a preventable cause of infertility and adverse reproductive outcome. Antibiotic-resistant strains of *Chlamydia* are emerging, which will make eradication of the disease extremely difficult as the number of effective antibiotics reduces over time. Treatment with antibiotics requires a high level of compliance to reduce the incidence of emerging resistant strains.

The Uterus

The functions of the uterus are to prepare to receive the fertilized ovum, to provide a suitable environment for growth and development of the fetus and to assist in the expulsion of the fetus, placenta and membranes at delivery. In the nonpregnant state, the pear-shaped uterus is situated within the true pelvic cavity. Normally the uterus is anteverted (tilted forwards) and anteflexed (curved forward), situated in a superior position to the urinary bladder (Fig. 2.10). A uterus in an abnormal position, such as a retroverted uterus, is not in an optimal position to expand in pregnancy and intervention may be required to adjust its position to allow the pregnancy to proceed so the growing uterus does not impact on the posterior edge of the pelvic brim. The anatomical position of the uterus is maintained by the uterine ligaments, which are important in supporting the weight of the uterus, particularly during contractions (Fig. 2.11). Its blood supply is shown in Fig. 2.12.

The nonpregnant uterus weighs ~50 g with a cavity of approximately 10 mL and is composed of three layers (Fig. 2.13). The inner layer of the uterus is the endometrium. This layer is markedly different in the body of the uterus compared with the cervix. The cells of the endometrium

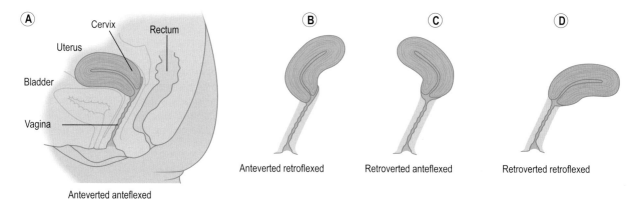

Fig. 2.10 The anteverted and anteflexed position of the nonpregnant uterus: (A) normal position and (B-D) abnormal positions. (Reproduced Herring W, *Learning radiology: recognizing the basics*, 4 ed, Elsevier 2020, Fig 19.16.)

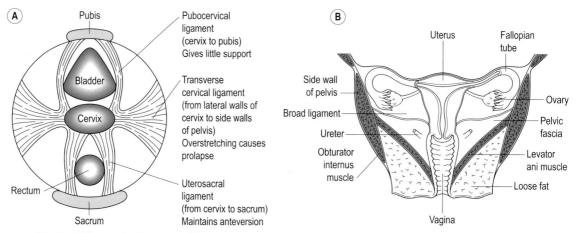

Fig. 2.11 The uterine ligaments: (A) transverse and (B) coronal sections. (Reproduced with permission from Sweet, 1996.)

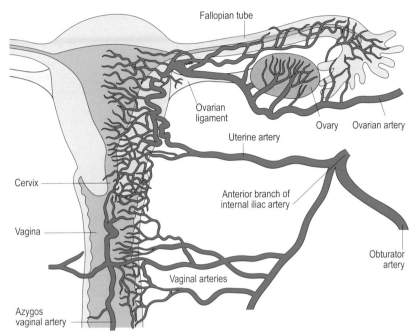

Fig. 2.12 The uterine and ovarian blood supply.

are ciliated and the entire cell layer undergoes considerable growth changes during the menstrual cycle; the superficial decidual layers are shed in menstruation at the end of the cycle (see Chapter 4). The vascular connective tissue, or stroma, contains many glands that secrete alkaline mucus into the uterine cavity.

The middle layer is called the myometrium and predominantly composed of smooth muscle arranged in three muscle layers (Box 2.7). In the nonpregnant state, these layers are not very distinctive but they become more distinct during pregnancy. The myometrium has inherent spontaneous contractile activity; this myogenic property means it regularly contracts without hormonal or nervous input whether the woman is pregnant or not. During early pregnancy, hormones suppress the spontaneous contractions.

The uterus has an outer layer of peritoneum that drapes over the uterus anteriorly to form a fold between the uterus and bladder, and over the uterine tubes to cover the myometrium. This is referred to as the perimetrium; it forms the broad ligament, thus maintaining the anatomical position of the uterus. The body of the uterus is ~5 cm in both length and width (excluding the dimensions of the cervix).

Arterial blood to the uterus is supplied by left and right uterine arteries, which branch along their length giving rise to arcuate arteries, which penetrate into the myometrium. Branches of the arcuate arteries anastomose freely ensuring that the blood supply to the uterus is robust. Radial

arteries branching from the arcuate arteries supply the tissue towards the lumen of the uterus. The radial arteries branch at the myometrial–endometrial boundary into the basal arteries that supply the myometrium and continue as spiral arteries. The spiral arteries are tightly coiled in the basal layer of the uterine lining but markedly narrow as they near the uterine lumen and divide into smaller straighter branches before terminating in capillary beds under the uterine surface and surrounding the uterine glands. The walls of the spiral and radial arteries are rich in smooth muscle and are innervated by the autonomic nervous system, so they are responsive to adrenergic stimuli, particularly the segments of the spiral arteries close to the myometrial–endometrial junction. The spiral arteries undergo transient vasoconstriction prior to menstruation (Maybin and Critchley, 2015); this is thought to induce hypoxia, which may provoke endometrial breakdown and subsequent repair, and limit blood flow. Menstrual blood loss is usually dark red in colour. Any bright red blood loss from the uterine cavity should be viewed with suspicion and investigated as it indicates fresh active bleeding, regardless of when it occurs in the menstrual cycle.

The uterus is innervated by both parasympathetic nerves (arising from the second, third and fourth sacral segments) and sympathetic nerves via the presacral nerve (branching from the aortic plexus) and branches from the lumbar sympathetic chain. Both types of innervation to the uterus are via

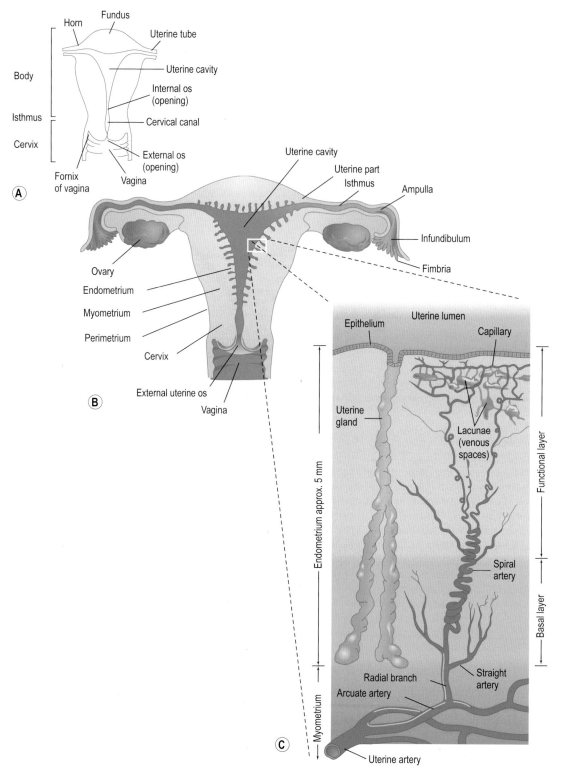

Fig. 2.13 (A) Parts of the uterus and vagina; (B) frontal section of the uterus, uterine tubes and vagina; (C) enlargement of section of the endometrium shown in box. (Reproduced from Moore KL, Persaud TVN, Torchia MG: *The developing human: clinically oriented embryology*, 11 ed, Elsevier 2020, Fig. 2.6.)

BOX 2.7   The Uterine Muscle Layers

1. *Inner layer*: fibres in the longitudinal plane that run from the anterior cervix, up over the fundus and back to the posterior edge of the cervix
2. *Middle layer*: interlaced spiral fibres concentrated in, and originating from, the fundal region of the uterus and getting less dense approaching the cervical region; the circular arrangement of the fibres is accentuated at the junctions with the uterine tubes and the cervix (internal os), thus providing closures to the expanding pregnant uterus
3. *Outer layer*: combination of longitudinal and circular fibres

---

the Lee–Frankenhäuser plexus, which is situated in the lower region of the pouch of Douglas, the posterior and lowest part of the peritoneal cavity (posteriorly inferior to the uterus).

The Cervix

The cervix is the neck of the uterus at the top of the vagina. It has an important role in protecting the uterus from infection and undergoes important changes preceding labour (see Chapter 13). The isthmus, an indistinct layer of tissue from which the lower uterine segment is formed in the last trimester of pregnancy (see Chapter 13), separates the body of the uterus and the cervix. The cervix is ~2.5 cm in length and is composed of dense collagenous circular fibres. The cervix is spindle-shaped with an os (smooth muscle arrangement forming a constriction) at the top and bottom. The internal os forms the inner opening of the cervix at the junction with the body of the uterus. The external os is located at the bottom of the cervical canal where it projects into the vagina. Two different types of cell meet at this junction: the columnar cells of the cervical canal and the squamous epithelial cells of the outer cervix. Abnormal precancerous cells are most likely to arise at this junction. Cervical cancer is one of the more common cancers affecting women of reproductive age; the risk of cervical cancer correlates with number of sexual partners. Conventional cervical screening utilizes the Pap smear (named after Georgios Papanikolaou), which is a cervical swab that samples cells and allows checking for precancerous changes. Liquid-based cervical cytology improves the diagnostic reliability of the smear test because the cells are rinsed in preservatives which remove the debris and allow better preparation of the sample. About 5–7% of cervical smears identify abnormal results such as dysplasia indicating the need for increased vigilance and further examination. The smear test is usually used in conjunction with the HPV (human papilloma virus) test, which identifies the presence of any type of HPV and is able to detect early cervical intraepithelial neoplasia. The rates of cervical cancer have fallen markedly with primary protection from HPV vaccination which began in 2006.

The observation that early cervical changes resemble cutaneous warts led to the identification of papillomaviruses in the aetiology of cervical cancer (DiMaio, 2015). The involvement of HPV, particularly the HPV16 and HPV18 strains, in cervical cancer was confirmed by the presence of antibodies to HPV and the finding that almost all cervical cancers express HPV oncogenes (that inactivate tumour suppressor genes), which are required for proliferation of the cancer cells. HPV itself is benign but it is thought to trigger changes in the cells of the cervix such as cervical dysplasia. HPV is one of the most common sexually transmitted viruses and is thought to infect the majority of sexually active women. Vaccination of girls and young women (usually aged 9–25 years) against certain types of high-risk HPV in many countries has reduced the incidence of cervical cancer, some genital cancers and genital warts. One recent review and meta-analysis reported a decrease in the prevalence of HPV16 and HPV18 by 83%, after 5–8 years of vaccination (Drolet et al., 2019). To be effective, vaccination must be used before infection can occur, therefore before girls or their partners are sexually active (Box 2.8). It is essential that males are also vaccinated, not just to reduce the spread of HPV to their partners but also because HPV is associated with other types of cancer including cancer of the vagina, vulva, penis, anus and mouth. It is estimated if the WHO immunization goal for HPV of a minimum of 70% coverage (take-up rate for the vaccine) was met, the rates of *all* cancers in those countries that achieved this level of herd immunity would decrease by 10%. There are many options for the treatment of precancerous and cancerous cells of the cervix, for example laser treatment, diathermy, cone biopsies and surgery. Trauma to the cervix from medical intervention can result in cervical weakness or incompetence, which may result in premature loss or premature delivery. Abnormal scarring could also potentially cause cervical dystocia (failure to dilate).

The lining of the cervix does not undergo cyclical changes in growth rate although its glandular activity changes. The inner tissue lies in folds that appear branched, giving it the name arbor vitae. These folds allow dilation during delivery. Occasionally, extensions of glandular cells that line the cervix extend through the cervical os and colonize the exterior surface of the cervix. These are described as cervical ectropion (or cervical erosions), which produce mucus and bleed easily at the same time as the menstrual cyclical rhythm of bleeding. These are harmless and often discovered when mid-cycle bleeding associated with coitus is investigated. If cervical ectropion causes problems such as heavy or painful bleeding or a discharge, it can be treated

BOX 2.8   Human Papilloma Virus (HPV) Vaccination

Most HPV-related cancer is caused by a few of the 170 strains of HPV, particularly HPV16 and HPV18. The different types of vaccine have slightly different protective effects against different strains; all vaccines protect against HPV16 and HPV18 and the newer vaccines protect against additional high-risk strains of HPV. The vaccines are prepared from the particles of the protein shells of the virus and do not contain any viral DNA so they cannot cause infection but are extremely effective and long-lasting. The reported side-effects from HPV vaccination are minor; pain and inflammation at the injection site.

To be effective, vaccination has to be given before a young woman (or young man) is sexually active and exposed to possible HPV infection; there is negligible benefit in vaccinating someone who is already infected. As the penetrance of HPV in the sexually active population is high, the optimal age for vaccination is 9–13 years. At this age, parental consent for vaccination is usually required; the surprisingly low take-up rate for safe and effective vaccination against a virus that has such extraordinary implications may be because parents do not like to consider their daughters in the target age may become sexually active in the relatively near future.

by laser, diathermy (cauterization with an electric current), cryocautery (cauterization with a cold spray) or by using silver nitrate.

The Vagina

The vagina is a distensible fibromuscular tube, about 8–10 cm long, situated within the true pelvic cavity, extending through the pelvic floor from the cervix to the vulva. The vagina is described as a potential tube because its walls are in contact but easily separated, but the walls of the vagina are not uniform. It was thought that the distal and the proximal parts of the vagina have different embryonic origins because the vaginal epithelial cells are different to the uterine epithelial cells. However, studies using knockout rodent models now suggest that the entire vagina is formed from the Müllerian ducts (Cai, 2009) (see Chapter 5).

The cervix protrudes into the vagina, normally pointing to the posterior wall of the vagina because of the anteverted and anteflexed position of the uterus. The recesses between the cervix and the upper portion of the vaginal wall are referred to as the anterior, lateral and posterior fornices (singular: fornix). The vagina has three main functions: the facilitation of coitus, as a passage for the release of the menses and as the route for the baby to be born, commonly referred to as the birth canal. It also helps to support the uterus and prevent ascending infection through the release of antibacterial secretions favouring the growth of commensal bacteria. If there is a weakness in the pelvic floor muscles, the structures that the pelvic floor supports such as the uterus, bladder, urethra, rectum or the vagina itself may droop into the vagina; this is referred to as a prolapse. Anterior prolapses usually involve the bladder, whilst posterior prolapses affect the rectum.

The vagina is host to a broad range of microorganisms, which form a complex ecosystem unique to humans. This seems to be dominated by one of four strains of lactobacilli (Nunn and Forney, 2016) but there are marked ethnic differences. The vaginal microbiome constitutes the first line of defence and inhibits the growth of pathogenic organisms through a range of mechanisms. The production of lactic acid by the microorganisms maintains a low pH of about 3.5–4.5, which creates a hostile environment for many potentially opportunistic and pathogenic species of bacteria, preventing infection. In addition, the lactobacilli may produce other bactericidal components; the effect is greater than that due to the lower pH. The pathogens that are suppressed by the protective environment created by the vaginal microorganisms include those involved in sexually transmitted and urinary tract infections, and yeast infections. The prevalence of lactobacilli is higher in white and Asian women; it is possible that differences in microbial colonization of the vagina might be responsible for the slightly higher vaginal pH in black and Hispanic women and their higher risk of preterm delivery (Fettweis et al., 2014). Dysbiosis, particularly deficiencies in the vaginal lactobacilli species, is also implicated in adverse reproductive and sexual health outcomes such as miscarriage and PID.

Although the lactobacilli that inhabit the female reproductive tract lack the required enzymes to metabolize glycogen, vaginal secretions appear to have amylase-like activity (Nunn and Forney, 2016), which can break down glycogen so the lactobacilli can use the glycogen breakdown products as well as sloughed-off vaginal cells as metabolic substrates. The profile of vaginal microorganisms changes markedly at various stages in a woman's life after the species are introduced at birth; the most significant changes occur with the fluctuations in oestrogen levels in childhood, puberty, pregnancy and menopause, which affect glycogen production. The clinical syndrome, bacterial vaginosis (BV), which is the most common vaginal disorder in women of reproductive age, is thought to be due to disruption of the normal 'healthy' vaginal microbiome (Ravel and Brotman, 2016). The vaginal microbiome interacts with the immune cells that are associated with the vaginal tissue and have immunomodulatory effects. The importance of the vaginal microbiome raises issues about the effects of hormonal contraceptives, use of antibiotics and other medications, vaginal lubricants and deodorant sprays, douching and intercourse on the stability of the ecosystem. There is also potential for deliberate manipulation of the vaginal microbiota to promote the health of women and their infants.

The vagina is lined by a layer of moist epithelial cells folded into ridges (called 'rugae') that distend during intercourse and childbirth, thus facilitating the stretching of the vagina. There is also a lining of smooth muscle, which maintains the tone of the vagina. The opening of the vaginal canal, the introitus, is protected by the external genitalia. The introitus lies below the urethral opening, which is situated below the clitoris (Fig. 2.14). The vagina does not

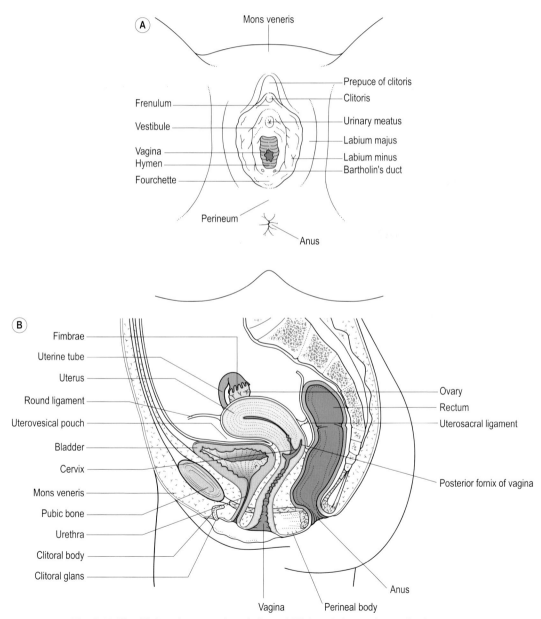

Fig. 2.14 The (A) female external genitalia and (B) female internal reproductive organs.

have glands but is maintained in a moist state by secretions from the cervical glands and transudate of fluid from the blood vessels that lie below the vaginal lining. This cervicovaginal fluid adds to the protection of the lower female reproductive tract, which is vulnerable to ascending infection; it is acidic and acts as a lubricant, traps exogenous microorganisms and is rich in antibodies and defensins (Aldunate et al., 2015). The vaginal mucus and sloughed-off epithelial cells facilitate the adhesion of the vaginal microorganisms.

The External Genitalia

The external genitalia (collectively known as the vulva) are those structures that can be seen (see Fig. 2.14). In recent years, there has been increased awareness and interest in the appearance of the external genitalia. The exchange of images on the internet, both socially and related to pornography, has increased. Complete removal of pubic hair is common for aesthetic reasons, and surgical procedures to alter the appearance of the vulva, such as labiaplasty, are one of the fastest growing areas of plastic surgery (Triana and Robledo, 2015).

The structures of the vulva can be classified as erectile (labia minora, clitoris and clitoral bulbs) or nonerectile components (mons pubis, labia majora and the vaginal vestibule). Most of the structures are well innervated; therefore, they are very sensitive and are a source of sexual arousal responses. The external genitalia are well vascularized, which means they bleed easily if subjected to trauma but also heal rapidly. It is becoming more common for women to have genital piercings; if present, these should be assessed and women advised to remove them prior to delivery to prevent further trauma at birth.

The mons veneris (or mons pubis) is a pad of subcutaneous fat covered by skin lying over the pubic bone; it provides support to the clitoris and urethra and functions as a cushion during intercourse. At puberty it becomes covered with a triangular area of pubic hair, which is coarse and curly because of the unusually oblique hair follicles. The labia majora (singular: labium majus) are two prominent fatty folds of tissue extending from the mons veneris in which the round ligaments terminate. The labia majora narrow where they unite between the vagina and anus. The outer surface is pigmented and covered in pubic hair; the inner surface is pink, smooth, hairless and rich in sebaceous and sweat glands. The labia majora enclose and protect the urogenital cleft. The labia minora are two smaller longitudinal fleshy folds of tissue; they are erectile, well-vascularized and rich in sensory receptors. They are pigmented, hairless and have some sweat and sebaceous glands. The labia minora enclose the clitoris anteriorly and unite posteriorly at the fourchette, which is commonly torn at the first delivery (first-degree tear). The labia minora are erectile tissue; the blood vessels are organized in a similar fashion to those of the corpus spongiosum of the penis. The functions of the labia minora are to contribute to sexual stimulation and arousal, to increase the depth of the vaginal canal during intercourse and to increase retention of the ejaculate following intercourse.

The clitoris is a highly sensitive erectile body (Fig. 2.15) that is composed of six components: glans clitoris, the suspensory ligament, body or corpora, root, a pair of crura and vestibular bulbs (Pauls, 2015). It is a complex structure, rich in sensory nerves, and is important to sexual arousal and orgasm. The external part (glans) is ~1.5–2.5 cm long and the internal components are longer but project internally. The external part of the clitoris, the clitoral glans, is a short cylindrical structure covered and protected by a fold of skin called the clitoral hood, or prepuce, which is homologous with the foreskin in males. The internal structures, the body, paired crura and vestibular bulbs, are embedded deep into the labia minora. The body of the clitoris is ~2–4 cm long and has a boomerang shape, which divides into two narrower arms (crura), ~5–9 cm long. The body, crura and vestibular bulbs are erectile bodies, analogous to the spongy tissue structures of the penis, which become erect and engorged on stimulation. The suspensory ligament restricts the movement of the clitoris so it does not straighten. The clitoris is an important source of sexual arousal, generating reflex lubrication responses from the surrounding tissue. When the labia are held open, the vestibule (the area from the glans clitoris to the fourchette) can be seen. It contains the external orifice of the urethra (meatus), the vaginal introitus (opening), the clitoral bulbs and the openings of the Bartholin's glands. The urinary

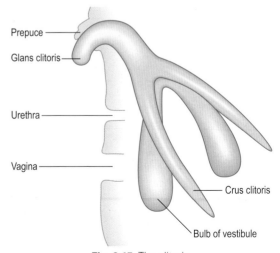

Prepuce

Glans clitoris

Urethra

Vagina

Crus clitoris

Bulb of vestibule

Fig. 2.15 The clitoris.

orifice or meatus lies ~2.5 cm below the clitoris, superior to the vaginal opening, and is a characteristic vertical slit with prominent margins formed by a horseshoe-shaped arrangement of the erectile tissue of the clitoral bulbs. It is important to precisely identify the urinary orifice in women requiring catheterization of the bladder.

To each side, slightly behind the urinary meatus, are the dimple-like mouths of the Skene's (or paraurethral) ducts, which are analogous to prostate glands; they have the same embryonic origin and resemble male prostate glands prior to puberty (Dwyer, 2012). The Skene's ducts are useful landmarks for the urinary orifice. They produce mucus-rich lubricatory secretions in states of sexual arousal and orgasm. The fluid is sometimes called female ejaculate and its production is known as 'squirting'. The biochemical analysis suggests the fluid may be secretions from the Skene's ducts and/or dilute modified urine (Pastor, 2013). It contains higher levels of glucose and lower levels of urea and uric acid than urine and also contains prostate-specific antigens (PSA), prostatic acid phosphatase and antimicrobial substances.

The vaginal introitus is almost closed in children but, in adult women, it is extremely elastic; it can stretch to allow the passage of the baby's head and subsequently return to a small size of ~3 cm. The vaginal introitus is partly occluded by the protective hymen, which is probably most important in preventing ascending infection before puberty when the pH of the vagina is less acidic. Once ruptured, the skin tags are referred to as hymen remnants or carunculae myrtiformes. The appearance of an intact hymen can have important significance in some societies as it is considered to be proof of virginal status. However, the hymen can be damaged by tampon use, medical use of a speculum to examine the vagina and cervix, athletic activity and horse riding.

The Bartholin's (or greater vestibular) glands lie posteriorly, one on each side of the vagina. These mucus-producing glands are analogous to the bulbourethral or Cowper's glands of the male. The Bartholin's glands are the size and shape of haricot beans and, unless inflamed, cannot normally be seen. Their rate of secretion of lubrication and mucus increases with the erection of the clitoris. If mucus builds up in the glands, cysts or abscesses may occur.

There is ongoing discussion about the existence of the Gräfenberg or G-spot (Pan et al., 2015). Descriptions of an erogenous zone in the anterior wall of the vagina have been reported over many centuries but little anatomical evidence for a discrete structure or region exists. Despite this, a huge industry around the G-spot has built up, which includes movies, books, toys and surgical interventions.

Box 2.9 describes an example of problems caused by mutilation of the external genitalia (female genital mutilation, Fig. 2.16).

BOX 2.9 Female Genital Mutilation

Female genital mutilation (FGM; 'female circumcision' or 'cutting') is an ancient cultural practice, which encompasses a range of ancient procedures that damage or remove a woman's external genital organs for no medical reason and have no health benefits. In the UK, FGM is illegal and it is mandatory for health professionals to report FGM to the police.

Many ethnic groups, particularly those of Muslim origin in Africa, Asia, the Middle East and other regions, regard FGM as essential to moderate sexual desire or to increase hygiene. Data collected by the WHO suggest that 200 million women in the world have experienced FGM. With increased immigration, healthcare professionals in countries such as the UK, Europe, Australia, New Zealand and the USA will encounter and need to care for women affected by FGM more often.

FGM is classified as a form of violence against women by Internal Human Rights Law and the UN has identified 6th February as the annual international day of zero tolerance to FGM. However, it is important to note that pressure for women to undergo FGM may be considerable and that many women who have undergone FGM consider it normal practice and could be offended by the term 'mutilation'. The surgery, performed in infancy, early childhood or puberty, may involve removal of the prepuce of the clitoris, removal of the labia minora and clitoris or removal of most of the labia and clitoris (Fig. 2.16). FGM can have severe and long-term consequences for physical and psychological health. The procedures are usually carried out without anaesthetic and often under unclean conditions for instance using thorns to form stitches on the vaginal walls, which increases the risk of infection, scarring and infertility. Genital mutilation may be accompanied by infibulation, the surgical closure of the labia majora (apart from a small opening for urine and menses) to ensure chastity. Although the practices are unacceptable and illegal in Western Europe, they may be undertaken illicitly or girls may be mutilated in other countries. At delivery, the urogenital tissue is extremely vulnerable to trauma, which can be minimized by anterior and mediolateral episiotomy incision. Failure to deliver vaginally may result in the rejection of the woman from her family. Infibulation will require surgical division to facilitate vaginal birth and although there may be pressure from the woman and her family to have the infibulation restored, this is illegal in many countries. Following division of infibulations, the introitus is restored by the suturing of the skin edges on the same side together.

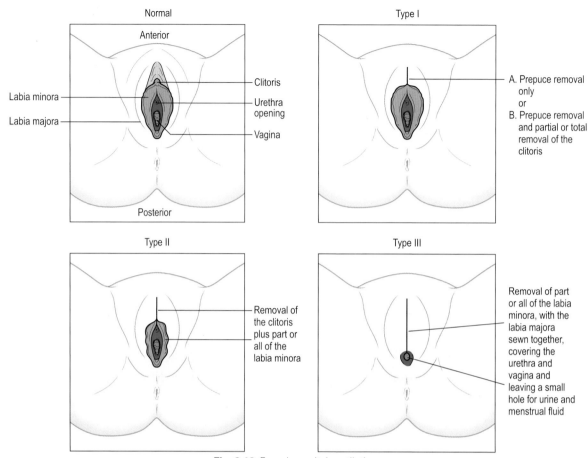

Fig. 2.16 Female genital mutilation.

The Pelvic Floor

The pelvic floor is composed primarily of the muscle fibres of the levator ani and the coccygeus muscle plus the connective tissues suspended within the outlet of the pelvis, forming a sling-like sheet of tissue that encloses and supports the pelvic contents (Box 2.10; Fig. 2.17). This sling arrangement is important in facilitating human birth by allowing rotational manoeuvres of the presenting fetal denominator. In women, the main characteristic distinguishing it from that of the pelvic floor of the man is that there are three openings instead of two. As well as the anal canal and urethra, the woman also has a vaginal opening. This is why women are much more likely to suffer from PID as there is a direct route from the external environment via the genital tract, uterine cavity and uterine tubes to the internal pelvic cavity lined by the peritoneum.

Pelvic Shape and Adaptation

The pelvis is a girdle composed of a number of bones held together by ligaments and cartilaginous and fused joints (Fig. 2.18). The dimensions of the inlet, cavity and outlet affect the passage of the fetus. The fetus has to negotiate the pelvic cavity by undergoing a rotational manoeuvre. The sling-like arrangement of the gutter-shaped pelvic floor muscles means that the fetus is forced to rotate in a forward position (see Chapter 13). The emergence with head flexed usually in the occiput anterior position (facing the mother's back and buttocks) is the most favourable presentation for spontaneous birth. This arrangement has evolved because of humans adopting an upright stance. The different and conflicting demands of locomotion and childbirth on the pelvis of humans and other primates have been described as the 'obstetric dilemma' (Trevathan, 2015). Bipedal posture, which evolved 5–7 million years

---

BOX 2.10   Functions and Characteristics of the Pelvic Floor

- Its muscles are arranged in two layers: superficial (perineal muscles) and deep (levator ani muscle) (Fig. 2.17).
- It supports and maintains the anatomical position of the internal female reproductive organs, the bladder and intestine.
- It provides voluntary muscle control for micturition and defecation.
- It contributes to maintaining optimal intra-abdominal pressure; damage to the pelvic floor can cause urinary or faecal incontinence and/or prolapse of the pelvic organs.
- It is involved in gait and movement.
- It has an essential role in delivery and facilitates birth by resisting descent of the fetal head and shoulders, so forcing the fetus to rotate forward in the presence of strong regular uterine contractions. This is particularly important in a bipedal species like the human, because the morphology of the pelvis is influenced by the evolution of our upright stance.
- Risk factors for pelvic floor damage or dysfunction can be considered as predisposing (such as gender, racial, environmental); inciting (such as childbirth, muscle or nerve damage); promoting (such as constipation, obesity, smoking, occupational or recreational, infection); and decompensating (such as ageing, disease, medication) (Hilde and Bo, 2015).

---

ago, means the abdominal contents including the pregnant uterus are supported by the muscles of the pelvic floor, unlike four-legged animals where the uterus is primarily supported by the abdominal wall. Efficiency of locomotion is facilitated by a narrower rigid pelvis and ischial spines (which support the pelvic floor muscles but restrict the birth canal), which are closer together. However, women with wider pelvis and birth canals have easier births (see Chapter 13) but if the ischial spines are further apart, the pelvic floor muscles are more easily weakened, which can contribute to the risk of pelvic organ prolapse. It has been suggested that there is a complex relationship between pelvis shape, stature (height) and head circumference (Fischer and Mitteroecker, 2015) due to natural selection processes, which may alleviate the obstetric dilemma to some extent. The shape of the pelvis is associated with head circumference and body height. Individuals with larger heads tend to have rounded pelvic inlets (gynoid shape); women with larger heads have offspring with larger heads so this facilitates delivery. Shorter individuals also tend to have

rounder pelvic inlets; shorter women may be more challenged by cephalopelvic disproportion, the most common cause of obstructed labour.

The female pelvis is larger, wider and shallower than the male pelvis. Each half of the pelvis is formed from the innominate or hip bone, which is composed of the ilium, ischium and pubic sections. These sections are the result of the fusion of three separate bones during puberty. Traditionally, pelvic morphology has been classified by four major categories (Fig. 2.19) in an attempt to identify risk of delivery problems. In practice, there is a continuum in pelvic form and many women have a pelvis, which combines features from all four categories. There are also recognized abnormalities of the pelvis including justo minor pelvis (normal shape but the overall dimensions are smaller than normal), Nägele's pelvis (asymmetrical due to abnormal bone formation on one side) and Robert's pelvis (similar to Nägele's pelvis but the abnormal bone formation is bilateral). Pelvic shape can also be affected by disease, for example rachitic pelvis due to childhood rickets, which is an extreme form of the platypelloid pelvis (has reduced anterior–posterior diameter). The shape of the pelvis affects the mechanism of labour (see Chapter 13); abnormal pelvic shape is associated with problems at delivery as the rotation of the presenting part may be suboptimal. Ultrasound and MRI of the pelvis before birth allows assessment of the diameters of the birth canal and relative size of the head enabling prediction of risk of problems at delivery. However, a fetal malpresentation, such as a deflexed posterior occipital presentation with asynclitism (lateral tilting of the head), could still present problems even if medical imaging identified the pelvis to be of normal size and shape.

THE MALE REPRODUCTIVE TRACT

The male reproductive tract comprises a number of structures that permit gamete formation (spermatogenesis) to occur below body temperature and provide conditions that allow sperm maturation and ejection/ejaculation (Fig. 2.20). It is estimated that healthy fertile men produce 45 million sperm per testis/day (Griswold, 2016); equivalent to over 1000 sperm per second! Spermatogenesis, from making to ejaculating sperm, takes about 74 days on average with a broad variation (42–76 days) (Neto et al., 2016). The testes also produce and secrete 3–10 mg testosterone/day.

The Testes

The testes, which are each about 30 mL in volume, are suspended within the scrotal sac or scrotum. Optimal spermatogenesis in humans is achieved 2–3°C below the body's core temperature. There are a number of mechanisms to

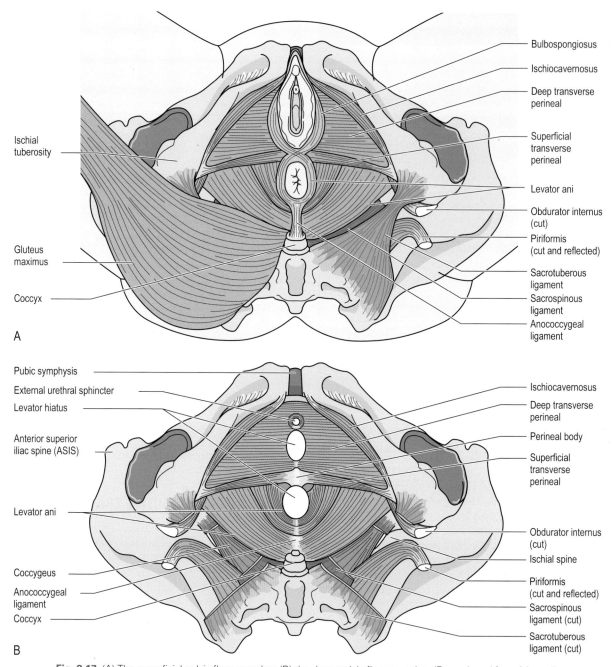

Fig. 2.17 (A) The superficial pelvic floor muscles; (B) the deep pelvic floor muscles. (Reproduced from Muscolino JE: *The muscular system manual: the skeletal muscles of the human body*, 4 ed, Elsevier 2017, Fig 19.38.)

regulate the temperature of the testes. The testes are suspended outside the abdominal cavity but can be retracted upwards towards the warmth of the body by contraction of the cremaster muscle, which covers the testes. This muscle will also reflexly raise the testes towards the body if the inner thigh is stroked, poked or scratched. This cremaster reflex is used as a neurological test to identify motor neuron or spinal disorders; it is also abnormal if there is testicular torsion. The pigmented skin of the scrotum lies in rugae (folds), which increase the surface area. The scrotum

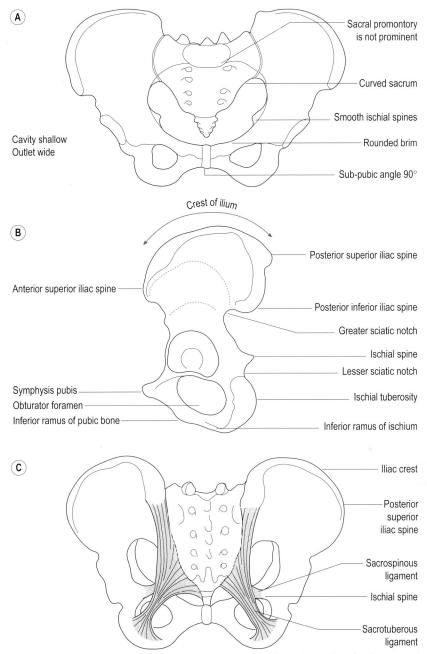

(A)

Sacral promontory
is not prominent

Curved sacrum

Smooth ischial spines

Rounded brim

Sub-pubic angle 90°

Cavity shallow
Outlet wide

Crest of *ilium*

(B)

Posterior superior iliac spine

Anterior superior iliac spine

Posterior inferior iliac spine

Greater sciatic notch

Ischial spine

Lesser sciatic notch

Symphysis pubis

Obturator foramen

Inferior ramus of pubic bone

Ischial tuberosity

Inferior ramus of ischium

(C)

Iliac crest

Posterior
superior
iliac spine

Sacrospinous
ligament

Ischial spine

Sacrotuberous
ligament

Fig. 2.18 The pelvic girdle: (A) the normal female pelvis; (B) innominate bone showing important landmarks; (C) posterior view of the pelvis to show ligaments. (Reproduced with permission from Bennett and Brown, 1999.)

is well vascularized but has no insulating hair or subcutaneous fat. It is lined by the dartos muscle, which contracts in response to cold. Blood flow to the testes allows heat to be transferred from the descending testicular arteries to the ascending pampiniform venous plexus forming a counter-current heat-exchange mechanism, which helps to maintain the lower temperature of the testes relative to the body.

The testes are a pair of glandular organs, analogous to the ovaries, that produce gametes (spermatozoa) and

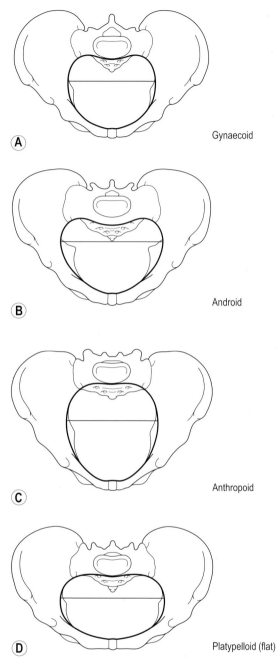

Fig. 2.19 Characteristics of the four categories of pelvic shape: (A) gynaecoid or 'normal' female pelvis, which is well-proportioned and spacious with an oval or round inlet and backwards inclination; (B) android pelvis has some masculine characteristics such as a prominent sacrum and triangular sacrum forming a heart- or wedge-shaped inlet, which may cause problems in childbirth; (C) anthropoid pelvis has an oval shape and widely spaced spines; (D) platypelloid (flat) pelvis is usual but wide and flat with a short sacrum resulting in reduced diameter of the lower pelvis, which is associated with transverse arrest.

male sex hormones. Within the scrotum, the testes are surrounded by a thick fibrous capsule called the tunica albuginea, which penetrates internally dividing the testes into lobules. Each testis has ~200–300 lobules, each containing about one to three loops of seminiferous tubules, ~0.2 mm in diameter and 70–80 cm long (Fig. 2.21). The seminiferous tubules are the site of spermatogenesis (sperm production). Within the tubules are spermatogenic cells (germ cells) and their supporting Sertoli cells, which cordon off the spermatogenic cells and the developing sperm into distinct compartments. Between the tubules are the interstitial cells of Leydig, which produce testosterone. Leydig cells also express the microsomal P450 aromatase enzyme, which converts testosterone to oestradiol, a step essential in the induction of spermatogenesis (note that this enzyme is also produced by adipose tissue, which is one of the reasons why obesity in men is associated with altered sex hormone profiles). Peritubular myoid cells are flattened cells surrounding the Sertoli cells; they contribute to the blood testes barrier and generate contractile waves, under the influence of oxytocin from Leydig cells, which propel testicular fluid containing immotile immature spermatozoa towards the rete testis (Neto et al., 2016) (see Fig. 2.12).

The epididymis is a comma-shaped convoluted tube, ~6 cm long, leading into the vas deferens. The sperm produced from the seminiferous tubules are stored in the epididymis where they are concentrated, via oestrogen action on the vasa efferentia, which promotes fluid absorption. In the epididymis, the sperm are matured and become motile; oxytocin stimulates epididymal motility. The vas deferens provides the conduit for sperm delivery during emission and ejaculation. It is a thick-walled tube leading from the tail of the epididymis to the ejaculatory duct. The vas deferens dilates into a storage reservoir, or ampulla, just before it joins with the exit of the seminal vesicle to form the ejaculatory duct. The vas deferens, blood vessels and cremaster muscle lie closely together forming the spermatic cord.

The testis is an immunoprivileged site, like the uterus in pregnancy (see Chapter 10), the eye and the brain (Chen et al., 2016). This means normal systemic immune system responses are suppressed; the unique immune environment protects the germ cells from detrimental damage by the immune cells whilst still allowing an appropriate response to the pathogens (such as bacteria, viruses, fungi and parasites) that could infect the testes. The testis is host to many types of immune cells, which include macrophages, lymphocytes, mast cells and dendritic cells. Inflammation of the testis is called orchitis. It can be unilateral or bilateral and can be caused by microbes, physical trauma, chemical toxins or tumours. Orchitis can be a cause of male infertility (see Chapter 6). Causes of infection include sexually

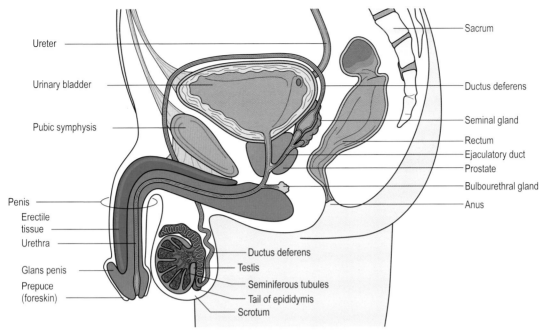

Sacrum

Ureter

Urinary bladder

Ductus deferens

Pubic symphysis

Seminal gland

Rectum
Ejaculatory duct
Prostate

Bulbourethral gland

Penis

Anus

Erectile
tissue

Urethra

Ductus deferens

Glans penis

Testis

Prepuce
(foreskin)

Seminiferous tubules

Tail of epididymis

Scrotum

Fig. 2.20 The male reproductive system. (Reproduced from Moore KL, Persaud TVN, Torchia MG: *The developing human: clinically oriented embryology*, 11 ed, Elsevier 2020, Fig. 12.12.)

transmitted infections such as *Neisseria gonorrhoeae* and *Chlamydia trachomatis* or viruses such as the mumps virus, which can cause infertility in adult men. Just as infection or trauma can cause blockage of the uterine tubes, the male reproductive capacity can also be affected by blockage, of the epididymis or vas deferens for instance, impeding the passage of spermatozoa.

The seminal vesicles are two pyramid-shaped membranous sacs, ~4 cm long, lying between the base of the bladder and the rectum. They produce semen, a viscous fluid rich in fructose, citric acid and lipids, which facilitates sperm transport and nourishment. The fluid component of semen is principally produced by the seminal vesicles and the prostate gland. Secretory activity of the seminal vesicles depends on the level of testosterone. The ejaculatory ducts begin at the base of the prostate gland and terminate in the single prostatic urethra. These muscular ducts carry sperm and seminal fluid through the prostate gland. The prostate gland is a walnut-sized exocrine gland lying just below the neck of the bladder, between the rectum and pubic bone. It is a compound gland, formed of ~20–40 smaller glandular units each with its own exit into the ejaculatory duct. Prostatic fluid is a thin alkaline lubricating secretion that mixes with the sperm and seminal fluid. The prostate gland can be palpated through the rectal wall. In elderly men, the prostate gland may undergo hypertrophy causing

benign prostatic hyperplasia, which can compress the urethra and impede micturition. Prostatitis or inflammation of the prostate gland can affect men of all ages. Prostatic carcinoma is one of the most common cancers affecting older men in developed countries; it is a major cause of death if it is not detected early. Prior to ejaculation, the bulbourethral glands (or Cowper's glands) secrete clear lubricating fluid into the urethra just below the prostate gland.

The penis carries the urethra, which provides a shared passage for sperm and urine, and allows intromission: the delivery of sperm into the vagina. Unlike other mammalian species, the human penis does not have an erectile bone (or baculum) and relies entirely on venous engorgement to achieve erection; it also cannot be withdrawn into the groin. Other primates have a baculum; it is suggested it is not required in humans because the male spends a lot of time with the female to endure paternity of offspring, which means there is frequent and short copulatory activity. It is also speculated that the lack of baculum means erection is more dependent on healthy blood vessels and control of blood pressure and may therefore have a role in sexual selection of a mate by the female.

Humans have one of the largest penis:body size ratios. The penis has three columns of erectile tissue: two lateral corpora cavernosa and a ventromedial corpus spongiosum

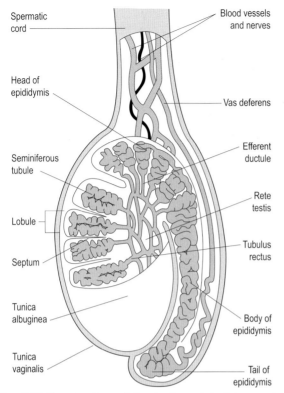

Fig. 2.21 The structure of the testis and ducts conveying sperm from the seminiferous tubules to the urethra. (Reproduced with permission from Brooker, 1998.)

(Fig. 2.22). The corpus spongiosum contains the urethra and does not engorge as much as the corpora cavernosa. This prevents trauma to the urethra and generates an appropriate angle for intromission. The expanded cone-shaped end of the corpus spongiosum forms the glans penis where the urethra opens. The penis is covered with a fold of skin or prepuce (foreskin), which can be retracted in an adult and older child to expose the glans penis. If the foreskin is too tight, it may not be able to be retracted past the glans penis; this condition is known as phimosis and may cause the child to have problems urinating or result in pain during an erection. A skin infection under the foreskin is termed 'balanitis'; the condition can cause urination to be painful and can be worsened by the use of perfumed soaps and topical agents.

The foreskin attaches to the underside of the penis at a small fold of tissue called the frenum. The prepuce and shaft skin are not attached to underlying tissue so they are free to glide along the shaft of the penis, which reduces friction, abrasion and loss of lubricating fluid during intercourse. On the underside of the penis, there is a small

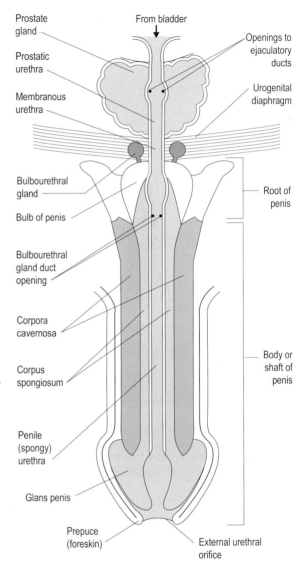

Fig. 2.22 Internal structure of the penis.

ridge called the raphe, which runs from the opening of the urethra across the scrotum to the perineum (between the scrotum and anus) in the midline. The spongy bodies of the penis become distended with blood during an erection (see Chapter 6).

GAMETOGENESIS

The process of gametogenesis is achieved through a specialized form of cellular division called meiosis (Fig. 2.23). (The stages of meiosis are reviewed in Chapter 7.)

Normal gametogenesis

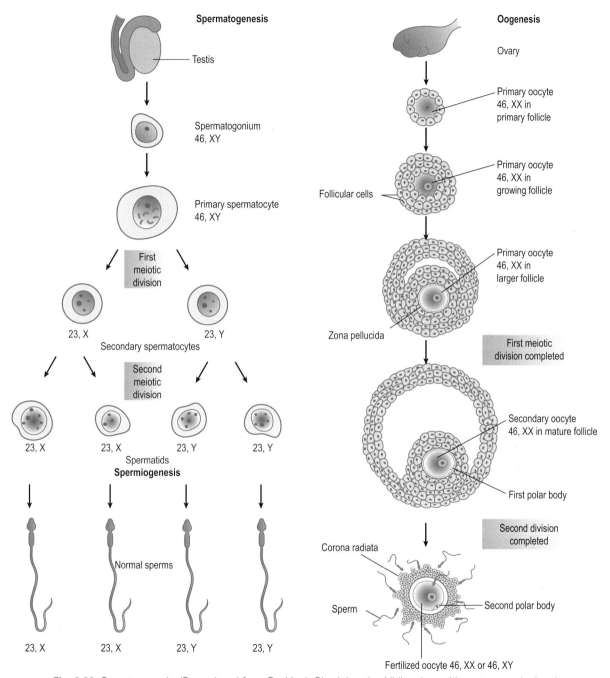

Fig. 2.23 Gametogenesis. (Reproduced from Rankin J: *Physiology in childbearing: with anatomy and related biosciences*, 4 ed, Elsevier 2017, Fig. 9.1.)

Gametogenesis is remarkably different in the male and female reproductive systems, both representing adaptation of the process of meiosis to facilitate reproduction. Gametes are specialized sex cells that contain half the genetic material (and, therefore, half the number of chromosomes) of the normal cell content. (Their fusion, referred to as fertilization, is described in detail in Chapter 6.)

The production of spermatozoa begins at puberty in the male and results in the continual production of millions of sperm each day. Spermatozoa have completed all the meiotic divisions prior to ejaculation and fusion with the oocyte. In this sense, they are true gametes containing the haploid number of chromosomes. (These terms are explained in Chapter 4.)

The differences between male and female gamete formation have evolved with the development of sexual reproduction and internal fertilization. Oocytes are relatively protected within the abdominal cavity and it is not necessary for a large number to be produced. Movement of oocytes is passive, influenced by the structure of the uterine tube. Sperm, in contrast, must become highly motile in order to travel along the female reproductive tract. Many are lost and, of the millions contained within the ejaculate, only a few hundred will make it to the vicinity of the oocyte. In addition, sperm have to survive relocation into the female reproductive tract, which is effectively equivalent to a foreign host, in order to perform their physiological role of fertilizing the oocyte. Thus, they have to be adapted to evade the innate immune defence mechanisms that protect the female reproductive tract such as the complement cascade (see Chapter 10), which is present in the secretions; both sperm and seminal fluid have immune system regulators, which enhance sperm survival (Chen et al., 2016).

Spermatogenesis

Spermatogenesis begins at puberty and continues into senescence, albeit less efficiently. It is a complex process, well-organized temporally and spatially, which takes place in the epithelium of the seminiferous tubules; groups of cells progress in clearly defined stages of cell division within a particular tubule, which is described as a 'spermatogenic wave'. There are three processes involved in spermatogenesis: (1) the renewal of the spermatogonial stem cell population and the formation and expansion of undifferentiated progenitor germ cells (spermatogonia) around the inner circumference of the seminiferous tubule, which divide and replicate by a process called mitosis (see Chapter 4), forming many spermatogonia (Fig. 2.24); (2) the reduction of the number of chromosomes in each progenitor cell by meiosis; and (3) the differentiation of the haploid cells into spermatozoa (spermiogenesis). During spermatogenesis, 13 distinct stages of developmental forms of human germ cells can be identified from spermatogonia to spermatocytes and spermatids (Neto et al., 2016). Each spermatogonium first divides into two diploid primary spermatocytes. The primary spermatocytes then undergo meiosis producing two genetically diverse secondary spermatocytes and then, after the second meiotic division, four haploid spermatids. For each cell undergoing meiosis, therefore, four gametes are produced. The round spermatids undergo spermiogenesis (nuclear and cytoplasmic changes) producing the characteristic morphology (shape) of a spermatozoon. As meiosis progresses, the immature sperm are supported within Sertoli cells, which regulate spermatogenesis (Griswold, 2016), which then release the sperm into the lumen of the seminiferous tubule by degrading the cell–cell junctions. Sertoli cells synthesize and secrete a number of glycoproteins involved in Sertoli-germ cell interactions including bioprotective proteins, proteases and protease inhibitors involved in tissue remodelling processes, glycoproteins that form the basement membrane and other regulatory glycoproteins including anti-Müllerian hormone and androgen-binding protein (ABP) (Box 2.11). Each Sertoli cell can support 30–50 spermatogonia at different stages of development.

The spermatozoa are stored in the epididymis, where they mature acquiring both motility and the capability for fertilization, for 2 weeks and may stay for up to 6 months. The shortest time between the initial meiosis and ejaculation is about 10 weeks, which is therefore the critical preconception period in men. Spermatogenesis is regulated by gonadotrophins and steroid hormones, the interaction of these hormones with the somatic cells of the testis (Leydig and Sertoli cells) and by retinoic acid (vitamin A) (Neto et al., 2016). It is affected by temperature, malnutrition, alcohol, cottonseed oil (a potential source of contraception), some drugs and heavy metals.

Steroidogenesis

The interstitial cells of Leydig interspersed between the seminiferous tubules produce 90% of the circulating testosterone (the remainder has an adrenal origin). Testosterone is responsible for the development of male secondary sex characteristics (see Chapter 3) and, together with follicle-stimulating hormone (FSH), controls production of sperm. Testosterone production is stimulated by luteinizing hormone (LH) from the pituitary gland (Fig. 2.25). Testosterone binds to ABP in the seminiferous tubules, which means that testosterone levels within

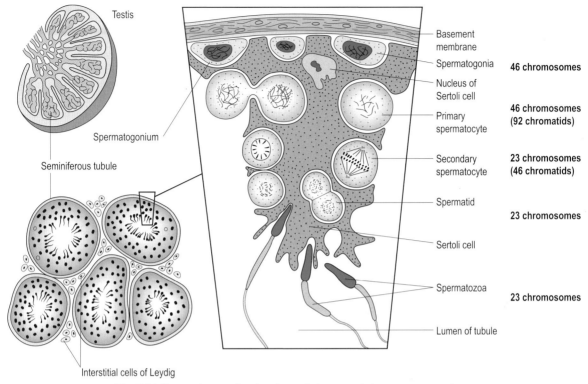

Fig. 2.24 Spermatogenesis, showing cell stages and chromosome numbers.

BOX 2.11   The Role of Sertoli Cells

- Control spermatogenesis. Support ('nurse') spermatogenic cells and migrate them inwards to the lumen of the seminiferous tubule as they develop
- Provide nutrients to spermatocytes and spermatids (hence their former name of 'nurse cells')
- Secrete fluid to aid release of sperm into lumen
- Contribute to the blood testes barrier
- Act as a barrier between sperm-producing areas of the seminiferous tubule and its lumen, forming environmentally distinct compartments of the seminiferous epithelium. The interior of the Sertoli cells forms compartments because of the intricate framework of cytoskeleton (Neto et al., 2016).
- Macrophagic activity; engulf and digest cellular debris left from spermiogenesis limiting the release of noxious cellular components from dead cells that could adversely affect spermatogenesis
- Produce inhibin B and activin A, which regulate follicle-stimulating hormone (FSH) secretion from the pituitary gland. The concentration of inhibin B in the blood reflects the number of functional Sertoli cells and spermatogenic effectiveness

- Produce androgen-binding protein (ABP, also known as testosterone-binding globulin), which increases seminiferous tubule (intratesticular) testosterone concentration and thereby spermiogenesis
- Produce anti-Müllerian-inhibiting hormone, which affects sexual differentiation (see Chapter 5) by inducing regression of the Müllerian ducts thus preventing the development of female internal genitalia
- Produce glial cell line-derived neurotrophic factor (GDNF), a small protein, which promotes neuronal survival and regulates kidney development and spermatogenesis
- Produce Ets-related molecule (ERM), a member of the Ets transcription factor family essential for spermatogonium stem-cell maintenance and self-renewal
- Synthesis and secretion of several proteins found in serum including the iron and copper-binding proteins, transferrin and ceruloplasmin, which are involved in spermatogenesis (Johnson, 2018)

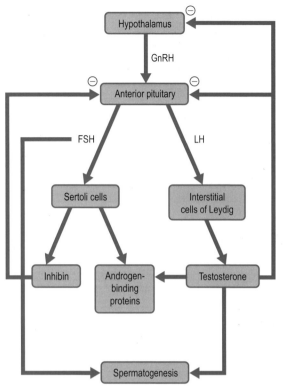

Fig. 2.25 Production of testosterone.

the tubule can be very high (100 times serum levels) while maintaining a concentration gradient that drives diffusion from outside to inside. Testosterone exerts a negative feedback mechanism on the hypothalamic–pituitary axis in a manner analogous to the feedback control by oestrogen in the female cycle (see Chapter 4). FSH stimulates the production of ABP by the Sertoli cells. Inhibin B produced from the Sertoli cells inhibits FSH production. Illness and stress can affect male reproductive capacity probably via the hypothalamic–pituitary axis.

Control of Gametogenesis

The control of gametogenesis and steroidogenesis in males and females has some similarities. The hypothalamus regulates reproduction by secreting gonadotrophin-releasing hormone (GnRH; see Fig. 2.25). This stimulates both FSH and LH production from the anterior pituitary gland. FSH stimulates gametogenesis: spermatogenesis in men and follicular development in women. LH plays a pivotal role in steroidogenesis: increasing testosterone production from the Leydig cells in men and stimulating the increases in progesterone and oestrogen secretion in the second half of the menstrual cycle in women (see Chapter 4).

KEY POINTS

- The renal system regulates water and electrolyte balance and is important in the maintenance of pH and the regulation of blood pressure. Waste products and foreign chemicals are excreted by the kidneys. The kidneys also have an endocrine role such as the regulation of the number of circulating erythrocytes.
- Glomerular filtrate is formed from continuous processing of plasma and contains water and substances such as amino acids and glucose that are small enough to be filtered.
- The filtrate is modified in the nephron by reabsorption of substances into the blood and secretion of waste products into the filtrate. Reabsorption and secretion are regulated by hormones and many systems have transport maxima that can be exceeded in pregnancy, leading to urinary excretion of substances not usually present in the urine.
- Micturition (urination) is stimulated by bladder stretch receptors and controlled by learned inhibitory pathways.

- The female reproductive system produces female gametes, receives male gametes and provides the optimum environment for fertilization, implantation and nurture of the fetus. The uterus remains quiescent during pregnancy and generates the forces required for delivery at the end of gestation. The system is quickly restored to a fertile state at the end of pregnancy.
- Gametogenesis begins with mitosis of the primordial germ cells followed by meiosis, which reduces the chromosome number and creates infinite variation in the genetic complement of the gametes.
- The male gonads produce gametes from the seminiferous tubules and testosterone from the Leydig cells. Gametogenesis has a relatively short time span in the man.
- The hypothalamus regulates reproduction by secreting GnRH, which stimulates production of FSH and LH from the anterior pituitary, which in turn has effects on the gonads. The sex steroids produced by the gonads exert negative feedback inhibition at the hypothalamic–pituitary axis.

APPLICATION TO PRACTICE

Why is an in-depth knowledge of the female genitalia required by the midwife and how will this knowledge affect the decisions made by the midwife within practice?

You might consider what the midwife needs to know in order to suture the peritoneum, to catheterize a woman during labour or to recognize the sex of a baby at birth and identify that anomalies are present (see Chapter 5).

There are many signs and 'symptoms' in pregnancy that are indicative of changes occurring within the renal system; knowledge of this will help the midwife to explain these fully to the woman.

Women with pre-existing renal disease need careful monitoring and maternity care should be integrated with specialist expert renal care. For some women, underlying renal disease may only become apparent in pregnancy when a woman fails to have the normal expected physiological fall in blood pressure in the first trimester and subsequently develops hypertension during the pregnancy. The earlier the hypertension develops, the higher is the risk for long-term problems for the mother. The fetus is also at increased risk of severe intrauterine growth retardation.

Women who have had a kidney transplant may become pregnant; however, the risk to the pregnancy must be carefully managed against the risk of reducing or modifying anti-rejection medication. It is important to consider that the anatomical placement of the donor kidney is usually much lower in the abdominal cavity. This is particularly important should the woman require surgical intervention for delivery to ensure that the donor kidney is not damaged during the procedure.

During routine antenatal check-ups, the midwife routinely performs urinalysis. Are you able to explain the significance of the findings as a whole or do you think it is appropriate that midwives just observe for evidence of proteinuria?

The hormones of pregnancy affect muscle tone and relax ligaments, so bladder control is often less effective in pregnancy and these effects may continue after pregnancy. In such cases, muscle tone can be improved by encouraging pelvic floor exercises to promote optimal continence following childbirth. Displacement of the pelvic organs resulting in anterior and posterior prolapses becomes increasingly common, as the parity due to the loss of effective muscle tone and ligament support is higher, and so pelvic floor exercises should be encouraged to minimize these problems.

ANNOTATED FURTHER READING

Cropp G, Armstrong J: Female genital mutilation and reporting duties for all clinical personnel, *Br J Hosp Med (Lond.)* 77:419–423, 2016.
A short article that considers the health professional's role in dealing with FGM and meeting the requirements of the UK legislation.
Elson CJ, Salim R, Potdar N, et al.: on behalf of the Royal College of Obstetricians and Gynaecologists: Diagnosis and management of ectopic pregnancy, *BJOG* 123:e15–e55, 2016.
Evidence-based best practice guidelines from the RCOG on the diagnosis and management of ectopic (or tubal) pregnancies. Note that the RCOG also provides an excellent and well-illustrated patient information booklet on ectopic pregnancy, which can also be accessed from their website: www.rcog.org.uk.
Fritsch H, Zwierzina M, Riss P: Accuracy of concepts in female pelvic floor anatomy: facts and myths!, *World J Urol* 30:429–435, 2012.
A description of the pelvic floor, illustrated with photographs, which describes the anatomical structures, identifies important landmarks, clarifies terminology and explains common misconceptions.
Gruss LT, Schmitt D: The evolution of the human pelvis: changing adaptations to bipedalism, obstetrics and thermoregulation, *Philos Trans R Soc Lond B Biol Sci* 370:20140063, 2015.
Illustrated review of the changing shape of the primate pelvis under evolutionary selection processes.

Jannini EA, Buisson O, Rubio-Casillas A: Beyond the G-spot: clitourethrovaginal complex anatomy in female orgasm, *Nat Rev Urol* 11:531–538, 2014.
Well-illustrated description of the gross anatomy and physiology of the clitourethrovaginal (CUV) complex.
Johnson MH: *Essential reproduction*, ed 8, Oxford, 2018, Wiley-Blackwell.
An integrated and well-organized research-based textbook that covers the fundamentals of reproduction using a multidisciplinary approach and explores comparative reproductive physiology of mammals, including anatomy, physiology, endocrinology, genetics and behavioural studies.
Jones LJ, Horton-Szar D: *Crash course: renal and urinary systems*, ed 4, St Louis, 2015, Mosby.
This well-illustrated book (with downloadable eBook) provides a useful reference text for students requiring more details of the renal and urinary systems.
Puppo V: Female genital mutilation and cutting: an anatomical review and alternative rites, *Clin Anat* 30:81–88, 2017.
An illustrated review, written for health professionals, which describes the cultural background surrounding the practice of FGM, the four WHO-classified types of procedures used, complications and proposes alternative rites of passage.
Puppo V, Puppo G: Anatomy of sex: revision of the new anatomical terms used for the clitoris and the female orgasm by sexologists, *Clin Anat* 28:293–304, 2015.

An interesting (and somewhat passionate and controversial) argument about the use (and misuse) of anatomical terms for the female reproductive tract, which includes discussion of the embryological origins and male homologues of the structures.

Trevathan W: Primate pelvic anatomy and implications for birth, *Philos Trans R Soc Lond B Biol Sci* 370:20140065, 2015.

Interesting review about the implications of the bipedal birth canal for encephalized (large brained) primates and the development of rotational birth manoeuvres.

Yeung J, Pauls RN: Anatomy of the vulva and the female sexual response, *Obstet Gynecol Clin North Am* 43:27–44, 2016.

A comprehensive review of the anatomy of the female reproductive tract with detailed description of the vascularization and innervation of the structures.

Readers are recommended also to read chapters on the renal and reproductive systems in a physiology textbook, such as those listed at the end of the Chapter 1.

REFERENCES

Aldunate M, Srbinovski D, Hearps AC, et al.: Antimicrobial and immune modulatory effects of lactic acid and short chain fatty acids produced by vaginal microbiota associated with eubiosis and bacterial vaginosis, *Front Physiol* 6:164, 2015.

Bennett VR, Brown LK: *Myles' textbook for midwives*, ed 13, Edinburgh, 1999, Churchill Livingstone, pp 940–942. 949.

Birder L, Wyndaele JJ: From urothelial signalling to experiencing a sensation related to the urinary bladder, *Acta Physiol (Oxf)* 207:34–39, 2013.

Brooker CG: *Human structure and function*, ed 2, St Louis, 1998, Mosby, pp 344. 345, 363, 470, 471, 473, 476, 483.

Cai Y: Revisiting old vaginal topics: conversion of the Müllerian vagina and origin of the 'sinus' vagina, *Int J Dev Biol* 53:925–934, 2009.

Castro RA, Arruda RM, Bortolini MA: Female urinary incontinence: effective treatment strategies, *Climacteric* 18:135–141, 2015.

Chan PA, Robinette A, Montgomery M, et al.: Extragenital infections caused by Chlamydia trachomatis and Neisseria gonorrhoeae: a review of the literature, *Infect Dis Obstet Gynecol* 2016:5758387, 2016.

Chen Q, Deng T, Han D: Testicular immunoregulation and spermatogenesis, *Semin Cell Dev Biol* 59:157–165, 2016.

DiMaio D: Nuns, warts, viruses, and cancer, *Yale J Biol Med* 88:127–129, 2015.

Drolet M, Bénard E, Pérez N, et al.: on behalf of the HPV Vaccination Impact Study Group: Population-level impact and herd effects following the introduction of human papillomavirus vaccination programmes: updated systematic review and meta-analysis, *Lancet* 394:497-509, 2019.

Dwyer PL: Skene's gland revisited: function, dysfunction and the G spot, *Int Urogynecol J* 23:135–137, 2012.

Fettweis JM, Brooks JP, Serrano MG, et al.: Differences in vaginal microbiome in African American women versus women of European ancestry, *Microbiology* 160:2272–2282, 2014.

Fields L, Hathaway A: Key concepts in pregnancy of unknown location: identifying ectopic pregnancy and providing patient-centered care, *J Midwifery Women's Health* 62:172–179, 2016.

Fischer B, Mitteroecker P: Covariation between human pelvis shape, stature, and head size alleviates the obstetric dilemma, *Proc Natl Acad Sci USA* 112:5655–5660, 2015.

Griswold MD: Spermatogenesis: the commitment to meiosis, *Physiol Rev* 96:1–17, 2016.

Hilde G, Bo K: The pelvic floor during pregnancy and after childbirth, and the effect of pelvic floor muscle training on urinary incontinence - A literature review, *Current Women's Health Reviews* 11:19–30, 2015.

Hughes RG, Brocklehurst P, Steer PJ, et al.: on behalf of the Royal College of Obstetricians and Gynaecologists: Prevention of early-onset neonatal Group B Streptococcal disease (Greentop Guideline No. 36), *BJOG* 124:e280–e305, 2017.

Johnson MH: *Essential reproduction*, ed 8, Oxford, 2018, Wiley-Blackwell.

Knight M, Nair M, Tuffnell D, on behalf of MBRRACE-UK, et al.: *Saving lives, improving mothers' care - lessons learned to inform maternity care from the UK and Ireland Confidential Enquiries into Maternal Deaths and Morbidity 2013–15*, Oxford, 2017, University of Oxford, National Perinatal Epidemiology Unit.

Maybin JA, Critchley HO: Menstrual physiology: implications for endometrial pathology and beyond, *Hum Reprod Update* 21:748–761, 2015.

Neto FT, Bach PV, Najari BB, et al.: Spermatogenesis in humans and its affecting factors, *Semin Cell Dev Biol* 59:10–26, 2016.

NICE: *Ectopic pregnancy and miscarriage: diagnosis and initial management (Clinical guideline)*, National Institute for Health and Care Excellence, 2012.

Nunn KL, Forney LJ: Unraveling the dynamics of the human vaginal microbiome, *Yale J Biol Med* 89:331–337, 2016.

Pan S, Leung C, Shah J, et al.: Clinical anatomy of the G-spot, *Clin Anat* 28:363–367, 2015.

Pastor Z: Female ejaculation orgasm vs. coital incontinence: a systematic review, *J Sex Med* 10:1682–1691, 2013.

Pauls RN: Anatomy of the clitoris and the female sexual response, *Clin Anat* 28:376–384, 2015.

Ravel J, Brotman RM: Translating the vaginal microbiome: gaps and challenges, *Genome Med* 8:35, 2016.

Sweet B: *Mayes' midwifery*, ed 12, London, 1996, Baillière Tindall, p 29.

Trevathan W: Primate pelvic anatomy and implications for birth, *Philos Trans R Soc Lond B Biol Sci* 370:20140065, 2015.

Triana L, Robledo AM: Aesthetic surgery of female external genitalia, *Aesthet Surg J* 35:165–177, 2015.

Virant-Klun I: Postnatal oogenesis in humans: a review of recent findings, *Stem Cells Cloning* 8:49–60, 2015.

Wesnes SL, Lose G: Preventing urinary incontinence during pregnancy and postpartum: a review, *Int Urogynecol J* 24:889–899, 2013.

Wira CR, Fahey JV, Rodriguez-Garcia M, et al.: Regulation of mucosal immunity in the female reproductive tract: the role of sex hormones in immune protection against sexually transmitted pathogens, *Am J Reprod Immunol* 72:236–258, 2014.

Endocrinology

LEARNING OBJECTIVES

- To introduce the basic concepts and terminology used in endocrinology.
- To discuss the different types of hormones, their functions, main sites of production and mechanisms of action.
- To describe the role of the sex steroids.

- To relate endocrinology to the physiological process of reproduction.
- To outline how hormones, synthetic analogues and hormone-like drugs can be used to manage clinical conditions affecting reproductive health.

INTRODUCTION

This chapter presents an overview of endocrinology and summarizes the role of hormones in the regulation of human physiology. Throughout the chapter, links to reproductive physiology will be highlighted and referenced to other chapters in the book, where the relevant interactions will be described more specifically.

The endocrine system, in conjunction with the nervous system, coordinates, regulates and adjusts physiological processes in the body in response to changes in the internal and external environment. The nervous system tends to react in situations where an immediate response is required, whereas the endocrine system is involved in sustaining body functions over a longer period (Table 3.1).

For example, shivering is induced by neuromuscular activity to counteract a fall in the environmental temperature, whereas many body cycles, such as the menstrual cycle, are almost entirely orchestrated through the endocrine system. However, the two systems interact extensively with each other and some rapid responses also have a hormonal component. For example, the release of the hormone adrenaline (epinephrine) from the adrenal glands in the fight-or-flight response begins in the amygdala of the brain and acts via a neuronal pathway to the hypothalamus to regulate hormone secretion. The advantage of the endocrine system over the nervous system is that it can instigate a much more diffuse response in multiple body tissues at about the same time and can therefore coordinate and integrate responses.

TABLE 3.1 Characteristics of the Nervous and Endocrine Systems

	Nervous System	Endocrine System
Source of signal	Brain	Endocrine glands or cells
Signal	Neurotransmitter and action potential	Hormone
Usual route	Efferent nerve	Blood
Response rate	Fast	Slow
Specificity	Specific	Diffuse
Target	Single	Multiple
Type of effect	Immediate effect	Long-term control and integration

Chapter Case Study

Zara is just 6 weeks' pregnant. She feels concerned about feeling increasingly nauseated, especially late in the evening; she vomited last night. Zara rings you, as her midwife, the next day expressing her concern, especially as her sister has told her that this is not the typical morning sickness of pregnancy.

- What explanations could you give Zara about the likely cause(s) of her nausea and what advice should you give to help her cope with her nausea?
- How is nausea and vomiting of pregnancy differentiated from hyperemesis gravidarum?
- What are the possible complications of hyperemesis gravidarum and what specific treatment is required to minimize complications?
- Later on in her pregnancy, Zara has a routine appointment at 26 weeks' gestation with her midwife who undertakes routine urinalysis and discovers that Zara has glucosuria.
- What are the possible causes for this, what further investigations need to be undertaken and what advice and treatment may be required?
- Can these findings be useful in predicting and preventing health complications later on in Zara's life?

WHAT IS ENDOCRINOLOGY?

The endocrine system was classically considered to be a relatively simple system of discrete glands (Fig. 3.1) that secreted chemical messengers, or hormones, into the blood where they were carried to specific target cells at a distant site, inducing a reaction. However, it is now clear that the endocrine system is more complex. Some hormones are secreted into ducts and not into blood; for instance, androgens are secreted into the seminiferous tubules. Some organs that have other functions also produce hormones. For example, the atrium of the heart produces atrial natriuretic peptide (ANP), which inhibits reabsorption of sodium chloride in the kidneys and hence affects blood pressure. Some hormones are produced by several different glands, for instance somatostatin, which is produced by the hypothalamus, pancreas, stomach and intestine. Although the trophoblast in early pregnancy is the prime site of human chorionic gonadotrophin (hCG) production, hCG can also be produced by other tissues, albeit in very low concentrations and can be used as a biomarker of pituitary disorders, ovarian cysts or cancers of the bladder or ovary (Duffy, 2013). The placenta appears to synthesize a very broad range of hormones and releasing factors that interact with both maternal and fetal physiology. Some

substances such as noradrenaline (norepinephrine) can act as both a hormone and a neurotransmitter, depending on their mode of delivery and whether they are released from a gland or as a neurotransmitter from neurons. The many functions of the hypothalamus include it serving as an interface between the endocrine and nervous systems, producing neurohormones important in this interaction. Finally, hormones are also produced by single cells, which are dispersed in body tissues such as the gut epithelium, rather than being integrated into discrete glands. Their existence as single dispersed cells has made their identification and isolation technically demanding and thus their functions much more difficult to study.

Overall, the endocrine system (in partnership with the nervous system) has numerous functions, for example it:

- coordinates homeostasis
- regulates various physiological systems that control essential body functions such as digestion, metabolism, reproduction, growth and feeding
- facilitates differentiation of the sexes at the embryonic stage and the manifestation of the secondary sexual characteristics at puberty
- modifies and induces behavioural changes within the individual
- prepares an organism to respond and react to changes within the external environment
- interacts with the immune system.

THE EVOLUTION OF ENDOCRINOLOGY

The evolution of the endocrine system has its origins within the activity of single-cell (unicellular) organisms. Although unicellular organisms did not require intercellular messengers, they developed the ability to sense the environment and to be attracted to chemicals, exhibiting a chemotactic response, or to chemicals that were vital for the functioning of the organism, exhibiting a chemotrophic response. Equally, these organisms developed the ability to recognize noxious chemicals (toxins) and were thus able to avoid them. The ability of unicellular organisms to react to chemical signals interacting with receptor sites on the cell membrane and within the cytoplasm led to the evolution of active cellular mobility.

As multicellular organisms evolved, the group of unicellular organisms that were the prototypes of multicellular organisms developed chemical communication as an extension of the chemotrophic response. As multicellular evolution progressed further, the cells became more differentiated and specialized. Regulation therefore became the function of more specialized types of cells. This is reflected in the developmental sequence of a fetus, beginning with the division of a single cell (see Chapter 7). With each successive division,

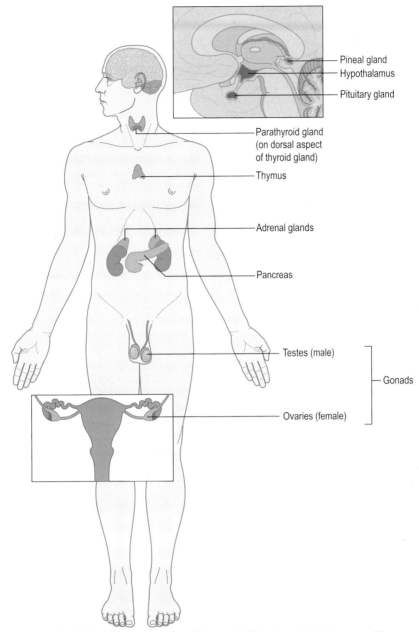

Fig. 3.1 The endocrine glands. (Reproduced from Soames R, Palastanga N: *Anatomy and human movement: structure and function*, 7 ed, Elsevier 2019, Fig. 4.119.)

the resulting cells are slightly different from the original fertilized egg or zygote. This process termed 'differentiation' begins during the early cell divisions of the embryo and is induced by the selective transfer of maternally derived factors from the cytoplasm of the zygote into daughter cells. Further differentiation as development continues is primarily under genetic control and is achieved through a process of induction from chemical signals produced by one cell type that influences the division and function of other neighbouring cells. The altered gene expression of the dividing cells results in a changed morphology and function as part of the developmental pathway.

As organisms became larger and more complex, cell-to-cell communication became more important and more complex. It evolved in three ways: the endocrine system (of chemical transmission via the circulating blood); the neural system (via transmission of an action potential; see Chapter 1); and the immune system (in which many aspects of signalling result from specific cell–cell contact; see Chapter 10). Under the traditional approach to biological science, the endocrine and neural systems were always considered in isolation; however, they are now considered to be extensions of the same system that are highly interactive. Many endocrine responses are initiated by a neural trigger. Many neurotransmitters and neuromodulators have also been found to be endocrine hormones.

CLASSIFICATION OF HORMONES

Hormones regulate metabolism, activate or inhibit the immune system, stimulate or inhibit growth, induce or suppress apoptosis (see below) and prepare the body to respond (such as fleeing or fighting) or undergo transition to a new stage of life such as puberty, pregnancy or menopause. Hormones are produced by almost every organ and type of tissue; they function as signals or messengers between cells. The action of hormones depends on the responses of the target cells and the pattern of hormonal secretion. Some hormones are circulated in the blood bound to a vehicle such as a binding protein; the ratio of the free (biologically active form) to the bound (inactive) hormone determines the amount of hormone available to act on the receptor. The effect of the hormone on its target cells will also depend on the extent of its degradation in the circulation or tissues; some hormones are rapidly broken down by enzymes and have particularly short half-lives.

Endocrine means 'secreted inwards' and is applied to hormones that fit the classical description of being synthesized and secreted from one organ into the bloodstream and having effects on distant target cells. There are also a small number of exocrine hormones, which are 'secreted outwards' into ducts. These include hormones that are secreted into the vas deferens and uterine tubes as well as pheromone secretion.

A number of hormones also have a local or paracrine effect, diffusing short distances to act on neighbouring cells or cells separated only by extracellular fluid. Paracrine hormones tend to have very short half-lives. Examples of paracrine responses are the effects of testosterone and anti-Müllerian hormone (AMH; also known as Müllerian-Inhibiting Hormone or Substance; MIH or MIS) on sexual differentiation (see Chapter 5). If the hormone produced acts upon the same cell that produced it, it is described as autocrine. For example, an autocrine hormone may induce cellular division or signal the process of programmed cell death (apoptosis). If it affects adjacent cells and has a very localized action, it is described as a 'juxtacrine' hormone. Therefore, the effect of a hormone depends on how and where it is secreted, the mode of transport (e.g. whether it is soluble or carried by a binding protein) and how quickly it is metabolized or inactivated.

Neuroendocrine hormones are synthesized in specialized neurons, and their effects can also be paracrine in nature (these are usually described as neurotransmitters and neuromodulators). Oxytocin is an example of a neuroendocrine hormone. It is released from the posterior lobe of the pituitary gland and stimulates contraction of the uterine myometrium (see Chapter 13) and myoepithelial cells in the breast (see Chapter 16). In these respects, oxytocin has an endocrine effect, but in many mammals it also has a neuroendocrine affect and modifies adult social behaviour by influencing maternal behaviour, social recognition and bonding, communication and aggression (Hammock, 2015). Oxytocin and antidiuretic hormone (ADH; also known as vasopressin) are both small (nine amino acid) polypeptide hormones, which are thought to influence the successful transition to parenthood and other aspects of human social behaviour such as social bonding, social recognition and communication (Hammock, 2015). Parental engagement may be expressed differently in the infant's parents; maternal behavioural changes tend to influence affectionate behaviour and emotional bonding and paternal parenting behaviour tends to affect play and social interaction with their infants. Furthermore, the infant's own production of oxytocin is affected by parental engagement. Both oxytocin and vasopressin affect infant brain development and have a long-term programming effect described as 'hormonal imprinting' (Hammock 2015). It is suggested that disruption of the early brain development and parent–infant engagement could have an impact on the risk of a wide range of conditions including mental illness (such as parental detachment disorder), depression and anxiety, eating disorders and possibly autism (Swain et al., 2014). The administration of oxytocin (or synthetic analogues) in labour and the peripartum period is common practice around the world to obstetrically manage clinical situations; it is used to induce and augment labour and to promote uterine contractions after delivery to control postpartum bleeding. Whilst the physiological advantages of these interventions have been widely researched and are clear, the possible psychological or neurological impact on both mother and baby have yet to be established.

A pheromone is a hormone or chemical signal secreted externally, that has evolved for communication with other members of the same species (Wyatt, 2015) and causes a change in behaviour or development. Pheromones are thought to be involved in a variety of phenomena such as identification of kin and gender, pair bonding, sexual attraction, parental attachment, marking territory and to assist in territorial defence. Pheromones elicit an innate and specific outcome, even under inappropriate circumstances; these responses are classified as releaser effects (stereotypical behaviour) or primer effects (developmental processes). Pheromones were originally identified in insects; there is some evidence that other mammals use pheromones but their existence and role in humans remains controversial. No single chemical nor combination of chemicals eliciting the outcomes expected of pheromones have been identified in humans. The putative pheromone or chemosensory receptor system, the vomeronasal organ located at the base of the nasal cavity, is vestigial in humans and appears not to have neural connections to the brain (Doty, 2014). In the 1970s, McClintock (1971) reported that the menstrual cycles of women living in close proximity became synchronized, a phenomenon referred to as 'Menstrual synchrony' or the 'McClintock effect'. This finding has been heavily criticized, however, particularly for methodological and statistical flaws (see a review by Harris and Vitzthum, 2013). The suckling and nipple-searching behaviour of infants in response to secretions from the Montgomery's glands of lactating women (see Chapter 16) is possibly a pheromone effect (Doucet et al., 2009).

Secretion of hormones is influenced by a number of factors, including the nervous system, hormone-binding proteins, plasma concentrations of nutrients and ions, environmental changes and other hormones, such as stimulating and releasing hormones.

Hormone Structure

Hormones can be classified according to their structure (Table 3.2). Steroid hormones and eicosanoids (the prostaglandin family of hormones) are lipids. The other classes are protein/ polypeptide hormones and hormones derived from amino acids.

Steroid Hormones

The steroid group of hormones consists of the sex steroids (progestagens, androgens and oestrogens), the glucocorticoids, mineralocorticoids and 1,25-dihydroxyvitamin D_3. Steroid hormones are derived from cholesterol, which is synthesized from acetate (Fig. 3.2). As well as being the

TABLE 3.2	Classification of Hormones and Examples	
Lipid hormones	Steroid hormones	Sex steroids, e.g. androgens, oestrogens and progestagens
		Glucocorticoids, e.g. cortisol
		Mineralocorticoids, e.g. aldosterone
		1,25-Dihydrovitamin D_3
	Eicosanoids	Prostaglandins (local hormones)
		Leukotrienes (local hormones)
Protein hormones	Gonadotrophic glycoproteins	Follicle-stimulating hormone (FSH)
		Luteinizing hormone (LH)
		Human chorionic gonadotrophin (hCG)
		Thyroid-stimulating hormone (TSH)
	Somatotrophic polypeptides	Prolactin (PRL)
		Human placental lactogen (hPL)
		Growth hormone (GH)
	Cytokines	Activins and inhibins
		Anti-Müllerian hormone (AMH)
		Interferons
		Growth factors
Small peptides		Gonadotrophin-releasing hormone (GnRH)
		Oxytocin (OXY)
		Antidiuretic hormone (ADH or vasopressin)
		β-Endorphin
		Vasoactive intestinal peptide (VIP)
Amino acid derived	Catecholamines	Adrenaline, noradrenaline and dopamine
		Melatonin
		Thyroid hormones (T_3 and T_4)

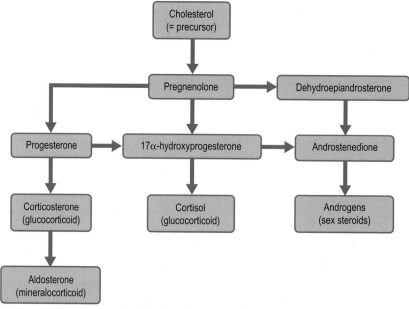

Fig. 3.2 Steroid hormone production.

precursor for the steroid hormones, cholesterol is also an important structural component of cell membranes where it regulates membrane fluidity.

The first and common step in the biosynthesis of sex steroids is the formation of pregnenolone, which is rate-limiting, and therefore important in controlling production of sex steroids. Pregnenolone is produced on the inner mitochondrial membrane whereas subsequent steps in steroid synthesis take place in the smooth endoplasmic reticulum (SER).

The three classes of sex steroids are structurally related, which provides the opportunity for interconversion. This means that a genetic defect in one of the steps can result not only in a deficiency in the normal amount of the product but also in an excess of another sex steroid. For example, a genetic deficiency of the enzyme that converts 17α-hydroxyprogesterone to the precursor of cortisol results in increased levels of 17α-hydroxyprogesterone, which is converted into androstenedione and then into androgens. Such unusually high levels of androgens can cause masculinization of the female fetus. These structural similarities mean that the steroid hormones can affect the activity of other steroid hormones by exerting agonistic and antagonistic effects at the receptor level. However, the effects of the hormones vary depending on their structure (Table 3.3).

The main role of androgens is in the development and maintenance of masculine characteristics and fertility.

Similarly, the dominant role of oestrogens is in development and maintenance of feminine characteristics and fertility. The key role for progesterone is the preparation for, and maintenance of, pregnancy. However, all of the steroid hormones are produced in men and women but with varying profiles; therefore, for instance, men produce more androgens than women but also produce some oestrogen. Although androgens are primarily associated with the development and maintenance of male sex characteristics, they also affect sexual behaviour and motivation (libido) in women (Johnson, 2018).

As steroid hormones are lipid-soluble, they are able to diffuse freely across the cell membrane and have their effect on their specific receptors within the target cell. After entering the cytoplasm, steroid hormones may also be chemically modified. The receptors for thyroid hormones are also located within the nucleus or cytoplasm of target cells. Thyroid hormones are not lipid-soluble and are transported into target cells by a family of iodothyronine transporters, before binding to their receptors to regulate gene expression. The receptors for steroid hormones are also either located within the nucleus or bind to their agonist in the cytosol before the steroid-receptor complex moves into the nucleus. Binding usually results in cleavage of smaller 'heat-shock' proteins from the receptors. Steroid hormones exert their effect by altering gene expression, RNA synthesis and subsequent protein synthesis (Box 3.1). The steroid-receptor complex binds to specific segments of

TABLE 3.3 Biological Activity and Effects of the Sex Steroids

Sex Steroid	Family Members (and Approximate Biological Activity)	Main Effects
Androgens	5α-dihydrotestosterone (100%) Testosterone (50%) Androstenedione (8%) Dehydroepiandrosterone (4%)	Differentiation of male embryo Secondary sex characteristics Spermatogenesis Male secondary sex characteristics Sexual and aggressive behaviour Growth promoting, protein anabolism, ossification and erythropoiesis Regulation of testosterone secretion Anticorticosteroid effects (DHEA)
Oestrogens	Oestradiol-17β (E_2) (100%) Oestriol (E_3) (10%) Oestrone (E_1) (1%)	Female secondary sex characteristics Prepares uterus for reception of sperm, ovulation and fertilization Vascular effects – increased blood flow, neovascularization Growth-promoting effects on endometrium and breasts Primes endometrium for progesterone action Mildly anabolic Increases calcification of bones May be associated with sexual behaviour
Progestagens	Progesterone (100%) 17α-hydroxyprogesterone (17α-OHP) (40–70%) 20α-hydroxyprogesterone (5%)	Prepares uterus for pregnancy Maintains pregnancy Stimulates glandular growth of breasts (but suppresses milk secretion) Affects sodium and water excretion Mildly catabolic Relaxes smooth muscle tone Affects appetite and thirst, metabolic rate, sensitivity to carbon dioxide

Modified from Johnson, 2018.

BOX 3.1 Action of Steroid Hormones

- Transported in plasma bound to binding protein
- Hormone released and diffuses into target cell
- Hormone diffuses into nucleus
- Hormone binds to a specific receptor either located in the nucleus or within the cytosol before movement of the hormone-receptor complex into the nucleus
- Affects DNA transcription
- Affects mRNA synthesis
- Affects protein synthesis
- Altered functional response of cell

DNA, called steroid response elements (SRE) in the promoter regions of target genes, affecting the rate of transcription and gene expression. Protein synthesis can be increased (or decreased) on a timescale of 30 min to days,

and the effects of steroid hormones are therefore relatively slow compared with those of protein and amino acid-based hormones. The term 'anabolic steroids' describes the effect of steroid hormones in influencing tissue growth

The other class of compounds sometimes described as lipid hormones is the eicosanoids (prostaglandins, thromboxanes and leukotrienes), which have an important role in reproduction. Eicosanoids are formed from the polyunsaturated fatty acid, arachidonic acid, which is generated by the activity of either phospholipase C and diacylglycerol lipase or phospholipase A_2 (Fig. 3.3). Arachidonic acid production appears to be the rate-limiting step. Most tissues of the body synthesize prostaglandins, including the myometrium, cervix, ovary, placenta, fetal membranes and prostate. Eicosanoids have local paracrine actions, rather than being secreted by glands into the bloodstream, so are strictly speaking 'local hormones' acting on the same tissue that secretes them. They have a short half-life

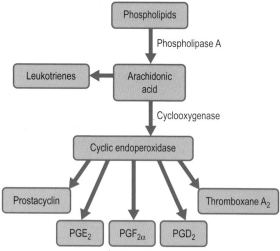

Fig. 3.3 Formation of eicosanoids.

and are metabolized quickly. Cyclooxygenases (COX-1 and COX-2) catalyse the production of prostaglandins by sequential oxidation of lipid precursors. COX-1 maintains baseline prostaglandin levels, whereas levels are increased by COX-2 during inflammation, pain and fever. Nonsteroidal anti-inflammatory drugs (NSAIDs) such as aspirin inhibit cyclooxygenase and are used clinically to reduce pain and inflammation whereas selective COX-2 inhibitors have been developed to avoid the gastrointestinal side-effects of nonselective COX-1 and COX-2 inhibition. Prostaglandins have an important role in amplifying signals at the onset of labour and can prevent closure of the ductus arteriosus, a shunt present in fetal life between the aorta and the pulmonary artery to bypass the nonfunctional lungs. Synthetic prostaglandins can be used clinically to trigger parturition and also to prevent closure of ductus arteriosus in newborns with certain cyanotic heart defects (see Chapter 13).

Leukotrienes are also synthesized from arachidonic acid by the enzyme 5-lipoxygenase in leukocytes and macrophages. They are involved in inflammatory reactions particularly in asthma and allergy and also seem to be important in pregnancy.

Protein, Peptide and Amino Acid-derived Hormones

These hormones are hydrophilic, polar molecules, which are membrane-impermeable and produce their biological effects by binding to specific receptors on the outer surface of target cells. They initiate a variety of cellular responses including plasma membrane depolarization, generation of second-messengers inside the target cell and protein phosphorylation, which regulate cellular activities with a faster

time-course than steroid hormones. These hormones have both stimulatory and inhibitory effects upon their target cells and often act via one of a large family of G-protein coupled receptors (GPCRs), which initiate various chemical reactions (Box 3.2). GPCRs can generate intracellular signals (second-messengers) such as cyclic adenosine monophosphate (cAMP) or a rise in intracellular calcium ion (Ca^{2+}) concentration and may also open ion-selective channels in cell membranes. These differences in the signalling pathways that are activated differ with the class of G-proteins with which the GPCR interacts. $G_\alpha s$ activates the enzyme adenylyl cyclase to generate the intracellular signalling molecule cAMP from ATP, whereas the $G_\alpha q$ G-proteins are linked to the activations of phospholipase Cβ (PLCβ), which generates the intracellular signal inositol trisphosphate (IP_3) from phospholipids in the inner leaflet of the membrane bilayer. IP_3 triggers the release of Ca^{2+} ions from their storage site in the endoplasmic or sarcoplasmic reticulum so that cytosolic Ca^{2+} ion concentrations ($[Ca^{2+}]$) are increased. These intracellular signals (second-messengers) stimulate different classes of protein kinase enzymes to phosphorylate (attach phosphate groups to) specific intracellular proteins. Attachment of a phosphate group alters the structure and therefore the activity of proteins, which control target cell function. Often, one protein kinase will activate a second protein kinase and so on, generating a signalling cascade, which ultimately results in thousands of target molecules becoming activated in response to a single hormone binding to a single receptor protein. Many amino acid-derived hormones (derivatives of tryptophan or tyrosine) also function as neurotransmitters in the brain.

Gonadotrophic Glycoproteins

This group includes thyroid-stimulating hormone (TSH), follicle-stimulating hormone (FSH), luteinizing hormone (LH) and hCG, all of which are structurally similar. Their structure is a globular protein, which is a heterodimer formed from two polypeptide chains; an alpha subunit, which is identical in all these hormones; and a unique beta subunit. The beta subunit has unique carbohydrate side-chains that bestow stability and biological activity. hCG is produced by placental tissue (the cytotrophoblasts produce the alpha subunit and the syncytiotrophoblast produces the beta subunit), whereas the other gonadotrophic glycoproteins are produced by the anterior pituitary gland.

Somatomammotrophic Polypeptides

This group of hormones includes prolactin (PRL), human placental lactogen (hPL; also known as human placental somatomammotrophin) and growth hormone (GH; also known as somatotrophin), which has marked effects on tissue growth. These hormones have a single polypeptide chain. PRL and hPL are involved in lactation whereas GH has a role in puberty including breast development. Although PRL and GH are pituitary hormones, the placenta also produces them in addition to hPL during pregnancy. However, the activity of the placental hormones is often not exactly the same as that of the pituitary hormones. For instance, placental GH has a higher affinity than pituitary GH has for the PRL receptor. The somatomammotrophic polypeptide hormones affect growth, including angiogenesis, functioning of the immune system and metabolism.

Cytokines

Cytokines are small polypeptides and comprise a large group of signalling molecules, which includes inhibin, activin, epidermal growth factors and AMH (see Chapters 5, 13; Box 3.3). Cytokines have a broad range of activities. They are synthesized in a variety of cell types rather than in a specific gland. Cytokines also act on many different cell types, often interacting with and modulating each other's responses. Several cytokines have similar and overlapping functions. Like eicosanoids, they usually have paracrine effects on nearby cells, and often modulate or mediate the actions of other types of hormone. Cytokines act by binding to their specific receptors on the target cell membrane; typically, these receptors are also tyrosine kinase (enzymes that catalyse the addition of a phosphate group to a tyrosine residue of a target protein or the receptor itself (autophosphorylation), which modifies its own activity and, in turn, regulates the activity of other enzymes).

Polypeptide Hormones

This group of hormones includes gonadotrophin-releasing hormone (GnRH), a decapeptide (i.e. a chain of 10 amino acids) from the hypothalamus, and other releasing hormones, oxytocin, ADH (also known as vasopressin), β-endorphin (described in Chapter 13) and vasoactive intestinal peptide (VIP). Most of these small polypeptide

---

BOX 3.3 Anti-Müllerian Hormone

A good example of the range of activity demonstrated by cytokines is AMH, which has long been known for its role in promoting regression of the Müllerian ducts in the male embryo (see Chapter 5). The female embryo does not produce AMH, so the Müllerian ducts develop into female internal genitalia. AMH is secreted from the Sertoli cells of the testes and continues to be produced in male children but declines throughout adulthood. Women produce AMH from the granulosa cells of the ovary, from puberty onwards; the role of AMH in the ovary is to limit excessive follicular recruitment by FSH, so it controls the number of primary follicles formed. It seems that puberty is preceded by a rise in AMH in girls and by a fall in AMH in boys. The changing levels of AMH also affect brain development via AMH receptors and are thought to mediate gender-specific behaviour. AMH is not present in the ovary after menopause. In women, AMH seems to be one of the best markers for ovarian reserve (the number of remaining follicles in the ovaries) and can be used to predict menopause and also the likely effectiveness of assisted reproductive technologies (Pilsgaard et al., 2018).

Recombinant human (synthetic) AMH analogues are emerging as potential therapy for a broad range of applications, including reversible nonsteroidal contraception, chemoprotection for preserving fertility in women receiving treatment for cancer, delaying menopause and treatment of polycystic ovarian syndrome and several cancers related to the reproductive system (Kushnir et al., 2017).

---

hormones are initially produced in the form of pre-prohormones (large inactive polypeptide precursors). The 'pre' sequence of the polypeptide hormone is involved in targeting the molecule to a particular biosynthetic route and is processed in the endoplasmic reticulum to form a prohormone. The processing may involve glycosylation (addition of carbohydrate groups) or removal of the N-terminal signal sequence. Prohormones often contain redundant sequences of amino acids required to direct the folding of the molecule into its active configuration before the 'pro' amino acid sequence is released by endopeptidases to form the active hormone. These connecting peptide sequences may have no further function and the active hormone is typically stored in membrane-bound secretory vesicles until a signal is received to trigger hormone release. Some of the 'pro'-fragments of the prohormones also exert a biological effect. The identification of secondary sites of hormone production, such as GnRH being produced in the placenta and ovary and oxytocin being produced in the testes and uterus, suggests that these small peptide hormones have diverse roles and may also function as neurotransmitters (Johnson, 2018).

Amino Acid-derived Hormones

This group includes catecholamines (dopamine, adrenaline and noradrenaline) and melatonin, all of which are derived from tyrosine (an amino acid) and may have a role in neuroendocrine control mechanisms. The medulla of the adrenal gland is a modified sympathetic ganglion; its cell bodies release adrenaline and noradrenaline (in the ratio 4:1) into the blood. Its effects, therefore, augment sympathetic nervous system activity. Dopamine is synthesized from tyrosine and then can be sequentially modified to form noradrenaline and then adrenaline. Dopamine released from the hypothalamus affects prolactin secretion (see Chapter 16). Melatonin, from the pineal gland, may have a role in seasonal and environmental influences on reproductive behaviour, particularly important in species other than humans, where breeding is dependent upon day length.

HORMONE TRANSPORT

Peptide, protein and amino acid-derived hormones are water-soluble and are delivered to target cells dissolved in the blood, whereas steroid hormones circulate bound to plasma proteins. When hormones are secreted into the blood supply, a large proportion become protein-bound, leaving only a small proportion free (unbound and able to access the target cell) and physiologically active. There are many types of hormone-binding proteins, all of which are colloidal in nature. Some hormones bind with great affinity to specific proteins. Other proteins may bind to numerous different hormones with different affinities that may be affected by the concentration of the hormone. Therefore, the amount of hormone present may affect its activity. For instance, oxytocin at high concentrations binds to ADH (vasopressin) receptors within the renal tubule. During labour, levels of oxytocin do not normally rise until the end of the first stage. However, exogenous oxytocin can be administered to augment uterine contractions. If the administration of oxytocin is high and prolonged, however, water retention can occur because oxytocin also stimulates ADH receptors in the kidney. This overlap in the biological activity of hormones is described as promiscuity.

HORMONAL REGULATION

One of the most important functions of the endocrine system is maintenance of the internal environment. This 'steady' state is described as homeostasis (see Chapter 1).

Homeostatic mechanisms buffer the effects of changes in both internal and external environmental conditions. Mammals have evolved to be homeothermic (warm-blooded) so that the chemical processes essential for physiological function proceed under optimal conditions of temperature. Fluctuations in temperature are monitored and the homeostatic mechanisms ensure that body temperature is held within a narrow range. Homeostasis is achieved through the integration of the nervous system with the endocrine system and these usually function as negative-feedback systems.

As mentioned above, hormonal release is often instigated by neurological stimulation. However, hormone release may also be stimulated by another hormone referred to as a trophic hormone, since it acts indirectly (via the second hormone) on the final target cell. The negative feedback tends to slow down a process and maintain homeostasis (stability), whereas positive feedback tends to speed up a process and generate rapid change.

Positive Feedback (or Feed-Forward)

Positive feedback describes a specialized chain of events involving one or more hormones in which there is a cycle of positive effects, greatly amplifying the original signal (Fig. 3.4). An example of positive feedback is the maintained production of PRL secretion from the anterior pituitary gland during lactation. Suckling of the infant stimulates PRL secretion, which maintains lactation. If suckling decreases or stops, then the amount of stimulation decreases and PRL production is reduced. PRL production is reduced and milk production for breastfeeding stops. This positive feedback is optimized by initiating feeding within an hour of birth and promoting demand feeding. Other examples of positive feedback include

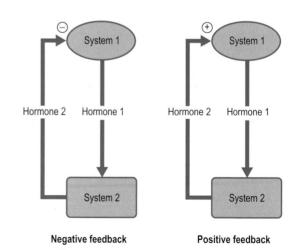

Fig. 3.4 Negative and positive feedback.

coagulation of blood and several aspects of the hormonal control of parturition. For example, corticotrophin-releasing hormone (CRH), released from the hypothalamus, stimulates the release of adrenocorticotrophic hormone (ACTH) from the pituitary, which, in turn, triggers cortisol release from the adrenal cortex. Together, these hormones comprise the hypothalamic–pituitary–adrenal (HPA) axis response to stress. To keep this response within limits, cortisol feeds back to negatively affect both CRH and ACTH secretion to maintain its own levels within an appropriate range. Trophoblastic, decidual and fetal membranes however, secrete increasing amounts of CRH as pregnancy proceeds but the negative feedback effect of cortisol is not seen with placental CRH secretion. Instead, increasing cortisol levels further increase placental CRH secretion in a positive feed-forward loop to drive the late stages of pregnancy leading to parturition as well as placental CRH stimulating the maternal HPA axis (Vannuccini et al., 2016) (see Chapter 13).

Negative Feedback

Negative feedback describes a similar specialized chain of events involving one or more hormones, except that here there is a cycle of negative influence (Fig. 3.4). An example of negative feedback is that the anterior lobe of the pituitary gland produces TSH, which stimulates the thyroid gland to produce thyroid hormone. TSH production is, however, inhibited by the presence of thyroid hormone, reducing the further production of thyroid hormones and setting an upper limit on their levels in plasma.

Activation and Deactivation

Hormone secretion may be triggered by the presence of a certain stimulus. For example, insulin release from pancreatic β-cells is increased by a rise in plasma glucose levels following carbohydrate consumption. Many specific metabolic pathways are activated by the build-up of specific metabolites within the internal environment. Similarly, secretion of some hormones may be inhibited by the presence of a signal. This may be another hormone, such as adrenaline, neural stimuli such as light stimulation inhibiting melatonin release from the pineal gland, or chemical, such as insulin inhibiting the release of glucagon. Labour is often observed, in humans and most mammals, to be suppressed if females are exposed to stressful situations resulting in high levels of adrenaline. This may underpin the finding that many alternative therapies used in labour may benefit women as they promote relaxation and calmness.

HORMONE ACTION

Hormones have their effects by interacting with a specific receptor. The hormone (or 'ligand') binds specifically to the receptor so that the two fit together in a way which is often described as analogous to 'a lock and key'. The interaction of the hormone and its receptor triggers intracellular signalling pathways resulting in the hormone-induced change in target cell function. The effects of hormones depend on a number of factors including affinity of the hormone for the receptor, effects of agonists or antagonists and receptor number and hormone levels. Receptor number is important in the selection of the dominant follicle (see Chapter 4) and the increased sensitivity of the uterus to oxytocin in early labour where receptor numbers are increased (see Chapter 13). A lack of receptor expression can cause abnormal development, such as testicular feminization in the absence of androgen receptors (see Chapter 5). Genetic variations in the structure of receptors, for instance caused by single nucleotide polymorphisms (where a single base change in a gene causes a single amino acid change in the receptor protein), can influence the binding of the hormone to its receptor and affect an individual's sensitivity and responses to the hormone (Johnson, 2018). Hormone levels are also affected by local circulation, stability, metabolism and excretion. An example of this is Sheehan syndrome, which manifests after severe and prolonged hypovolaemic shock resulting in the destruction of the anterior pituitary gland. Early signs are failure to establish lactation, later signs include amenorrhoea and lethargy (due to reduction in thyroid activity and body atrophy). If not recognized this condition is potentially fatal. Many hormones are inactivated within the blood, liver and by their specific target cells. The breakdown of hormones is achieved by the action of various enzymes.

Many hormones show temporal patterns of secretion. For instance, secretion of testosterone and prolactin exhibit circadian rhythms (characteristic patterns of change during a 24-h period), whereas GnRH, FSH, LH and PRL are released in a pulsatile fashion (in regular bursts). A continuous infusion of these hormones would diminish their effects on target tissues since the constant occupancy of the receptors can uncouple them from their second-messenger system or result in a decrease in receptor number (down-regulation), effectively reducing the ability of the cell to respond (an example of this is the use of an oxytocin infusion to augment labour occupying ADH receptors in high doses and in prolonged situations). A high blood flow increases dissipation of hormones and is likely to increase a systemic endocrine response but decrease paracrine responses.

Levels and metabolism of binding proteins will also affect the activity of hormones. The protein-bound hormone complex renders the bound hormone inactive but also protects the hormone from enzymatic degradation and, in some cases, is involved in the interactions of hormones with their target receptors. Hormone turnover may be affected by multiple sites of production. Different tissues may have different feedback mechanisms controlling hormone production. Replication of hormone production occurs physiologically during pregnancy when placental cells also secrete a range of hormones, but also pathologically from tumours. Hormones and their metabolites may be excreted via the kidney during the formation of urine. As the rate of excretion of many hormones is proportional to their concentration in plasma and therefore their rate of secretion, excretion rate in urine can be used as an indicator of secretion rate. Generally, peptide hormones are readily metabolized either by enzymes in blood or liver and are easily excreted, so their half-life in the blood is short compared with that of protein-bound steroid hormones.

Levels of hormones may change within the tissues themselves, as hormones can be converted to a form with a higher biological activity. For instance, the enzyme 5α-reductase in many of the target tissues for testosterone converts testosterone to 5α-dihydrotestosterone, which has twice the biological activity. A deficiency of this enzyme can cause poor development of the male external genitalia (Box 3.4). Also, the target cell may metabolize a hormone, for example, some peptide hormone/receptor complexes are endocytosed so that the hormone is broken down and the receptor is recycled.

Agonist and Antagonist Effects

An agonist is a ligand or substance that binds to a receptor on the cell membrane or within the cytoplasm or nucleus of the target cell to trigger a response. An antagonist also binds to the receptor often partially and does not therefore activate it, thus blocking or inhibiting both the binding of the agonist and the physiological response. By occupying the receptor site, a competitive antagonist blocks the action of the specific hormone (agonist) that normally binds to the site; antagonists can also be noncompetitive. A partial agonist activates a receptor to a lesser degree and elicits a smaller physiological response. The physiological overlap of oxytocin and ADH is an example of an agonist effect. The molecular structures of oxytocin and ADH are similar. Oxytocin can elicit the same biological response as ADH because it can bind to the same receptor sites. Therefore, oxytocin is agonistic to the ADH receptor and may be described as an ADH agonist. Also, progesterone acts as a glucocorticoid receptor agonist with effects on metabolism (see Chapter 11).

Many natural and environmental chemicals can mimic the effects of hormones and act as antagonists or agonists. These are detailed in Box 3.5.

BOX 3.4   5α-Reductase Deficiency

In the Dominican Republic, there is an increased incidence of an autosomal recessive condition resulting in 5α-reductase deficiency, which creates some interesting and challenging ethical issues (Byers et al., 2017). 5α-Reductase is the enzyme that converts testosterone to the more biologically active 5α-dihydrotestosterone within the target cell. The lack of enzyme means that there is a diminished response to testosterone during fetal sexual development (see Chapter 5), so an affected baby may have small and ambiguous genitalia, appearing female at birth (testicular feminization). However, at puberty the surge in testosterone production is adequate to stimulate the cells; therefore, the child then develops male external genitalia. This condition is known as 'Guevedoces'.

BOX 3.5   Environmental Influences on Hormonal Expression

A number of environmental chemicals, such as phthalates (plasticizers) and polychlorinated biphenyls (PCBs), exert hormone-like effects. The chemicals may mimic or antagonize endogenous hormones, disrupt synthesis and metabolism of endogenous hormones and/or affect receptor expression. These oestrogenic contaminants were initially linked to abnormal sexual development in wild animals and fish but effects on humans, such as reproductive abnormalities in male fetuses and effects on male fertility, are also under investigation. The pesticide DDT has been associated with reduced sperm counts and decreased libido. Chemicals used in plastics have been demonstrated to have oestrogenic properties. Degradation of alkylphenols used in detergents releases oestrogenic compounds. These environmental chemicals have been implicated in the increased incidence of testicular cancer, hypospadias (incomplete fusion of the urogenital folds of the penis), cryptorchidism (undescended testicles), breast cancer and endometriosis. It has also been suggested that fetal development, particularly of reproductive organs, may be affected by exposure to these compounds. The protective effect of phytoestrogens may be related to interaction with environmental contaminants. Phytoestrogens, such as genistein from soy protein, may affect the length of the menstrual cycle and have similar protective effects on cardiovascular health and bone mineralization as endogenous oestrogen.

ENDOCRINE GLANDS, HORMONES AND REPRODUCTION

Hormones can influence the ability of the target cell to respond by regulating the number of hormone receptors. Prolonged exposure to a low concentration of hormone may increase the number of receptors expressed by the cell (described as 'up-regulation'). Conversely, prolonged exposure to a high concentration of hormone might decrease the number of receptors for that hormone (described as 'down-regulation'). For example, the expression of oxytocin receptors is down-regulated on prolonged exposure to oxytocin; this may explain the lack of response to exogenous oxytocin in induction of labour (see Chapter 13). If labour is established, ongoing administration of oxytocin is required; often in prolonged labour, increasing doses are also required to achieve and maintain effective uterine contractions. Initial high doses of oxytocin can stimulate prolonged, intense uterine contractions, which can be potentially harmful to the fetus. Therefore, oxytocin infusions are gradually titrated against the manifestation of effective regular contractions balanced against the manifestation of signs of fetal distress throughout the augmentation of labour. Hormones can also affect receptors for other hormones, increasing or decreasing their effectiveness. When one hormone must be present for another to have its full effect, it is described as permissive.

The endocrine glands and their main functions are summarized in Table 3.4.

TABLE 3.4 The Endocrine System

Endocrine Gland	Main Function(s)
Hypothalamus	Regulates homeostasis Controls pituitary function Integrates nervous and endocrine systems Regulation of food intake and body weight homeostasis Produces antidiuretic hormone and oxytocin for release by pituitary Produces releasing hormones to act on pituitary
Pituitary	'Master gland' Stimulates other endocrine glands
Pineal body	Produces melatonin during nocturnal period Involved in biological rhythms and body 'clock'
Thyroid	Affects metabolism and growth
Parathyroid glands	Maintenance of calcium homeostasis
Thymus	Produces hormones that control T-cell development and function

Adrenal glands	Medulla:
	    Secretion of catecholamines (adrenaline and noradrenaline)
	Cortex:
	    Secretion of corticosteroids
	    • glucocorticoids affect metabolism and responses to stress
	    • mineralocorticoids affect electrolyte and fluid homeostasis
	Sex steroids

Pancreas	Insulin and glucagon control plasma glucose levels. Insulin controls glucose uptake and the metabolism of glucose, proteins and fat. Somatostatin: growth hormone-inhibiting hormone
Gonads (testes or ovaries)	Produce sex steroids that affect reproductive cycles and gamete formation
Kidney	Produces erythropoietin, which regulates erythrocyte production released by fetal liver and adult bone marrow
Heart	Atrial natriuretic peptide lowers blood pressure
Adipose tissue	Secretes leptin, which suppresses long-term appetite Secretes cytokines (adipokines), e.g. adiponectin Affects steroid hormone metabolism

The Pituitary Gland

The pituitary gland is a pea-sized gland at the base of the brain, which is connected to the hypothalamus via the tuberoinfundibular pathway. It is often described as a 'master' gland since it secretes hormones, which regulate a broad range of body activities. These include both trophic hormones, which regulate the secretion of a second hormone from endocrine glands to bring about the final effects on the target tissue and nontrophic hormones, which act directly on target tissues. The pituitary gland has two main lobes, the anterior lobe (or adenohypophysis) and the posterior lobe (or neurohypophysis) (Fig. 3.5). The anterior lobe originates from the primitive oral cavity, whereas the posterior lobe is a projection of the hypothalamus. The anterior lobe produces hormones such as LH and FSH that regulate gametogenesis and act trophically to stimulate steroidogenesis by the gonads (see Chapter 4). Exogenous administration of LH and FSH can be used artificially to mimic the reproductive cycle in assisted reproductive technology (ART) to promote and increase the number of viable oocytes. The maintenance of lactation is achieved through the production of PRL, which acts directly (nontrophically) on the breast (see Chapter 16). The anterior lobe also produces TSH, GH, ACTH and endorphins. GH is unique amongst pituitary hormones in having both trophic effects (via stimulating

insulin-like growth factor secretion) and having direct (nontrophic) effects on tissues including adipose tissue. The posterior lobe of the pituitary gland does not produce hormones but stores and secretes the hormones oxytocin and ADH (vasopressin), which are produced in neurons, which originate in the hypothalamus and are released by the posterior pituitary. The tiny intermediate lobe of the human pituitary gland, which is almost indistinguishable from the anterior pituitary, produces melanocyte-stimulating hormone (MSH).

The Thyroid Gland

The thyroid gland is butterfly-shaped and is the largest endocrine gland. It lies in front of the trachea, posterior to the larynx, and produces thyroid hormones. Thyroid hormones affect all tissues in the body and regulate metabolic rate, growth, brain development and function. The thyroid hormones, which contain iodide, are thyroxine (T_4), which is circulated and converted to the active form, triiodothyronine (T_3), within the target tissues. Essentially T_4 is the prohormone and T_3 is 5–10 times more active than T_4. More than 99% of circulating T_4 and T_3 are bound to binding proteins in the blood. During pregnancy, the fetus initially utilizes maternally derived thyroxine, so the maternal thyroid gland increases in size (hypertrophy) to compensate

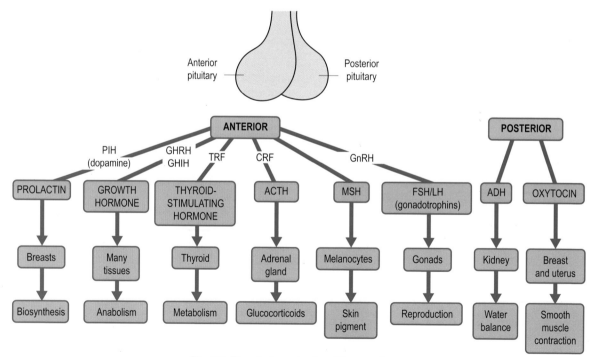

Fig. 3.5 The pituitary gland and its secretions.

for this (referred to as the goitre of pregnancy). This is achieved by the thyrotrophic effect of hCG and a placentally derived hormone called 'human chorionic thyrotrophin'. Thyroid hormones are essential for development and maturation of the fetal brain. Low levels of thyroid hormones may result in congenital hypothyroidism, which requires clinical intervention in the neonatal period to prevent irreversible neurological damage. Maternal thyroid gland activity is stimulated by oestrogens and hCG and these changes contribute to optimizing glucose provision for the fetus (see Chapter 11). The increase in thyroid activity increases the basal metabolic rate of the pregnant woman, resulting in an increase of maternal and fetal oxygen consumption (see Chapter 11). The parafollicular cells of the thyroid gland produce calcitonin, which is involved in the metabolism of calcium and phosphorus, in response to hypercalcaemia (high levels of calcium in the blood). Calcitonin promotes the uptake of calcium by bone; levels increase in pregnancy and it is suggested that this may protect the maternal skeleton from excessive bone resorption. Hyperthyroidism is an overactive thyroid gland and hypothyroidism is an underactive thyroid gland; both conditions can affect fertility and treatment of either condition can be affected by pregnancy. Thyroid conditions need careful monitoring during pregnancy as drug requirements may change as pregnancy progresses. 'Euthyroidism' is the term used to describe a normally functioning thyroid gland.

The Parathyroid Glands

Humans have four tiny (3–4 mm) parathyroid glands, closely associated with the thyroid gland, that produce parathyroid hormone to maintain calcium homeostasis. Parathyroid hormone (PTH) levels increase in response to a fall in serum calcium; it causes a decrease in urinary calcium excretion, increased mobilization of calcium from bone and, indirectly (via an increase in vitamin D), causes an increase in calcium absorption in the gut. Although parathyroid hormone is the primary regulator of 1,25-dihydroxyvitamin D synthesis in the nonpregnant state, it may not be important in pregnancy as levels do not change much in pregnancy, and women without functioning parathyroid glands still have a raised level of circulating 1,25-dihydroxyvitamin D during pregnancy (Fig. 3.6). As seen with other 'paired' hormone responses, the opposing effects of PTH and calcitonin work together to maintain plasma calcium levels within the normal physiological range.

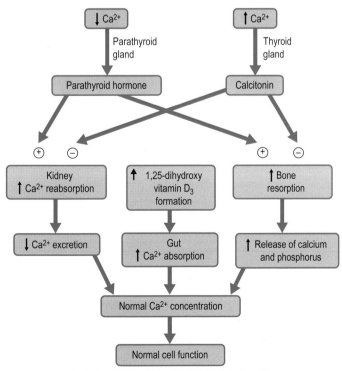

Fig. 3.6 Maintenance of calcium homeostasis.

The Adrenal Glands

The adrenal glands are triangle-shaped glands situated on top of the kidneys that regulate the response to stress by synthesizing corticosteroids from the cortex (outer layers) of the gland and catecholamines from the medulla (central region) of the gland. Glucocorticoids, such as corticosterone and cortisol, are involved in the regulation of carbohydrate metabolism, the body's responses to stress and the regulation of the immune system. Carbohydrate metabolism is altered during pregnancy but it would appear that the fetal–maternal interaction relating to carbohydrate metabolism is mediated through the action of other hormones (see Chapter 11). CRH from the hypothalamus controls the release of ACTH from the anterior pituitary gland, which regulates the production of hormones from the adrenal cortex; this is described as the hypothalamic–pituitary–adrenal (HPA) axis. During pregnancy, ACTH levels double and cortisol levels increase. The adrenal glands also produce steroid hormones and mineralocorticoids such as aldosterone, which are principally involved in the regulation of the electrolyte balance of the body (see Chapter 2). Aldosterone levels increase in pregnancy as a response to increased renin and angiotensin II levels.

The Gonads

The gonads are responsible for the production of the sex steroids. In men, the testes predominantly produce testosterone. In women, the ovaries produce oestrogens and progesterone. The endocrine cells of the gonads lack the enzymes to produce mineralocorticoids and glucocorticoids. (The gonadal function of the regulation of reproduction is discussed in Chapter 4.)

FETAL ENDOCRINOLOGY

Many of the endocrine and metabolic changes of pregnancy are results of hormonal signals originating from the fetal–placental unit (FPU), which is a major site of protein and steroid hormone production and secretion. The interactions of neuronal and hormonal factors mediated by the FPU are critical in directing the initiation and maintenance of pregnancy, maternal adaptations to pregnancy, fetal growth and development, coordination of the timing of parturition and preparation for lactation. Production of oestradiol involves cooperation between the maternal and fetoplacental systems (see Chapter 11). The fetal endocrine system is also involved in the differentiation and development of the sexes (see Chapter 5).

KEY POINTS

- The endocrine system and the nervous system interact and are involved in communication and maintenance of the internal environment.
- The classic description of a hormone as a substance released from a gland and transported in the blood to its target organ(s) cannot be applied to all hormones.
- Hormones can be classified structurally as amino acid-derived, protein/polypeptide or lipid hormones.
- The major group of lipid hormones, steroid hormones, are produced from cholesterol precursors and include mineralocorticoids (such as aldosterone), glucocorticoids (such as cortisol) and sex steroids (oestrogen, progesterone and testosterone).

- Steroid hormones circulate bound to plasma proteins and exert their effect by binding to intracellular receptors to alter gene expression and protein synthesis in their target cells.
- Peptide hormones and catecholamines circulate in the plasma and act via plasma membrane receptors and signal transduction pathways in their target cells.
- Hormonal effects are modulated by binding proteins, receptor expression, hormone metabolism and agonist–antagonist effects.
- Testosterone and oestrogen are responsible for the development and maintenance of sexual characteristics and fertility. Progesterone is involved in preparation for and maintenance of pregnancy.

APPLICATION TO PRACTICE

During pregnancy, apart from the growth of the fetus, there is also increased maternal tissue growth and development that is controlled by the action of hormonal changes within the maternal system and interactions with hormones produced by the fetal–placental complex.

Throughout the entire antenatal, perinatal and postnatal periods, the midwife should be able to observe these physiological changes and use them to form an assessment of the progression and wellbeing of the pregnant woman and fetus.

Some conditions may only manifest during pregnancy, for example gestational diabetes results from maternal hyperglycaemia and a reduced capacity to increase insulin secretion to compensate for the increase in plasma glucose availability to the fetus; orchestrated by placental hormones. In severe cases, insulin therapy may be required to minimize the risks to the fetus, for example from fetal overgrowth (macrosomia). Women with type 1 diabetes may require significantly more insulin during pregnancy to compensate for the pregnancy induced hyperglycaemia. A marginal ability to regulate maternal plasma glucose during pregnancy may also indicate an increased likelihood of type 2 diabetes in later life.

Other endocrine disorders are also complicated by pregnancy, for example hypothyroidism, resulting in an increase in the amount of thyroxine required as the pregnancy progresses. All pregnant women with disease states relating to hormonal balances and interactions require careful specialist management in coordinated and integrated medical and obstetric clinics.

ANNOTATED FURTHER READING

Carlson NR, Birkett MA: *Physiology of behavior*, ed 12, New York, 2016, Pearson.

An interesting and comprehensive exploration of how physiological processes regulate and influence the behaviour and psychology of an organism; this textbook and supporting interactive material describes sexual behaviour in depth, relating it to endocrine and neurological interactions.

Greenstein B, Wood D: *The endocrine system at a glance*, ed 3, Oxford, 2011, Wiley-Blackwell.

Introduces the study of endocrinology including principles and mechanisms in a clear and easy-to-understand way, enhanced by good illustrations, clinical scenarios and information about interpretation of diagnostic tests.

Johnson MH: *Essential reproduction*, ed 8, Oxford, 2018, Wiley-Blackwell.

An integrated and well-organized research-based textbook that covers the fundamentals of reproduction using a multidisciplinary approach, which explores comparative reproductive physiology of mammals, including anatomy, physiology, endocrinology, genetics and behavioural studies.

Rees M, Levy A, Lansdown A: *Clinical endocrinology and diabetes at a glance*, Oxford, 2017, Wiley-Blackwell.

This book provides a clear, illustrated guide to clinical endocrinology focusing on diabetes. Although, primarily intended as a medical textbook, it is useful for all healthcare professionals.

Strauss III JF, Barbieri RL, Gargiulo AR: *Yen & Jaffe's reproductive endocrinology: physiology, pathophysiology, and clinical management*, ed 8, Edinburgh, 2018, Elsevier.

This well-established text is an excellent reference book for all aspects of reproductive endocrinology.

REFERENCES

Byers HM, Mohnach LH, Fechner PY, et al.: Unexpected ethical dilemmas in sex assignment in 46,XY DSD due to 5-alpha reductase type 2 deficiency, *Am J Med Genet C Semin Med Genet* 175:260–267, 2017.

Doty RL: Human pheromones: do they exist?. In Mucignat-Caretta C, editor: *Neurobiology of chemical communication*, Chapter 19, Boca Raton, 2014, CRC Press, pp 535–560.

Doucet S, Soussignan R, Sagot P, et al.: The secretion of areolar (Montgomery's) glands from lactating women elicits selective, unconditional responses in neonates, *PLoS One* 4:e7579, 2009.

Duffy MJ: Tumor markers in clinical practice: a review focusing on common solid cancers, *Med Princ Pract* 22:4–11, 2013.

Hammock EA: Developmental perspectives on oxytocin and vasopressin, *Neuropsychopharmacology* 40:24–42, 2015.

Harris AL, Vitzthum VJ: Darwin's legacy: an evolutionary view of women's reproductive and sexual functioning, *J Sex Res* 50:207–246, 2013.

Johnson MH: *Essential reproduction*, ed 8, Oxford, 2018, Wiley-Blackwell.

Kushnir VA, Seifer DB, Barad DH, et al.: Potential therapeutic applications of human anti-Müllerian hormone (AMH) analogues in reproductive medicine, *J Assist Reprod Genet* 34:1105–1113, 2017.

McClintock MK: Menstrual synchrony and suppression, *Nature* 229:244–245, 1971.

Pilsgaard F, Grynnerup AG, Lossl K, et al.: The use of anti-Müllerian hormone for controlled ovarian stimulation in assisted reproductive technology, fertility assessment and counseling, *Acta Obstet Gynecol Scand* 97:1105–1113, 2018.

Swain JE, Kim P, Spicer J, et al.: Approaching the biology of human parental attachment: brain imaging, oxytocin and coordinated assessments of mothers and fathers, *Brain Res* 1580:78–101, 2014.

Vannuccini S, Bocchi C, Severi FM, et al.: Endocrinology of human parturition, *Ann Endocrinol (Paris)* 77:105–113, 2016.

Wyatt TD: The search for human pheromones: the lost decades and the necessity of returning to first principles,, *Proc Biol Sci* 282:20142994, 2015.

4

Reproductive Cycles

- To describe follicular development, oogenesis, ovulation and subsequent events in the ovary.
- To describe the hormonal changes in the nonfertilized menstrual cycle.
- To outline the principles of hormonal regulation of reproduction and to identify factors that affect this regulation.
- To describe the effects of the hormonal changes on the female reproductive system.

- To relate the cyclical fluctuation in hormone levels to other changes in female physiology.
- To describe the hormonal changes leading to menopause and how they affect fertility and wellbeing.
- To discuss how an understanding of the human reproductive cycle can be used to prevent fertilization (contraception) or to enhance fertilization (e.g. natural conception and assisted reproductive technologies).

INTRODUCTION

The function of the ovaries is to release female gametes or ova (singular: ovum or 'egg'; Box 4.1) and to produce steroid and peptide hormones, which regulate the hypothalamic control of reproduction. Relatively few oocytes are produced during a woman's reproductive life compared with the number of gametes (spermatozoa) produced by a man. The ovarian follicles produce oocytes, steroid hormones (oestrogen and progesterone) and cytokines such as the inhibins, which inhibit synthesis and secretion of follicle-stimulating hormone (FSH). The cyclical pattern of hormone release during the menstrual cycle has cyclical effects on the whole body, and behaviour, of the woman. The effects are particularly pronounced on the reproductive tract, facilitating its functions in gamete transport and the implantation and development of the conceptus. The first part of the cycle, the follicular phase, is dominated by the release of oestrogen produced by the developing follicles (Fig. 4.1). This oestrogen-dominant phase prepares the woman for ovulation, receipt of the sperm and fertilization of the oocyte. The oestrogens are synthesized by the follicular cells, which is why this stage of the menstrual cycle is called the follicular phase. In the second half of the cycle, the effects of progesterone are dominant. The physiological changes in this phase of the cycle prepare the woman's body for pregnancy and

promote implantation and nurture of the conceptus, should fertilization be successful. Progesterone is produced by the corpus luteum and has marked effects on the secretory activity of the secretory glands of the endometrium; this phase of the cycle is known as the luteal or secretory phase. Follicular development prior to ovulation encompasses three distinct phases: from a primary (preantral) follicle to a secondary (antral) follicle and then to a tertiary (preovulatory) follicle. After ovulation, follicular cells remaining in the ovary form the corpus luteum.

BOX 4.1   Note about Terminology

Although the terms are often used interchangeably, the term 'oocyte' refers to the developing gamete within the ovary, whereas the term 'ovum' (plural 'ova') refers to the gamete after ovulation had occurred. Oogenesis refers to the process of formation (mitotic division) of oocytes from oogonia (formed from the primordial germ cells). The primary oocyte is an oocyte that has undergone mitosis and entered meiosis and is arrested in the prophase of meiosis I from the 7th month of gestation). By the time the female infant is born, all her oogonia are primary oocytes in meiotic arrest. The secondary

Continued

BOX 4.1 Note about Terminology—cont'd

oocyte is formed (together with the first polar body) when the first meiotic division is completed each month (after menarche) in response to the LH surge, just before ovulation. So the ovum is the egg after the first meiotic division, which gives rise to the secondary oocyte arrested in metaphase II of meiosis and the first polar body. Meiosis II will be completed only if fertilization occurs giving rise to the fertilized ovum (zygote) and the second polar body. Once the chromosomes from the egg and sperm are united, the fertilized ovum is known as a zygote, which will begin a series of cleavage divisions to form the developing embryo. At the 16-cell stage, the embryo is called a 'morula' and at this stage, the cells begin to specialize (differentiate) towards either embryonic or extra-embryonic tissues. They are therefore no longer totipotent, and are referred to a pluripotent (see Chapter 6). When the fluid-filled cavity (blastocoele) forms in the embryo separating the trophoblast cells from the inner cell mass, the embryo is called a 'blastocyst'.

CHAPTER CASE STUDY

Following a routine 12-week scan, Zara contacts her midwife as she thinks the information noted on the scan is incorrect. Zara was very sure of her dates; she always had a regular cycle of 29–30 days and has kept a diary as part of her conception planning. The ultrasonographer has marked Zara's estimated date of delivery (EDD) as a week later than the midwife's calculation.

How should the midwife explain the difference in the dates and is this anything to be concerned about?

Which estimation should the midwife base the EDD on and what would be the consequences if the wrong date was referred to as a basis for delivery planning?

Ovulatory cycles usually have a duration of 24–32 days; the follicular phase is 10–14 days and the luteal phase between 12 and 15 days. Cycles tend to decrease in length as women get older; longer cycles usually have a prolonged follicular phase and delayed ovulation. The convention is to consider the first day of menstruation (LMP; last menstrual period) as the beginning of the menstrual cycle. The LMP is used clinically for predicting the expected date of delivery (EDD; see Box 6.5) and as the baseline for the commencement of oral contraceptive regimes.

The ovary contains oocytes (the germ cells or gametes), granulosa cells, which support the oocytes, steroidogenic (thecal and granulosa) cells, which produce steroids,

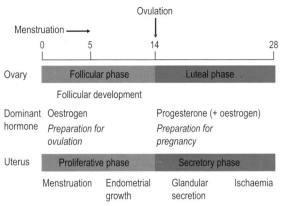

Fig. 4.1 Phases of the menstrual cycle.

ovarian stromal cells and ovarian surface epithelial cells. The ovarian surface epithelial cells form the outer covering of the ovary. They are a single layer of flat to slightly cuboidal cells, which confer a grey colour to the ovary. Their role is not entirely clear, but they appear to be involved in the follicular rupture, which occurs when the ovum is released at ovulation and the subsequent repair of the follicle wall. They are implicated in the development of most ovarian cancers (though some probably originate from the uterine tube tissue); the incessant ovulation theory suggests that the repeated breakdown and repair of the ovarian surface epithelium after each ovulation or recurrent exposure to factors in follicular fluid increase the risk of DNA damage leading to carcinogenesis (Webb and Jordan, 2017). The first phase of the menstrual cycle (follicular phase) covers follicular development in the ovary; the dominant hormone secreted by these developing follicles is oestrogen, which prepares the uterus for impending implantation. The ovum is released from the dominant follicle. After ovulation, the dominant follicle becomes the corpus luteum (hence luteal phase) and the dominant hormone secreted by the follicular cells of the corpus luteum is progesterone, which prepares the uterus (and body) for pregnancy.

Developmental Stages

The stages of cell division leading to the production of the female gametes begin early in fetal life (see Chapter 5). Meiotic cell division of these primary oocytes is arrested in prophase-1. After puberty, meiosis of one primary oocyte is completed each month in response to the luteinizing hormone (LH) surge, until ovulation ceases at menopause (which means there can be up to 50 years between the arrest of meiosis during fetal life and resumption of meiosis before ovulation). Cell division of this secondary oocyte is also arrested, this time at the metaphase-II stage, and meiosis-II is not completed until fertilization occurs.

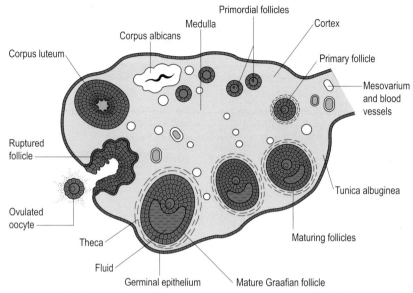

Fig. 4.2 Ovarian follicles. (Reproduced with permission from Brooker, 1998.)

Oogenesis, the development of the female gametes, can be split into several phases: oocytogenesis describes the mitotic proliferation resulting in the formation of oogonia (diploid cells with two chromatids) during fetal development; ootidogenesis describes meiosis I and II, which will result in haploid cells being produced; and finally, oogenesis proper in which the mature ovum develops. Folliculogenesis describes the changes in the cells of the follicle, which surround and support the developing oocyte. It begins with the recruitment of primordial follicles from the ovarian pool; the signals, which initiate recruitment are unknown. At the beginning of the cycle, several primary follicles are recruited to undergo initial development, stimulated by LH. These secondary follicles express FSH receptors. One follicle is selected to continue development as the dominant follicle.

In the female fetus, the primordial germ cells (PGC) migrate from the endoderm of the yolk sac to the developing gonads at around 21 days postfertilization and become germ stem cells (GSCs) or oogonia. The GSCs proliferate by mitotic division and then differentiate into primary oocytes; by 20 weeks' gestation, in each ovary, there are more than 5 million primary oocytes ready to enter meiotic division (see Chapter 5). Follicle formation begins at approximately weeks 16–18 of gestation; somatic epithelial cells surround the oogonia to form primordial follicles, mitosis stops and meiosis begins. Oocyte numbers decrease dramatically from about week 27 due to continual apoptosis through the remainder of fetal and postnatal life. The female neonate is born with a finite number of about

1 million oocytes (Herbert et al., 2015). Degeneration of these oocytes continues throughout postnatal life and there are fewer than 300,000 oocytes left at puberty and numbers continue to fall more gradually with age. By menopause there will only be about 1000 oocytes remaining (Herbert et al., 2015). However, if one assumes a reproductive life of about 35–40 years and usually a single ovum being released in each cycle, the maximum number of ova maturing to ovulation between puberty and menopause will be 300–400. The established dogma, that the capability for human germ cell renewal is lost during fetal development, was challenged by the demonstration of follicular renewal in postnatal mice (Johnson et al., 2004) and it is now suggested that some ovarian oogonia still unassociated with follicular cells persist from the fetal period and can undergo mitosis, thus acting as a stem cell source of oocytes in postnatal life (Virant-Klun, 2015). This controversy is still disputed.

The developing female gamete is called an oocyte; it differentiates into a mature haploid ovum (or egg). Although dramatic progress in the development of an oocyte takes place during the follicular phase, significant development of the follicle begins about 3–4 months prior to the menstrual cycle, in which it is released at ovulation (Fig. 4.2). Folliculogenesis begins with the recruitment of primordial (or primitive) follicles from the ovarian pool; the signals that initiate this recruitment remain unknown but probably include cytokines. From puberty, a few primordial follicles are recruited each day to join the cohort of developing follicles; this means there is a continuous trickle of primordial follicles starting development (Johnson, 2018). Each primordial follicle is made up of an oocyte surrounded by a single layer of granulosa cells, which are flattened resting somatic cells (Monniaux et al., 2014). At this stage, the chromosomes are arrested at the dictyate (resting) stage of meiosis (see Chapter 8) within the germinal vesicle of the oocyte, which is enclosed by the nuclear membrane. When the primordial follicles are activated by the signals from the ovarian cortex, the granulosa cells become cuboidal and start proliferating, forming multiple layers, and the oocyte becomes metabolically active and enlarges so the diameter of the follicle increases 10- to 20 fold. Thus, the primordial follicles are transformed into preantral follicles.

At the beginning of each menstrual cycle, a number of preantral (or primary) follicles are recruited to undergo initial development to antral (secondary) follicles. The preantral follicles express receptors for FSH and their development is driven by FSH secreted from the anterior pituitary gland. The granulosa cells of the preantral follicles become cuboidal and divide into two distinct layers: the external thecal and the inner granulosa layers, each of about 3–6 layers of cells. The oocyte continues to expand and secretes the components of the zona pellucida; tiny cytoplasmic processes extend from the oocyte through the zona pellucida to communicate with the granulosa cells (Box 4.2).

BOX 4.2 Two-cell Model: Cell Cooperation (Two-cell, Two-gonadotrophin Hypothesis)

The production of oestrogen from the follicular cells requires cooperation between the granulosa and thecal cells. The outer thecal cells of the follicle synthesize androgens from cholesterol and acetate precursors; this is stimulated by LH. The thecal cells have very limited ability to convert the androgens into oestrogens. The inner granulosa cells cannot synthesize androgens but do express the aromatizing enzymes required to convert androgens into oestrogens; these reactions are stimulated by FSH. LH stimulated thecal cell production of androgens, which are aromatized by the granulosa cells, under the influence of FSH, to form oestrogens. In addition to being the substrate for oestrogen formation, the androgens (together with oestrogens) stimulate the proliferation of granulosa cells and stimulate aromatase activity (Johnson, 2018). This means there is a positive feedback system for oestrogen production.

The developing preantral follicles start to produce follicular fluid, which accumulates in small extracellular cavities in the granulosa layer. This stage of development is particularly vulnerable; most of the preantral follicles undergo atresia rather than continuing to develop. The small preantral cavities coalesce to form a single fluid-filled antrum, which separates the follicular cells into two distinct groups; the mural granulosa cells, which make up the bulk of the follicular wall and a smaller group of follicular 'cumulus' cells, which surround the oocyte (see Fig. 4.3) The mural granulosa cells stop proliferating and differentiate into mature follicular cells, which produce oestrogen and express receptors for LH. Within the follicle, the oocyte completes its growth and prepares to resume meiosis.

One 'dominant' follicle is selected from the pool of secondary (or antral) follicles to continue development as the preovulatory (or tertiary) follicle, which secretes oestrogen as it matures and then releases the ovum at ovulation. Occasionally two dominant follicles continue development and dizygotic twins may eventuate. After ovulation, the remnants of the follicle then become the corpus luteum, which secretes both progesterone and oestrone until it undergoes luteolysis after about 14 days.

Arrested Meiosis

Meiosis is a specialized cell division involved in the production of gametes. There are two successive cell divisions (see Chapter 7, p. 172, for a detailed description). The sperm and the egg (both haploid) have to contribute one copy of each chromosome for a diploid embryo to be produced at fertilization. In meiosis, the number of chromosomes is reduced from 46 (the diploid number) to 23 (the haploid number). In the first part of meiosis, the DNA replicates, so each chromosome is copied resulting in a pair of chromatids. The homologous chromosomes (one maternal and one paternal) align and pair up along their long axes and are joined together ('zipped') by a protein structure called the 'centromere synaptonemal complex'. This stabilizes the homologous pairing and promotes crossing over so the chromosomes exchange genetic material. In humans, two or three exchanges of DNA occur per chromosome pair ensuring that the combination of genes making up each will be unique (Box 4.3). This is achieved by areas of fusion (called chiasmata) forming between adjacent chromosomes (see Chapter 7). The new chromatids thus have segments of paternal and maternal genetic material.

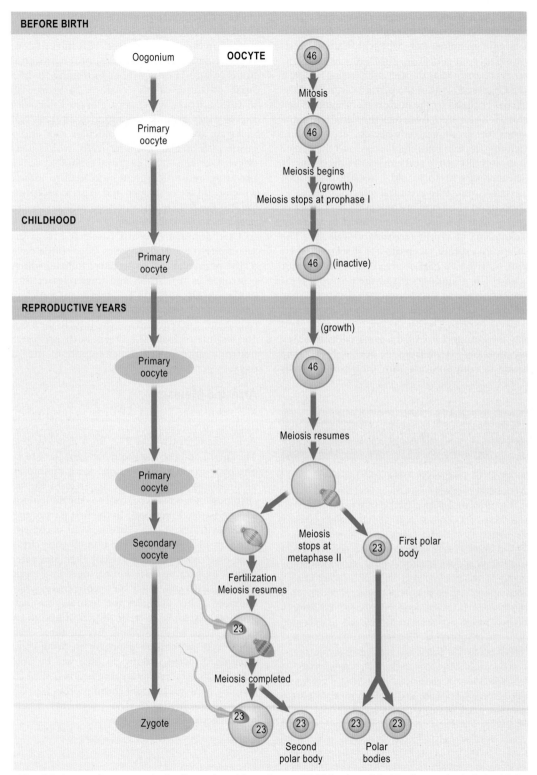

Fig. 4.3 Arrest of oocyte meiosis. (Reproduced from Patton KT, Thibodeau GA: *The human body in health & disease*, 7 ed, Elsevier 2018, Fig. 23.11.)

BOX 4.3 Summary of Gametogenesis

- In the early fetus, primordial germ cells become oogonia in the primitive gonads.
- Oogonia divide by mitosis to produce millions of oocytes most of which degenerate (atresia). In contrast, mitosis in spermatogonia continues throughout life.
- Some of the oogonia will develop into primary oocytes and arrest in prophase of meiosis I. Of ~1–2 million primary oocytes present at birth, only 40,000 will remain at puberty and only approximately 400 will be ovulated during a woman's life.
- Each month, the LH surge triggers completion of meiosis I in a primary oocyte giving rise to two very different cells, a secondary oocyte arrested in meiosis II (prior to ovulation) and the first polar body.
- Penetration by the sperm causes the final stages of meiosis to occur.

BOX 4.4 Oogenesis Compared with Spermatogenesis

- Mitosis: fetal stage in females; after puberty in man
- Meiosis: arrested gametogenesis in woman can last many years
- Relatively few (300–500) oocytes released
- Release is episodic at ovulation; not a continuous stream
- Organization is comparable with testis (stromal tissue containing primordial follicles, tubules) and glandular tissue (interstitial glands, Leydig cells)
- Mitotic proliferation is less
- Time course of gamete production is much longer

The oocyte remains arrested in dictyate in the prophase stage of division I of meiosis for a number of years until sexual maturity at puberty (Fig. 4.3); the LH surge just before ovulation triggers meiosis to resume. Thus, most oocytes in the ovary are in the dictyate state. Arrested meiosis provides a specialized mechanism to allow the oocyte to grow while it contains duplicate copies of chromosomes and, therefore, twice as much DNA is available to direct synthesis of RNA compared with a somatic cell. Dictyate also allows damaged DNA in the future gamete to be repaired.

The increasing oestrogen levels drive the mature LH surge, which will release the oocyte from the first meiotic block; this process is called oocyte maturation. The oocyte resumes division I of meiosis. During this time, the primary oocytes synthesize the extracellular matrix and the secretory vesicles. The chromosomes recondense, the nuclear envelope breaks down and the meiotic spindle forms. The chromosomes then segregate into the two daughter nuclei. The cytoplasm divides asymmetrically to form a large secondary oocyte and a small polar body (which is expelled), each of which contains 23 chromosomes as pairs of chromatids. Meiotic division then arrests for a second time, so the oocyte released at ovulation has still not completed meiosis. Activation of the oocyte and release from the second meiotic block occurs at fertilization. In the second meiotic division, the sister chromatids finally segregate into two nuclei and the cytoplasm again divides asymmetrically, thus forming the mature ovum and a second polar body, each with 23 chromosomes. Because both divisions of the cytoplasm are asymmetrical, the ovum is large. Effectively, the polar bodies are small packages of cytoplasm, which contain discarded chromosomes and cytoskeleton. During *in vitro* fertilization

(IVF), observing the presence of the second polar body indicates that fertilization has occurred (see Chapter 6).

In the female, mitosis of the gametes stops in the fetal period (when the germ cells enter meiosis to become primary oocytes), whereas in the male, mitotic division of gametogenesis begins at puberty and continues until senescence (Box 4.4). The termination of mitosis in the female, and entry into meiosis, is under the regulation of retinoic acid (Feng et al., 2014). Although it occurs with a different time course, retinoic acid (RA) is also the driver of entry into meiosis in male germ cells. RA is derived from the oxidation of vitamin A (retinaldehyde) by retinaldehyde dehydrogenases and is essential in the development of many organ systems. The bioavailability of RA depends on the balance between its production and its degradation. *STRA8*, the gene STimulated by Retinoic Acid 8, is required for the RA-signalling pathway in humans leading to the initiation of meiosis. In the fetal ovary, RA-induced expression of Stra8 is maintained so meiosis takes place in fetal life whereas in the fetal testis, RA signalling is attenuated because it is actively degraded as soon as it is formed; meiosis in the male begins at puberty.

Both premature arrest at the end of oocyte maturation and parthenogenic release from meiotic arrest are thought to cause infertility. As women age, the extended duration of arrested meiosis, which may last for over 50 years, probably results in the meiotic spindles (see Fig. 7.11, p. 174) becoming increasingly fragile; this leads to an increased incidence of failure to separate chromatids (nondisjunction) and of abnormalities such as Trisomy 21 (Down syndrome) and failed implantation. Chromosomes often fail to segregate correctly in human meiosis, particularly as women age, which results in oocytes with abnormal numbers of chromosomes (Webster and Schuh, 2017). If they are fertilized, the aneuploid embryos usually fail to implant but can also continue to develop resulting in increased rates of infertility, miscarriage and congenital abnormalities.

Primordial (Primitive) Follicles

Development of a mature female gamete depends on complex interactions between the developing gamete and the surrounding cells forming the outer layers of the follicle. Mitosis is completed during fetal development. During the first meiotic prophase, the PGC drive the organization of the surrounding cells to form the granulosa cells (flattened cuboidal epithelial cells), which condense and encircle them, forming the primordial follicles. The follicular cells secrete a basement membrane around the outside forming a cellular unit (Fig. 4.4). These granulosa cells are connected to the oocyte by gap junctions through which nutrients can be transported. The primitive oocyte therefore has two layers and is about 18–20 μm in diameter. A few follicles may resume development spontaneously and incompletely throughout fetal and neonatal life. However, regular recruitment of the primordial follicles into the pool of growing follicles begins at puberty when levels of FSH increase, so the primordial follicles containing oocytes may stay arrested in meiosis for decades.

Preantral (Primary) Follicles

From puberty, a few primordial follicles spontaneously resume their development each day, forming a continuous stream or trickle of growing preantral or primary follicles. Most of these early follicles fail to develop fully and undergo atresia (fail to develop any further); less than 0.1% of follicles will go on to ovulate and subsequently develop into a corpus luteum. The granulosa cells of follicles undergoing atresia accumulate lipid droplets and reduce protein synthesis. Both the granulosa cells and the oocyte become apoptotic (undergo 'programmed cell death'). White blood cells invade the dying follicular cell mass and scar tissue forms.

As most of the follicles regress rather than progress through development, the ovary has a dense population of atretic follicles resulting in the irregular corrugated outer surface of the ovary. The development of primordial follicles into primary or preantral follicles takes about 85 days; the preantral phase is the longest phase of development of the oocyte. Initiation and progress through this early follicular development is independent of pituitary hormones (LH and FSH) but there may be paracrine regulation by cytokines (see Chapter 3), such as epidermal growth factor (EGF; Box 4.5). These developing follicles do not secrete significant amounts of steroid hormones. Further follicular development requires pituitary support (secretion of FSH and LH). During the preantral phase of development, which has a duration of about 120 days in humans, the size of the follicles increases by about 10-fold, predominantly due to the increase in size of the primary oocyte, which, despite being in meiotic arrest, synthesizes proteins and intracellular organelles.

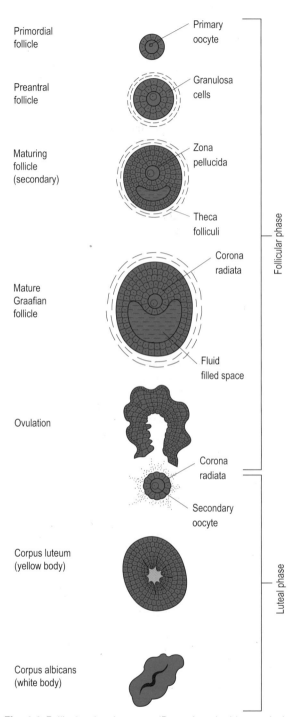

Fig. 4.4 Follicular development. (Reproduced with permission from Brooker, 1998.)

BOX 4.5 Cytokines and Growth Factors

Inhibin and Activins

The gonadotrophins (FSH and LH) stimulate the production of the cytokines, activin and inhibins. The cytokines modulate actions of steroid hormones and gonadotrophins. Inhibins appear to affect only reproduction (see Fig. 4.7), whereas the closely related activin affects cell growth and differentiation in other tissues. Inhibin is produced by the granulosa cells of small antral follicles in response to FSH and suppresses FSH secretion. It is also produced by the Sertoli cells of the testis. Levels peak mid-cycle but remain high in the luteal phase, because the corpus luteum produces inhibin in response to LH. Inhibin production in the pituitary has a local inhibitory effect on FSH release. Inhibin stimulates androgen output by the thecal cells and moderates aromatizing activity of the granulosa cells. Activin is produced by granulosa cells, which also secrete follistatin, which may modulate the effects of activin. The thecal cells of the dominant follicle also produce activin. The anterior pituitary gland produces activin, which is co-secreted with the gonadotrophins and enhances FSH production. It inhibits pituitary production of growth hormone (GH), adrenocorticotrophic hormone (ACTH) and PRL. It may also have a role in embryogenesis. Activin is present in follicular fluid but is inhibited by follistatin. Activin suppresses the androgen output by thecal cells but stimulates aromatizing capacity of granulosa cells. It therefore inhibits progesterone production. Activin is present early in the cycle, and inhibin later in the cycle, thereby producing a balance between androgen output and conversion.

Follistatin

Follistatin is an inhibitor of FSH secretion, which is synthesized in the ovary and inhibits activin activity by acting as an activin-binding protein.

Interleukins

Interleukins are a diverse group of cytokines (secreted signalling proteins) that communicate between different immune system cells, and with other cell types. They are usually secreted by immune cells and usually have a local action. Interleukins include histamine, prostaglandins, tumour necrosis factor (TNF), IL-1 and IL-6. IL-1 is a polypeptide cytokine, usually produced by activated macrophages, which induces an acute phase reaction in the liver in response to inflammation. However, it is also produced by granulosa cells in a hormone-dependent manner with a peak production mid-cycle. IL-1 affects follicular maturation and a number of aspects of ovulation, including increasing production of prostaglandins, collagenase, nitric oxide and hyaluronic acid (Gérard et al., 2004) and steroidogenesis. It is not known whether other members of the interleukin family are involved in follicular development.

Epidermal Growth Factor

The epidermal growth factor (EGF) family is comprised of 11 proteins including EGF, TGF-α, amphiregulin (AREG) and epiregulin (EREG) with similar structures and functions. EGF-like peptides play crucial roles via their signalling pathways in granulosa and cumulus cells in driving oocyte meiotic maturation and developmental capacity. Secretion of EGF-family proteins by granulosa cells in response to the LH surge explains the powerful effects of LH on oocyte maturation and ovulation, despite the absence of LH receptors on preovulatory oocytes (Richani and Gilchrist, 2018).

Transforming Growth Factors

Transforming growth factors (TGFs), TGF-α and TGF-β, have been identified in thecal cells. TGF-α has similar properties to EGF and suppresses granulosa cell differentiation. It also regulates differentiation of other cell types including fetal ovaries and ovarian carcinoma cells. Members of the TGF-β family are structurally similar to inhibin and increase FSH receptor expression, positively modulating granulosa cell proliferation and differentiation.

Insulin-like Growth Factors

Insulin-like growth factors (IGFs) stimulate mitotic division and cell differentiation. Their effects are mediated by two insulin-like growth factor receptors (IGFR1 and IGFR2) and also by a family of seven IGF binding proteins (IGFBPs). In follicular development, they appear to coordinate the production of steroid hormones from the granulosa and thecal layers of the follicle. IGF-1 enhances follicular development and hormone production. IGF-2 enhances the response to insulin. IGFBPs bind to the IGFs decreasing the concentration of free growth factor. Decreased levels of binding proteins are associated with follicular growth and increased concentrations of binding proteins are found in atretic follicles. The large follicles from women with polycystic ovaries have lower concentrations of growth factors and higher concentrations of binding proteins. IGFs seem therefore to have an important role in follicular growth, maturation and ovulation. In pregnancy, IGFs and their binding proteins play essential roles in modulating fetal growth and development (see Chapter 9).

Tumour Necrosis Factor

Tumour necrosis factor (TNF) was initially identified as having a role in inflammation and in inhibiting tumour growth. It is produced by follicular cells and stimulates steroidogenesis, and may have a role in ovulation.

Early in the cycle in which the follicle will release its ovum, the concentration of FSH is sufficient to support the further development of some preantral follicles. The preantral follicles that are optimal for further development are of the appropriate size and maturity to respond and have adequate FSH receptors. Recruitment of the follicles is related to the interaction between the FSH concentration and the number of FSH receptors on the developing follicles. Therefore, the number of follicles surviving is related to the amount of FSH present. The antral development phase, ovulation and luteal phase comprise one cycle in humans. In other mammalian species, antral expansion occurs in the luteal phase of the previous cycle, thus shortening nonfertile cycles.

Antral (Secondary) Follicles

Usually ~15–20 preantral follicles are rescued from atresia each month and undergo initial stages of development and marked enlargement in response to the increasing FSH concentration at the beginning of each cycle. Several components contribute to the growth of the follicle: the oocyte enlarges, the follicular cells divide and further stromal cells are recruited to form the expanded outer layers of the follicle. The oocyte itself increases in diameter to 60–120 µm. It synthesizes large amounts of ribosomal RNA (rRNA) and messenger RNA (mRNA) to increase synthesis of protein stores ready for the maturation of the oocyte and fertilization, but does not resume meiosis. The follicular cells divide into several layers of granulosa cells, which secrete an amorphous and acellular translucent jelly, the zona pellucida. The zona pellucida is formed from condensation of different glycoproteins and accumulates between the granulosa cells and the oocyte, acting as the extracellular coat of the oocyte. It has an important role in sperm binding and penetration during fertilization (see Chapter 6). Although the zona pellucida acts to separate the oocyte from the avascular granulosa cells, cytoplasmic processes (transzonal projections) penetrate the zona pellucida forming gap junctions at the oocyte surface. These allow delivery of low molecular weight substrates, such as nucleotides and amino acids, and cellular signalling molecules into the oocyte to support its metabolism and regulate its differentiation. Gap junctions also exist between granulosa cells.

The third component of follicular growth is condensation of ovarian stromal cells on the basement membrane (membrana propria) of the follicle. These recruited cells form a loose matrix of spindle-shaped cells around the follicle, known as the thecal layer. The cells differentiate into two layers: the theca interna, an inner layer of highly vascular glandular cells, and the theca externa, a poorly vascularized fibrous capsule.

There is critical bidirectional paracrine and juxtacrine communication between the oocyte and the surrounding somatic or follicular cells of the ovary, the granulosa and thecal cells. FSH is required both for granulosa cell differentiation and division (Richards et al., 2018). The granulosa cells acquire receptors for FSH and oestrogen and the theca interna cells acquire receptors for LH. Synthesis of steroid hormones by the follicle requires cell cooperation (Fig. 4.5; Box 4.2). Interstitial glands lie within the stroma and between the developing follicles. They are formed of steroidogenic cells and produce androgens for secretion and aromatization to oestrogen in follicles. LH stimulates the theca interna cells to synthesize androgens (testosterone and androstenedione) from acetate and cholesterol but these cells initially have limited capacity to synthesize oestrogens. Androgens from the theca interna cells diffuse to the avascular granulosa cells. The granulosa cells are unable to synthesize androgens but can aromatize androgens to oestrogens (oestradiol-17β and oestrone). The enzyme aromatase (CYP19) is involved in the steroid biosynthesis pathway leading to increased oestrogen production. FSH stimulates production of insulin-like growth factor 1 (IGF-1), which stimulates aromatase activity and hence oestrogen production. Activins and oestradiol enhance the actions of FSH. Small amounts of LH are required to amplify follicular oestrogen production. The steroids are secreted into the bloodstream, where they have a systemic effect, and into the follicular fluid, where they may have a paracrine role. Androgens also stimulate aromatase. Oestrogens stimulate granulosa cells to proliferate and express further oestrogen receptors. Therefore, oestrogen further stimulates oestrogen output, an example of positive feedback. This increases the amount of circulating oestrogen from the most advanced or 'dominant' follicle (therefore, monitoring oestrogen output is a guide to the maturity of the most mature follicles). The dominant follicle, which undergoes the most growth, will enlarge from 20 to 200–400 µm in diameter. The dominant follicle produces oestradiol, which inhibits FSH secretion. However, the dominant follicle develops exquisite sensitivity to FSH and can continue to respond to the decreasing concentration of FSH. The smaller follicles, destined to become atretic, lose their responsiveness to FSH and do not develop LH receptors.

Early in the antral phase under the influence of FSH, the granulosa cells produce inhibin B and activin, which suppresses androgen output and increases the aromatizing capability of the granulosa cells, thus promoting oestrogen synthesis. Later in the antral phase under the influence of both FSH and LH, the granulosa cells switch to producing inhibin A, which stimulates androgen output and attenuates the aromatizing activity. Thus, androgen output is

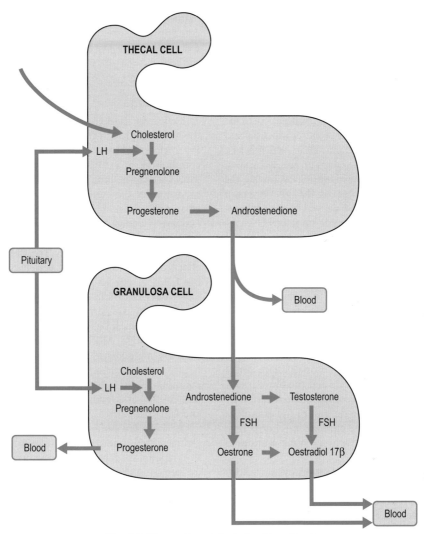

Fig. 4.5 'Two-cell model' of steroid synthesis.

regulated by activin and inhibins so the ratio of inhibin A:inhibin B and output of oestrogen act as a marker of follicular growth and development indicating ovulation is near.

The Dominant Antral Follicle

The single follicle emerging as dominant undergoes pre-ovulatory growth. This dominant follicle produces more oestrogen, which inhibits production of FSH from the pituitary gland. This is an example of negative feedback where a product limits its own production. The effect of oestrogen inhibiting production of FSH is that further development of the other follicles is limited. These follicles with fewer FSH receptors exposed to a diminishing supply of FSH are least able to respond to FSH and therefore undergo a downward spiral and become atretic. The dominant follicle continues to produce inhibin A, which stimulates androgen production by the thecal cells and aromatization by the granulosa cells, thus leading to the surge of oestrogen. The dominant follicle also has a high ratio of insulin-like growth factor 2 (IGF-2) to IGF-BP, which mediates LH-stimulated androgen output and FSH-dependent aromatization.

Angiotensin II (A-II), the product of the renin–angiotensin system (RAS, see Chapter 2), may be involved in oocyte maturation and ovulation. There is a RAS that is specific to the ovary and A-II occurs in high concentrations in preovulatory follicles. This ovarian RAS is implicated in the pathogenesis of ovarian tumours, ovarian hyperstimulation syndrome, ectopic pregnancy and hypertension (Palumbo et al, 2016). Symptoms of ovarian hyperstimulation syndrome include serious metabolic and fluid disturbances, which are associated with abnormal control of the RAS (note that ovarian hyperstimulation syndrome is a recognized complication of IVF treatment; see Chapter 6). It has also been suggested that A-II may have a role in the formation and maintenance of the corpus luteum, regulation of progesterone production and angiogenesis. The biggest or dominant follicle, which is best able to respond to FSH, further develops on the pathway to expansion and ovulation. Oestrogen and FSH stimulate the mid-cycle expression of LH receptors on the outer layers of granulosa cells of the dominant follicle, which means that it will be able to respond to the mid-cycle surge of LH secretion. Entry into the preovulatory phase depends on both the expression of these receptors and a surge of LH from the anterior pituitary gland.

The granulosa cells continue to divide and increase in size. However, most of the increase in follicular size is due to accumulation of follicular fluid formed from mucopolysaccharides, secreted from granulosa cells, and serum transudate. The fluid coalesces forming an antrum (or cleft) filled with follicular fluid. The antrum separates the granulosa cells into two regions: the corona radiata (a rim of granulosa cells) around the oocyte and the outer membrana granulosa. The oocyte becomes isolated and suspended in the fluid connected to the rest of the granulosa cells by a thin strand of cells, the cumulus oophorus (egg stalk). The oocyte does not increase in size but continues to synthesize RNA and protein.

Follicular development is dependent on pituitary support. Removal of the pituitary gland (hypophysectomy) results in the cessation of follicular growth and the death of the oocyte. This can be halted by adding back LH and FSH, which stimulate further growth. It takes 8–12 days for the primary follicle to grow into the antral follicle. Failure of follicular growth for any reason results in a restarting of the cycle of follicular development, and hence both a longer first phase of the cycle and a longer cycle. It seems likely that women who regularly have a longer than normal menstrual cycle have either a slow rate of follicular development and increasing oestrogen secretion or the dominant follicle starts developing but fails, so the next most appropriate follicle takes over the role as the dominant follicle.

Although the increasing concentration of oestrogen (predominantly oestradiol, E_2) initially has a negative feedback on the hypothalamus and pituitary, there is a critical concentration of oestrogen (2- to 4-fold higher than that of the early phase of the cycle) that is stimulatory (i.e. has a positive feedback effect on secretion of LH and FSH), provided it lasts for a critical duration (~48 h). When the diameter of the follicle is 18–22 μm and the oestradiol concentration reaches 600–1200 pmol/L, there is positive feedback on the anterior pituitary gland leading to a sudden increase or 'surge' of LH release (Johnson, 2018; Fig. 4.6).

The LH Surge

The effect of the LH surge is twofold. First, it stimulates the terminal growth phase of the preovulatory follicle and the meiotic and cytoplasmic maturation of the oocyte, culminating in expulsion of the oocyte from the ovary. These effects include reinitiation of oocyte meiosis and expansion of the cumulus cell–oocyte complex (Richards et al., 2018). Second, it causes luteinization, a series of endocrine changes within the follicular cells that result in a progesterone-dominant hormone secretory profile in the second half of the cycle. The LH surge has powerful effects on oocyte maturation as well as triggering ovulation but LH does not act directly on the oocyte since preovulatory oocytes do not express LH receptors. The LH surge acts indirectly via stimulating the theca and mural granulosa cells of the follicle to produce several growth factors, including EREG, AREG and BTC (see Box 4.5). These peptides are members of the epidermal growth factor (EGF) family and switch on gene expression in granulosa and cumulus cells to trigger oocyte maturation followed by follicle rupture and formation of the corpus luteum (Richani and Gilchrist, 2018).

Within a few hours of the LH surge, there are dramatic changes in the oocyte, which resumes meiotic division. Progression through the remainder of the first meiotic division results in half the chromosomes (as paired chromatids) and almost all the cytoplasm being enclosed in the secondary oocyte, which is destined to become the ovum. The remaining chromosomes and very little cytoplasm are enclosed in a membrane forming a very small defunct cell, known as the first polar body (see Fig. 4.3). Thus, the secondary oocyte keeps the bulk of the materials that were synthesized earlier in follicular development so that these are conserved for the zygote and early cleavage divisions. As the cell divisions are not even, the ovum retains almost all of the contents of the 'mother' cell prior to meiotic division including the mitochondria. The only contribution from the fertilizing sperm is its DNA; sperm mitochondria are marked with ubiquitin and are destroyed. So mitochondrial DNA is inherited exclusively from the mother and can be used to trace maternal lineage (the female line from mother to grandmother to great-grandmother, etc.) (see Chapter 6).

The chromosomes of the secondary oocyte enter the second meiotic division and go on to the next stage of division, called the metaphase (see Fig. 7.11), where they

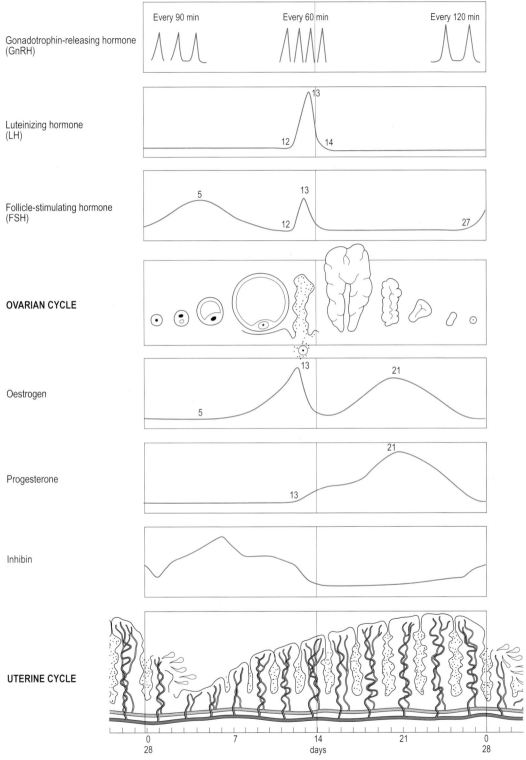

Fig. 4.6 The reproductive cycle and hormone levels.

align on the spindle. However, meiosis is then immediately arrested for a second time; this is regulated by cytostatic factors. Meiosis, resulting in the production of a mature female pronucleus, will not resume until successful fertilization following ovulation. By this time, the oocyte will already contain the sperm nucleus. Thus, there is actually no time when the oocyte is a true gamete in the sense of being a cell with only 23 chromosomes, as is the case of a spermatozoon. Failure of the oocyte to jettison one set of female chromosomes into the second polar body results in digynic or gynogenetic triploidy (where the fertilized ovum contains three sets of chromosomes: one from the sperm and two from meiotic division of the ovum) (Johnson, 2018; Box 4.6).

BOX 4.6   Triploidy

Triploidy (or triploid syndrome), although rare, is one of the most common chromosomal disorders in humans. Instead of being diploid (having two sets of chromosomes), the triploid fetus has three copies of each chromosome (total of 69). It can result from three possible mechanisms: an extra set of paternal chromosomes because two sperm have fertilized the egg (dispermy), an extra set of paternal chromosomes because the egg was fertilized by a sperm with two sets of chromosomes, or an extra set of maternal chromosomes because of abnormal meiosis (digynic trisomy). In the latter case, the extra set of maternal chromosomes usually results from none being packaged into the second polar body after fertilization. Triploidy can also be mosaic where some cells are triploid and other cells are diploid (normal); this has less severe outcome. Triploidy affects all organ systems but the effects are most marked in the skeleton and nervous system. Common defects include abnormal development of the brain and central nervous system including neural tube defects, cleft lip and palate, club foot, syndactyly (fused fingers), congenital heart defects, intrauterine growth restriction, oligohydramnios (abnormally low volume of amniotic fluid), placental abnormalities including enlargement and abnormally high levels of alpha-fetoprotein (which can be used diagnostically). Triploidy affects about 1–2% of pregnancies but most triploid fetuses fail to develop, and miscarry (accounting for ~10% of all spontaneous abortions); or termination is offered. It is rare for triploid fetuses to survive to birth; those who do, usually die shortly afterwards. Diandric triploidy (where the extra set of chromosomes is paternal in origin) is associated with partial hydatidiform mole (p. 256).

Concurrently, the LH surge promotes maturation of the cytoplasmic compartment of the oocyte. The cytoplasmic processes between the oocyte and the granulosa cells withdraw and contact is lost. The Golgi apparatus (see Table 1.1) synthesizes lysosome-like cortical granules, which align under the surface of the oocyte. Protein synthesis continues but the profile of the proteins synthesized changes as the oocyte prepares for fertilization. The gonadotrophin surge stimulates the cumulus cells surrounding the oocyte (see Fig. 4.4) to secrete hyaluronic acid, which disperses the cumulus cells embedding them in a mucus-like matrix.

Ovulation

Ovulation is triggered by the mid-cycle surge of LH, which occurs in response to sustained high levels of oestrogen released from the developing dominant follicle. The single mature preovulatory follicle has a diameter of 2–2.5 cm in an ovary that is approximately 3 cm long. It was this structure that Regnier de Graaf identified and named in 1672. The increased size and changed position of the follicle mean that it protrudes from the surface of the ovary (see Fig. 4.2). This contributes to the thinning of the layer of epithelial cells between the wall of the follicle and the peritoneal cavity. As expansion continues, the wall becomes thinner and avascular, and the cells appear to dissociate.

At ~36 h after the LH surge, ovulation occurs and the oocyte is expelled from the ovary (see Fig. 4.2). The LH surge stimulates the production of a cascade of proteolytic enzymes, including renin and other trypsin-like enzymes from thecal cells, which digest the follicle wall. The biochemical changes, including generation of reactive oxygen species (free radicals), that precede ovulation, are similar to those seen in inflammation. Plasminogen activator, which converts procollagenase to collagenase, is produced by granulosa cells resulting in the breakdown of the connective tissue. Production of progesterone and 17α-progesterone rises immediately after the LH surge and this preovulatory increase in progestogens may be important in follicular rupture as it decreases formation of collagen. Prostaglandins increase vascular permeability, which maintains the intrafollicular pressure as fluid begins to leak through the eroded follicular wall. Small contractile waves also ripple across the ovary, increasing the intrafollicular pressure. The force is cushioned by the follicular fluid, so the pressure generated is targeted at the weakened ovarian surface, causing it to rupture. Some women experience lower abdominal and pelvic pain around the time of ovulation on the same side as the ovary producing the ovum. This is referred to as Mittelschmerz (derived from German 'middle pain'), which is sometimes mistaken for appendicitis. As the follicle ruptures and the ovarian surface is breached, the fluid washes out the oocyte, which is surrounded by the granulosa (cumulus) cells, from the ovary to the exterior. The oocyte is swept into the uterine tube by the fimbria. It is then propelled towards the uterus by peristaltic muscular activity and ciliary movements on the epithelial cells lining the tube. Having taken 12–50 years to complete the maturation process, the oocyte is then viable and fertilizable for only 1 day.

THE LUTEAL PHASE

Within ~2 h of the LH surge, there is a transient rise in the oestrogen and androgens secreted by the follicle as the thecal layers become stimulated and hyperaemic. The outer granulosa cells with their newly expressed receptors for LH no longer convert androgens to oestrogen but synthesize progesterone instead. The cells no longer bind oestrogen or FSH. The result is a marked increase in progesterone secretion, which begins several hours before ovulation.

The Corpus Luteum

After ovulation, the residual parts of the follicle remaining in the ovary collapse into the space and form the corpus luteum ('yellow body'; see Fig. 4.4), which is a temporary endocrine structure. Initially, there is some bleeding and fibrotic activity in the cavity, which drives the formation of a fibrin core around which the remaining granulosa cells congregate. The structure is enclosed by a capsule of fibrous thecal cells. The basement membrane between the granulosa cells and thecal cells breaks down allowing vascularization of the interior. This allows increased transport of cholesterol precursors to the luteinizing granulosa cells to maintain a high rate of progesterone synthesis and secretion. A few of the thecal cells disperse to the stroma tissue. The granulosa cells first luteinize, then stop dividing and hypertrophy into large luteal cells. The luteal cells are rich in mitochondria, endoplasmic reticulum and Golgi and have numerous lipid droplets and lutein, a yellow carotenoid pigment.

Hormonal Changes

Luteinization is associated with a progressive increment in secretion of progesterone and 17α-progesterone from the corpus luteum. The outer thecal cells form a stem cell population of smaller luteal cells, which have numerous LH receptors and produce progesterone and androgens. Levels of progesterone rise until the middle of the luteal phase (see Fig. 4.6). The corpus luteum produces oestrogen and inhibin A as well as progesterone. All three hormones inhibit secretion of FSH from the anterior pituitary gland and therefore prevent further development of follicles.

It has been suggested that a cause of fertility problems may be inadequate production of progesterone at the time of ovulation and during the subsequent luteal phase. However, exogenous administration of progesterone or human chorionic gonadotrophin (hCG) has had limited success in clinical practice. It appears that many women have a proportion of their cycles with a low progesterone output without their fecundity (capacity to conceive) or fertility (number of live births) being affected and that women in nonindustrialized countries typically have lower progesterone associated poorer nutritional status and higher physical activity without any negative effect on reproductive success (Vitzthum et al., 2004). A shortened luteal phase associated with low progesterone is associated with intermenstrual bleeding, premenstrual 'spotting' and short cycles.

The corpus luteum also synthesizes relaxin, a peptide that is structurally similar to insulin (Marshall et al., 2017). Other reproductive organs such as the uterus also produce some relaxin. Relaxin is not a well-characterized hormone; not all of is roles are understood and there are also species-specific differences in its synthesis and activity. The secretion of relaxin peaks in the middle of the luteal cycle (Marshall et al., 2017), probably regulated by LH. Relaxin has a uterotrophic effect; it stimulates growth and structural changes in the uterus including remodelling of the extracellular matrix and adaptations of the uterine vasculature. Inadequate relaxin production is associated with an increased risk of preeclampsia, miscarriage, endometriosis and uterine fibrosis (Marshall et al., 2017).

Effectively, the corpus luteum is a ephemeral endocrine gland producing oestrogen and progesterone. The LH surge stimulates its growth and activity. Unless fertilization occurs, the life of the corpus luteum is very short, and it undergoes spontaneous luteolysis (degeneration and regression) after about 6–8 days after the LH surge. The corpus luteum appears to have an age-related decrease in responsiveness to LH (Devoto et al., 2017) and so requires progressively more LH for survival. Following the LH surge, the LH concentration in the luteal phase is low, so luteolysis will occur. Blood flow to the corpus luteum falls and the follicular tissue becomes ischaemic. The concentrations of oestrogen and progesterone begin to fall as the degenerating corpus luteum ceases hormone production. Thus, luteolysis terminates a nonfertile cycle. As the level of oestrogen falls, the inhibition on the hypothalamus will be abrogated and FSH secretion will resume, ready for the next cycle. The atrophying corpus luteum loses its yellow pigment, so it becomes known as a corpus albicans ('white body'). It gradually contracts over a period of months, leaving white scar tissue, which is absorbed into the stromal tissue of the ovary.

Changes on Fertilization

If fertilization occurs, then hCG, which has structural similarities to LH, rescues the corpus luteum from luteolysis, stimulating its further growth and production of steroid hormones up to the 10th week of pregnancy when placental endocrine function becomes established. hCG has a longer half-life than LH, so it provides a sustained and more intense stimulus. If fertilization occurs, then the concentration of relaxin also continues to rise until the end of the first trimester.

REGULATION OF GONADOTROPHIN SECRETION

The brain controls and regulates the ovarian cycle. The gonadotrophs in the anterior pituitary secrete the glycoprotein hormones LH and FSH (which together are known as gonadotrophins). There appear to be two distinct populations of cells in the anterior pituitary, each producing one particular type of hormone; however, fluorescent labelling techniques (immunocytochemistry) show that some cells contain both hormones. Synthesis and secretion of both LH and FSH are dependent on gonadotrophin-releasing hormone (GnRH) from the hypothalamus, which acts as the common mediator of influences via the central nervous system (CNS). (GnRH is also known as luteinizing hormone releasing hormone, or LHRH.) The hypothalamus releases GnRH into the hypophysial portal circulation that runs to the pituitary gland. This pathway means that the control of reproduction can be modulated by other inputs from the higher brain centres. The GnRH neurons convert neural signals into endocrine signals. Stress, nutritional status and environmental influences, for instance, affect the timing and success of the reproduction. Ovulation appears to be seasonally regulated in populations experiencing seasonal variation in food availability; suspending reproductive function when nutrition is poor favours maternal health and the outcome of pregnancy. There are two levels of regulation: the GnRH neurons of the hypothalamus have an inherent pulsatile activity. The steroid hormones, the gonadotrophins (LH and FSH) and GnRH feedback on the hypothalamic–pituitary axis (HPA) to exert a second level of endocrine control. Prolactin (PRL) also has an effect on the control of reproduction.

GnRH and gonadotrophins are released in a pulsatile manner (Box 4.7). The cells releasing GnRH appear to be widely and diffusely distributed but are remarkably synchronized to produce pulses of GnRH. During the follicular phase, the pulses are of low amplitude and high frequency, occurring about every 60 min. In the luteal phase, they are more irregular and have high amplitude

and occur with a low frequency of about 1 pulse every 2–6 h. The output of the gonadotrophins, LH and FSH, is changed by increasing or decreasing the amplitude or frequency of the pulses or by modulating the response of

---

BOX 4.7   Biological Rhythms

The study of biological rhythms is termed 'chronobiology'. All living cells, organs, organisms and groups of individuals demonstrate rhythmical changes within their internal (endogenous) physiology that can also result in external changes in behaviour. The rhythms can be categorized according to the length of the cycle or period of oscillation.

- *Ultradian*: the rhythm is less than 1 day, e.g. rapid eye movement in sleep.
- *Circahordal*: the period of oscillation is around 1 h.
- *Circadian*: the period of oscillation is about 1 day; levels of many hormones such as cortisol fluctuate on a daily basis.
- *Infradian*: the rhythm is repeated in a cycle >1 day, e.g. menstrual and oestrus cycles.
- *Circaseptram*: the period of oscillation is about 1 week.
- *Circatidal*: the rhythm relates to tidal movement of water.
- *Circalunar (synodic)*: the rhythm relates to the cycle of the moon.
- *Circannual*: the rhythm has a cycle of about 1 year.

These fluctuations are often affected by the external environment and appear to enable the individual to respond to forthcoming changes within the environment. Factors that influence or reset the cycle are described as entraining the cycle. In the human brain, the suprachiasmatic nuclei (SCN) of the hypothalamus may influence daily fluctuations. The pineal gland secretes the hormone melatonin at night and is entrained by signals from the retina, independent of visual perception by rods and cones and their signalling via the optic nerve. Melatonin secretion by the pineal gland is inhibited when light is detected by photosensitive retinal ganglion cells containing the photopigment melanopsin, which signal to the circadian pacemaker located in the SCN. Efferent neurons from the SCN signal the light-induced suppression of melatonin secretion. Therefore, within temperate zones, light acts as an entrainer on a daily basis and, because of the fluctuation of the photoperiod (length of daylight exposure), entrainment of annual cycles can also be achieved. In relation to reproduction, this is observed in animals with seasonal breeding behaviour.

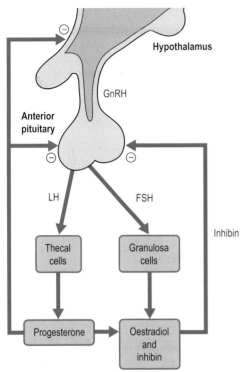

Fig. 4.7 Hormonal regulation of the menstrual cycle. (Reproduced with permission from Johnson and Everitt, 1995.)

is involved in the negative feedback of FSH secretion. However, the dominant follicle is exquisitely sensitive to even a diminishing concentration of FSH and continues to produce oestrogen, which markedly increases by 2- to 4-fold. These concentrations are maintained for about 48 h, which produces a positive feedback effect resulting in the dramatic surge of LH and FSH release seen in mid-cycle prior to ovulation. The effect of oestradiol is very sensitive: a low concentration has a marked and rapid effect that is evident within 1 h and maximal within 4–6 h. During the luteal phase, increased progesterone concentrations reinforce the negative feedback effects of oestradiol. The production of both LH and FSH secretion is very low; therefore, the positive effect of oestradiol is blocked.

CYCLICAL EFFECTS OF OESTROGENS AND PROGESTERONE

Effects on the Uterus

Organs that respond to hormonal changes have cellular receptors for the hormones. Responses can change because hormone levels fluctuate or because receptor density on the target cells changes. The principal actions of oestrogen and progesterone during the monthly cycle are on the endometrium, which is one of the tissues most sensitive to ovarian steroid hormones. The endometrium undergoes cyclical changes with the growth of the uterine wall in expectation of an embryo, and then degenerates if fertilization does not take place. In the first half of the cycle, the uterus goes through a proliferative phase. Oestrogen stimulates the epithelial cells of the basal layer of the endometrium to divide and proliferate, forming a thick mucosal wall with numerous endometrial glands (Fig. 4.8). Oestrogen also stimulates proliferation of the stroma and glands and angiogenesis (growth of new blood vessels): extensive vascular tissue, spiral arteries and veins develop within the endometrium. Within the space of a few days, the effect of oestrogen is to increase the height of the wall from 0.5 to 5 mm, a remarkable 10-fold increase. The thickness of the endometrium is monitored by ultrasound in assisted conception (see Chapter 6) to assess whether it is optimal for implantation; the insertion of embryos into a uterine cavity with an endometrium <5 mm thick is unlikely to be successful. The myometrium does not grow extensively during the menstrual cycle. During the proliferative phase, oestrogen primes the endometrial cells by inducing the synthesis of progesterone receptors.

After ovulation, the cells of the enlarging corpus luteum begin to secrete progesterone, which has a dramatic effect on the secretory activity of the endometrial glands. In this secretory phase, the effects of progesterone are dominant,

the gonadotrophs to the pulses. Prior to the LH surge, gonadotroph GnRH receptor density increases and the cells become more sensitive to GnRH. Inhibin A and activin affect secretion of FSH without affecting secretion of GnRH. Two phenomena are observed: first, a depressant effect on output of gonadotrophins by increased oestrogen, progesterone and inhibin A; and second, an increased surge of LH and FSH secretion induced primarily by oestradiol (Fig. 4.7). The pattern of pulsatile secretion of GnRH is regulated by a complex mechanism that allows multiple signals, such as neurotransmitters and sex steroids, to determine ovulation. Both oestrogen and progesterone have a negative feedback effect on the anterior pituitary production of gonadotrophins; oestrogen also reduces the pulse amplitude of GnRH production by the hypothalamus whereas progesterone reduces the pulse frequency (Johnson, 2018).

In the early part of the follicular phase, rising levels of FSH stimulate oestrogen production from the developing follicles. Rising concentrations of oestradiol have a negative feedback effect on gonadotrophin production from the anterior pituitary, so FSH secretion falls. Inhibin A

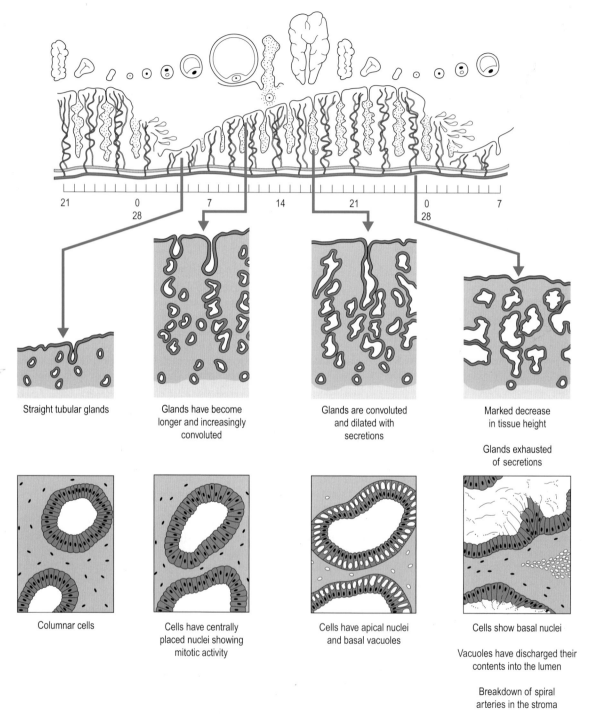

Fig. 4.8 Cyclical effects on the endometrium.

although oestrogen is still secreted from the corpus luteum. The spiral arteries continue growing and thus become more prominent and coiled as the height of the endometrium remains unchanged. The endometrial glands become dilated and convoluted with secretions rich in glycogen, mucus, proteins, sugars, amino acids and enzymes. The secretory products are important for the survival and nutrition of the zygote and blastocyst prior to implantation. Failure of conception results in atresia of the corpus luteum and decreased steroid hormone production. By the 7th postovulatory day, the secretory process ceases and the glands become exhausted and regress.

Cyclical effects are particularly evident within the female reproductive tract. Activity of the myometrium is inversely related to progesterone secretion. During menstruation, when progesterone levels are low, the uterine contractions, mediated by prostaglandins, have a higher frequency and strength than in labour. These uterine contractions are responsible for dysmenorrhoea (period pains). Nonsteroidal anti-inflammatory drugs (NSAIDs) such as aspirin inhibit prostaglandin synthesis, and are therefore effective in reducing period pain. After menstruation, there is a slow decline in myometrial activity during the follicular phase; it reaches negligible activity mid-cycle. Thus, the uterus is at its most quiescent (still) at the time of implantation. Uterine quiescence is maintained until the late luteal phase when levels of progesterone fall. If pregnancy intervenes, levels of progesterone remain high and the myometrium remains inactive. Uterine blood flow, on the other hand, correlates positively with the pattern of oestrogen secretion. Because of low levels of oestrogen, blood supply to the endometrium during menses and early follicular phase is reduced. A marked increase occurs just prior to ovulation followed by a slight nadir. A secondary peak occurs in the luteal phase, which mirrors the rise in oestrogen production. This means that endometrial blood flow is relatively high at the time of implantation but lower at menstruation, which helps to limit the blood loss at the latter time.

Uterine contractile activity varies with the stage of the menstrual cycle. The periovulatory waves of muscle contraction are directional, moving inwards from the cervix to the fundus, encouraging the semen to travel towards the egg (Kuijsters et al., 2017). In the preovulatory period, uterine peristaltic activity within the uterine tube also directs sperm transport preferentially to the uterine tube lateral to the ovary containing the dominant follicle. The uterine activity is relatively quiescent in the late luteal phase, which favours implantation. However, there are still some gentle peristaltic waves that may promote high fundal implantation. It is thought that uterine peristalsis may cause some retrograde menstruation, which may be

of evolutionary benefit and help to preserve body iron. Dysfunction of uterine activity may be involved in the development of endometriosis (Box 4.8), uterine adenomyosis and infertility.

BOX 4.8 Endometriosis

Endometriosis is a condition in which endometrial tissue, usually located inside the uterine cavity, has 'escaped' and established outcrops of endometrial tissue outside the uterus, usually on the surrounding tissue such as the ovaries or uterine tubes or on the internal wall of the abdominal cavity. Endometriosis affects around 8% of women. The main symptom is recurrent pelvic pain (although about 25% of women with endometriosis are pain free), which changes cyclically during the menstrual cycle and worsens at menstruation as the endometrial tissue is hormonally responsive and thickens and bleeds. In severe cases, back and abdominal pain may also be present. Endometriosis is often associated with infertility; about 40% of women with endometriosis are infertile and about a third of infertile women are diagnosed with endometriosis. The cause is not known. The current dominant theory is that endometriosis is caused by retrograde menstruation (some of the endometrial debris flowing inwards via the uterine tubes to the peritoneal cavity) but not every woman with retrograde menstrual flow develops endometriosis. Furthermore, endometriosis can occur in other parts of the body such as the brain and has been reported in men, prepubertal girls and fetuses. Other theories suggest stem cells or Müllerian duct tissue may be involved or that endometriosis is due to oxidative stress, immune cell dysfunction or environmental toxins.

In severe cases, this abnormally located endometrial may cause localized swelling and subsequent formation of fibrous tissue (scarring). This can lead to the formation of pelvic adhesions, resulting in abnormal positioning of the abdominal organs, and stuck together in abnormal ways. Severe endometriosis can contribute to infertility as the patency of the uterine tubes can be affected by adhesions and scarring. Treatment options can be hormonal, using combined oral contraceptives and hormone impregnated coils, to suppress the cyclical hormonal responses but these treatments only reduce the symptoms of endometriosis and are not a cure. Surgical intervention to realign tissue by excising the adhesions may reduce pain and restore fertility. Laparoscopic laser therapy and diathermy may be used to destroy the endometriotic tissue to reduce symptoms in severe cases. In extreme cases, bowel resection and partial bladder resection may be required.

Effects on the Uterine Tubes, Cervix and Vagina

Uterine Tubes

Oestrogen stimulates epithelial cell activity, increasing the number of cilia and their movement, as well as fluid secretion. This facilitates the movement of the ovum along the uterine tubes following ovulation. These effects are reversed by progesterone, which inhibits the peristaltic activity of the uterine tube smooth muscle and suppresses ciliary movement and uterine tube secretion.

Cervix

Oestrogen relaxes the myometrial fibres supplying the cervix and increases stromal vascularization and oedema. Collagenase is activated, which causes some dispersal of the tightly bound collagen bundles into a looser matrix. The result is that the cervix becomes softer to touch. The external os everts prior to ovulation. Progesterone causes the cervical muscle to retract and the stroma to become more compact as the collagen matrix reforms. The external os becomes tighter. The change in texture of the cervix is used as part of natural family planning (Box 4.9). The cervix is softer at ovulation and a few days before, coinciding with the fertile period. At this stage, it has the consistency of lips compared with the harder 'nose-like' cartilaginous consistency of the cervix later in the cycle when the effects of progesterone are dominant.

The cyclical changes in blood flow are reflected by the composition of cervical mucus, which is copious and receptive to sperm penetration in mid-cycle (Table 4.1). When progesterone levels are high, small volumes of thick cervical mucus are secreted that are hostile to, and impenetrable by, sperm. The increased viscosity of the mucus in the latter half of the menstrual cycle reduces the risk of ascending infection at the time of implantation.

Both oestrogen and progesterone are secreted from the corpus luteum in the second half of the cycle. The concentrations of oestrogen and progesterone will continue to rise if successful fertilization results in secretion of hCG and consequent survival of the corpus luteum. Therefore, the effects of the hormones on the female body in the second half of the cycle portend the changes that would take place in pregnancy.

Vagina

Oestrogen increases mitotic activity and secretion in the vaginal epithelial cells. It is important when examining cervical cells, obtained from a smear, to relate the morphological characteristics to the stage of a woman's menstrual cycle. Stimulation by progesterone results in an increased size of the nucleus of vaginal epithelial cells. Earlier in the cycle, cells appear flatter, whereas under the influence of progesterone they tend to become clumped and folded. There are also cyclical changes in the pH of the vagina as oestrogen stimulates the growth of commensal lactobacilli (Döderlein's bacilli). These lactobacilli metabolize glycogen from the cervical secretions producing lactic acid as a metabolic by-product, which decreases pH to a level that protects the reproductive tract from opportunistic pathogenic microorganisms.

The resident flora of the vagina also produce volatile aliphatic acids, which have distinctive odours. The profile of acids changes throughout the cycle under the influence of the changing hormones, and may result in changed sexual behaviour. Sexual desire, sexual activities and sexual

---

BOX 4.9 Concepts of Natural Family Planning

- On the basis of periodic abstinence
  - also known as the 'rhythm method' or 'safe period'
  - assumes that the interval between ovulation and menstruation is constant
  - probably most effective for birth spacing
- On the basis of recognition of signs of ovulation and fertile phases of menstrual cycle
  - temperature rise after ovulation
  - increased cervical mucus and watery vaginal secretions (Spinnbarkeit)
  - softer consistency of cervix

TABLE 4.1 Changes in Cervical Mucus

Proliferative Phase (Follicular)	Secretory Phase (Luteal)
'E' MUCUS	'G' MUCUS
Oestrogen	Progesterone
Network of long parallel bundles	Meshwork of polypeptide chain strands
Carbohydrate side chains	Increased carbohydrate side chains
Forms channels 5 µm	Smaller space between wide molecules
High water content (98%)	Lower water content
Copious volume	Scanty volume
Clear	Cloudy
Acellular	Cells present
Spinnbarkeit = 10–20 cm	Spinnbarkeit ~3 cm (stretching between glass plates)
Dehydration: ferning	No ferning
Assists transport of sperm	Forms mucus plug to protect against infection

satisfaction are all reported to increase around ovulation (see Chapter 5). It is suggested that male responses to their partners are affected by these cyclical fluctuations in olfactory stimuli stimulating sexual responsiveness and interaction. These olfactory signals do not seem to be consciously perceived in humans and may possibly be examples of pheromones. Although it was thought that women who live together could demonstrate menstrual synchrony (i.e. a tendency to ovulate and menstruate at the same time) or that menstrual cycles are affected by the lunar phase, there is negligible scientific evidence to support either of these theories (Harris and Vitzthum, 2013).

Other Effects

There are additional effects and benefits of oestrogen on women's health. Oestrogen appears to protect the cardiovascular system; thus, women of reproductive age and normal endocrine function have a lower incidence of hypertension and a reduced risk of cardiovascular disease owing to higher levels of high-density lipoproteins (HDL), which lower circulating levels of cholesterol. Oestrogens stimulate osteoblasts, the cells involved in bone formation, thereby maintaining bone mass. Oestrogens may depress appetite and are mildly anabolic. There is a preovulatory drop in food intake; this decrease in female 'foraging' behaviour is hypothesized to allow the woman more time for activity, including 'shopping' for alternative mates (see Chapter 5). This hypothesis is also supported by the suggestion that because ovulation is concealed in humans, the woman is able to select her mate at ovulation. Increased consumption of food is observed in the late luteal phase.

Postovulatory levels of progesterone are high, causing a slight increase in the basal metabolic rate. The basal body temperature rises owing to the influence of progesterone on the thermoregulatory centre of the hypothalamus. A temperature rise of 0.2–0.6°C confirms ovulation has taken place but does not predict it. In the second half of the cycle, the skin may appear more pigmented and acne may worsen as progesterone increases the constriction of sebaceous glands. Progesterone also increases appetite and energy intake during the luteal phase (Hintze et al., 2017).

Most ovulatory women experience and recognize symptoms indicating impending menstruation but, in some women, these are significant and affect the quality of their lives. Reproduction and behaviour are intimately linked (see Chapter 5); it is understandable that swings in reproductive steroids, which are powerful neuroregulators, have significant effects on many aspects of mood and behaviour (Schiller et al., 2016). Women with premenstrual syndrome (PMS) or the more severe premenstrual dysphoric disorder (PMDD) often report cravings for carbohydrate, which may be associated with feelings of depression (Box 4.10).

BOX 4.10 Premenstrual Syndrome (PMS)

PMS is very common, with cyclic physical and psychological symptoms occurring prior to menstruation; if affects about 50% of women of reproductive age during their lifetime. Premenstrual dysphoric disorder (PMDD) is a more severe form of PMS that is also associated with the luteal phase of the menstrual cycle. PMDD is recognized as a depressive disorder by the American Psychiatric Association and affects about 3–5% of women. It is characterized by anxiety, anger and severe irritability. It is more severe than PMS and usually requires treatment to allow an affected woman to function normally in her environment. Both PMS and PMDD are characterized by mood swings, including depression, but clinical depression occurs in PMDD. Some women have been acquitted of crimes conducted when they were affected by PMS and PMDD.

The cause of PMS is not clear. It may be due to a hormonal imbalance and low progesterone secretion in the luteal phase, abnormal neurotransmitter responses, disorganized aldosterone function leading to water retention, deficient adrenal hormone secretion due to abnormal hypothalamic–pituitary–adrenal function, carbohydrate intolerance, a nutrient deficiency, stress or a combination of these factors. Women may be prescribed antidepressants such as serotonin reuptake inhibitors. Many women select lifestyle modification and complementary or alternative medicine approaches rather than conventional medicine. Women with PMS tend to consume more dairy products, refined sugar and high-sodium foods, so some clinicians recommend reducing the intake of these. As fat contributes to oestrogen levels and fibre helps to reduce the effects of oestrogen on gut microbiota, high-fibre low-fat diets may be recommended. Reducing caffeine intake, from coffee, tea and caffeinated soft drinks, can also be helpful. Vitamin B_6 can affect neurotransmitter release but the evidence that it improves PMS symptoms is inconclusive. As excess vitamin B_6 can cause nerve damage before symptoms of toxicity are evident, the daily dose should be limited. There is some evidence that calcium and/or vitamin D supplements can be beneficial. Of the herbal preparations more commonly used to relieve symptoms, the evidence is stronger for chasteberry (Vitex) and ginkgo than for black cohosh, kava and St John's wort; the effects of evening primrose oil are thought to be a placebo effect. Exercise, such as yoga, helps reduce depression and anxiety symptoms. Many women find that keeping a symptom diary helps to identify exacerbating and relieving strategies.

It is frequently reported by women who are more sensitive to the hormonal changes in the menstrual cycle that common medical and mental health disorders are exacerbated at specific phases of the menstrual cycle (Reid and Soares, 2018). The prevalence of affective disorders is higher in women than in men. Patterns of fluctuations in energy intake, appetite and depression may be associated with low serotonin or dopamine activity or other hormonally induced alterations in the brain, which influence responses to pleasure and desire and thus affect food ingestion; it is hypothesized that increasing carbohydrate intake might influence serotonin levels (Wurtman and Wurtman, 2018). The changes in appetite and cravings, which influence energy intake, may predispose to obesity. Ovarian steroid hormone fluctuations during the menstrual cycle can affect exercise performance (Williams and Ruffing, 2018). Metabolism of drugs and alcohol may also alter cyclically during the menstrual cycle.

Oestrogen and progesterone affect connective tissue oedema and hyperaemia and can cause increased breast size and tenderness. Progesterone binds to renal aldosterone receptors, causing natriuresis (sodium excretion) and competitively blocking aldosterone binding. Aldosterone is normally increased to restore sodium retention, so there is a net effect of sodium retention. Oestrogen stimulates angiotensinogen production, which also tends to enhance sodium retention. Thus, in the luteal phase of the cycle, salt and water retention may be increased causing generalized weight gain and premenstrual feelings of feeling bloated. The fluctuations in oestrogen and progesterone throughout the menstrual cycle affect the skin including skin structure (thickness, collagen production and breakdown and fluid retention), dermal water content (hydration), pigmentation, elasticity, barrier function, improved wound healing and vasodilation. There are also cyclical changes in conditions such as acne and eczema (Raghunath et al., 2015). Thermoregulation, immune function and sleep patterns also exhibit a cyclical pattern in parallel with hormonal changes. In addition, reproductive hormones impact on psychoneurological processes affecting cognitive, emotional and sensory functions, even at the level of hormone fluctuations that occur during the menstrual cycle.

MENSTRUATION

Menstruation is the loss of most of the decidual (superficial) layers of the endometrium accompanied by some blood loss that occurs after withdrawal of steroid hormones, particularly progesterone, at the end of each menstrual cycle. Regression of the corpus luteum results in a sharp drop in progesterone levels, which triggers a local inflammatory response in the endometrium. This involves the activation of matrix metalloproteinases, infiltration of leukocytes, oedema and cytokine production causing the breakdown of the endometrial tissue. During the menstrual cycle, the spiral arteries supply the endometrial stroma in preparation for implantation of the blastocyst; they have a remarkable ability to vasoconstrict during menstruation in order to limit blood loss. In humans, menstrual loss usually lasts about 5–7 days. Humans, and other 'old-world' primates, together with elephant-shrews and fruit bats, are the only animals that menstruate. In these species there is a marked progesterone-related proliferation of the endometrium and implantation is invasive. In most other species, regression of the endometrium is accompanied by reabsorption of tissue debris.

It was suggested that menstruation evolved as a protective mechanism (cleansing process) against sperm-borne pathogens by shedding any infected endometrial tissue and delivering immune cells to the uterine cavity. It has also been suggested that cyclical menstruation protects the uterine tissue from hyperinflammation and oxidative stress associated with deep placentation (Macklon and Brosens, 2014). An alternative hypothesis is that cyclical regression and proliferation of the endometrium is energetically more economical in terms of reproductive costs, than constantly maintaining a receptive endometrium (Maybin and Critchley, 2015). However, the spontaneous decidualization hypothesis is currently favoured. After ovulation, progesterone causes the oestrogen-primed endometrium to decidualize. The endometrial stromal cells become more spherical and secretion of glycogen, PRL and insulin-like growth factor binding protein increase. In menstruating species such as the human, decidualization is extensive and occurs before implantation whereas in those species, which do not menstruate, the changes in the endometrium are triggered by the embryo being in contact with the endometrium at the time of implantation. Spontaneous decidualization before implantation is positively correlated with a high level of trophoblastic invasion during implantation. It is suggested that spontaneous decidualization confers maternal immunotolerance to the allogeneic embryo, facilitating controlled and extensive trophoblastic invasion. It also may provide a selection mechanism by which genetically abnormal embryos can be screened and rejected. Indeed, it is thought that some cases of recurrent miscarriage may be due to implantation of a poor-quality embryo into a poorly decidualized endometrium (Macklon and Brosens, 2014). Repeated shedding and then regeneration of the denuded endometrial surface allows complete repair. Many women who experience recurrent miscarriage do have a successful pregnancy eventually. This concept by which decidualization is involved in embryo selection is known as the 'choosy uterus'; effectively the endometrium acts as a sensor of embryo quality.

Menstruation is an inflammatory process, which results in extensive tissue remodelling and a remarkable degree of repair. The endometrial wall is described as being in a state of 'secretory exhaustion' and begins to breakdown because there is no embryonic signal (i.e. hCG). The mechanism of menstruation is thought to be tissue destruction following necrosis and a self-limiting inflammatory response (Maybin and Critchley, 2015). The degeneration of the corpus luteum results in a fall in oestrogen and progesterone levels, which causes a modest but significant decrease in endometrial tissue height so the spiral arteries are coiled more tightly and compressed. This results in a reduced blood flow, ischaemia and denudement of the endometrial tissue and interstitial haemorrhage. The withdrawal of progesterone stimulates the production of prostaglandins, which are released by the spiral arteries stimulating vasoconstriction and vasodilatation resulting in rhythmic waves of contraction and relaxation in the latter. (The effect is like breaking a wire by rhythmically bending it backwards and forwards.) The waves become longer and more profound causing the decidual endometrium to break away along the natural plane of cleavage. The straight arteries in the basal layer maintain the blood supply. It is from these that new spiral arteries will regenerate. Menstruation also involves an inflammatory response. The fall in progesterone, which is an anti-inflammatory steroid, causes an increased production of cytokines as well as prostaglandins. This results in an influx of leukocytes, particularly neutrophils, and the activation of matrix metalloproteinases, which have the capacity to degrade the extracellular matrix of the tissue. Prostaglandins are also involved in stimulating uterine contractions, which aid the removal of endometrial debris and blood.

Within 12 h, the height of the endometrium falls from 4 to 1 mm. At the end of the secretory phase, there is an ischaemic phase followed by the menstrual phase, leading to the next proliferative phase. Endometrial repair is very rapid and occurs without scarring. Regrowth of the epithelium begins on day 2 and is completed by day 6. The mechanisms involved in endometrial repair following menstruation probably include proliferation of epithelial cells from stem cells at the base of the epithelial glands, mesenchymal cells from the stroma of the endometrium undergoing transition and differentiating into epithelial cells and the regeneration of tissue from endometrial stem cells.

The copious menstrual bleeding in humans may be related to the relatively large size of the uterus and the organization of the microvasculature. Menstrual flow is usually between 35 and 95 mL and consists of endometrial debris and blood. Menstrual blood has been identified as a potentially valuable source of easily harvested stem cells (MenSCs) for regenerative medicine (Lv et al., 2018). Blood loss is limited by vasoconstriction of the spiral arteries and formation of thrombin–platelet plugs in the terminal portions of the straight arteries. When oestrogen secretion resumes at the beginning of the next cycle, it stimulates healing and new tissue growth, including angiogenesis. Menstrual blood does not coagulate in the pattern seen normally. The damaged endometrial cells secrete proteolytic and fibrinolytic enzymes, which inhibit the formation of fibrin and therefore clot formation. The average volume of blood loss per month is 26–60 mL (which is equivalent to about 0.5–0.7 mg of iron, a loss that is just matched by dietary iron absorption (Coad and Conlon, 2011). Blood loss is lower in women using oral contraceptives and higher in women using intrauterine contraceptive devices. Women of late reproductive age, prior to menopause, tend to have higher blood loss (average 60 mL/month), which may sometimes be excessive (>200 mL). Heavy menstrual blood loss (>80 mL per cycle, menorrhagia) is associated with iron loss, which is difficult to replace from a normal diet. Women who have high menstrual blood loss may have less vascular smooth muscle in their spiral arteries and/or an imbalance of vasoconstrictive prostaglandins (Maybin and Critchley, 2015).

Case study 4.1 gives an example of calculating the length of gestation from the date of the LMP.

HORMONAL CAUSES OF INFERTILITY

Hormonal causes of infertility account for about one-third of the known causes (Box 4.11).

Hypogonadotrophic Hypogonadism

Hypogonadotrophic hypogonadism (HH) is caused by malfunction of the HPA. It can be due to problems with either the hypothalamus (lack of GnRH) or the anterior pituitary gland (lack of gonadotrophins: FSH and LH) and is characterized by low levels of oestrogen. There are two

---

CASE STUDY 4.1

Martha is expecting her third baby. Her previous pregnancies ended at term +7 days with normal uncomplicated deliveries. Martha reports that she always has regular menstrual cycles of 35 days. Martha informs the midwife that she thinks that this baby will arrive 1 week later than the EDD that the midwife has given her. Following a routine antenatal scan, her EDD is revised and 1 week is added onto the calculated EDD. Is Martha right to be confident in her EDD and can you explain why the ultrasound resulted in the recalculation of the EDD?

forms: congenital HH (due to genetic abnormalities and abnormal migration of the GnRH neurons in embryonic development, which affects pubertal development) or acquired HH (usually due to tumour production of hormones, which interfere with the HPA).

Women with HH and normal pituitary functions can be successfully treated with pulsatile exogenous GnRH from a small infusion pump. The hypothalamus is entrained by the pump so normal rhythms of pulsatile secretion continue after the pump is removed. Alternatively, women can be treated with exogenous gonadotrophins. Human menopausal gonadotrophin (hMG) extracted from the urine of postmenopausal women (the effects of ovariectomy or the menopause is decrease oestradiol concentrations, which results in raised circulating levels of FSH and LH) is used because it contains both FSH and enough LH to stimulate synthesis of androgenic precursors for oestrogen production. Ultrasound monitoring of follicular development is important to assess the development of excess follicles and the risk of multiple pregnancy. Ovarian stimulation can cause iatrogenic ovarian hyperstimulation syndrome (OHSS), which has serious implications because vascular permeability can suddenly increase resulting in fluid imbalance, which can be life-threatening (Kwik and Maxwell, 2016). In many respects, HH resembles menopause.

Anorexic States and Weight Fluctuations

Weight loss can also disrupt the HPA. Anorexic patients often have disrupted menstrual cycles, but acute weight loss or disruptions in energy intake (such as those associated with 'crash' dieting) even within a normal body weight range may also affect hormone secretion. A body mass index (BMI) >19 kg/m^2 and at least 22% fat as a proportion of body weight seem to be necessary for the maintenance of normal ovulatory cycles. It has been suggested that the critical fat mass for fertility is equivalent to the energy requirements of pregnancy (Frisch, 1990). Low body fat delays puberty and the menarche. Weight loss particularly affects LH secretion and can result in an abbreviated luteal phase.

BOX 4.11 Hormonal Causes of Infertility

- Hypogonadotrophic hypogonadism
- Anorexic states
- Weight fluctuations
- Obesity
- Hormonal anomalies that affect ovulation including hyper- and hypothyroidism
- Hyperprolactinaemia
- Polycystic ovary syndrome (PCOS)

Appetite is stimulated by the hormone ghrelin, secreted by the stomach in response to hunger, which signals via orexigenic neuropeptide Y (NPY) neurons in the hypothalamus to stimulate food intake. NPY has both stimulatory and inhibitory effects at the pituitary gland. In the well-nourished state, NPY release is acute and intermittent, a mode of secretion that potentiates GnRH-induced LH release. However, fasting stimulates ghrelin secretion and decreases plasma glucose concentrations and, as with extremes of exercise, results in chronic secretion of NPY and continuous NPY receptor activation, which is inhibitory to LH release and thus fertility.

Eating increases storage of triacylglycerides in adipose cells, which stimulates the cells to release leptin. Leptin is a satiety signal that, like insulin (which is elevated after carbohydrate consumption), inhibits NPY neurons in the hypothalamus and inhibits food intake. In starvation, leptin and insulin levels are low and ghrelin levels are high, stimulating NPY levels, which inhibits GnRH. The nutritional control of reproduction probably had an important evolutionary role in suppressing fertility at times of poor food supply. Suspending reproductive function at times of food shortage is protective.

Case study 4.2 looks at the problem of underweight in the calculation of gestation.

CASE STUDY 4.2

Mona, a 16-year-old primipara, presents herself at the midwives' clinic, giving a vague history and saying that she thinks she might be pregnant. Mona is pale and appears extremely underweight and, during the past 6 months, has been homeless due to a disagreement with her parents. On palpation and abdominal examination, Mona seems to be about 26 weeks' pregnant and this is supported by a fundal height of 26 cm as measured by the midwife. The auscultation of fetal heart sounds confirms that Mona is indeed pregnant.

On questioning Mona, the midwife discovers that Mona has had only two scanty periods in the last 2 years and does not know the date of her last menstrual period. Mona smokes 60 cigarettes a day and often consumes excessive amounts of alcohol.

- Can you identify any possible reasons why Mona might have irregular periods?
- Why must the midwife not assume that Mona is 26 weeks' pregnant?
- Are there any clues that the midwife may investigate (or refer for further investigation) to estimate more precisely the actual gestation of Mona's pregnancy?

Obesity

Paradoxically, since a low BMI has negative effects, fertility is also affected by obesity; obese women are over-represented in fertility clinics and have an increased incidence of menstrual abnormality and a higher risk of miscarriage. The effects of obesity may persist even after weight loss has occurred. One of the reasons is that the adipose tissue is metabolically active, producing altered ratios of oestrogens and androgens. Obesity also affects insulin secretion and obese individuals are more likely to exhibit insulin resistance with effects on leptin production and therefore on hypothalamic signalling.

Hyperprolactinaemia

Hyperprolactinaemia can result from PRL-secreting tumours, which are usually benign. However, other factors including stress, breast stimulation or examination, hypothyroidism, polycystic ovary syndrome (PCOS) and dopaminergic antagonists can also raise circulating PRL levels. Hyperprolactinaemia can cause oestrogen deficiency, amenorrhoea and galactorrhoea (milk production not associated with pregnancy or childbirth). The management of hyperprolactinaemia is usually by administration of bromocriptine, a dopamine agonist (see Chapter 16), although tumours may be surgically removed.

Polycystic Ovary Syndrome

The prevalence of PCOS suggests that approximately 5–10% of women are affected by this disorder, although uncertainties about the correct diagnostic criteria might make this an underestimate. As such, PCOS is one of the most common endocrine and metabolic disorders in premenopausal women and is one of the leading causes of infertility. It is usually suspected from clinical signs and symptoms; diagnosis is confirmed by ultrasound examination that shows enlarged ovaries containing more than 10 large cysts. Some women exhibit symptoms of disrupted cycles, central obesity and hyperandrogenism, which can cause acne, alopecia and hirsutism. The aetiology of PCOS remains uncertain but is thought to reflect a genetic predisposition with dietary, lifestyle and epigenetic factors also involved. The endocrine causes are hypersecretion of LH, glucose intolerance and increased levels of testosterone, insulin and PRL. Oestrogen levels are high but not cyclical and frequently ovulation does not occur. Studies using animal models have also implicated prenatal exposure to excess androgen levels leading to a permanent PCOS-like phenotype (Escobar-Morreale, 2018). A characteristic of PCOS is that the follicles retain the oocyte, forming ovarian cysts, which may take on a 'string-of-pearls' appearance. Weight loss often improves the hormonal profile and alleviates the symptoms. Women with PCOS are at greater risk of developing insulin resistance, impaired glucose tolerance and type 2 diabetes; when pregnant, they are at greater risk of developing gestational diabetes.

Clomifene citrate (Clomid) is an anti-oestrogenic drug that can be used to re-establish a normal pattern of ovulation in women with PCOS; however, its use is associated with an increased risk of multiple pregnancies. In cases where women fail to respond to clomifene citrate, especially if the BMI is >25 kg/m^2, combined treatment with metformin and clomifene citrate improves ovulation and pregnancy rates (NICE, 2013).

ARTIFICIAL CONTROL OF FERTILITY

Oral Contraceptives

The most common form of contraception is the oral contraceptive pill. The first oral contraceptives were extracts from yam. Although yams are rich in progesterone-like compounds, the active ingredient was actually mestranol, an oestrogenic agent. The combination of progestogen and mestranol was essential for good cycle control; mestranol comprised the oestrogenic component of many of the first oral contraceptive pills. Natural progesterone and most other steroid hormones are digested in the gastrointestinal tract and are usually effective only if injected. Chemically modified analogues of the hormones are resistant to digestion in the gut but retain their biological activity. Many synthetic steroid hormones have been developed that have similar biological activity to the naturally occurring hormones and are metabolized very slowly by the liver, increasing their half-life. The term 'progestogens' is used to describe the family of natural and synthetic progesterone-like compounds.

The first contraceptive pills, used in Britain since 1961, were combined oral contraceptive (COC) pills, combinations of an oestrogen and a progestogen. Currently, the most common progestogen and oestrogen combinations used are norethisterone and ethinyloestradiol, respectively (Fig. 4.9). A course of COC pills is taken for 21 days followed by 7 pill-free (or placebo) days when hormone levels fall, simulating natural hormonal cycles and allowing a withdrawal bleed. Monophasic pills have a constant concentration of the active agents whereas biphasic and triphasic preparations attempt to mimic the characteristic fluctuations in oestrogen and progesterone throughout the cycle. Monophasic pills can be taken for extended cycles, e.g. for 3 months if the placebo pills are skipped or as a 3-month pack.

Progesterone-only preparations (POP), known as 'mini-pills', containing small doses of only progesterone

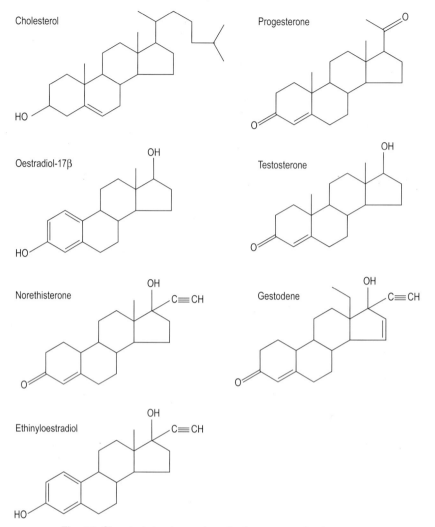

Fig. 4.9 Chemical structures of synthetic contraceptive hormones.

are taken on a continuous basis. Progesterone can also be administered as a depot injection or as a slow-releasing preparation from a subcutaneous or uterine source. It takes at least one complete menstrual cycle for the pill to become effective. Some drugs reduce the effect of the pill and can cause breakthrough bleeding, or even permit pregnancy. These include barbiturates, rifampicin-like antibiotics (but not other antibiotics), some antiepileptic and antiretroviral drugs and St John's Wort (*Hypericum perforatum*; a herbal medicine used as a treatment for depression).

There are two methods of emergency contraception: emergency postcoital/hormonal contraceptive pills (ECPs; 'the morning-after pill') or intrauterine devices (IUDs). ECPs contain higher doses of combinations of oestrogen and progesterone or progesterone only than are used in regular oral contraceptive pills. They are taken after contraceptive failure, rape or unprotected sex and may prevent pregnancy, but are more effective when taken close (within 12 h) to intercourse. In the UK, the ECPs (Levonelle and ellaOne) can be purchased from pharmacies or obtained free of charge from various organizations (such as GP surgeries, sexual health clinics, NHS walk-in centres, and some pharmacies and accident and emergency departments of hospitals). In many countries (e.g. the UK), a prescription is not required for girls over 16 years of age.

The IUD is more effective than ECPs and can offer ongoing contraception. Levonelle One Step (sold under several names, e.g. Plan B) is a progesterone-only preparation containing levonorgestrel, which is taken within 72 h of unprotected sex. Levonorgestrel is a progestogen (an agonist of the progesterone receptor), which inhibits ovulation and promotes the thickening of cervical mucus. The ellaOne pill contains ulipristal acetate, which is a selective progesterone receptor modulator (or antiprogestin) that blocks or delays ovulation and/or delays the maturation of the endometrium. It has to be taken within 120 h of unprotected sex (and is also used to treat uterine fibroids).

ECPs have stronger side-effects than regular contraceptive pills (such as headache, abdominal pain, nausea, breast tenderness and fatigue) and relatively low reliability so they are not recommended as the main method of birth control; they also do not protect against sexually transmitted diseases (STDs). ECPs are contraindicated in known or suspected pregnancy; they are not abortifacients. Mifepristone (RU-486) is a synthetic steroid used as an abortifacient for the medical abortion of early pregnancy.

Effects of Oral Contraceptives on the Reproductive Cycle

Synthetic oestrogens will feedback on the hypothalamus during the antral phase of the menstrual cycle, reducing the levels and the rate of pulsatile secretion of GnRH. Therefore, the release of FSH is inhibited and follicular maturation and expression of LH receptors do not occur. The oestrogens also prevent the LH surge and subsequent ovulation. Production of endogenous oestrogen is reduced.

Synthetic progestogens interfere with the pulsatile secretion of GnRH and decrease the production of LH. Small doses of progesterone may not suppress ovulation but large doses inhibit maturation of follicles and ovulation. Norethisterone also slows down the breakdown of natural progesterone by the liver. It can be used in low doses because it specifically binds to the progesterone receptors, rather than to androgen receptors as well. Progestogens also reduce secretory activity of the endometrium, so it is not favourable to implantation. Under the influence of progestogens, the cervical mucus is thick and tenacious and so is unreceptive to sperm. The peristaltic muscle activity and ciliary movement of the uterine tube become uncoordinated, so transport of the ovum and sperm are affected; this may directly affect successful fertilization. This effect on tubal motility is the reason why there is a slight increase in the risk of ectopic pregnancy (implantation in the uterine tube) associated with progesterone preparations.

COCs have their effect by inhibiting ovulation (interrupting feedback on the hypothalamic–pituitary–ovarian axis and reducing FSH and LH), preventing follicular development and maturation, reducing sperm penetrability of the mucous by increasing its viscosity and affecting endometrial growth and receptivity. The progestogen-only pill works by reducing sperm penetrability of the mucous, slowing motility of the uterine tubes, reducing endometrial thickening and receptivity and reducing ovulation. It is well tolerated but has a higher pregnancy rate as timing of pill taking is more important.

Side-effects

Reported side-effects of oral contraceptives include weight gain, headaches and nausea, depression, vaginal infection or discharge, urinary tract infection, breast changes, skin problems and gum inflammation. Oestrogens affect coagulation factors and promote intravascular coagulation so they increase the risk of vascular thrombosis. They also tend to increase plasma lipid levels. Therefore, they can be used safely in young, healthy, motivated women who have no history of circulatory disease. However, smoking and obesity significantly increase the risk of side-effects, particularly thromboembolic complications. Although chemical contraceptive agents have been linked to an increased risk of breast cancer, the doses of synthetic hormone used in current contraceptive preparations are now extremely low, so it is difficult to assess their risk. Contraindications to COC use include arterial disease, smoking, hypertension, migraine, stroke, venous thromboembolism and some cancers. Although hormonal treatment has known thromboembolic health concerns, the morbidity complications from pregnancy and labour far outweigh the risks of using oral contraceptives. Women using oral contraceptives excrete oestrogens into their urine, which enters the water systems and may cause endocrine disruption to fish populations inhabiting streams contaminated with treated sewage effluent.

Non-oral Contraception

The popularity of non-oral hormonal contraception is increasing because it is convenient and efficient and safer for women at risk. Methods include the vaginal ring and contraceptive patches, which contain sustained release oestrogen preparations. Progestogen-only methods include contraceptive implants and injectable depo-preparations. Intrauterine methods such as the copper IUD and long-lasting plastic devices such as the T-shaped levonorgestrel intrauterine system are also effective. Barrier methods of contraception include male and female condoms, diaphragms, caps and spermicides. Sterilization for both men and women is used in many countries as a permanent method of contraception and worldwide is the most common method of contraception. Female sterilization is more common, although male sterilization is safer, more effective and cheaper. Regret following sterilization is reported to be rare, particularly when individuals are at an older age at sterilization, but requests for reversal following vasectomy are fairly commonplace and usually related to new partnerships or death of children.

Puberty

Puberty describes the morphological, physiological and behavioural changes that occur as the gonads change from infantile to the adult condition. The most obvious ('definitive') sign of sexual maturation in women is menarche (the first menstrual cycle), which indicates that the levels of oestrogen and progesterone are adequate to induce development of the uterus. The equivalent step in boys is the first ejaculation, which is often nocturnal. However, menarche or the first ejaculation do not necessarily mean that the adolescent body is able to reproduce; early menstrual cycles are frequently anovulatory and the ejaculate of pubertal boys may be mostly seminal plasma, lacking sperm. The underlying hormonal changes are initiated 2–4 years before menarche and the first ejaculation. The sequence of pubertal changes is constant in that the changes occur in the same order (described as the harmony or 'consonance' of puberty) but the starting age and the time for the changes to take place vary. The hormonal changes at puberty lead to a growth spurt and attainment of adult height. In girls, the pubertal growth spurt occurs early in puberty, whereas in boys the growth spurt occurs late in puberty (Fig. 4.10). There is thought to be an evolutionary advantage to the differential timing of adult appearance (attainment of adult height) and sexual development (fertility). Bigger girls may be treated as equals by other females in society and taught 'female life-skills' before they are able to ovulate and conceive, whereas smaller males will not be construed as competitive by other males in society while they are undergoing physical development despite being able to produce fertile gametes; indeed, becoming fertile while not having an adult appearance may allow an adolescent male to sneakily mate (Bogin, 1999a).

Physical Changes

Physical changes include the development of secondary sex characteristics, the adolescent growth spurt and marked changes in height, psychological states and fertility. All muscle and skeletal dimensions change and the body composition also alters. The earliest changes are measurable in young girls from the age of 6 years. Secondary sex characteristics become evident as secretion of oestrogen (from ovaries) and androgens (from ovaries and adrenal glands) increases. Changes are seen in the breasts, genitalia, pubic hair and voice.

Hormonal Changes

The hypothalamic–pituitary–gonadal axis, which has been developing since fetal life, is activated in early

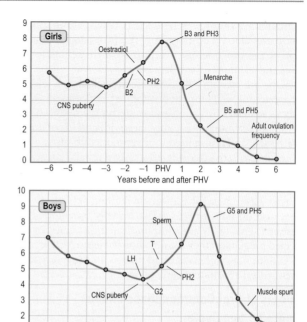

Fig. 4.10 Order of sexual maturation events for girls and boys during the adolescent growth spurt. CNS puberty represents the changed activity of the hypothalamus and nervous system controlling the pubertal changes; stages prefixed B, G and PH represent the development of the breasts, male genitalia and pubic hair, respectively, on a 5-point scale. Note that sexual maturation in girls (marked by menarche) follows the peak height velocity (PHV), but in boys (marked by sperm production) occurs before the peak height velocity. (Reproduced with permission from Bogin, 1999b.)

infancy but inhibited in childhood before being reactivated ('re-awoken') at puberty. Immediately after birth, levels of hCG and placental steroid hormones fall. LH and FSH levels increase and they are released in a pulsatile pattern, with nocturnal dominance, throughout infancy and childhood. FSH levels are higher in females and LH levels are higher in males. In the prepubertal period, FSH levels are relatively high compared with LH levels.

At puberty, the pulse amplitude of GnRH increases, resulting in dramatically increased magnitude and frequency of LH secretion, particularly during sleep. In late puberty, day-time secretion of LH also increases until the adult pattern of higher basal LH levels is reached. The 'on' switch for puberty is unknown but may be related to body mass, energy metabolism, leptin secretion or other nutritional factors. There is a progressive change in pituitary responsiveness to GnRH, and a lifting of the restraint on the hypothalamus, which may be related to maturation of the central nervous system and hypothalamus. One of the important signals appears to be activation of the kisspeptin system (Tena-Sempere, 2012). Kisspeptins are a family of peptides, which bind to the kisspeptin receptors in the hypothalamus, which are closely associated with the GnRH neurons. They have recently been identified as essential neuropeptide regulators of reproductive maturation, which influence the onset of puberty, ovulation and the metabolic regulation of fertility. Adrenal function matures independently before gonadal function and adrenal secretion of sex steroids increases. Adrenal androgens stimulate pubic and axillary hair growth and have a small effect on growth and bone development. The timing of gonadal maturity and the onset of puberty correlate more closely with bone development than with chronological age. The central nervous system can restrain the onset of puberty by affecting the pattern of hypothalamic GnRH secretion.

Delayed puberty may result from Kallmann syndrome, a form of hypogonadotropic hypogonadism, which is a genetic abnormality arising from mutations in a number of genes that results in a deficiency of GnRH release from the hypothalamus. Precocious puberty, when puberty is initiated at a very early age, is usually unexplained and probably due to natural variation but it can also be a result of brain injury or a tumour such as a hypothalamic or pituitary tumour and unusually high production of GnRH or gonadotrophins. Whatever the cause, precocious puberty has serious consequences for social and psychological development and can influence adult height (as the pubertal hormone surges cause the early closure of the bone epiphyses and the cessation of subsequent growth). The increasing incidence of childhood obesity has tended to result in girls entering puberty earlier and boys entering puberty later. It has been suggested that the earlier timing of puberty over the last few decades has resulted in a dissociation between biological maturity, which occurs at an earlier age and psychosocial maturity, which lags behind and that this mismatch of modern puberty is instrumental in some of the social issues faced by adolescents today (Gluckman and Hanson, 2006).

Age of Menarche

Over half of early menstrual cycles are anovulatory and do not result in the release of an ovum. Ovulation usually first occurs about 10 months after menarche. After a period of 5 years, the incidence of anovulatory cycles decreases to ~20%. There are secular trends in the age of menarche, which has become progressively earlier, particularly in the early to mid-20th century. The average age of menarche in Europe is currently 12–13 years compared with 14–15 years a century ago. However, with the marked increase in childhood obesity over the last 20 years, the age of menarche has fallen in parallel with increased body size. Accelerated pubertal development may be associated with increased morbidity and mortality in later life. Early age at menarche has been linked to metabolic disorders such as obesity, type 2 diabetes and cardiovascular disease and to other health problems such as breast cancer, impaired fertility, psychological disorders and behavioural issues (Yermachenko and Dvornyk, 2014).

Various influences on the age of menarche have been investigated and both genetic and environmental factors have been identified. Although the effect of genetics is strong, environmental factors are potentially modifiable but the effect varies in different populations. Age at menarche is particularly influenced by factors, which affect growth in the prenatal and early childhood years such as body weight, intake of animal protein, levels of physical activity and family stressors (e.g. single parenting) (Yermachenko and Dvornyk, 2014).

The Frisch hypothesis suggested that women have a critical body mass or critical fat mass for successful reproduction; if their body mass falls <48 kg or body fat is <22%, the menstrual cycle becomes erratic and stops (Frisch and Revelle, 1971). Anorexic women have lower levels of FSH and LH (see p. 104). Moderate obesity is associated with earlier menarche but severe obesity delays it. The combination of heavy exercise and undernutrition is synergistic, as can be observed in ballet dancers and athletes (see Chapter 12). Chronic illness or stress can also delay menarche but the exact mechanisms involved are unknown. An alternative view is that there are genetic factors influencing the rate of development and that body fatness and age at menarche are both driven by the 'blueprint' or genetic plan, rather than age at menarche being a consequence of fat deposition. Children who are taller tend to have earlier pubertal development and the age at menarche correlates better with height than with weight.

Sequence of Changes at Puberty

The normal sequence in females (Fig. 4.10) is breast budding (at 8–13 years), growth of pubic hair, peak growth velocity (9.5–14.5 years) and then menarche (10–16.5 years). The pattern in boys is testicular growth, pubic hair growth, penile growth and growth spurt. These characteristic changes in pubic hair distribution and breast development in girls and external genitalia in boys have been classified as Tanner stages, which are used to assess pubertal development (Table 4.2).

From about 6 months of age, childhood growth depends on adequate growth hormone (GH) secretion. Growth declines progressively and reaches its slowest velocity just

TABLE 4.2	Tanner Stages of Pubertal Development		
Stage	Pubic Hair	Breast Development in Females	External Genitalia in Males
1	None	Prepubertal; no breast tissue and papilla elevated	Pre-adolescent stage
2	Sparse growth of long downy hair along labia	Areolar enlargement with breast bud	Scrotum and testes enlarged (>4 mL); changes texture/colour of scrotal skin
3	Coarser and curly pigmented hairs	Enlargement of breast and areolar as a single mound	Further growth of testes (6–10 mL) and scrotum; increase in penis size
4	Small adult configuration	Projection of areolar above breast as a double mound	Further enlargement of testes (10–15 mL), scrotum and penis; glans penis development
5	Adult pubic hair distribution	Mature adult breast as a single mound	Adult stage

before the onset of the pubertal growth spurt. In boys, the growth spurt starts slightly later, and is faster (9.4 cm/year compared with 8.3 cm/year in girls) with delayed fusion of the epiphyseal plates, so men attain a higher adult height. The pubertal growth spurt depends on sex hormones secreted from the gonads. Optimal growth depends on both GH levels, which are highest in the pubertal period, and on sex steroids. Lack of GH during development can cause dwarfism, whereas abnormally high levels of GH before the epiphyseal plates have fused can cause gigantism, the most extreme example of which resulted in an adult height of 2.72 m.

MENOPAUSE

Women continue to have menstrual cycles until the finite population of oocytes in the ovary is exhausted; when the number of oocytes dwindles to about 1000, the hormonal drive is inadequate and ovulation ceases (Herbert et al., 2015). The term 'menopause' is literally the cessation of menstrual cycles. It is defined as permanent cessation of menstruation due to loss of ovarian follicular activity after 12 consecutive months of amenorrhoea without another cause and, hence, can only be determined retrospectively 12 months after the final menstrual period. However, the term 'menopause' is frequently applied to the climacteric (perimenopausal phase), which is the transitional decline of reproductive activity over a period of 2–3 years leading up to the final menstrual period, usually occurring between the ages of 45 and 55 years (median 50–51 years). Age at menopause is extremely consistent among different populations and over time, despite longevity having increased. The climacteric begins when fertility is already rapidly declining and continues until the ovaries cease secreting oestrogen. Ovarian senescence is actually a gradual process beginning from around 35 years of age; it is marked by a progressive decline in fertility and increased rate of menstrual irregularity, miscarriage and birth defects such as trisomy 21 from the mid-30s onwards.

The hormonal changes of menopause affect particularly the tissues that have a high density of oestrogen receptors such as skin, epithelium of the vagina and bladder, neuronal tissue (changes in neurotransmitter release affect libido, irritability, mood, sleep, concentration and memory) and factors, which influence cardiovascular and bone health. Thermoregulation is also affected.

The decline in oestrogen production is related to the follicular reserve: the number of remaining primordial follicles, the number recruited in each cycle and the proportion of follicles that reach maturity before ovulation (Davis et al., 2015). As the pool of oocytes gets smaller, hormonal changes occur; these precede the final depletion of follicles. Defective follicular phases result in fewer granulosa cells in the follicle and therefore reduced oestrogen production. As oestrogen exerts a negative feedback effect on the HPA, the decrease in oestrogen level causes FSH level to rise from about 35 years onwards. The first notable hormonal change preceding the climacteric is a decrease in inhibin B secretion, which results in a lowering of the negative feedback on the hypothalamic–pituitary–gonadal axis. Inhibin B is produced from the small antral follicles and so peaks in the first half of the menstrual cycle; it is a marker of the size and growth of the antral follicle cohort. As fewer follicles are recruited the level of inhibin B falls so its inhibitory effect on the HPA decreases. Therefore, FSH secretion increases, which means more follicles are recruited at this early stage of the climacteric.

The increased level of follicular development results in enhanced oestrogen production from the greater number of follicles; twin ovulations (and pregnancies) are more common. This, paradoxically, means that fertility towards the end of reproductive life is increased (reflected in an increased rate in twinning in older women) but it also increases the rate at which the dwindling pool of oocytes are depleted. So, the hormonal changes move from being compensated to decompensated as the follicles are rapidly depleted below a critical number. The compromised hormonal status then results in a decreased follicular phase of the cycle and a shorter cycle length. Functioning of the ovary becomes more erratic with a variable cycle length and an increased number of anovulatory cycles. Luteinization does not occur; there is no increase in progesterone secretion but oestrogen drives endometrial proliferation, which can be excessive, as can be menstrual loss when there is a cycle with successful luteinization. Eventually, as the follicles are depleted, oestrogen and progesterone levels fall and menstrual cycles cease. The loss of steroid hormone negative feedback results in a gradual rise in FSH secretion, which tends to fluctuate from cycle to cycle.

The loss of follicles means that there is no oestrogen production from granulosa cells and no recruitment of thecal cells that produced androgens. Although the postmenopausal ovary no longer synthesizes oestradiol, there is some peripheral conversion of androstenedione by adipose tissue providing a source of oestrone. Thus, body fat essentially acts like inbuilt hormone replacement therapy (HRT). The adrenal gland produces a small amount of progesterone and some testosterone. Dehydroepiandrosterone production by the ovaries falls, which means ovarian androstenedione production falls (although some is still produced by the adrenal gland), so testosterone levels fall. The secretion of sex hormone binding globulin (SHBG) from the liver diminishes because its production is stimulated by oestrogen and inhibited by androgens (and obesity). Postmenopausally, levels of SHBG fall and bioavailability of free testosterone is enhanced. However, overall the net effect is one of androgen deficiency, which can affect sense of wellbeing, muscle mass and strength, sexual desire and sexual receptivity, sexual arousal and orgasm, memory and cognition, and cause depression, adding to the effect of oestrogen deficiency.

Premature menopause is defined as menopause before 40 years of age; it is usually a result of autoimmune disorders, genetics or problems with ovarian development or chromosomal abnormalities. Menopause can also be induced, for instance by surgery (removal of ovaries usually with a hysterectomy) or by treatment for cancer. With recent increases in longevity, an average woman may spend about 35–40% of her lifespan in the postmenopausal period. Menopause is a complex and natural process of ageing and is thought to have an evolutionary advantage. There are advantages to the species in preventing late childbearing and ensuring that the dependent human offspring are more likely to have the care and protection of their mother (and she to have the support of her mother; Kim et al., 2019). The 'Grandmother Hypothesis' suggests that the presence of postmenopausal women is beneficial for the species; human infants are altricial (very helpless and dependent); maturation is delayed (because childhood is an important learning time for a species with a big brain); infant mortality rates are high and inter-birth intervals are short. Grandmothers are socially established, reliable and skilled, possess specialized knowledge and have a vested interest in the survival of their grandchildren. Indeed, there are examples of grandmothers (who have their own infants), being able to take over the breastfeeding of their grandchildren (Scelza, 2009).

A number of factors affect the age of menopause. These include leanness and nutritional status, ethnicity and genetics. Smokers, women who have not had children and women of lower socioeconomic status tend to have an earlier menopause, as do women who have shorter menstrual cycle length. There is no relationship between age at menarche and age at menopause.

Effects on the Reproductive System

Morphologically, the ovaries at menopause appear smaller and relatively devoid of follicles. There is a finite number of ova; however, hormonal changes precede the depletion of follicles. There are about 1000 follicles remaining at the time of menopause. One of the earliest changes is a decrease in inhibin production by the granulosa cells. This results in decreased negative feedback at the HPA and an increase in the GnRH level, which promotes secretion of FSH and follicular development. This is the reason for the paradoxical increase in twinning rate that is observed in women conceiving late in reproductive life. After this brief increase in follicular development, the menstrual cycles tend to become shorter, particularly in the follicular phase. This results in oestrogen secretion diminishing, so the production of androgens increases. Menstrual cycles become increasingly erratic with variable cycle lengths and an increase in anovulatory cycles. Anovulation is associated with progesterone deficiency, which is associated with prolonged or irregular vaginal bleeding. As the cycles become less frequent, there is increased time for endometrial proliferation, which can lead to excessive menstrual blood loss. Ultimately, oestrogen and progesterone levels decrease and cycling ceases.

From menopause onwards, levels of FSH and LH are high and levels of oestrogen and inhibin are decreased. FSH increases because of the lack of a negative feedback from oestrogen influencing the anterior pituitary gland. The postmenopausal ovary continues to produce considerable amounts of androgens and some progesterone; thus, natural menopause is not equivalent to the effects of a surgically induced menopause following oophorectomy (removal of ovaries). There is some oestrogen production by the adipose tissue; this (and the protective cushioning provided by fat) is the reason why fatter women are protected, at least partially, from osteoporosis (however, note that increased inflammation associated with marked obesity is detrimental to bone health).

Effects on Other Physiological Systems

In addition to the reproductive tract itself, there are many other target organs bearing oestrogen receptors, which respond to the fall in circulating oestrogen levels. The resulting vasomotor instability produces symptoms of hot flushes (or 'hot flashes'), sweats and palpitations. The thermoregulatory centre in the hypothalamus falsely signals that body temperature is too high. It is thought that the decreased oestrogen level abrogates the catecholamine–oestrogen inhibition of tyrosine hydroxylase so noradrenaline levels are increased. This results in physiological processes such as increased peripheral vasodilation that attempt to reduce core body temperature. Hot flushes are not always visible but may be extreme; skin temperature may increase by as much as 7–8°C for a few minutes accompanied by a rapid increase in heart rate. Emotional and psychological problems such as anxiety, depression, loss of libido and mood swings may occur. Insomnia is also a frequently cited problem.

All the tissues of the female reproductive tract have a high density of oestrogen receptors and are profoundly affected by oestrogen withdrawal. The uterus shrinks. The vaginal epithelium diminishes and becomes less elastic. The vaginal cells decrease production of glycogen, affecting lactobacillus colonization, so the pH increases, resulting in increased susceptibility to vaginal infections. Vaginal atrophy causes vaginal secretions to diminish, which may result in painful intercourse. Menopausal women have an increased frequency of urinary problems, which is probably related to oestrogen withdrawal as there are many oestrogen receptors in the urinary tract (which shares the same embryonic origin as the lower reproductive tract). The walls of the lower bladder and urethra become thinner and the urethral muscles weaken, which increases the risk of stress incontinence.

Oestrogen protects the cardiovascular system; the risk of cardiovascular disease doubles in women following menopause. The incidence of coronary heart disease in premenopausal women, and in postmenopausal women treated with HRT, is much lower than in men. Oestrogen inhibits the uptake and degradation of low-density lipoprotein (LDL) by the coronary blood vessel endothelium. It may also inhibit coronary vasospasm. Oestrogen has been shown to decrease vascular resistance (and therefore blood pressure), increase cardiac output and increase synthesis of nitric oxide (NO, a potent locally acting vasodilator). Postmenopausal women have significantly higher levels of serum cholesterol and triacylglycerides. Oestrogen inhibits endothelial hyperplasia, smooth muscle cell growth and platelet activation. Oestrogen withdrawal is associated with raised levels of certain blood-clotting factors and an increased tendency for thrombosis, and thus with increased risk of myocardial infarction and cerebrovascular accident (stroke). Insulin resistance is more common in postmenopausal women.

Skeletal changes occur as the decrease in oestrogen results in increased bone resorption, increasing the tendency to stoop and the likelihood of fractures. Osteoblasts (bone-producing cells) have oestrogen receptors. Osteoclast activity increases postmenopause and osteoblast activity decreases. Oestrogen deficiency uncouples bone formation and bone resorption. This effect is increased by changes in the hormones controlling calcium balance. Levels of calcitonin fall in parallel with oestrogen levels. Calcitonin inhibits the activity of osteoclasts (bone-absorbing cells). The progressive loss of calcium from the bones and the long postmenopausal lifetime mean that a woman can lose about half of her trabecular bone mass and about one-third of her cortical bone and is therefore predisposed to osteoporosis. Collagen is also lost from the skin, tendons and bones.

There are also changes in metabolism and body composition postmenopause. Women tend to gain fat, especially visceral fat, and to lose muscle mass.

Hormone Replacement Therapy

HRT aims to reduce the diverse symptoms and adverse effects of the menopause (Box 4.12). HRT provides low doses of various combinations of hormones. It is effective during its use but not in the long term. Oestrogen on its own is mitogenic and promotes endometrial hyperplasia (which is associated with an increased risk of cancer). Oestrogen with progesterone is safer as progesterone abrogates cell division and increases endometrial secretory activity. The Women's Health Initiative (WHI) studies in the United States looked at long-term health outcomes of women taking HRT using randomized controlled primary-prevention trials. The WHI studies found that HRT increased the risk of heart disease, stroke, deep vein thrombosis, pulmonary embolism and some types of cancer. This was at odds with previous studies, which tended to select healthy women as subjects and excluded women who smoked or might be at increased risk of vascular disease. However, the figures need to be considered in context; although the risk of disease was increased significantly, the actual numbers of women affected were very low. Rather than being a panacea for all menopausal problems, there are benefits and risks to HRT, which need to be assessed, as for all medications. Some women have extreme menopause symptoms, which have a negative influence on their quality of life.

BOX 4.12 Hormone Replacement Therapy (HRT)

- Exogenous oestrogen and progesterone analogues are administered to replace ovarian steroids
- Effective during use but not long term (no longer than 5 years before the age of 60 is the usual recommendation)
- Oral route or directly to genital tract or systemically (transdermal patch or subcutaneous implant, which minimize hepatic oestrogen metabolism)
- Abrogates flushing and sweating, vaginal atrophy and dryness, dyspareunia, decreased libido
- Stimulates replication of, and secretion from, vaginal epithelial cells
- Progesterone is required as 'unopposed' oestrogen has a mitogenic effect and promotes endometrial hyperplasia (which could lead to cancer)
- Progesterone is given to induce menstruation (and prevent endometrial hyperplasia)
- Progesterone-withdrawal bleeding is a major reason for noncompliance
- HRT decreases the risk of bone fracture (hip and vertebral) and colon cancer but increases the risk of cardiovascular disease and stroke, breast cancer and dementia; the changed risk is small
- The effects of HRT are variable and depend on dose of steroids, type of steroid analogue used, timing of the dose in relation to menopause and the age of the woman

KEY POINTS

- The ovary produces the female gametes (ova) and steroid hormones, oestrogen and progesterone.
- Relatively few female gametes are released by the ovaries (ovulated) during a woman's reproductive life, between puberty and the menopause.
- The meiotic division of the ovum begins in the female fetus and is suspended until ovulation, then halts again, and is completed at fertilization.
- Follicular development begins about 3 months prior to ovulation but key stages in development of the follicles are stimulated by FSH in the first half of the menstrual cycle in which the ovum is released. The developing follicles produce oestrogen; usually a single dominant follicle matures and ovulates.
- The first half of the menstrual cycle (follicular phase) is dominated by oestrogen and prepares the reproductive system for ovulation, for instance by stimulating growth of the endometrial lining.
- Ovulation is triggered by the surge of LH. The ovum surrounded by a rim of cumulus cells is released and swept into the uterine tube.
- Follicular cells remaining in the ovary become the corpus luteum, which produces progesterone and oestrogen.

- The second half of the cycle (luteal phase) is dominated by the effects of progesterone, which prepare the body for pregnancy.
- LH promotes steroid hormone secretion (predominantly progesterone) from the corpus luteum. However, the effect is short-lived, so the corpus luteum regresses, unless rescued by hCG from the dividing cells of the embryo, and menstruation ensues.
- Pituitary secretion of FSH and LH is under the control of pulsatile GnRH release from the hypothalamus. Oestrogen and progesterone exert negative feedback effects on the hypothalamic–pituitary axis except at mid-cycle, when a sustained high concentration of oestrogen exerts positive feedback leading to the LH surge and ovulation.
- The hypothalamus integrates other signals regulating reproductive function. Fertility can be disrupted by abnormal endocrine activity such as abnormal production of GnRH and hyperprolactinaemia, abnormal follicular development and extremes of weight loss or gain.
- Understanding the hormonal regulation of reproduction has allowed manipulation of fertility using chemical analogues of the steroid hormones in contraceptives.

APPLICATION TO PRACTICE

There are many environmental influences, both internal and external, that may affect the regulation of reproductive cycles. There is increasing evidence that many pollutants and chemicals in the environment can have negative effects upon human reproduction and possibly contribute to subfertility.

It is important to realize that the menstrual cycle starts to prepare women for pregnancy. The physiological changes, in preparation for and support of pregnancy, are initiated prior to ovulation and conception.

An understanding of the variance in the menstrual cycle is important when considering the estimated due date.

Knowledge of the reproductive cycles is essential in understanding the various methods of birth control.

Birth control medications are effective as they interrupt the normal hormonal control of the reproductive cycle. Midwives must be able to discuss and advise women on the use of contraceptive medicines to enable women to make informed choices on how they may wish to control their own fertility.

Most infertility and subfertility treatments involve therapies that augment and promote reproductive cycles to optimize fertilization and implantation. Some of these regimes are intense, with potential harmful effects, so women undergoing these treatments require close clinical monitoring.

ANNOTATED FURTHER READING

Balen AH, editor: *Infertility in practice*, ed 4, London, 2014, Informa.
A practical guide, based on the author's clinical practice, which provides an overview of human infertility problems, their aetiology and assessment together with evidence-based approaches to selecting possible interventions.

Bednarska S, Siejka A: The pathogenesis and treatment of polycystic ovary syndrome: what's new? *Adv Clin Exp Med* 26:359–367, 2017.
A review of the current state of knowledge about PCOS, which includes the pathogenesis, diagnostic criteria, genetic factors, clinical implications and possible treatments.

Cameron ST, Li H, Gemzell-Danielsson K: Current controversies with oral emergency contraception, *BJOG* 124:1948–1956, 2017.
A recent and considered review, which aims to address some of the myths and misconceptions about emergency contraception by considering the evidence base.

Chester RC, Kling JM, Manson JE: What the Women's Health Initiative has taught us about menopausal hormone therapy, *Clin Cardiol* 41:247–252, 2018.
A discussion about the WHI, the largest randomized placebo-controlled trial in the world, intended to objectively evaluate the use of HRT, which considers the study findings and their practical implications.

Foster R, Kreitzman L: *Circadian rhythms: a very short introduction*, Oxford, 2017, OUP.
An explanation of how the earth's rotation affects living organisms, which includes a broad range of topics related to chronobiology such as jet-lag, schizophrenia and obesity.

Foxcroft L: *Hot flushes, cold science: a history of the modern menopause*, London, 2010, Granta.
A fascinating and scholarly account of the social and cultural aspects of menopause throughout the last 2000 years.

Guillebaud J: *Contraception today*, ed 8, Oxford, 2016, CRC press.
This popular pocketbook provides an evidenced-based guide to all forms of contraception available and discusses the pros and cons of each method. This latest edition includes sections on special considerations such as contraceptive use in the older women and emergency contraception.

Johnson MH: *Essential reproduction*, ed 8, Oxford, 2018, Wiley-Blackwell.
An integrated and well-organized research-based textbook that covers the fundamentals of reproduction using a multidisciplinary approach and explores comparative reproductive physiology of mammals, including anatomy, physiology, endocrinology, genetics and behavioural studies.

Leung PCK, Adashi EY: *The ovary*, ed 3, London, 2019, Academic Press.
A detailed and scholarly description of ovarian structure and function at the cellular and molecular level, including normal development and pathophysiology.

McVeigh E, Guillebaud J, Homburg R: *Oxford handbook of reproductive medicine and family planning*, ed 2, Oxford, 2013, OUP.
A concise handbook about reproductive medicine, which includes the physiological basis and practical guidelines about all aspects of family planning and sexual health including topics such as infertility, contraception, recurrent miscarriage, PCOS and hirsutism.

Monteleone P, Mascagni G, Giannini A, et al.: Symptoms of menopause – global prevalence, physiology and implications, *Nat Rev Endocrinol* 14:199–215, 2018.
A detailed review of the biology of menopause, its symptoms, individual factors and impact on the woman.

REFERENCES

Bogin B: Evolutionary perspective on human growth, *Ann Rev Anthropol* 28:109–153, 1999a.

Bogin B: *Patterns of human growth*, ed 2, Cambridge, 1999b, Cambridge University Press.

Brooker CG: *Human structure and function*, ed 2, St Louis, 1998, Mosby, pp 480, 488, 489.

Coad J, Conlon C: Iron deficiency in women: assessment, causes and consequences, *Curr Opin Clin Nutr Metab Care* 14:625–634, 2011.

Davis SR, Lambrinoudaki I, Lumsden M, et al.: Menopause, *Nat Rev Dis Primers* 1:15004, 2015.

Devoto L, Henriquez S, Kohen P, Strauss III JF: The significance of estradiol metabolites in human corpus luteum physiology, *Steroids* 123:50–54, 2017.

Escobar-Morreale HF: Polycystic ovary syndrome: definition, aetiology, diagnosis and treatment, *Nat Rev Endocrinol* 14:270–284, 2018.

Feng CW, Bowles J, Koopman P: Control of mammalian germ cell entry into meiosis, *Mol Cell Endocrinol* 382:488–497, 2014.

Frisch RE: The right weight: body fat, menarche and ovulation, *Baillieres Clin Obstet Gynaecol* 4:419–439, 1990.

Frisch RE, Revelle R: Height and weight at menarche and a hypothesis of menarche, *Arch Dis Child* 46:695–701, 1971.

Gérard N, Caillaud M, Martoriati A, et al.: The interleukin-1 system and female reproduction, *J Endocrinol* 180:203–212, 2004.

Gluckman PD, Hanson MA: Evolution, development and timing of puberty, *Trends Endocrinol Metab* 17:7–12, 2006.

Harris AL, Vitzthum VJ: Darwin's legacy: an evolutionary view of women's reproductive and sexual functioning, *J Sex Res* 50:207–246, 2013.

Herbert M, Kalleas D, Cooney D, et al.: Meiosis and maternal aging: insights from aneuploid oocytes and trisomy births, *Cold Spring Harb Perspect Biol* 7:a017970, 2015.

Hintze LJ, Mahmoodianfard S, Auguste CB, et al.: Weight loss and appetite control in women, *Curr Obes Rep* 6:334–351, 2017.

Johnson J, Canning J, Kaneko T, et al.: Germline stem cells and follicular renewal in the postnatal mammalian ovary, *Nature* 428:145–150, 2004.

Johnson MH: *Essential reproduction*, ed 8, Oxford, 2018, Wiley-Blackwell.

Johnson MH, Everitt BJ: *Essential reproduction*, ed 4, Oxford, 1995, Blackwell Science, pp 64, 65, 108, 109.

Kim PS, McQueen JS, Hawkes K: Why does women's fertility end in mid-life? Grandmothering and age at last birth, *J Theor Biol* 461:84–91, 2019.

Kuijsters NPM, Methorst WG, Kortenhorst MSQ, et al.: Uterine peristalsis and fertility: current knowledge and future perspectives: a review and meta-analysis, *Reprod Biomed Online* 35:50–71, 2017.

Kwik M, Maxwell E: Pathophysiology, treatment and prevention of ovarian hyperstimulation syndrome, *Curr Opin Obstet Gynecol* 28:236–241, 2016.

Lv H, Hu Y, Cui Z, Jia H: Human menstrual blood: a renewable and sustainable source of stem cells for regenerative medicine, *Stem Cell Res Ther* 9:325, 2018.

Macklon NS, Brosens JJ: The human endometrium as a sensor of embryo quality, *Biol Reprod* 91:98, 2014.

Marshall SA, Senadheera SN, Parry LJ, Girling JE: The role of relaxin in normal and abnormal uterine function during the menstrual cycle and early pregnancy, *Reprod Sci* 24:342–354, 2017.

Maybin JA, Critchley HO: Menstrual physiology: implications for endometrial pathology and beyond, *Hum Reprod Update* 21:748–761, 2015.

Monniaux D, Clement F, Dalbies-Tran R, et al.: The ovarian reserve of primordial follicles and the dynamic reserve of antral growing follicles: what is the link? *Biol Reprod* 90:85, 2014.

NICE: *Fertility problems: assessment and treatment (Clinical guideline 156)*, London, 2013, National Institute for Health and Care Excellence.

Palumbo A, Avila J, Naftolin F: The ovarian renin-angiotensin system (OVRAS): a major factor in ovarian function and disease, *Reprod Sci* 23:1644–1655, 2016.

Raghunath RS, Venables ZC, Millington GW: The menstrual cycle and the skin, *Clin Exp Dermatol* 40:111–115, 2015.

Reid RL, Soares CN: Premenstrual dysphoric disorder: contemporary diagnosis and management, *J Obstet Gynaecol Can* 40:215–223, 2018.

Richani D, Gilchrist RB: The epidermal growth factor network: role in oocyte growth, maturation and developmental competence, *Human Reprod Update* 24:1–14, 2018.

Richards JS, Ren YA, Candelaria N, et al.: Ovarian follicular theca cell recruitment, differentiation and impact on fertility, *Endocr Rev* 39:1–20, 2018.

Scelza BA: The grandmaternal niche: critical caretaking among Martu Aborigines, *Am J Hum Biol* 21:448–454, 2009.

Schiller CE, Johnson SL, Abate AC, et al.: Reproductive steroid regulation of mood and behavior, *Compr Physiol* 6:1135–1160, 2016.

Tena-Sempere M: Deciphering puberty: novel partners, novel mechanisms, *Eur J Endocrinol* 167:733–747, 2012.

Virant-Klun I: Postnatal oogenesis in humans: a review of recent findings, *Stem Cells Cloning* 8:49–60, 2015.

Vitzthum VJ, Spielvogel H, Thornburg J: Interpopulational differences in progesterone levels during conception and implantation in humans, *Proc Natl Acad Sci USA* 101:1443–1448, 2004.

Webb PM, Jordan SJ: Epidemiology of epithelial ovarian cancer, *Best Pract Res Clin Obstet Gynaecol* 41:3–14, 2017.

Webster A, Schuh M: Mechanisms of aneuploidy in human eggs, *Trends Cell Biol* 27:55–68, 2017.

Williams NI, Ruffing KM: The menstrual cycle and the exercising female: Implications for health and performance. In Forsyth J, Roberts C-M, editors: *The exercising female: science and its application*, London, 2018, Routledge, pp 19–29.

Wurtman J, Wurtman R: The trajectory from mood to obesity, *Curr Obes Rep* 7:1–5, 2018.

Yermachenko A, Dvornyk V: Nongenetic determinants of age at menarche: a systematic review, *Biomed Res Int* 2014:371583, 2014.

5

Sexual Differentiation and Behaviour

LEARNING OBJECTIVES

- To describe and discuss the advantages of sexual and body dimorphism.
- To describe how sexual differentiation occurs during embryo development.
- To describe possible causes and aid identification of indeterminate sex.

- To outline the phases of gonad development.
- To identify the main differences in gonadal function between the male and female.
- To briefly identify factors affecting sexual behaviour.

INTRODUCTION

Evolutionary biologists have long questioned why evolution has led to sexual dimorphism: the differentiation of the sexes into male and female forms. Hermaphroditism remains limited to lower life forms, such as the annelids (worms) and molluscs (slugs and snails), although it is widespread throughout the plant kingdom. It is widely accepted that the development of sexual reproduction increased the speed of evolution resulting in the wide diversity of life forms upon the planet. The essential characteristic of sexual reproduction is that the new individual is produced from two distinct packages of genes: half from the male gamete (spermatozoon) and half from the female gamete (oocyte). The meiotic division that produces the gametes not only halves the normal (diploid) number of chromosomes but also increases genetic variability within each chromosome by exchange of parts of homologous chromosomes (see Chapter 7). Fertilization results in the gametes combining to form a genetically unique zygote (see Chapter 6).

Most animals reproduce sexually. Sexual reproduction involves segregation and recombination of genetic material (see Chapter 7) resulting in genetically variable progeny and thus a wide diversity of genetic material within a species. The advantage of this diversity and maintenance of variation is that the species is more likely to exhibit rapid evolutionary response to shifts in the environment so the population is more resilient to environmental challenges. Asexual reproduction, however, is less flexible as genetic adaptation can only occur by mutation; under certain circumstances, this clonal reproduction may be advantageous as the entire genome is passed on intact to the next generation, conserving favourable gene combinations. The question as to why higher life forms evolved a reproductive strategy involving dimorphism remains unanswered. However, mammalian gametes are morphologically different, which lessens the potential for same-sex fertilization, which is not far removed from self-sex fertilization, thus ensuring optimal mixing of genes. The gametes have distinct male or female forms and are made in morphologically different male and female gonads, which produce a distinct pattern of sex hormones.

CHAPTER CASE STUDY

Zara and her husband, James, are very keen to know the sex of their babies and had been informed by one of their friends, who is a doctor they met while in Africa, that they would be able to find out the sex when they have the 12-week ultrasound scan.

- When Zara informs you that they wish to be told the sex of the babies when the scan is performed, what do you think would be important to discuss with Zara and her husband regarding the identification of the sex of the babies?
- Are there any situations where it can be justified to identify the sex of the baby at the 12-week scan?
- What should the midwife do if a woman requests a termination of pregnancy solely because she knows the sex of her baby?
- Is it possible to identify the sex of the embryo earlier in pregnancy? If so, why would it be appropriate to do this?

The gametes control both the development of the distinct male and female phenotype and affect behaviour and physiology thus ensuring that the gametes have an optimal chance of delivery and that mating occurs at the optimal time for fertilization. The sex hormones also prepare the female to carry the developing embryo throughout pregnancy and to nurture it through the period of lactation and dependency.

DIFFERENTIATION INTO MALE AND FEMALE

In humans, biological sex is determined by five factors: genes carried on the Y chromosome, the gonads, the profile of steroid hormones, the internal reproductive anatomy and the external genitalia. Sexual ambiguity is not common in humans (1 in 1500–2000 live births); in most individuals, the five factors are either all female or all male. If an individual is born with a combination of male and female characteristics and does not fit the typical definition of either male or female, their assigned gender is intersex. There is ongoing controversy about whether intersex should continue to be categorized as a disorder of sex development (DSD), which it has been since 2006. The classification of intersex as a disorder legitimizes medical procedures on infants with ambiguous external genitalia, such as invasive and irreversible reassignment ('genital normalizing') surgery, to enforce them to fit socially accepted sex categories (Dickens, 2018). In some countries, intersex is included as a third gender on the infant's birth certificate.

Differentiation into either a male or female fetus is usually under genetic control, depending on whether the ovum is fertilized by a sperm carrying an X chromosome (gynosperm; female) or a Y chromosome (androsperm; male). However, events such as severe maternal pyrexia (over 40°C), maternal illness or exposure to toxins in the first trimester of pregnancy occasionally result in abnormal cell division and development (teratogenesis), in some cases contributing to indeterminate (ambiguous) sexual characteristics as well as other physical malformations. As in all mammals, the human female is the homogametic sex and usually carries the XX chromosome arrangement, whereas the male is the heterogametic sex and carries the XY arrangement for reproductive function to be successful. Therefore, it is the sperm that determines the sex of the fetus (Fig. 5.1). Rarely, mosaic individuals (carrying a patchwork of XX and XY cells) or those individuals with mutations in genes important for sex determination may express a phenotype opposite to their karyotype leading to XX males or XY females. If a Y chromosome is present, the individual develops testes (male gonads), regardless of the number of X chromosomes.

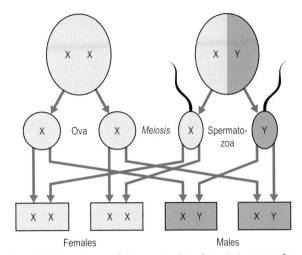

Fig. 5.1 Paternal genetic determination of sex in humans. Sex determination is genetically influenced by the SRY gene normally located on the Y chromosome; therefore it is fertilization by either a gynosperm or an androsperm that influences sexual dimorphism.

The Indifferent Embryo

The development of the fetus, both male and female, is initially the same. The gonads are formed from the mesenchymal tissue of the genital ridge primordia, which develop each side of the descending aorta. Until approximately the 4th week of gestation, the fetus is in a sexually undifferentiated state. If a Y chromosome is present, the fetus will normally develop a male phenotype (Jobling and Tyler-Smith, 2017). The differentiation process is initiated by the SRY (sex-determining region of the Y) protein, a transcription factor encoded by the SRY gene on the Y chromosome. SRY is the master regulator of male sex determination and triggers a cascade of gene networks by regulating the expression of SOX9; the outcome is differentiation of the precursor cells into Sertoli cells (rather than the granulosa cells of the ovary) and formation of the testes (She and Yang, 2017). There is a critical window for SRY expression; if it is delayed, the bipotential gonad differentiates into an ovary rather than a testis (Sekido, 2014). If the SRY gene is not expressed, alternative gene cascades are triggered, which result in the formation of female genitalia and ovarian development. The function of SRY can be lost by a gene deletion or point mutation so even though the genotype is XY, the phenotype might be female. Occasionally, the SRY gene and function may be translocated to another chromosome and result in a male phenotype despite an XX genotype. These unusual circumstances result in the rare outcomes of sex-reversed XX male and XY female individuals.

The human brain also exhibits sexual dimorphism, which has implications for gender-specific patterns of susceptibility to diseases and effects on behaviour. Brain imaging methodology such as MRI has identified sex differences in cortical thickness and sizes of various brain components. SRY is expressed in these brain structures. Sexual differentiation of the brain is regulated by a coordinated pattern of steroid hormone production, particularly aromatization of testosterone to oestrogen in particular regions of the brain. The steroid hormone production surges and spikes in critical windows of brain development: the organizational period of embryonic brain development and during the activational period in adulthood (Rosenfeld, 2017).

Abnormal numbers of sex chromosomes are often compatible with fetal development, and therefore occur with a relatively high birth frequency (Table 5.1). The major consequence of an aberrant number of X chromosomes is infertility. If there is an additional one or more X chromosome, as in Klinefelter syndrome (KS) (47 chromosomes, XXY), the fetus will differentiate along the male pathway, because the Y chromosome and SRY gene are present. The absence of a Y chromosome, as in normal female development (XX) or Turner syndrome (TS) (45 chromosomes, X0, where 0 indicates an absent sex chromosome), will result in the fetus developing as a female.

The Y chromosome is very small compared with the X chromosome and codes for about 70 proteins, whereas the genes of the X chromosome code for about 640 proteins. Much of the DNA of the Y chromosome is heterochromatin; it is tightly packed or condensed DNA (like the DNA of the inactive X chromosome) that is not accessible to polymerases so it cannot be transcribed to direct the synthesis of RNA.

The sex chromosomes evolved from autosomes about 160 million years ago and were therefore originally identical (Bellott et al., 2014). Since then, the Y chromosome has differentiated from the X chromosome and lost almost all of its genes. The Y chromosome undergoes high mutation rates due to the number of cell divisions in gametogenesis and because the sperm has few antioxidant defence mechanisms to protect it from the oxidative environment of the testes. Most of the regions of the Y chromosome, other than the tips of the chromosome, are unable to recombine with the X chromosome during meiosis, which protects it from losing the sex determining regions so the Y chromosome is passed from father to son intact. This means that the Y chromosome has accumulated repetitive non-coding 'junk' DNA from mutations and deletions, which cannot be edited out. However, the Y chromosome is able to recombine with parts of itself during meiosis using palindrome base-pair sequences, which code for genes that are crucial for male fertility. Effectively, these gene duplications act as a template for DNA checking and correction in the same way that the partners of autosomes and X chromosomes do. Although it was estimated that the Y chromosome may disappear completely within the next 10 million years (Aitken and Graves, 2002), it now seems that the Y chromosome is not shrinking at the rate originally estimated. Some smokers and older men have cells that lack Y chromosomes.

The SRY gene of the Y chromosome acts as a controller gene, which regulates other downstream genes involved in sex determination and testes formation; these genes are on the other autosomal chromosomes and the X chromosome. Effectively, the Y chromosome issues the instruction to 'make a testis' (Johnson, 2018). The SRY gene codes for a DNA-binding protein, which is a transcription factor (see Chapter 7) and upregulates other genes involved in the differentiation of Sertoli cells and the expression of androgen receptors. The effects of these androgens on tissue differentiation and development result in sexual dimorphism of the male during the embryonic phase. During the embryonic phase, female form develops in the absence of endocrine activity although oestrogen is required for puberty and fertility. Therefore, a genetic male may develop female characteristics if the SRY gene is either absent or not activated (Fig. 5.2).

The Undifferentiated Gonad

The early human embryo is bipotential (can become either male or female) at all levels of sexual differentiation; no morphological differences can be identified at the initial stages of embryonic development. The developmental switch, which drives the differentiation of the bipotential gonad to become a testis or ovum, is described as mammalian sex determination. The gonads are derived from three embryonic tissue sources: the coelomic epithelium, the underlying mesenchyme and the primordial germ cells (PGCs; Fig. 5.3). The coelomic epithelium develops into the genital ridge, which is found on the medial side of the mesonephros (which develops from the mesenchyme). The PGCs, which are ultimately responsible for the production of the gametes (spermatozoa and ova), originate from the yolk sac. Here, they undergo rapid mitosis before migrating from the yolk sac wall towards the genital ridge, about 4 weeks after fertilization. The genital ridges appear to produce chemotactic substances that attract the PGCs, stimulating them to develop pseudopodia and undergo amoeboid movement. Colonization of the primitive gonad by the PGCs is completed during the 6th week of embryonic development. The primitive sex cords develop from the gonadal ridges into the underlying mesenchyme forming the medulla and cortex of the gonad. In the testes, the

TABLE 5.1 Normal and Abnormal Sex Chromosome Complements

State	Karyotype	Phenotype (Expressed Sex)	Incidence per Live Births	Notes and Effects
Normal female	46, XX	Female		
Turner syndrome (TS)	45, X0	Female	0.1 per 1000 females	Females are usually short in stature, possibly with a broad chest, webbed neck, cubitus valgus (extreme outward displacement of the extended forearm) and autism. They are infertile (primary amenorrhoea) and sexually immature
'Super female'	47, XXX	Female	1.0 per 1000	Normal in female appearance and fertility, may have intellectually disability
Normal male	46, XY	Male		
Klinefelter syndrome (KS)	47, XXY (up to four X chromosomes have been found)	Male	1.3 per 1000 males	Affected males are tall and thin with long limbs and small testes. May be infertile (azoospermia) and have gynaecomastia (breast development). May have intellectually disability. More common in sons of older mothers
'Super male'	47, XYY	Male	1.0 per 1000 males	Affected males tend to be tall, have reduced IQ and often show 'antisocial' behaviour. Some studies show increased incidence (2–3%) in institutes for the criminally insane
Sex reversed	46, XXsxr	Male	1.0 per 20,000	Small piece of Y chromosome containing *SRY* gene is translocated on to an X chromosome

medulla develops and will go on to form Sertoli cells and the cortex regresses; this is reversed in the development of the ovary where the cells of the sex cords condense into clusters around the PGCs (oogonia) and go on to form the granulosa cells of the primordial ovarian follicles. The steroidogenic cells differentiate into Leydig cells in the male embryo or thecal cells in the female embryo (She and Yang, 2017). Two sets of primitive internal genitalia (gonads) begin to develop into testes or ovaries. Further development will follow either the male or the female route depending on the hormonal influences.

DEVELOPMENT OF MALE MORPHOLOGY

Embryological Development

The embryo has two sets of primitive unipotential internal genitalia, each of which has the potential to develop

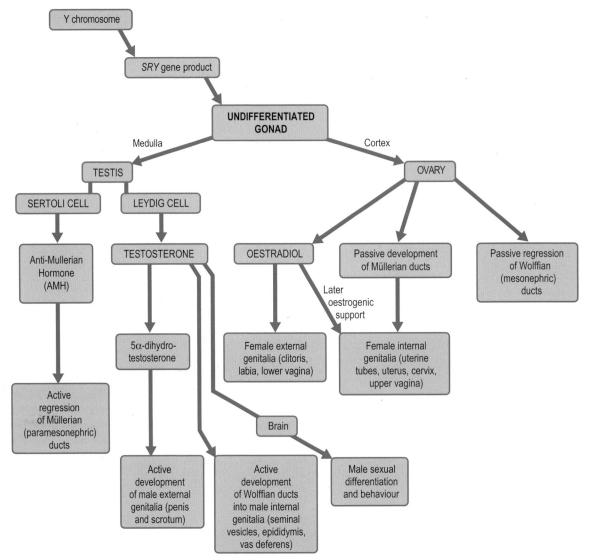

Fig. 5.2 Sex determination factors: activation and influence of the SRY gene. Activation of this gene instigates a number of endocrine influences that determine the male morphology. In the absence of SRY gene activation, female morphology develops under a genetic influence.

depending on the hormonal environment. The *SRY* gene and the male gonad are essential for the development of male morphology. The *SRY* gene stimulates the medulla of the undifferentiated gonad to develop into the testes and produce two hormones, testosterone and anti-Müllerian hormone (AMH; also known as Müllerian-inhibiting substance, MIS or Müllerian-inhibiting hormone, MIH), which promote male genital duct development. In the absence of AMH and testosterone secretion, female sexual differentiation occurs. AMH, from Sertoli cells, drives the

regression of the Müllerian structures (paramesonephric 'female' ducts) and testosterone, from Leydig cells, stimulates development of the Wolffian (mesonephric 'male') ducts into the male internal genitalia, the epididymis, vas deferens and seminiferous tubules. In the absence of testosterone, the Wolffian structures regress and the Müllerian ducts continue to develop into the uterus, uterine tubes and the upper part of the vagina. Sexual differentiation along the male pathway requires active diversion, whereas differentiation into a female embryo was historically considered

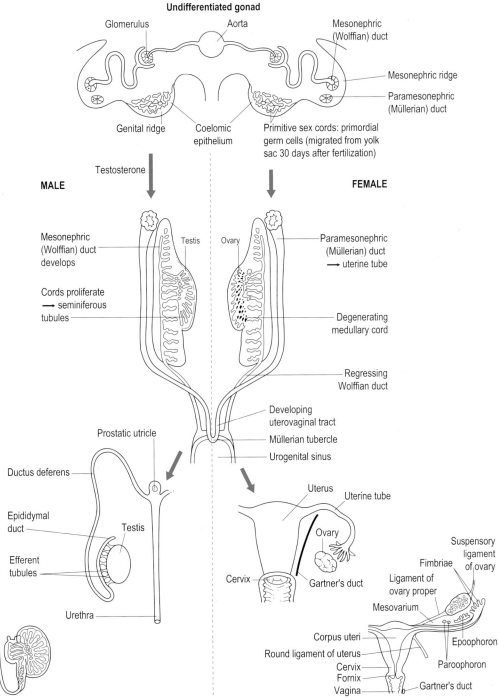

Fig. 5.3 Development of the internal genitalia. Once differentiation of the gonads has occurred, the resulting endocrine production coordinates the development of the internal genitalia. In the male, the reproductive tract is an evolutionary adaptation of a vestigial urological system.

to passively follow an inherent pattern or 'default pathway'. However, it is now appreciated that ovarian development involves active repression of the pathway leading to testicular development (Sekido, 2014).

The Wolffian, or mesonephric, ducts initially develop as part of the embryological renal system. The adaptation of the mesonephric ducts to form the male morphology is a significant development in sexual dimorphism, in evolutionary terms. Sexual differentiation at this stage is very efficient; it is extremely rare for individuals to have both testicular and ovarian tissues. These true hermaphrodites may have an internal testis on one side and an ovary on the other side (or a gonad with both ovarian and testicular characteristics known as an 'ovotestis'). The cause of ovotesticular disorder is not known but it may be due to translocation of the *SRY* gene to the X chromosome or an autosome, or gene duplication or mutation (Arboleda et al., 2014).

The phenotypic sex is determined by the sexual characteristics of the individual. The external genitalia are also bipotential and initially exist as a urogenital slit flanked by urethral folds, a genital swelling and a genital tubercle or bud. Steroid hormones directly influence the development of male external genitalia (unlike the female). Testosterone from the testes is converted into 5α-dihydrotestosterone (5α-DHT) within the target cells. Under the influence of this biologically more potent androgen, the tissues of the external genitalia form the penis and scrotum (Fig. 5.4). The urethral folds fuse, enclosing the urethral tube to form the shaft of the penis and genital swellings fuse to form the scrotum. The genital tubercle expands to form the glans penis. The testes, like the ovaries, initially develop within the abdominal cavity but the testes do not remain there. They descend to their normal position within the scrotal sac, suspended outside the abdominal cavity, just before or soon after birth. However, it is quite common (affecting 2–9% live-born males) for either one or both testes to fail to descend at this time and this condition is described as cryptorchidism. Spontaneous descent usually occurs within the first year of life. Testicular damage, potentially resulting in later failure of spermatogenesis and a higher incidence of malignant tumours, occurs if the testes remain within the abdominal cavity, so the testes are surgically lowered and fixed in the scrotum (orchiopexy or orchidopexy) if spontaneous resolution has not occurred. It has been suggested that the increase in male reproductive problems such as cryptorchidism, hypospadias and disorders of sex development is associated with exposure to environmental factors and endocrine disrupters such as pesticides and components of plastics (Skakkebaek et al., 2016).

The relative size of the male primary sex organs (testes and penis) has been used to characterize the ancestral human mating system. Human testes size is moderate compared with the highly promiscuous bonobos and chimpanzees but larger than the monogamous gorillas and gibbons. Chimpanzee males can ejaculate many times a day, which supports the suggestion that there is an association with frequency and volume of ejaculate and behaviour that is more promiscuous. The small size of human testes and ejaculate, and the nonexistence of clear sperm plugs blocking access to sperm from subsequent mates, suggest a moderate level of sperm competition in humans (van Schaik, 2016b). Overall, it appears that the ancestral mating system is most likely to have been pair bonding with some extra-pair mating (females having some polyandry); the relationship suggests long-term courtships and mate guarding.

Sexual Dimorphism of the Body

Adult men are heavier and taller on average than women. Men have more muscle and skeletal mass and women have more body fat with a different pattern of distribution. It is consistently observed, in nonhuman primates and other mammals, that if the species demonstrates sexual dimorphism in body size, it is never monogamous (the partners of the pair bond do not have only one mate at a time) (van Schaik, 2016a). Extra-pair copulations (sexual intercourse with another mate) can result in extra-pair paternity. As extra-pair paternity could result in a man investing in offspring not related to him, it is argued that men are likely to demonstrate mate guarding to prevent other males impregnating their partners or to desert their mate if extra-pair copulation is apparent.

Usually, there is a relationship between the size of the canine teeth and primate body size. However, this is not the case in humans; possibly bipedalism meant that weapons such as clubs and punching with fists became the predominant fighting style so the canines evolved to be less important and smaller. There is sexual dimorphism in the distribution of body hair. It is suggested that these differences may be a result of 'antithesis', traits that exaggerate the differences between the genders. Beards may be important as a signal of sexual maturity; facial hair grows after puberty and is more luxuriant in men with higher androgen levels. It has even been suggested that facial hair is more common during periods when men outnumber women and have to be more competitive for a mate and that being clean shaven is associated with a reduced tendency to violence (van Schaik, 2016b).

Sexual Dimorphism of the Brain

In the rat, testosterone from the testes crosses the blood–brain barrier and is aromatized into oestrogen within the brain. Oestrogen affects the size of the hypothalamic preoptic area (POA), the brain region that controls sexual

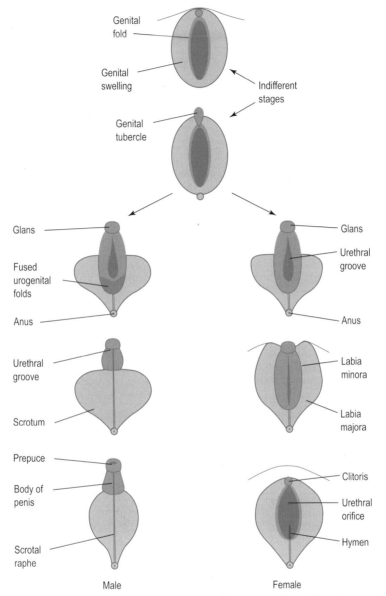

Fig. 5.4 Development of the external genitalia: formation of the external genitalia is hormonally influenced; absence of testosterone or functioning testosterone receptors will result in the female morphology developing regardless of genotype. (Reproduced from White BA, Harrison JR, Mehlmann LM: *Endocrine and reproductive physiology*, 5 ed, Elsevier 2019, Fig. 8.6.)

behaviour, which is distinctly larger in males. If developing rats are exposed to oestrogens, female-typical sexual behaviour is reduced and male-typical sexual behaviour is enhanced (Luoto and Rantala, 2018). For many years, it was assumed that similar responses to the presence of oestrogen, responsible for differentiation of certain brain structures in

a male pathway, also occurred in humans. However, the 'aromatization hypothesis' of male neural development in the rat does not apply to human males who do not convert testosterone to oestrogen in the brain and do not express receptors for oestrogen in the brain. Instead, sexual differentiation in the human brain is mediated by androgens binding to androgen receptors (Motta-Mena and Puts, 2017). In the developing rat brain, alpha-fetoprotein binds to oestrogen to prevent it from crossing the blood–brain barrier to masculinize the fetal brain. In humans, the fetal brain is protected from excess exposure to oestrogen by sex hormone-binding globulin (SHBG; see Chapter 3), which binds to oestrogens with high affinity (Luoto and Rantala, 2018). However, some reports suggest that female human fetuses exposed to the synthetic oestrogen diethylstilboestrol (DES), a drug used to treat recurrent miscarriage in the mid-20th century and prostatic cancer in men and to 'chemically castrate' homosexuals, were more likely to demonstrate bisexual or homosexual behaviour in adulthood. This suggests that DES (to which SHBG does not bind with high affinity) caused oestrogenic masculinization of behaviour, to some degree, in humans.

Sexual Behaviour

Humans, like other primates, have slow life histories; they reproduce at a relatively late age and at a modest rate, have relatively low fertility, long lives and a high level of parental investment in their offspring (Jones, 2011). They also live in social groups, demonstrating sexually differentiated behaviour (Motta-Mena and Puts, 2017). Additionally, humans have some unique behaviours. The juvenile period and lifespan are very long, even compared with other primates, allowing cultural learning and the acquisition of skills (Motta-Mena and Puts, 2017). Male investment in offspring is notably high and females demonstrate high levels of mating competition. In most nonhuman primates, female sexual activity is distinctive during the fertile period of the cycle. In women, ovulation is not evident; intercourse frequency shows little variation across the cycle and behavioural changes during the fertile cycle are difficult to detect. One suggestion is that this concealed or unpredictable ovulation prevents dominant males from monopolizing copulations during the fertile period and so facilitates parental investment by subordinate males, widening the gene pool. Women also demonstrate a high level of mating competition, which may be evident as aggressive behaviour or take the form of mate attraction. This is suggested to be a result of variation in male mate quality (Motta-Mena and Puts, 2017). Women demonstrate near continuous sexual receptivity even during pregnancy and lactation.

Humans form pair bonds, which confine the mating system and affect sexual behaviour but these two dimensions are also affected by cultural norms. Sexually mature women are unusual among primates in that the breasts and buttocks are permanent secondary sexual characteristics evident from puberty onwards. This indicates that these features evolved through sexual selection and are indicators of fertility and hence attractive to men. Both features are associated with the effects of oestrogen promoting fat deposition (van Schaik, 2016b). Similarly, a woman's fertility (and attractiveness to a male partner) is also associated with a low waist:hip ratio. Lower waist:hip ratios indicate higher oestrogen levels in the follicular phase and an increased likelihood of pregnancy. Compared with other primate species, human mating is remarkably frequent and is often discrete, for instance taking place during the night. The ventro-ventral (face-to-face) posture of human mating allows eye contact between mates and may strengthen the emotional bonds between them. It is a relatively common position of mating in primates and may reflect the long arms and flexible shoulder joints of apes. It is suggested that the most unusual aspect of human mating is the duration of copulation, which lasts for minutes compared with the few seconds of bonobos and chimpanzees.

Puberty

The Leydig cells in the testes of the male embryo produce testosterone from ~8–10 weeks' gestation with a transient peak of ~2 ng/mL at about weeks 13–15 (Johnson, 2018). Levels fall from then but reach about the same level ~3 months after birth. Thereafter levels fall but slowly increase from ~12 months. The prenatal peak is common in many mammals but the postnatal peak appears to be unique to primates, including humans. There may also be another smaller spike in testosterone levels at about 12 months. As in the female, puberty commences when the secretory pattern of follicle-stimulating hormone (FSH) and luteinizing hormone (LH), under the influence of gonadotrophin-releasing hormone (GnRH), becomes mature and receptors become sensitive. Initially, secretion of LH increases nocturnally, which explains the pattern of nocturnal sperm emission in pubertal boys. FSH and LH orchestrate spermatogenesis within the male (see Chapter 2). The testes gradually increase in size throughout childhood but at puberty, the increase in size is significant as the seminiferous cords canalize, the Sertoli cells increase in size, number and activity and the germ cells resume mitotic activity and spermatozoa develop. Unlike the ovarian cycle, spermatogenesis is a continuous process resulting in the production of many gametes. The testes produce testosterone from the Leydig cells, which influences the development of the male secondary sex characteristics (Box 5.1). Unlike the female, the male retains the capability of spermatogenesis indefinitely but failure to achieve an erection (erectile dysfunction) becomes more common with the progression of age, particularly for vascular reasons (Yafi et al., 2016). Production of testosterone gradually falls from the 4th decade and oestrogen increases, which promotes loss of muscle mass and an increase in body fat (Bribiescas, 2010).

BOX 5.1 Male Secondary Sex Characteristics

- Enlargement of the penis
- Pubic and axillary hair growth
- Deepening of voice (due to growth of larynx)
- Masculine pattern of fat distribution
- Development of the skeletal muscle (protein anabolism)
- Secretion of sebum from skin sebaceous glands (predisposes to acne)
- Bone growth and adolescent growth spurt (via growth hormone secretion)
- Male sexual behaviour and aggression

DEVELOPMENT OF FEMALE MORPHOLOGY

Embryological Development

As the X chromosome does not contain the *SRY* gene and there is an absence of the testicular AMH, the Müllerian ducts passively differentiate into the female internal genitalia, the uterine tubes and fimbriae, the uterus, cervix and upper part of the vagina. The lower part of the vagina is formed from the sinovaginal bulbs of the urogenital sinus (Roy and Matzuk, 2011). The undifferentiated gonad develops into the ovary; the cortex develops and the medulla regresses. This is the route of differentiation in the absence of testosterone and MIH. Female external genitalia form independently of any hormonal influences; therefore, the ovary has little endocrine activity until puberty. The genital tubercle becomes the clitoris and the urethral folds and genital swellings remain unfused, forming the labia minora and majora, respectively.

Common Abnormalities

During development, the body of the uterus, cervix and upper vagina are formed by the fusion of the two Müllerian (paramesonephric) ducts. Abnormalities may range from a simple uterine septum to the complete duplication of the reproductive system (two vaginas, cervix and lateral uterine horns; a rare condition due to abnormal embryonic development, which does not prevent a woman being able to conceive) (Fig. 5.5). The failure of one of the paramesonephric ducts to develop will result in a unilateral rudimentary horn.

Puberty: the Initiation of Fertility Cycles

In the female, the germ cells or oogonia cease mitotic division and enter their first meiotic division (becoming primary oocytes) *in utero* and most of them die before birth, so the number of oocytes a woman has is finite and determined before her birth. Meiotic division is then arrested until the oocyte is triggered to resume development. Recruitment of primordial follicles into the pool of developing follicles begins at puberty. Puberty commences with the activation of the hypothalamus to produce GnRH in a mature pattern of secretion. It is suggested that menarche is initiated when a critical mass of body fat, which may be genetically defined, is accumulated (Frisch, 1990). GnRH stimulates the anterior pituitary to produce FSH and LH, which orchestrate the reproductive cycles in the female (see Chapter 4). The ovaries begin to produce oestrogens, which influence the development of the female secondary sex characteristics. The breasts develop, the deposition of adipose tissue is responsible for the distinct female body curvature, and the growth of hair in the axilla and genital region commences.

Menopause

Menopause (see Chapter 4) marks the end of the ability of the female to reproduce. This midlife reproductive senescence results in follicular depletion and permanent cessation of the menstrual cycle. The ovaries atrophy and so there is a marked decrease in the amount of systemic oestrogen present in the postmenopausal woman. Modern fertility treatments can reverse the menopause to restore the menstrual cycle but not ovarian function. Hence, postmenopausal fertility treatment requires the donation of an ovum from a fertile, premenopausal woman, or cryopreserved ova, harvested and preserved before the loss of fertility. Menopause is notable in humans because fertility declines so much more rapidly than other ageing processes and so much of a woman's life is spent in the postreproductive stage.

INDETERMINATE SEX

Indeterminate, or ambiguous, sexual features at birth are usually attributable to genetic abnormality, endocrine dysfunction (see Fig. 5.6) or developmental failure. In cases of ambiguous genitalia, the karyotype of the individual is assessed to determine the chromosomal sex (i.e. the presence of a Y chromosome for a male or the absence of a Y chromosome for a female, regardless of the number of X chromosomes present within the karyotype).

Genetic Abnormalities

The aetiology of genetic disease is discussed in Chapter 7. There are genetic conditions that result in a range of variable sexual development, such as KS and TS (see above). These disorders have been useful in understanding the control of normal sexual development. In KS (47, XXY; normal number of autosomes but two X and one Y – there

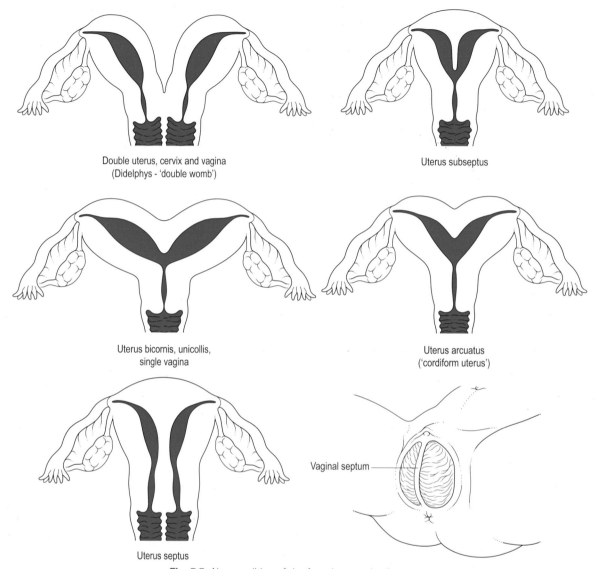

Double uterus, cervix and vagina
(Didelphys - 'double womb')

Uterus subseptus

Uterus bicornis, unicollis,
single vagina

Uterus arcuatus
('cordiform uterus')

Uterus septus

Vaginal septum

Fig. 5.5 Abnormalities of the female reproductive tract.

may be more than one extra X chromosome), which is the most common sex chromosome abnormality affecting 1 in 500 to 1 in 700 live-born males, the testes form normally but the germ cells die as they enter meiosis (Corona et al., 2017). Most patients with KS are azoospermic in adulthood because the low level of testosterone results in high FSH and LH, which cause extensive and progressive fibrosis (growth of fibrous tissue), and hyalinization (deposition of hyaline, an acellular protein-rich material) of the seminiferous tubules and hyperplasia of Leydig cells, preventing normal spermatogenesis. It is not clear whether the

germ cells are lost because of these changes or whether the fibrotic process occurs after the germ cells are destroyed. Conventional or microsurgical testicular sperm extraction (TESE), with possible cryopreservation of sperm, and intracytoplasmic sperm injection (ICSI) offer a route for men with KS to have children. Recent research has investigated the optimal time for TESE and found that the germ cell loss in KS starts early in life, probably in early childhood long before puberty in many cases (Van Saen et al., 2018). This presents challenges for fertility preservation strategies such as testicular stem cell banking, as many men with KS are not diagnosed before puberty. It is possible that hormone profiles may be predictive of changes in the testes; higher testosterone and lower LH levels are associated with a higher success rate of TESE. It is common in men with KS to develop breast tissue (gynaecomastia) and female patterns of fat distribution following puberty.

In TS (45, X0), which is the most common sex chromosome anomaly in women (occurring in about 1 in 2000 to 1 in 2500 livebirths), the single X chromosome initiates development of the ovary normally; there is a normal number of germ cells present in the early genital ridges in embryos. However, by mid-gestation, the numbers of germ cells are markedly reduced due to accelerated follicular apoptosis and the ovary regresses (ovarian dysgenesis). The ovary at birth forms a streak ovary, similar to a postmenopausal ovarian structure. Embryos with a 45,X karyotype have a high rate of uterine death. Women with TS have a very high risk of primary ovarian insufficiency and infertility; most have no spontaneous pubertal development and 90% have primary amenorrhoea.

Some women with TS are born with a small residual pool of primordial follicles. It is thought this may reflect variable rates of follicular atresia or may be due to sex chromosome aneuploidy or mosaicism (see Chapter 7) in the ovarian tissue (which may not be evident in the leukocyte karyotype normally used to identify abnormalities in chromosome number). The ovary would then have a mixture of oogonia, 45,X and 46,XX (Oktay et al., 2016). This pool might be enough for a young woman to undergo menarche and normal stages of pubertal development. However, this small pool of primordial follicles is likely to be used up soon after puberty, leading to premature ovarian insufficiency and infertility. The size of the pool can be monitored by the production of AMH (see Chapter 4); AMH is more likely to be detected in girls with TS who have a mosaic karyotype. Spontaneous conception is rare in women with TS; 2–5% of women with TS conceive spontaneously but these pregnancies are probably in women with mosaic karyotypes and spontaneous menarche (Bernard et al., 2016); these are associated with a high rate of chromosomal abnormalities and miscarriage. Most women with full TS will have the ovarian reserve depleted before puberty, if not before birth. Oocyte (or embryo) cryopreservation is a possible approach to preserve fertility in those women born with some follicular reserves. Cryopreservation of ovarian tissue, removed early in childhood and auto-transplantation later in life, is a possible option but is still at the research stage. Other strategies to permit parenting include oocyte or embryo donation, adoption or use of gestational surrogacy (Oktay et al., 2016). Maternal mortality is high in women with TS because of the increased likelihood of cardiovascular, renal and endocrine complications; the more serious of these are contraindications to pregnancy.

Endocrine Dysfunction

Fetal Endocrine Dysfunction

It is thought that an increasing number of infants are born with intersex variations such as sexual ambiguity (Rich et al., 2016), possibly because of the increasing exposure of embryos to endocrine-disrupting chemicals (EDCs) at critical times of development. The dissociation of gonadal and genital sex is usually due to failure of appropriate endocrine communication (Johnson, 2018). The embryonic stage of male sexual differentiation is under endocrine influence. This may be disrupted by the failure, total or partial, of production of, or response to, the necessary hormones (Fig. 5.6). Therefore, the genetic male may fail to develop male genitalia, and appear female at birth. As described previously, the activation of the *SRY* gene on the Y chromosome results in the formation of the testes, which produce testosterone. However, if the androgen receptor is defective, the response to testosterone will be ineffectual so the Wolffian ducts will fail to develop into the male reproductive tract. The defective receptor may also be present on other tissues so the external genitalia will also be unable to respond to testosterone and the infant will appear female. AMH will continue to inhibit the growth of the female internal reproductive tract. Thus, the child will be born with the external appearance of a female but lack both male and female internal structures. The testes remain within the abdominal cavity and as a result become dysfunctional.

Sufficient amounts of testosterone may be produced, but if the target cells lack the functional androgen receptors, or if the enzyme (5α-reductase) required to convert the testosterone into 5α-DHT is lacking, then virilization will not occur. In XY-individuals with complete androgen insensitivity syndrome (CAIS) or testicular feminization, the gonads develop as testes, which produce normal to high levels of androgens and remain undescended in the abdomen. The androgen receptors (ARs) are nonfunctional so androgens do not control gene transcription in the target tissues and the external genitalia appear female. XY-individuals with CAIS have female gender identity, demonstrate feminine behaviour and are sexually attracted to men, which suggests functional ARs masculinize the brain and control prenatal sexual differentiation. The lack of normal endocrine communication between the gonads and genitalia causes secondary or pseudo-hermaphroditism, a disparity between the gonadal sex (having testes or ovaries) and the phenotypic sex (appearing male or female).

Müllerian duct syndrome can occur if the AMH receptor is defective (persistent Müllerian duct syndrome) or if production of AMH is inadequate. Both the Wolffian and

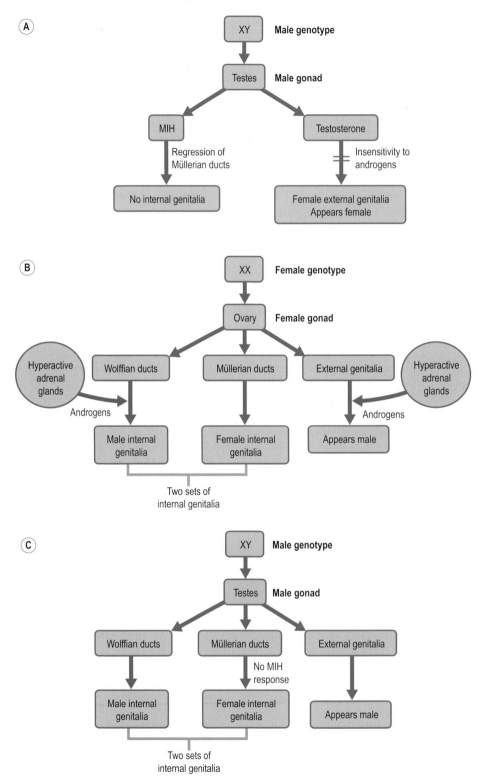

Fig. 5.6 Aetiology of indeterminate sex at birth. (A) Testicular feminization – insensitivity to androgens; (B) androgenital syndrome – excess androgens; (C) Müllerian duct syndrome – insensitivity to AMH (MIH or MIS).

Müllerian ducts develop simultaneously, which results in the development of both the male and female internal genitalia. The baby is genetically and gonadally male but retains the female internal structures, which developed from the Müllerian ducts. Men undergoing surgery for unrelated problems are sometimes found to have an unusual development of female internal genitalia without it causing any problem.

If a female embryo is exposed to elevated androgens during development, the internal and external genitalia may develop via the male pathway. Congenital adrenal hyperplasia (CAH) is an autosomal recessive disease usually caused by a defect in the 21-hydroxylase enzyme, resulting in underproduction of corticosteroid and overproduction of other steroid hormones, including androgens. CAH can cause early masculinization of males and causes the majority of cases of female virilization (androgenital syndrome), accounting for most cases of ambiguous genitalia at birth. In the female fetus with CAH, androgens stimulate the development of the Wolffian ducts and stimulate the external genitalia to resemble the male form. The Müllerian system remains because there is no AMH. Although the baby is genetically and gonadally female (XX with ovaries), it has the internal genitalia of both sexes and male external genitalia. With high androgen concentrations, the sex of the baby may not initially be questioned and thus the problem may be evident only because there are no testes to descend. XX-individuals with CAH report greater attraction to females and less satisfaction with female sex assignment (Motta-Mena and Puts, 2017), suggesting that early exposure to androgens affects gender behaviours.

In the 1950s and 1960s, high levels of progestogenic drugs were given to mothers who had previously had a mid-term spontaneous abortion to prevent miscarriage in subsequent pregnancies. It was thought that the pregnancies failed because of inadequate production of progesterone. However, progestogens are androgenic and can stimulate testosterone receptors causing pharmacological virilization of the fetus ('progestogen-induced hermaphrodites').

In response to rulings from the European Court of Human Rights, the UK passed the Gender Recognition Act in 2004. This allows a transsexual individual to have a gender recognition certificate, which means that their 'acquired' gender can be legally reassigned to be different to the one on their original birth certificate, which was assigned at birth. To request gender reassignment, the person is required to have psychiatric assessments and proof of living for 2 years in their preferred gender. In other European countries, the process is simpler and is based on a system of self-identification.

Case study 5.1 is an example of possible endocrine dysfunction.

CASE STUDY 5.1

Milly, who is 43, has had an uncomplicated third pregnancy. Following a chorionic villus sample, she was informed that her baby appeared to have a normal female karyotype. As Milly's other children are boys, she was thrilled to be expecting a daughter because she had decided that this was to be her last pregnancy, regardless of the outcome. Milly spontaneously went into labour at 39 weeks' gestation and, following a rapid and uncomplicated delivery, a 4.2 kg male infant, of normal appearance, was presented to her.

- What are the possible reasons to explain this?
- Do you think there is a need for any further investigations and, if so, what should they be?

Developmental Failure

The physiological processes resulting in the development of the reproductive tracts are complex, arising from the induction and differentiation of embryonic tissue. If the tissues, such as the pronephros upon which the gonads develop are missing, then the gonads fail to develop because essential induction factors produced by the pronephros are lacking.

Induction, differentiation and growth of tissues are also affected by several other factors. Optimal development occurs at body core temperature. Maternal pyrexia at critical stages of embryonic development may severely disrupt the process. Many pathogens produce chemicals or toxins that can also severely affect embryological development (Box 5.2). There is growing concern

BOX 5.2   Teratogens and Endocrine Disrupters

- Teratogens are chemical substances that are known to interfere with embryological development and so result in the manifestation of fetal abnormalities.
- Teratogens may be produced by pathogens, ingested by the mother either intentionally or unintentionally, or may be present within the external environment.
- Many drugs such as thalidomide (used in the late 1950s as an antiemetic agent in early pregnancy) are now known to produce physical deformities.

among environmentalists over the increasing amounts of manmade chemical pollutants within the environment (see Box 3.5, p. 76). Many of these chemicals may disrupt endocrine function in a variety of ways, not only by inhibition but also by mimicking the effects of endogenous hormones.

Case study 5.2 describes an example of ambiguous genitalia.

CASE STUDY 5.2

The midwife examines a newborn baby and is concerned over the appearance of the genitalia. Initially, the parents were congratulated upon the birth of a daughter but, on closer examination, the labia appear fused and the clitoris seems unusually large and so a referral to a paediatrician is made.

- What are the possible causes for this ambiguity?
- What investigations will be performed to establish the true sex of the baby?
- Why is it important to confirm the sex of the baby before registering the birth?
- What are the implications of assigning the wrong sex at birth?

SEXUAL BEHAVIOUR

Hormonal control of sexual dimorphism results not only in physical differences between the male and female, but also in behavioural differences. There are many brain structures that are sexually dimorphic (different in males and females). Males have slightly larger brains and tend to perform better in visuospatial skills; they tend to show more physical aggression and display more sensation-seeking and risk-taking behaviour. Females, however, perform better in verbal skills, memory tasks, language and emotional processing and seem to have greater communication between the two halves of the brain. The differentiation of certain brain structures, together with biochemical differences, is thought to explain the differences in sexual behaviour between the sexes. However, it is important to acknowledge that social construction also influences the development of sexual behaviour in humans (Carlson and Birkett, 2017). It is generally accepted that gonadal steroids induce brain sexual dimorphism but there may also be a direct genetic influence. Testosterone acts either directly or via local conversion into oestradiol and appears to stimulate formation of neural circuits involved in masculine behaviour.

Young children appear to demonstrate gender-related patterns of energy expenditure, parental rehearsal, explicit sexual behaviour and attentiveness to personal appearance. It is suggested that children recognize their own gender identity by the time they are about 2.5 years old and ambiguity may have long-term developmental consequences. It is not clear whether there is any link between transsexualism and biological or social gender ambiguity. The correct assignment of sex at birth was thought to be important in gender development, sexual orientation and attitudes later in life but this is now challenged and it is suggested 'intersex' should be a gender category on a birth certificate (see above).

Gender Identity and Sexual Orientation

Gender identity refers to an individual's self-conception of being female, male, both or neither. Sexual orientation refers to the relative sexual attraction that an individual has for men, women or both (Bailey et al., 2016). Differences in morphology underpin the biological explanations for behavioural patterns differing between the sexes. Male sexual activity appears to depend on the presence of testosterone above a critical threshold. Female sexual activity in the human may be cyclical in response to changes in male behaviour. There are cyclical changes in the organic acid content of vaginal secretions (derived from normal bacterial flora), which may be a mechanism of olfactory communication to the woman's sexual partner (see Chapter 4).

Gender identity and sexual orientation are not explained by gender socialization (the typical environment and gender-related culture that a child is exposed to) alone. Historically, gender reassignment occurred in hormonally male infants who were born with cloacal exstrophy (resulting in abnormal development of the penis and abdomen) or whose penises were irreversibly damaged during circumcision. It was believed that the best option was to medically reassign (surgically and socially) these male infants as female, however in adulthood the individuals affected usually retained male gender identity and sexual attraction to females (Bailey et al., 2016).

Human sexuality is complex; sex appears to serve a social, as well as reproductive, function. There is a wide diversity of sexual behaviour patterns within humans, ranging from complete homosexuality, to bisexuality, to complete heterosexual behaviour (see Case studies 5.3 and 5.4). Traditionally, in Western cultures, heterosexual behaviour has always been regarded as normal and any other variation as being abnormal. This assumption was based upon many animal observations where copulation appeared to be involved only in reproduction. Justification of such behavioural patterns has been argued from a sociological perspective.

CASE STUDY 5.3

Lisa is a 20-year-old primigravida who has conceived by donor insemination. The biological father of the baby is Lisa's brother's partner and Lisa has agreed to act as a surrogate mother for the two men.
- Would Lisa's care by the midwife be any different than to a woman who had conceived normally?
- How could the midwife include Lisa's brother and his partner in her care and facilitate the couple's preparation for parenthood?
- Are there any legal considerations that Lisa needs to consider over the parenting of the child and if so how can the midwife facilitate this?

CASE STUDY 5.4

Joan and Pippa are in a civil union and are both pregnant. They present themselves to the midwives' clinic where they inform the midwife that the babies have the same biological father who is an anonymous sperm donor. Joan and Pippa are very excited over the prospect of becoming parents.
- How should the midwife manage this situation and how would she plan the care of both these women?
- Why is it not correct to call the babies 'twins'?

The causes of differences in sexual orientation and gender identity are controversial and still not understood. It is assumed that sexual differences in behaviour may be due to differences in the brain but there is no scientific basis for a 'female brain' and a 'male brain'. Consistent differences have been identified such as the size of the brain and various brain structures, the organization of neurons, neurotransmitter concentrations and number of receptors (Fisher et al., 2018) but the brains of males and females are extremely similar and the magnitude of the differences is very small. Sexual differences may depend on life experience and epigenetic modification. It is usually assumed that sexual orientation is determined during early development through the interaction of steroid hormones and genetics with the developing brain (organizational effects) and then becomes evident at puberty and subsequently (activational effects).

Sexual orientation, defined as sexual attraction, sexual behaviour and self-identification, can be markedly different.

The majority of men are sexually attracted to women (gynaephilic) and majority of women are sexually attracted to men (androphilic). Research in this field can be affected by issues about disclosing sexual orientation and fears about homophobia. The early investigation of sexual behaviour by Kinsey and co-workers in the 1940s suggested nearly half of the population studied reacted to people of both genders and engaged in both heterosexual and homosexual activities. The distribution in sexual behaviour is different in men and women. Men are mostly attracted to one sex or the other in a bimodal distribution; few men are similarly sexually attracted to both sexes (Ngun et al., 2011). Whereas a smaller proportion of women is exclusively attracted to the same sex but women are more likely to report sexual fantasies involving both sexes. It is hypothesized that this greater human female sexual fluidity evolved to increase harmony in polygamous marriages (Kanazawa, 2017).

Clinical studies of individuals with CAH, where the female fetus is exposed to abnormally high androgen levels and is more likely to develop masculine behaviour, suggest prenatal androgens influence sexual orientation. Similarly, individuals with CAIS (46, XY), who do not have functioning androgen receptors, tend to have typical female behaviour, suggesting androgens are important in the development of male behaviour. Indirect measures of prenatal androgen exposure have also been investigated such as biological markers for prenatal androgen exposure including finger ratio (the length of the index finger compared with the ring finger; 2D:4D) and otoacoustic emissions (weak sounds emitted by the inner ear, which are stronger in females).

There may be a genetic component to homosexuality (nature) but sexual orientation is also affected by social, familial, environmental (nurture) and endocrine factors. If homosexuality is due to gene(s) in the population, it appears to create a Darwinian paradox; genes that promote nonreproductive behaviour should not survive. However, the 'maternal fertile female hypothesis' suggests that ascendants in the maternal line of homosexual males were significantly more fecund than ascendants in the maternal line of heterosexual males (Jannini et al., 2010). It has also been noted that there is a fraternal 'birth order effect'; homosexual men are more likely to have a greater number of older brothers possibly due to a maternal immune effect (maternal anti-male antibodies crossing the placenta) during fetal development (Bogaert and Skorska, 2011). These theories have engendered much controversy (Gavrilets et al., 2018). Finding genetic differences between homosexual and heterosexual brains may increase social acceptance of homosexuals; alternatively, it could provide a pseudoscientific rationale for discrimination and homophobia. Although a number of candidate genes have been investigated, the role of genetics in gender identity is not clear.

The emergence of genetic fingerprinting has enabled the identification of parents. Many biologists formerly accepted that many animals pair bonded, reproduced and then cooperated to bring up their young, sometimes on a seasonal basis or for life. However, recent genetic studies have revealed that the offspring of many animals were conceived outside the pair-bonding arrangement. Promiscuity appears to be widespread throughout the animal kingdom. The human male is often portrayed as sexually promiscuous but females are more likely to seek other partners, particularly close to the time of ovulation. This has a clinical significance in relation to family history-taking because as many as one in six children may be fathered outside of a relationship. Animal studies have also revealed that some animals use sex as a means of providing social stability. Studies of the Bonobo (pygmy chimpanzee) show that sex is used as a form of greeting, bonding and submission and that a full range of sexual behaviour from homosexuality to heterosexuality is present (de Waal, 1995).

The programming of sexual behaviour may occur by endocrine organizational influences during the embryological period. However, reproductive behaviour may also be influenced by the endocrine system on a cyclical basis. Human females copulate throughout the menstrual cycle, but sexual motivation appears to increase during the ovulatory period and to decrease during the luteal phase.

Some animal studies have shown that the presence of sex steroids is required for positive sexual behaviour to be initiated. An example of this is the female rat that is receptive to the male only at certain times. During the fertile period, the female will adopt a specific position for mating called lordosis, which is induced by the presence of oestrogens and progesterone. The sex steroids also appear to make the female chemically attractive to the male by the production of pheromonal substances. Therefore, sexual behaviour in the female rat can be described in three ways:

1. Receptive: develops an ability to copulate
2. Proceptive: increase in sexual motivation
3. Attractive: physiological changes that arouse sexual interest in the male.

Some animals have a visual signal to the attractiveness component, such as the female baboon who advertises her sexual receptiveness by developing swollen genitalia. These components of female sexual behaviour are most clearly evident in animals that have an oestrus cycle, where ovulation is stimulated by copulation to maximize the chance of fertilization. In the human female, it appears that all three components are present throughout the cycle, which suggests that sexual activity in humans has evolved to have a social role. In many animals, it appears that various forms of stimuli produced by the female influence male reproductive behaviour that promotes successful reproduction. Human male sexual behaviour, however, may have developed to be more responsive to the social aspects of sex.

KEY POINTS

- Females have two X chromosomes, whereas the presence of the *SRY* gene on the Y chromosome causes maleness. If there is an abnormal number of sex chromosomes, the presence of a Y chromosome leads to the phenotypic expression of maleness.
- If the embryo has a Y chromosome, the indifferent gonads differentiate into testes, which produce testosterone and anti-Müllerian hormone. Testosterone promotes male differentiation of the internal and external genitalia. Anti-Müllerian hormone causes the structures that would have formed the female internal genitalia to regress.

- The endocrine changes at puberty cause development of secondary sex characteristics and the start of reproductive maturity.
- Indeterminate or ambiguous sex at birth can be due to genetic, endocrine or developmental problems.
- An abnormality of sex chromosome number is frequently associated with effects on fertility and mental ability.
- Sexual behaviour has been associated with endocrinology, brain development and cultural factors.

APPLICATION TO PRACTICE

- Knowledge of sexual differentiation is essential in the examination of the newborn.
- Abnormalities of the sex organs and genitalia have their aetiology in the failure or dysfunction of the endocrine system. This may have a genetic origin or may be influenced by external factors such as pollutants.

An increasing number of individuals with restricted fertility due to genetic conditions are being offered assisted conception techniques to achieve pregnancy. The midwife must be able to support and understand the anxieties and stress related to these situations.

ANNOTATED FURTHER READING

de Waal F: *The bonobo and the atheist: in search of humanism among the primates*, London, 2014, W.W. Norton.
This book summarizes the ideas of the eminent primatologist, Frans de Waal, on the relationship between biological nature and morality. He suggests that moral behaviour in primates is a product of evolution and describes some wonderful case studies of chimpanzee and bonobo behaviour.

Dixson AF: Copulatory and postcopulatory sexual selection in primates, *Folia Primatol (Basel)* 89:258–286, 2018.
An extensive review of comparative aspects of primate reproductive anatomy and physiology covering a broad range of topics such as sperm competition, copulatory behaviour and cryptic female choice.

Domoney C: Psychosexual disorders, *Obstet, Gynaecol Reprod Med* 28:22–27, 2018.
This is a short practical review of the more common problems that affects psychosexual health, recognized by the World Health Organization as an important component of wellbeing; the ley points are well-illustrated by case study vignettes.

Graves JAM: Weird animals, sex, and genome evolution, *Annu Rev Anim Biosci* 6:1–22, 2018.
A delightful and thoughtful account of Jenny Graves' career investigating sex chromosomes, which includes her extraordinary personal story and work experience as a science researcher in Australia and elsewhere as well as a scientific review of sex chromosomes in different species.

Hatzichristou D, Kirana PS, Banner L, et al.: Diagnosing sexual dysfunction in men and women: sexual history taking and the role of symptom scales and questionnaires, *J Sex Med* 13:1166–1182, 2016.
A useful assessment and comparison of the tools used for evaluating sexual dysfunction with recommendations for clinical use.

Hegazi A, Pakianathan M: LGBT sexual health, *Medicine* 46:300–303, 2018.
A short review of issues and inequities affecting lesbian, gay bisexual and transsexual people.

Herbert S: Sexual history and examination in men and women, *Medicine* 46:272–276, 2018.
A succinct summary of the key points and clinical considerations to consider, including communication skills and ensuring a nonjudgemental approach, when taking a sexual history or undertaking a genital examination.

Hines M, Constantinescu M, Spencer D: Early androgen exposure and human gender development, *Biol Sex Diff* 6(3), 2015.
A well-written summary of the effects of androgens on sexual differentiation and gender development.

Hughes JF, Page DC: The biology and evolution of mammalian Y chromosomes, *Annu Rev Genet* 49:507–527, 2015.
An extensive and scholarly account of the history of the mammalian Y chromosome and the development of its unique features and the issues raised by selection processes driving these changes.

Johnson MH: *Essential reproduction*, ed 8, Oxford, 2018, Wiley-Blackwell.
An integrated and well-organized research-based textbook, recently updated, that explores comparative reproductive physiology of mammals, including anatomy, physiology, endocrinology, genetics and behavioural studies.

Okeigwe I, Kuohung W: 5-Alpha reductase deficiency: a 40-year retrospective review, *Curr Opin Endocrinol Diabetes Obes* 21:483–487, 2014.
A description of the discovery of 5-Alpha reductase deficiency and how it led to understanding the role that this key enzyme plays in the differentiation of the male external genitalia.

Sykes B: *Adam's curse: a future without men*, London, 2010, Bantam Press.
Written by Bryan Sykes, Professor of Human Genetics at the University of Oxford, this beautifully written book explores the biological and behavioural mysteries of the male sex and discusses the cannibalization of the Y chromosome by the X chromosome drawing the conclusion that men are headed for extinction.

Yang L, Comninos AN, Dhillo WS: Intrinsic links among sex, emotion, and reproduction, *Cell Mol Life Sci* 75:2197–2210, 2018.
A recent review about the links between sexual and emotional brain processes and how they affect reproduction.

REFERENCES

Aitken RJ, Graves JAM: Human spermatozoa: the future of sex, *Nature* 415:963, 2002.

Arboleda VA, Sandberg DE, Vilain E: DSDs: genetics, underlying pathologies and psychosexual differentiation, *Nat Rev Endocrinol* 10:603–615, 2014.

Bailey JM, Vasey PL, Diamond LM, et al.: Sexual orientation, controversy, and science, *Psychol Sci Public Interest* 17:45–101, 2016.

Bellott DW, Hughes JF, Skaletsky H, et al.: Mammalian Y chromosomes retain widely expressed dosage-sensitive regulators, *Nature* 508:494–499, 2014.

Bernard V, Donadille B, Zenaty D, et al.: Spontaneous fertility and pregnancy outcomes amongst 480 women with Turner syndrome, *Hum Reprod* 31:782–788, 2016.

Bogaert AF, Skorska M: Sexual orientation, fraternal birth order, and the maternal immune hypothesis: a review, *Front Neuroendocrinol* 32:247–254, 2011.

Bribiescas RG: An evolutionary and life history perspective on human male reproductive senescence, *Ann N Y Acad Sci* 1204:54–64, 2010.

Reproductive behaviour. In Carlson NR, Birkett MA, editors: *Physiology of behavior*, Harlow, 2017, Pearson Education, pp 310–343.

Corona G, Pizzocaro A, Lanfranco F, et al.: Sperm recovery and ICSI outcomes in Klinefelter syndrome: a systematic review and meta-analysis, *Hum Reprod Update* 23:265–275, 2017.

de Waal FBM: Bonobo sex and society, *Sci Am* 272(3):82–88, 1995.

Dickens BM: Management of intersex newborns: legal and ethical developments, *Int J Gynaecol Obstet* 143:255–259, 2018.

Fisher AD, Ristori J, Morelli G, et al.: The molecular mechanisms of sexual orientation and gender identity, *Mol Cell Endocrinol* 467:3–13, 2018.

Frisch RE: The right weight, body fat, menarche and ovulation, *Baillières Clin Obstet Gynaecol* 4:419–439, 1990.

Gavrilets S, Friberg U, Rice WR: Understanding homosexuality: moving on from patterns to mechanisms, *Arch Sex Behav* 47:27–31, 2018.

Jannini EA, Blanchard R, Camperio-Ciani A, et al.: Male homosexuality: nature or culture? *J Sex Med* 7:3245–3253, 2010.

Jobling MA, Tyler-Smith C: Human Y-chromosome variation in the genome-sequencing era, *Nat Rev Genet* 18:485–497, 2017.

Johnson MH: *Essential reproduction*, ed 8, Oxford, 2018, Wiley-Blackwell.

Johnson MH, Everitt BJ: *Essential reproduction*, ed 4, Oxford, 1995, Blackwell Science, p 10.

Jones JH: Primates and the evolution of long, slow life histories, *Curr Biol* 21:R708–R717, 2011.

Kanazawa S: Possible evolutionary origins of human female sexual fluidity, *Biol Rev Camb Philos Soc* 92:1251–1274, 2017.

Luoto S, Rantala MJ: On estrogenic masculinization of the human brain and behavior, *Horm Behav* 97:1–2, 2018.

Motta-Mena NV, Puts DA: Endocrinology of human female sexuality, mating, and reproductive behavior, *Horm Behav* 91:19–35, 2017.

Ngun TC, Ghahramani N, Sanchez FJ, et al.: The genetics of sex differences in brain and behavior, *Front Neuroendocrinol* 32:227–246, 2011.

Oktay K, Bedoschi G, Berkowitz K, et al.: Fertility preservation in women with turner syndrome: a comprehensive review and practical guidelines, *J Pediatr Adolesc Gynecol* 29:409–416, 2016.

Rich AL, Phipps LM, Tiwari S, et al.: The increasing prevalence in intersex variation from toxicological dysregulation in fetal reproductive tissue differentiation and development by endocrine-disrupting chemicals, *Environ Health Insights* 10:163–171, 2016.

Rosenfeld CS: Brain sexual differentiation and requirement of SRY: why or why not? *Front Neurosci* 11:632, 2017.

Roy A, Matzuk MM: Reproductive tract function and dysfunction in women, *Nat Rev Endocrinol* 7:517–525, 2011.

Sekido R: The potential role of SRY in epigenetic gene regulation during brain sexual differentiation in mammals, *Adv Genet* 86:135–165, 2014.

She ZY, Yang WX: Sry and SoxE genes: how they participate in mammalian sex determination and gonadal development? *Semin Cell Dev Biol* 63:13–22, 2017.

Skakkebaek NE, Rajpert-De ME, Buck Louis GM, et al.: Male reproductive disorders and fertility trends: influences of environment and genetic susceptibility, *Physiol Rev* 96:55–97, 2016.

Van Saen D, Vloeberghs V, Gies I, et al.: When does germ cell loss and fibrosis occur in patients with Klinefelter syndrome? *Hum Reprod* 33:1009–1022, 2018.

van Schaik CP: Human mating systems and sexuality. In *The primate origins of human nature*, Hoboken, 2016a, Wiley, pp 175–202.

van Schaik CP: Sex, sexual selection and sex differences. In *The primate origins of human nature*, Hoboken, 2016b, Wiley, pp 143–162.

Yafi FA, Jenkins L, Albersen M, et al.: Erectile dysfunction, *Nat Rev Dis Primers* 2:16003, 2016.

Fertilization

LEARNING OBJECTIVES

- To describe the physiological processes involved in coitus.
- To describe the morphology and characteristics of the male and female gametes and how they are adapted to their specific function.
- To discuss factors thought to be involved in the conception of a male or a female baby.
- To describe capacitance, the acrosome reaction and the cortical reaction in the stages of fertilization.

- To describe events in the first week after fertilization: the first mitotic divisions, cell compaction, hatching, implantation and maternal recognition of pregnancy.
- To outline the relevance and implications of parental imprinting.
- To outline common causes of subfertility and infertility.
- To discuss the approaches used in assisted reproductive technologies.

INTRODUCTION

Fertilization is a series of processes that culminate with the union of the haploid male gamete (the sperm) and the haploid female gamete (the oocyte) to form a diploid zygote. Following fertilization, the single-celled zygote progressively divides into the ~6 trillion differentiated cells (6×10^{12}) present at birth, forming a genetically unique individual in ~38–40 weeks. Understanding fertilization is important to our understanding of the events that follow during pregnancy and also to an understanding of some of the causes of infertility and failed pregnancy. Knowledge about fertilization has led to the development of sophisticated methods of *in vitro* fertilization (IVF) and, conversely, strategies for preventing fertilization (the basis for contraception).

Mammalian fertilization naturally occurs internally, usually within the ampulla section of one of the uterine tubes of the female reproductive tract. Only a few hundred of the 200–300 million sperm (spermatozoa) deposited in the vagina during intercourse (coitus) actually reach the oocyte (egg), a tiny fraction, which appears to be similar across different species (Dixson, 2009). The long journey through the female reproductive tract (equal to about 10,000 times the length of the sperm) presents the first of a series of challenges to successful fertilization. There is extensive and intricate crosstalk between the oocyte and

Chapter Case Study

Zara and James attended the local hospital for the 12-week scan and have been informed that there is now only one baby present in the uterus. It appears that one of the sacs, observed at Zara's earlier scans, has failed to develop further and the ultrasound scan could no longer detect any evidence of the sac or its remnants. Zara and James are understandably upset over the loss of one of their babies but are reassured that the other baby has an extremely low risk of having Trisomy 21 (Down syndrome), is developing well and appears normal.

- How would you explain to Zara and James the possible reasons for one of the embryos failing to develop?
- Is it more likely to occur in heterozygous or homozygous twins?

the fertilizing sperm, which leads to activation of both the sperm and the oocyte, which are essential to successful fertilization. Following the sperm oocyte fusion (syngamy) that occurs at fertilization, the female and male pronuclei fuse and the zygote undergoes the first cleavage divisions while travelling through the oviduct (fallopian tube) to the uterine cavity, where it implants in the endometrium (inner lining of the uterine wall).

COITUS (COPULATION)

Coitus in humans lasts on average 4 min, which is quite long compared with our closest primate relative, the chimpanzee, which averages 8 s. Masters and Johnson (discussed in Levin, 2017) described a four-phase model for sexual responses in humans. This is known as the EPOR model:

- E: excitement phase, when stimuli increase sexual arousal or tension.
- P: plateau phase, when arousal becomes intense; if the level of stimulation is inadequate, arousal subsides and there is no further progression to the next phase.
- O: orgasmic phase, which is a few seconds of involuntary climax during which sexual tension is relieved, usually accompanied by a wave of profound pleasure.
- R: resolution phase, when sexual arousal is dispersed; in males, it is believed that there is an absolute refractory period in which further sexual arousal and orgasm are impossible.

In the Male

The principal event necessary for a male to engage fully in coitus is acquisition and maintenance of penile erection to facilitate penetration and ejaculation. This is primarily a vascular phenomenon, initiated by neurological controls and facilitated by appropriate psychological and hormonal components. Initial stimulation of the penis can be both psychogenic (from erotic stimuli and sexual fantasy) and tactile (via touch receptors in the penis and perineum) and necessitates autonomic nervous system activity to coordinate increased blood flow into the vascular tissues (cavernous and spongiosum bodies, see Chapter 2). Centrally perceived sensual stimuli are relayed via the spinal thoracolumbar erection centre (T11–L2), and reflex erections, initiated by tactile stimuli to the genital area, activate a reflex arc involving the sacral erection centre (S2–S4; Yafi et al., 2016). Involuntary nonsexual nocturnal erections occur during rapid eye movement sleep. There are three components of erection: increased arterial blood flow, relaxation of the sinusoidal spaces and venous constriction. In the excitement phase, increased inflow of blood converts the low-volume, low-pressure vasculature to a large-volume, high-pressure system.

The arterioles and arteriovenous shunts dilate so there is an increase in blood flow, which engorges the erectile vascular tissues, the corpora cavernosa and corpus spongiosum. The corpus spongiosum does not increase in turgor as much as the two corpora cavernosa so the urethra is not compressed during erection and ejaculation is not impeded. Blood outflow is occluded by compression and constriction of the veins, so the sinusoids (blood-filled spaces) of the penis enlarge further. This results in hardening and erection of the penis as the blood volume is increased by ~50%.

The control of an erection is by stimulation of parasympathetic nerves, and probably simultaneous inhibition of sympathetic outflow, which reduces arterial smooth muscle tone causing vasodilation and increased blood flow. Many central and peripheral neurotransmitters are involved in mediating the erectile response. Centrally, dopamine, nitric oxide (NO), oxytocin and adrenocorticotrophic hormone (ACTH)/melanocyte-stimulating hormone (α-MSH) have a facilitatory role; serotonin may be either facilitatory or inhibitory, and enkephalins are inhibitory. Peripherally, the balance between vasoconstrictive factors (such as noradrenaline, endothelin and angiotensin) and vasodilatory factors (such as NO, vasoactive intestinal peptide (VIP) and prostanoids) controls the tone of the smooth muscle of the corpora cavernosa and determines the functional state of the penis. Other neurotransmitters implicated in the erectile response are acetylcholine and endothelins, also intracellular signalling via Rho-kinases. NO is considered the most important factor facilitating vasodilation, thus maximizing blood flow and penile erection. NO promotes the generation of cyclic guanosine monophosphate (cGMP), which triggers smooth muscle relaxation causing increased blood vessel diameter and increased blood flow. Detumescence (loss of erection) occurs because NO-induced vasodilation abates as cGMP is broken down, predominantly by the intracavernosal cGMP phosphodiesterase type 5 (cGMP–PDE5). Sildenafil citrate (Viagra) and related oral therapies for erectile dysfunction (ED), such as Vardenafil (Levitra) and Avanafil (Spedra), selectively inhibit the breakdown of cGMP by PDE5 causing increased vasodilation in the corpus cavernosum and penile erection. Side-effects of these drugs may include headache, flushing, rhinitis, urinary tract infections, visual disturbances, diarrhoea, dyspepsia and sudden hearing loss, and they may be contraindicated for men with cardiac and other medical conditions such as Peyronie's disease, which is a connective tissue disorder that results in abnormal scar tissue formation (affects ~9% of men).

Descending pathways can be either excitatory (such as those initiated by the perceived attractiveness of the partner) or inhibitory (such as anxiety or guilt). Testosterone, mediated by oestradiol, is required to maintain intrapenile NO synthase levels, which mediate local vasodilatation by increasing NO production. In hypogonadal men, testosterone therapy can restore libido and erectile function whereas, in contrast, anabolic steroid use can result in lower plasma testosterone levels, smaller testes and ED after the abuse of steroids is discontinued. Other hormones, such as prolactin, adrenal steroids and thyroid hormone, also contribute to male sexual function.

Erectile dysfunction ('impotence') is defined as the inability to regularly achieve and/or to maintain an erection for long enough to permit satisfactory sexual intercourse; it affects a considerable number of men, at least sporadically. It can be caused by penile trauma, infection, circulatory disorders or impaired neural inputs affecting the nervous control of erection. It can result from psychogenic, organic (endocrine or neurogenic causes such as spinal trauma, hormonal, vascular, cavernosal or be drug induced) or mixed causes. Most cases of ED have an organic origin, and are vasculogenic (affecting blood supply). Atherosclerosis results in endothelial damage, cellular migration and smooth muscle proliferation influenced by cytokines, thrombosis, growth factors, reactive oxygen species (ROS) and metabolic changes. Ageing affects NO production by the endothelium. Smoking is a risk factor for ED because it affects the vascular endothelium; nicotine both increases sympathetic tone leading to smooth muscle contraction in the corpora cavernosa and decreases the activity of the enzyme nitric oxide synthase. Failure of erection can be caused by damage to the spongy bodies, impaired flow in the vessels supplying the penis, drugs that interfere with neurotransmitter action or psychogenic factors. Local atherosclerosis can affect blood flow as can nicotine, which has vasoconstrictive properties.

ED is usually treated with lifestyle modification (exercise, diet and stopping smoking), nonsurgical interventions such as PDE5 inhibitors (such as Viagra), which are oral antagonists of cGMP–PDE5, vacuum erection devices, intraurethral suppositories (of prostaglandin E_2) and intracavernosal injection of vasoactive drugs (such as prostaglandin E_2, phentolamine and papaverine). PDE5 inhibitors competitively inhibit PDE5 so cGMP is not broken down and NO builds up. However, although ~66% of men respond to these drugs, many men do not like or cannot tolerate PDE5 inhibitors because of the side-effects. ED can also be treated by surgical interventions such as penile implants (insertion of rods) and penile revascularization treatment (microvascular arterial bypass surgery).

Neurogenic ED can also arise from lesions in the nervous system, such as peripheral and central nerve damage. At the cellular level, alterations in potassium efflux may lead to a state of hypercontraction and lack of erectile response. ED is a common age-related problem, so the incidence of ED will increase as human life expectancy increases; ageing is associated with a decline in testosterone, which may compromise the oestrogen–androgen ratio involved in the control of erection. Diabetes, particularly if coexisting with obesity, is a risk factor for ED and is related to accelerated atherosclerosis, alterations in erectile tissue, neuropathy and changes in hormone levels (Kouidrat et al., 2017). Diabetes-associated changes include smooth muscle degeneration, endothelial cell dysfunction, abnormal collagen deposition and high levels of advanced glycation end products (AGEs) that

reduce NO levels; these result in impaired relaxation of the corpus cavernosum smooth muscle. Medications for hypertension can contribute to ED; β-blockers can cause 'dry' ejaculation, which is probably due to retrograde ejaculation (RE) because β-blockers can cause bladder neck relaxation.

ED can also be a manifestation of underlying cardiovascular disease; hyperlipidaemia and hypercholesterolaemia affect the production of NO by the vascular endothelium. There may be an association between ED and vitamin D deficiency (Quilter et al., 2017). ED is a symptom not a disease; it may act as a barometer of cardiovascular health and be the first presenting (early warning) sign of previously undiagnosed hypertension, atherosclerosis or diabetes. Although the incidence of ED is high and increasing, it is underreported, underdiagnosed and undertreated, as many men are reluctant to seek help. The condition can have a considerable psychological and social impact on the affected man and his partner and their quality of life, causing depression, anxiety and loss of self-esteem.

As the penis becomes erect, the testes also increase their blood volume and are drawn up towards the perineum. The dartos muscle contracts so the scrotal skin thickens and contracts. As stimulation proceeds, the plateau phase of emission occurs, where the muscles of the prostate, vas deferens and seminal vesicle undergo coordinated responses that propel seminal fluid containing the spermatozoa into the urethra. Ejaculation, the orgasmic phase, is the process of ejecting sperm from the urethra following contraction of the urethral smooth muscle. This is accompanied by contraction of the pelvic floor muscles and the accessory muscles including the vesicular urethral sphincter, which prevents RE into the bladder. Orgasm, or contraction of the muscles, can occur without ejaculation. Oxytocin plays a key role in the regulation of erection and, together with endothelin-1, in coordinated contraction of the epididymis and tubules at orgasm; oxytocin responsiveness seems to be mediated by oestrogen. The composition of semen changes during ejaculation because the contractions are sequential and there is relatively little mixing of the components (Table 6.1). Premature or rapid ejaculation is the most common ejaculatory dysfunction

TABLE 6.1 Composition of Ejaculate During Orgasm		
Fraction	**Dominant Gland**	**Particularly Rich in**
Initial	Prostate	Acid phosphatase
Mid	Vas deferens	Sperm
Late	Seminal vesicles	Fructose

and is usually caused by anxiety or emotional stress; it is treated with behavioural therapy, pelvic floor muscle exercises, α-adrenoceptor antagonists ('sympathetic α-blockers'), topical anaesthetics such as lidocaine cream, tricyclic antidepressants and selective serotonin reuptake inhibitors (SSRI).

Neurological lesions, such as spinal cord damage or damage following injury or surgery to the colon or abdomen, can also cause ejaculatory dysfunction; the sympathetic nerves associated with control of sexual functioning can easily be damaged. Other problems, such as diabetes and multiple sclerosis, can cause ejaculatory problems. Drugs, such as medication for hypertension and the common cold, may also cause a lack of emission (deposition of the seminal fluid into the posterior urethra), resulting in failure of ejaculation. Bladder neck damage in men who have undergone prostate surgery (particularly, transurethral resection of the prostate) can result in RE. Blood in the ejaculate (haematospermia) is usually a benign and temporary condition caused by infection or inflammation of the seminal vesicles, colon or prostate gland, which is treatable with antibiotics.

In the Female

Women have similar responses in coitus to those of men. Tactile stimulation of the perineal region and the glans clitoris as well as psychogenic stimuli elicit these responses. The corpora of the clitoris and the labia undergo vascular engorgement. Increased blood flow to the vagina increases transudation and vaginal lubrication. The vagina increases in width and length and the uterus is elevated upwards, which lifts the cervical os to produce a 'tenting effect'. At orgasm, vaginal and uterine contractions increase in intensity. During orgasm, women may expel fluid produced by Skene's glands from the urethra. Sexual responses in the female tend to be more prolonged than in males. Detumescence of the female organs is similar to detumescence of the penis. Orgasm in women seems to be 'learnt' through experience, whereas in men, it is a reflex action and, unlike males, female orgasm is not essential for pregnancy.

Systemic effects occur in both males and females: heart rate and blood pressure increase, accompanied by peripheral vasodilatation. This is followed by the resolution phase.

THE GAMETES

Male Gametes

The sperm (Fig. 6.1) develop in the seminiferous tubules of the testes (see Chapter 2). At about 40–50 μm long, of which only approximately 5 μm is the head, the sperm cell

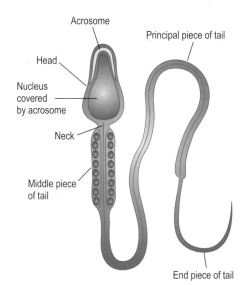

Fig. 6.1 The male gamete: the spermatozoon or sperm. (Reproduced with permission from Moore KL, Persaud TVN, Torchia MG: *The developing human: clinically oriented embryology*, 11 ed, Elsevier 2020, Fig. 2.5A.)

is one of the smallest human cells. It retains its ability to fertilize for 2–5 days once it has undergone capacitation in the female reproductive tract. The genetic material of the male gamete is carried in the head of the sperm at the tip of which is located the acrosome, a large vesicle containing digestive enzymes. The midpiece is located between the head and the tail and is packed with mitochondria, which generate the ATP required for movement. The tail or flagellum of the mature sperm has a whip-like action, which generates the propulsion for the sperm to swim at about 30 cm/h. Abnormalities in human sperm morphology (such as having no tail, two tails or a coiled tail, or no head, two heads or a small head) are very common. Table 6.2 summarizes these defects and their possible causes. Abnormal morphology of sperm, or impaired motility as seen, for example in primary ciliary dyskinesia (PCD), cause problems with fertilization and are thus associated with infertility. As well as the paternal haploid genome (23 paternal chromosomes), the sperm contributes the signal that initiates metabolic activation and cleavage division of the oocyte and also the centrioles, which is essential for the organization of microtubules to form the mitotic spindle necessary for cell division.

Sperm Competition

Female choice and male-to-male competition prior to copulation are examples of sexual selection (Lewis et al., 2008). However, it seems that in many species, females typically mate with more than one male during the time

TABLE 6.2 Abnormalities of Sperm

Type of Abnormality	Description	Possible Causes
Azoospermia (aspermia)	No sperm present within the ejaculate	Primary testicular failure; blockage to the vas deferens, that is, infection or trauma
Oligozoospermia (oligospermia)	Reduced numbers of sperm in the ejaculate (low sperm count)	Gonadotrophin insufficiency; drugs (social and medical, alcohol, toxins, etc.)
Idiopathic oligospermia	Low sperm count but physiological parameters normal	Unexplained
Teratozoospermia (teratospermia)	Abnormal morphology, for example, giant heads, double tails	Genetic, toxins, viral infection
Asthenospermia	Reduced (or lack of) mobility	Toxins, infection
Sperm agglutination	Sperm clump together in groups	Infection, production of an immune response against sperm (autoimmune response)

when they could conceive. Sperm competition is the competition between sperm from two or more males to fertilize an ovum. There are various mechanisms involved such as sperm number and sperm length, removal of rival sperm, switching off female receptivity to subsequent males and plugging the female reproductive tract. Comparative physiology predicts that mammalian species that have a large testis:body weight ratio are more likely to benefit from a promiscuous mating system in which sperm competition operates (because larger testes produce more sperm); by these criteria, men did not evolve to be promiscuous.

Female Gametes

The ovum, consisting of the oocyte surrounded by a layer of cumulus or granulosa cells (also termed the 'corona radiata'), is expelled from the dominant mature follicle of the ovary (see Chapter 4) and 'picked up' by the fimbria of the uterine tube. The human oocyte has a diameter of ~120 μm and therefore has the largest volume of any human cell type, making it just visible to the naked eye. In comparison, follicular cells are typical-sized human cells of about 10 μm diameter. A rim of these follicular cells forms the corona radiate, which surrounds the oocyte at ovulation. During follicular growth, the oocyte accumulates RNA and protein and numerous large mitochondria, which will provide for the needs of the early cell divisions of the fertilized egg. Primary oocytes arrest in prophase of meiosis I during fetal life and, after menarche (and possibly >40 years later), the luteinizing hormone (LH) surge in the female during each menstrual cycle triggers completion of meiosis I to form a secondary oocyte and a defunct daughter cell called the first polar body (1 PB). This secondary oocyte is also arrested in meiosis II prior to ovulation and, if fertilization occurs, penetration by the sperm causes the final stages of meiosis II to occur (see Chapter 7).

The Fertile Window

The lifespan of the human oocyte is thought to be ~6–24 h. Sperm have a viability of up to about 5 days in oestrogenized cervical mucus, so sperm, which arrive in the reproductive tract up to 5 days before ovulation, have a chance of fertilizing an oocyte. This means that the 'fertile window', when conception is possible, is ~4–5 days before ovulation until 1 day after.

Intercourse is most likely to result in pregnancy when it occurs within the 3-day interval ending on the day of ovulation. Peak fecundability was observed in one study when intercourse occurred during the 2 days prior to ovulation (Wilcox et al., 1995).

Sperm concentrations fall with increasing frequency of intercourse but not to an extent that daily intercourse reduces the likelihood of conception. Sperm counts are maximal after about 5 days of abstinence. Thus, daily intercourse during the fertile window optimizes conception because each day of intercourse increases the probability of pregnancy. The best outcome might be achieved by couples abstaining from intercourse for about 5 days prior to the fertile window and then aiming for daily intercourse.

Sex of the Zygote

In meiotic division, the cells have their genetic complement reduced from 46 to 23 chromosomes. Each normal oocyte will have 22 autosomes and an X sex chromosome, and each normal sperm will have 22 autosomes and either an X or a Y sex chromosome. If the oocyte is fertilized by a sperm bearing an X chromosome (a gynosperm), the zygote will be female, and if it has a Y chromosome (an androsperm), the offspring will be male (see Chapter 5). Theoretically, there will be equal numbers of gynosperm and androsperm since the alignment of two X and two Y spermatids on the cytoplasmic bridge during spermatogenesis ensures that equal numbers of male and female sperm are released. However, the sex ratio is not constant either during gestation or between birth and death. Recently, Orzack et al. (2015) monitored fetal male:female sex ratios using the largest dataset ever assembled. From conception (50:50), the ratio decreased in the first week due to excess male mortality, then increased for at least 10–15 weeks due to excess female mortality. The gender ratio levelled off after ~20 weeks, and declined slowly from 28 to 35 weeks (due to excess male mortality). Total female mortality during pregnancy exceeded total male mortality. The number of male babies born (typically ~51.3% of live births) exceeds the number of female babies all over the world. Following birth, the male:female ratio is 'all downhill' with 3–4 times more women than men reaching 100 years of age and close to 20 times more women reaching 110 years of age (Austad, 2015).

There are a number of methods that can be used by couples wishing to choose the gender of their baby before pregnancy. Of these, the most effective is preimplantation genetic screening (PGS), a variation on the powerful technique of preimplantation genetic diagnosis (PGD) (see Chapter 7). PGD is used to genetically screen early embryos resulting from IVF, either to identify their gender so that sex-linked diseases are not passed on to the offspring or, in an increasing number of diseases for which the gene-defect has been identified, to return to the uterus only those embryos that are not carrying the defective gene. PGS uses a similar approach to identify the gender of the embryos resulting from IVF so that only male or female embryos are returned to the mother's uterus. Use of PGS for 'family balancing' in this way is an expensive and ethically controversial technique, which nevertheless has become widely available in some countries.

Less costly but also less reliable are techniques to alter the androsperm:gynosperm ratio in semen and thus improve sex selection. The difference in mass of gynosperm and androsperm in some species is much more marked than it is in humans. Bovine sperm, for example, can be effectively separated by differential centrifugation. The bottom fraction in the tube will be enriched with the heavier gynosperm, which can be used to impregnate cows to increase their proportion in the herd. Separation of human androsperm and gynosperm seems more difficult but is practised albeit with questionable success rates. Separation of human androsperm from gynosperm is also possible using the technique of cell sorting (flow cytometric sperm sorting), the major provider of this technology being MicroSort. This technique distinguishes male from female sperm using a fluorescent DNA probe. Because the X chromosome is larger than the Y, gynosperm contain 2.8% more total DNA than androsperm, so that sperm can be sorted by detecting the fluorescence signal from the DNA probe in each individual sperm and used to direct the collection of male and female sperm into different samples. The MicroSort technique has been reported to allow enrichment of human sperm samples to 87.7±5% X-bearing sperm or 74.3±7% Y-bearing sperm, resulting in the ability to select IVF outcomes to produce either 93.5% females or 85.3% males, respectively (Karabinus et al., 2014). MicroSort has the disadvantage compared with PGD of a less predictable outcome, but the major advantage that sperm of the enriched gender can be delivered to the would-be mother by artificial insemination, without the greater personal demands and much greater expense of one or more rounds of IVF with PGD.

In addition, other less reliable techniques for gender selection are also used including the separation of the faster-swimming male sperm (Ericsson method) and the timing of intercourse to specific days of the menstrual cycle (Shettles and Whelan methods). Some environmental factors may also influence the ratio of X- and Y-bearing sperm (James, 2008). Although a number of practices may have no scientific foundation, an increased number of female babies are born as the father ages. In some parts of the world, selective abortion or infanticide is also reported. In many countries, sex selection is also evident in that couples who have both a male and a female child are less likely to have further children. Case study 6.1 looks at the question of sex determination.

CASE STUDY 6.1

Molly, who has four healthy daughters, is expecting her fifth child. She jokes with the midwife that she knows that this will be a girl as well. The midwife asks her why and Molly informs her that her husband works on an oil rig and is always home for 10 days and then away for 10 days. She laughingly states that every time she has conceived she has always started her period on the day her husband returns home.

- What factors in Molly and her husband's life may influence the sex of their children?
- How unusual is it to have five children all of the same sex?

STAGES OF FERTILIZATION

In the days (proliferative stage) leading up to ovulation, the epithelial cells lining the uterine tubes become more ciliated and smooth muscle activity increases. At ovulation, the fimbriae of the uterine tube move closer to the ovary and rhythmically stroke its surface. These sweeping movements, together with the currents generated by the moving cilia, facilitate the capture of the ovum released at ovulation. Ovum capture is remarkably efficient such that in women who have only one functional ovary and one functional uterine tube on opposite sides, pregnancy can still occur (because the uterine tube is mobile and can move to the functional ovary). The oocyte is transported towards the uterus by movements generated by peristaltic contractions of the uterine tube aided by the beating movement of the cilia. The oocyte has no inherent motility but is washed along by tubal fluid secreted by the epithelial cells and serum transudate. It takes 3–4 days to reach the uterus. Initially, the movement through the ampulla, where fertilization is most likely to occur, is slow, but the zygote travels faster through the isthmus into the uterus. The junction between the uterine tube and the uterus relaxes under the influence of progesterone and allows the oocyte through. If the oocyte has not been fertilized, it degenerates and is discarded within the menstrual bleeding.

Gamete Motility and Sperm Deposition

Spermiogenesis is the final stage of spermatogenesis (see Chapter 2) and occurs in the seminiferous tubules but, although the sperm are morphologically mature, they are not fully motile. The sperm develop swimming ability during a maturation phase of 4–12 days in the epididymis. At intercourse, about 200–300 million sperm are released in about 3 mL of seminal fluid (Box 6.1), which is deposited in the vagina. Repeated ejaculation normally results in a fall in sperm concentration, but the proportion of motile sperm decreases in men who are infertile, suggesting that impaired motility affects transport through the male genital tract. The sperm coagulate in the vagina, which appears to facilitate their retention and to buffer them against the normally unfavourable acidic environment (pH ≈4–5) of the vagina. The pH of the vagina is increased by the buffers in the seminal fluid favouring sperm motility and access to the cervix. The coagulum dissolves in about 20–60 min.

Between days 9 and 16 of the menstrual cycle, during the fertile period of the few days preceding and including ovulation, the watery composition of cervical mucus facilitates passage of sperm (see Table 4.1, p. 100). The cervical mucus interacts with the sperm and provides protection and nourishment. The acid environment of the female reproductive tract is inhospitable. The sperm that reach the oocyte have undertaken a remarkable journey; it is long, tortuous and filled with viscous fluid, dead ends and hostile immune cells. Cervical mucus offers an immunotolerant storage site and facilitates sperm transport and selection, filtering out sperm with abnormal morphology and motility (Suarez, 2016). It also acts as a reservoir keeping sperm alive for up to several days, temporarily inhibiting capacitance and releasing a few sperm at a time (Holt and Fazeli, 2015). Most sperm (99%) do not enter the uterus. A few hundred sperm reach the uterine tubes within a few hours of coitus; this first wave of rapid transport probably depends on rhythmic muscular contractions of the female reproductive tract. Muscular activity of the female genital tract does not seem to be essential for fertilization; some sperm will be stored in cervical crypts and then travel in a relatively slow second wave through the cervical mucus, reaching the uterine tube a few days after ejaculation. Sperm motility is regulated by the entry of calcium through the sperm-specific CatSper calcium channel to trigger a rise in the intracellular Ca^{2+} concentration. CatSper, in human sperm, is directly activated by progesterone, prostaglandins and odorants (Brenker et al., 2012) and functions as a chemosensor to guide sperm to these chemoattractants, released from the ovum and the surrounding cumulus cells.

Capacitation

Ejaculated sperm are already highly motile but have no ability to recognize or interact with the oocyte, processes that require sperm capacitation. On route towards the ovaries, sperm enter the isthmic region of the oviduct where they interact with the endosalpingeal epithelium to form a sperm reservoir. It is here that the process of capacitation takes place and the sperm remain here for up to 24 h until a signal, as yet unidentified, resulting from oocyte ovulation triggers their release from the reservoir in a hyperactivated state and primed to interact with the oocyte, undergo the acrosome reaction and bring about fertilization (Aitken and Nixon, 2013). The action of female hormones at ovulation triggers the biochemical and functional changes of capacitation. The changes include removal of cholesterol and adherent proteins from the sperm plasma membrane, changes in phospholipid content and unmasking of cell-surface receptors for zona pellucida binding, pulsatile release of Ca^{2+} from intracellular calcium stores, an increase in cyclic adenosine monophosphate (cAMP) and phosphorylation of sperm proteins (Aitken and Nixon, 2013). These modifications trigger hyperactivation of

---

BOX 6.1 Composition of Ejaculate

- 40–300 million sperm
- Prostatic fluid (30%): citric acid, acid phosphatase, magnesium and zinc ions
- Seminal fluid (60%): fructose (energy source for sperm), alkaline
- pH 7.0–8.3
- Volume: 2–6 mL

sperm motility resulting in whiplash-like movement of the flagellum so that sperm migrate along the oviduct towards the oocyte, guided by chemotaxis and thermotaxis.

The successful development of techniques for IVF by Bob Edwards and colleagues in the late 1960s relied entirely on the ability to mimic the process of sperm capacitation *in vitro* (Edwards et al., 1969). The pioneering research of Bob Edwards and Patrick Steptoe resulted in the birth of the first human baby from IVF, Louise Brown, in 1978 with >6 million IVF births recorded by 2018, 40 years later. Bob Edwards was belatedly awarded the Nobel Prize in Medicine in 2010, some 32 years later, but since the Nobel Prize is not awarded posthumously, Patrick Steptoe's contribution was not recognized, having died in 1988. Despite the presence of the mitochondrion-rich midpiece, there has been much speculation and disagreement about the relative importance of aerobic mitochondrial ATP production, versus the much less efficient anaerobic glycolytic ATP production, to supply the energy required for sperm motility. Some studies have demonstrated the importance of glucose (or fructose) to support the energy requirements of hyperactivated sperm, suggesting an important role of glycolytic ATP production, which may be essential, given the fructose-rich environment of oviductal secretions (Williams and Ford, 2001).

Access to the Oocyte

The ovulated oocyte is surrounded by two 'barriers' that need to be penetrated by the sperm in order for it to reach and fuse with the oocyte plasma membrane. The first barrier preventing access of the sperm to the oocyte plasma membrane is the outer layer of cumulus cells, the corona radiata, embedded in an extracellular matrix of carbohydrates, protein and hyaluronic acid. Hyaluronidase,

released from the sperm acrosome, breaks down the hyaluronic acid matrix between the follicular cells so sperm can pass through to reach the zona pellucida. The hyperactive swimming movements of the sperm aid penetration of the corona radiata. The gradual release of sperm from the reservoir of cervical mucus and their activation close to the oocyte means that the time limit of fertilization is extended. The second barrier is the zona pellucida.

Binding to the Zona Pellucida

The oocyte is surrounded by the zona pellucida, which is about 10–20 μm thick. It is an extracellular matrix composed of sulphated glycoproteins that were produced by the growing oocyte and is permeable to some molecules such as immunoglobulins and enzymes (and also to some viruses). The zona pellucida acts as a barrier that is species-specific, only allowing sperm of the same species to access the underlying oocyte membrane. One practical use of this species specificity is the Hamster Zona-Free Ovum (HZFO) test, which can be used as an indicator of male factor infertility. Once the zona pellucida is removed from hamster oocytes, these can be used to test if the capacitated sperm of the male partner are able to gain access to the oocyte cytoplasm. Although development will rapidly arrest, the HZFO assay provides a valuable test for male-factor infertility without wasting the precious human oocytes of the would-be mother.

The Acrosome Reaction

After binding to the zona pellucida (ZP), the sperm undergo the acrosome reaction (Fig. 6.2). The sperm binding to the ZP family of glycoproteins initiates a signal transduction cascade that causes a rise in intracellular Ca^{2+} concentration in the sperm. The outer acrosome membrane fuses

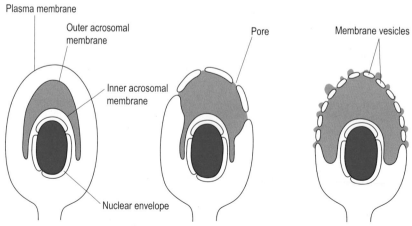

Plasma membrane

Outer acrosomal membrane

Inner acrosomal membrane

Pore

Membrane vesicles

Nuclear envelope

Fig. 6.2 The acrosome reaction.

with the plasma membrane of the sperm and small vesicles containing acrosomal enzymes are pinched off and their contents are released. The inner acrosomal membrane, which contains essential oocyte plasma membrane-binding proteins, is then exposed. A tunnel is digested through the zona pellucida by acrosin, a serine protease that remains bound to the inner acrosomal membrane, and the acrosomal enzymes released from the vesicles. The thrashing movements of the sperm flagellum propel the sperm forward through the zona pellucida, which is locally disrupted by the digestive secretions from the acrosome, a process termed the 'enzymatic drill'. The accentuated lateral head movements of the sperm also generate a boring action, which aids access through both the cumulus cells and the zona pellucida to the oocyte.

The human zona pellucida is composed of four glycoproteins ZP1, ZP2, ZP3 and ZP4 (Gupta, 2018), in contrast to the three found in the mouse (ZP1, ZP2 and ZP3), a commonly used experimental model for studies of human fertilization. ZP glycoproteins play crucial roles at several steps in fertilization. They provide a specific binding site for sperm to recognize and bind to the zona pellucida; their binding triggers the acrosome reaction in sperm and their modification following fertilization prevents further sperm–oocyte interaction providing the first block to polyspermy. In humans, sperm bind to all four glycoproteins but binding to ZP1, ZP3 and ZP4 has been implicated in induction of the acrosome reaction via different signalling pathways. Induction of the acrosome reaction by ZP3 can be blocked by pertussis toxin, a commonly used antagonist from the bacterium that causes whooping cough (*Bordetella pertussis*), which blocks binding of the Gi subunit to G-protein-coupled receptors (see Chapter 3) (Chakravarty et al., 2005). The ability of ZP1 and ZP4 to trigger the acrosome reaction is unaffected by pertussis toxin but does require a rise in intracellular cAMP, showing that these act via different signalling pathways to ZP3. All three of these glycoproteins require the presence of extracellular Ca^{2+} to trigger the acrosome reaction, suggesting that signalling pathways are complex. Human sperm bind to ZP2 only after they have undergone the acrosome reaction.

The Zona Reaction

The composition of the zona pellucida changes as a result of fertilization. Secretion of cortical granules by the oocyte is triggered by the oscillations in intracellular Ca^{2+}, which are triggered by sperm entry. The enzymic contents of these granules modify the structure of the ZP proteins to prevent further sperm from binding. This process, called the 'zona reaction', is an important block to polyspermy in humans but does not prevent oviductal secretions from reaching the oocyte during the early stages of cell division. All aspects of fertilization, including the mechanisms that prevent polyspermy (the production of polyploid, nonviable embryos), are difficult to study in human tissue for ethical reasons and the mechanisms involved are often different in animal models. Studies in transgenic mice have shown that ZP2 is cleaved by the protease ovastacin, released from cortical granules, and this may be an important component in the block to polyspermy at the level of the zona (Gupta, 2018). Other studies have implicated a role of ZP3 breakdown by cortical granule glycosidase.

The contents of the cortical granules (enzymes such as proteases and peroxidase, and polysaccharides) are released into the perivitelline space and diffuse through the zona pellucida to modify its structure and digest the ZP sperm receptors. The zona pellucida loses its ability to bind to sperm and to induce the acrosome reaction. The changed texture of the zona pellucida is described as 'zona hardening'. This zona reaction block to polyspermy prevents further sperm from accessing the oocyte but the exact mechanisms involved in humans remain unclear.

The zona pellucida has a number of vital roles in the reproductive process. It is essential for the production of oocytes in gametogenesis, for sperm recognition, for prevention of polyspermy and for the protection of the early cleavage-stage embryo prior to 'hatching' and implantation. The zona pellucida also has a role in preventing the blastocyst from prematurely implanting into the wall of the fallopian tube before it reaches the uterus. It is possible that an excessively thick zona pellucida can also cause problems with blastocyst hatching and subsequent implantation.

Interaction of sperm with the zona pellucida seems to occur in several stages. At first, the capacitated sperm adhere loosely and reversibly to the surface of the zona pellucida, then the sperm become strongly and irreversibly bound. Many sperm bind to the oocyte zona pellucida but usually only a few sperm penetrate into the perivitelline space and, ideally, only one will fuse with and gain access through the oocyte plasma membrane so that polyspermy, and the inevitable failure of fertilization that results, is avoided. The sperm then reaches the perivitelline space so that its head can now make contact with the oocyte plasma (vitelline) membrane. Anti-zona pellucida antibodies may be the cause of some cases of female infertility (Gupta, 2018) and the targeting of zona pellucida sperm-binding sites may be useful in the generation of novel contraceptive vaccines.

Gamete Fusion

The acrosome reaction triggers changes in the sperm membrane including the exposure of the posterior (postacrosomal) region of the sperm head that allow sperm–oocyte binding and then fusion to occur. Binding sites for oocyte-surface receptors are exposed on the sperm cell membrane by this process and one of these proteins, Izumo1, can interact with receptors on the outer surface of the oocyte membrane (Inoue et al., 2005). The receptor for this sperm protein has recently been identified (Bianchi et al., 2014) and named 'Juno', after the Roman goddess of marriage and fertility. Izumo1 on the sperm and its receptor, Juno, on the oocyte plasma membrane are essential for fertilization in several mammalian species, including humans, and female mice lacking Juno are infertile. Importantly, Juno has recently been shown to be responsible for another block to polyspermy since it is shed from the oocyte plasma membrane following fertilization, so that the sperm binding site is lost. Furthermore, additional sperm have their Izumo1 neutralized by binding to the shed Juno (Bianchi and Wright, 2014). This process constitutes the second block to polyspermy.

The surface of the oocyte is covered with microvilli, except in the region overlying the meiotic spindle. Oocyte microvilli surround the head of the sperm preceding fusion and then the sperm is incorporated into the oocyte. Various docking and recognition molecules on both the sperm head and the oocyte plasma membrane have been implicated in sperm–oocyte binding and fusion in addition to Izumo1 and Juno, including sperm ADAMs (a family of proteins with a disintegrin and metalloprotease domain) and CD9 and other proteins on oocytes (Bianchi and Wright, 2016). Whereas female mice lacking CD9 have reduced fertility, Juno-deficient mice are completely infertile. In human fertilization, the sperm tail remains motile and is incorporated into the oocyte. Paternal mitochondria entering the oocyte in the sperm midpiece are selectively degraded so that the zygote, fetus and postnatal individual have only maternal mitochondria. Since the mitochondrial genome (mtDNA) is always maternally inherited, this characteristic has been used for lineage tracing in anthropological studies of female ancestry. mtDNA mutations cause a range of debilitating and sometimes fatal diseases and recently, techniques have been developed to prevent the inheritance of mitochondrial diseases by the transfer of pronuclei from a fertilized oocyte from parents undergoing IVF to a 'third person' donor oocyte with normal mitochondrial DNA; a technique referred to as 'three-person embryos'. To overcome the ethical, theological and safety concerns that have been raised by this technique, novel methods of embryo-sparing donor-independent mitochondrial replacement therapies are being sought (Adashi and Cohen, 2018). Oocytes also seem to lose mitochondrial DNA (mtDNA) with increasing maternal age, a factor that may be important in infertility. One technique to deal with this is transfer of the cytoplasm from a younger woman's oocytes to 'rescue' oocytes from older women (Barroso et al., 2009).

The Blocks to Polyspermy

Polyploidy is usually fatal and is often detected in spontaneously aborted fetuses. Most human triploidy is due to polyspermic fertilization where two (or more) sperm fertilize a single oocyte. Only about one-millionth of the 200–300 million sperm deposited in the vagina actually reach the newly ovulated oocyte. This is both a reflection of the distance the sperm must travel relative to their size but is also regulated by sperm transit from reservoirs in the female reproductive tract. The relative importance of the plasma membrane versus the zona pellucida block to polyspermy varies between species. In most mammalian oocytes, the zona pellucida is thought to provide the most important block to polyspermy. The number of supernumerary sperm found in the perivitelline space between the ZP and the plasma membrane is usually 1–100 in humans, suggesting that the membrane block occurs almost simultaneously with the ZP block. As mentioned above, two key events are involved in preventing polyspermy in humans, the zona reaction involving modification of the zona pellucida by enzymes released from the cortical granules and the shedding of Juno from the oocyte plasma membrane preventing its binding to Izumo1 on the sperm membrane so that attachment of subsequent sperm does not take place. Failure of either of these steps results in polyspermy. Polyspermy results in nondiploid (polyploid) zygotes, which are usually not viable but, in some cases, can develop into gestational trophoblastic neoplasias and tumours such as the benign hydatidiform mole or the malignant choriocarcinoma (Hauzman and Papp, 2008). The incidence of nondiploid zygotes increases with alcohol use, drug use, anaesthesia and fertilization of 'aged' oocytes (i.e. aged in terms of hours after ovulation). Polyspermy may account for 2% of losses in normal conceptions and around 7% in IVF procedures. IVF using intracytoplasmic sperm injection (ICSI) does not trigger the membrane block to polyspermy, since it bypasses the interaction of the Juno and Izumo1 proteins. This is not important in the clinical scenario, since ICSI-fertilized eggs are directly injected with a single sperm, so the block to polyspermy is not needed.

The Ca^{2+} increase in the oocyte triggered by sperm binding evokes the fusion of cortical granules with the oocyte plasma membrane The Ca^{2+} signal starts from the site of sperm fusion and moves as an oscillating wave through the oocyte, sequentially activating the secretion of ~4000 cortical granules (Fig. 6.3). The trigger responsible for this Ca^{2+} rise has been extensively researched and the mechanisms involved are still not completely understood. The major pathway, however, is the release by the sperm of a novel phospholipase C, PLC-ζ (PLC-zeta), into the oocyte cytoplasm following cell fusion (Cox et al., 2002).

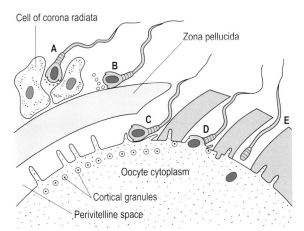

Fig. 6.3 Fertilization: (A) acrosome reaction; (B) binding to zona pellucida; (C) penetration of zona pellucida; (D) fusion of oocyte and sperm, and cortisol reaction; (E) fertilization.

This PLC-ζ hydrolyses a specific phospholipid (PIP$_2$) in the phospholipid bilayer membrane of cytoplasmic vesicles to release the cytosolic signalling molecule IP$_3$ which, in turn triggers the release of Ca^{2+} from the endoplasmic reticulum of the oocyte. PLC-ζ activity is directly stimulated by Ca^{2+} in a positive feed-forward mechanism that generates the characteristic Ca^{2+} oscillations that are essential for oocyte activation and early embryo development (Swann and Lai, 2016).

Direct introduction of PLC-ζ was demonstrated to mimic the pattern of Ca^{2+} oscillations evoked by ICSI (Fig. 6.4). During the ICSI procedure used in IVF (see below), it is common practice to immobilize the sperm by mechanical damage to the sperm tail just before injecting it into the egg. The extensive disruption of the sperm membrane wrought by this damage may help the sperm factor to be released, as there is a more rapid onset of calcium oscillations after ICSI. There is considerable interest in the possible role of PLC-ζ in male factor infertility and in its potential therapeutic use to improve the success rate of IVF. Although ICSI has proved to be an extremely effective form of IVF, up to 5% of ICSI cycles result in total fertilization failure, mostly due to a failure of oocyte activation. Assisted oocyte activation (AOA) is used to treat repeated failure and, most commonly, a Ca^{2+}-ionophore is used to provide a lipophilic pore in the oocyte plasma membrane through which Ca^{2+} ions can enter down their concentration gradient, mimicking the essential Ca^{2+} rise normally induced by sperm. Ionophore exposure causes a single and transient increase in Ca^{2+} (calcium ion) concentration, rather than the sustained Ca^{2+} oscillations, which result from sperm entry or PLC-ζ injection. It is not known whether these differences between normal

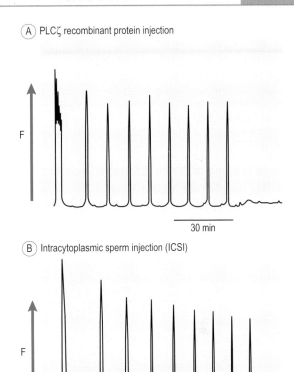

Fig. 6.4 A Ca^{2+}-sensitive fluorescent probe was loaded into oocytes from mice to allow intracellular Ca^{2+} concentrations to be monitored over time. (A) The oocyte was either microinjected with the human recombinant zeta isoform of phospholipase C (PLCζ) or (B) was subjected to intracytoplasmic sperm injection with a single mouse sperm. The patterns of Ca^{2+}-oscillations are similar suggesting that introduction of this sperm PLC into the oocyte at fertilization is responsible for triggering oocyte activation in mammals. (Reproduced with permission from Swann and Lai, 2016.)

fertilization, ICSI and ICSI/AOA have any consequences for normal embryo development but it is clearly preferable to develop an AOA protocol, which mimics as closely as possible the normal oocyte activation that results from sperm entry. To this end, several lines of evidence suggest that PLC-ζ may provide a better approach than current methods of AOA. Reduced levels of PLC-ζ in sperm have been shown to account for failure of egg activation and, in some cases, infertility due to failure of IVF and ICSI (Heytens et al., 2009). Possible adverse effects of current methods of AOA, such as exposure to ionophore, might also be avoided by injection of PLC-ζ, which mimics the repetitive Ca^{2+} oscillations seen in normal fertilization. The use of purified recombinant PLC-ζ might therefore provide a better approach to solving these problems (Nomikos et al., 2013).

Egg activation is triggered by the rise in intracellular calcium concentration; the earliest indicators are the resumption of meiosis and secretion of cortical granules. The rise in calcium subsequently initiates the first division of the zygote.

Events Leading to the First Mitotic Division
Possible Benefits of Arrested Meiosis

Prior to fertilization, the chromosomes of the oocyte had been arrested in metaphase of the second meiotic division (see Fig. 7.11, p. 174). It has been suggested that growth of the oocyte requires a diploid number of chromosomes. Meiotic arrest in the diplotene stage of metaphase means that both maternal and paternal alleles can be expressed during oocyte maturation. Observation of IVF has shown that the human meiotic spindle is unstable and very sensitive to external influences.

As a species, humans have a high frequency of aneuploidy – zygotes and embryos with the wrong number of chromosomes. Down syndrome is an example of trisomy where fertilization results in three copies of chromosome 21 (trisomy 21) with 47 chromosomes in total (see Table 7.1, p. 175). In most cases, this results from fertilization of an oocyte, which already contains two copies. Trisomy 21 is compatible with fetal survival and birth, whereas other trisomies are thought to be just as likely but lead to embryonic or fetal death or poor prognoses such as in Edwards syndrome (trisomy 18) or Patau syndrome (trisomy 13). Chromosome 21 and 22 are both small chromosomes; chromosome 21 has only 225 active genes, whereas chromosome 22 has 545 active genes. Therefore, trisomy 21 results in a relatively small number of genes in triplicate form, which may explain why trisomy 21 is often compatible with life. Genes on chromosome 21 are of particular interest because of their role in Down syndrome, which, for example, is associated with an early onset of Alzheimer's disease (AD) and several types of cancer such as leukaemia. Amyloid precursor protein (APP), coded for by a gene on chromosome 21, is the precursor of neurotoxic amyloid plaques, which are a major contributor to neurological dysfunction in AD. Having three rather than two copies of this gene is thought to explain the early-onset AD found in Down syndrome sufferers as early as 40 years old. These diseases and the small number of genes on chromosome 21 led to it being the second fully sequenced human gene in the Human Genome Project.

Aneuploidy in the embryo is mostly due to nondisjunction of chromosomes in either the first or the second meiotic division (see Fig. 7.11) (Webster and Schuh, 2017) and is associated with pregnancy loss. When the fetus survives, aneuploidy is the most common cause of mental retardation. The frequency of aneuploidy increases with increasing maternal age; ageing oocytes seem more prone to errors in meiosis and abnormal segregation of chromosomes, perhaps because the mechanisms responsible for normal chromosome disjunction have deteriorated during the more extended period of meiotic arrest. Studies have shown that Down syndrome more commonly results from fertilization of an oocyte that already contains two copies of chromosome 21 resulting from nondisjunction in oogenesis and giving rise to a trisomic zygote on single sperm entry. A lower incidence of Down syndrome results from fertilization by a disomic (two copies of chromosome 21) sperm. Also, this is less likely to be linked to increasing age of the male partner since male gametes are not suspended in meiosis I from their production in the fetus, a long period in which the meiotic process may cease to function normally. Gametogenesis in males is a continuous process throughout most of life.

Other factors such as alcohol abuse, chemotherapy and smoking have been found to disrupt meiosis. Arrest in the second meiotic division may help to prevent aneuploidy and the inclusion of an extra or absent chromosome in the oocyte.

Completion of the Second Meiotic Division

The Ca^{2+} rise that triggers the cortical reaction at sperm entry is also the stimulus for the oocyte to increase its metabolism. Calcium regulates the cell cycle in the oocyte and promotes resumption of meiosis, probably via activation of the M-phase-promoting factor and completion of second meiotic division (Fig. 6.5). The increase in oxidative metabolism is preceded by a rise in intracellular pH. The 23 paired chromatids then separate, half being expelled as the second polar body into the perivitelline space. A pronuclear membrane appears around the remaining 23 chromosomes forming the female pronucleus, thus completing the meiotic division.

Decondensation of the Sperm Nucleus

The chromatin or genetic material of the mature sperm is transcriptionally inert and compacted tightly in the head. After the head of the sperm enters the cytoplasm of the oocyte, it is affected by cytoplasmic factors that cause the chromatin threads of DNA to decondense and become transcriptionally competent. The decondensation takes place while the sperm pronucleus is moving towards the pronucleus of the oocyte. The centrioles that are both provided by the sperm radiate microtubules in a formation known as a 'sperm aster', which aids the movement of the two pronuclei. Then, oocyte histones begin to associate

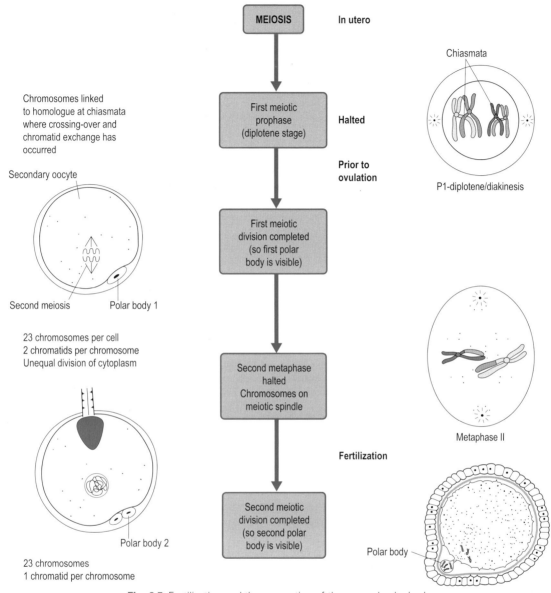

Fig. 6.5 Fertilization and the generation of the second polar body.

with the male chromosomal material (see Chapter 7). As the developing pronuclei near each other in the centre of the cell, they synthesize DNA in preparation for the first mitotic division and the chromosomes replicate into chromatids.

First Mitotic Division

In the first mitotic division, the membranes of both pronuclei break down and the male and female chromosomes become organized around a mitotic spindle ready for the first cell division. The combination of the male and female chromosomes is called 'syngamy'. It is at this point that conception has successfully occurred. Fertilization is complete about 18–24 h after fusion, and the fertilized oocyte becomes a zygote (the steps of fertilization are summarized in Box 6.2). A cleavage furrow then appears due to rearrangement of the cytoskeleton and the zygote divides into two identical cells (blastomeres).

During sperm and oocyte development (gametogenesis), the random distribution of chromatids between daughter

---

BOX 6.2 Sequence of Steps in Fertilization

- Deposition of sperm
- Sperm capacitation in the female reproductive tract
- Penetration of the corona radiata
- Binding of capacitated sperm to the zona pellucida
- Acrosome reaction
- Penetration of zona pellucida
- Fusion of sperm with oocyte plasma membrane
- Cortical reaction and prevention of polyspermy
- Increased respiration and metabolism by the oocyte
- Completion of the second meiotic division of the oocyte
- Extrusion of the second polar body
- Decondensation of the sperm nucleus
- Development and fusion of the male and female pronuclei

---

cells in meiosis and the random exchange of nuclear material between chromatids by crossing-over create new combinations of genes so that gametes are both haploid and genetically unique. Fertilization results in a unique combination of genetic material in the zygote, which is important in variation of the species (see Chapter 7). Whether the sperm carries an X or Y chromosome will determine the sex of the zygote so it will differentiate into either a female or male embryo (see Chapter 5). Fertilization restores the diploid number of chromosomes and initiates embryo development.

The mitochondria contained in the midpiece of the sperm enter the egg at fertilization but seldom survive beyond 2–3 days after fertilization. The number of mitochondria present in somatic cells ranges from a few hundreds to a few thousands depending on the energy requirements of the specific cell type. Each mitochondrion contains 5–10 identical, circular molecules of mtDNA, which codes for 13 proteins involved in the mitochondrial respiratory chain as well as ribosomal RNA (rRNA) and transfer RNA (tRNA) molecules. Mature oocytes are very large cells with high energy requirements and contain approximately 100,000 mitochondria. The fertilizing sperm introduces up to 100 mitochondria into the oocyte cytoplasm at fertilization. The sperm mtDNA are highly vulnerable to ROS and these highly reactive free radicals can cause mutagenesis during the lengthy process of spermiogenesis, storage, migration through the male and female reproductive tracts and fertilization, particularly as the sperm has little antioxidant capability. So, destruction of potentially defective sperm mitochondria is important to ensure that the developing embryo has a healthy stock of mtDNA. The mechanism by which sperm mitochondria, but not the mitochondria provided by the oocyte, are selectively destroyed relies on the tagging of spermatozoa with ubiquitin during spermatogenesis. Ubiquitin is a small (76 amino acids) polypeptide expressed in all eukaryotic cells (ubiquitous) where, among other functions, it is used to tag protein molecules that are destined for degradation by cellular protein complexes called proteasomes, a normal component of cellular protein turnover. After initial tagging, sperm mitochondrial ubiquitin is subsequently masked by disulphide bond formation during maturation and storage in the epididymis but following fertilization, the glutathione-rich environment of the early embryo exposes the ubiquitin-tagged sperm midpiece, which is then recognized by the oocyte's ubiquitin-proteasome-dependent proteolytic pathway so the sperm midpiece is lysed and its component mitochondria and their mtDNA are destroyed. The outcome of this efficient destruction of male-derived mitochondria and their mtDNA is that all mtDNA in human offspring is maternally derived (matrilinear). There is no change in the base pair sequence (of about 16,500 base pairs) when the mtDNA is passed on from mother to child so it is a useful tracking tool for tracing ancestry through the female line (Sykes, 2001). The relatively simple analysis of mtDNA from, for example, buccal smears, can therefore establish maternal ancestry (see Chapter 7). In forensic investigations, mtDNA rather than nuclear DNA is useful for very small tissue samples, since there are hundreds of copies of mtDNA per cell. mtDNA can also be used in lineage tracing of maternal ancestors, for example to identify members of the Russian royal family, descendants of Queen Victoria, who were murdered during the Russian revolution. Some convincing conclusions have been drawn, for example the 'Maori of Aotearoa share exactly the same mitochondrial DNA as their cousins in Polynesia' (Sykes, 2001). However, mtDNA has a high mutation rate and mtDNA mutations in all 13 protein-coding genes are responsible for a range of monogenic diseases (Koopman et al., 2012) and are also implicated in age-related disorders such as AD, since the juxtaposition of mtDNA to oxidative phosphorylation makes it a prime target for oxidative damage, which accumulates through the lifecycle (Wallace, 2010).

DEVELOPMENT BEFORE IMPLANTATION

The embryo spends about 4–6 days travelling to the uterine cavity. It is propelled through the uterine tube by the peristaltic action of the smooth muscle and the sweeping movements of the cilia and the fluid produced by the ciliated epithelium. Embryonic divisions initially occur approximately every 15 h; the division time becomes

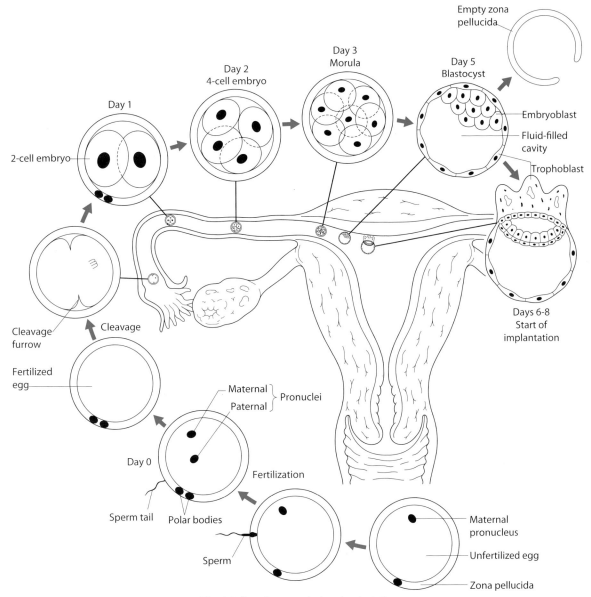

Fig. 6.6 Development before implantation.

progressively shorter. During the initial cleavage steps, the embryo is enclosed within the restraining zona pellucida and its total mass remains approximately constant to the original mass of the oocyte; the constant size of the embryo facilitates its free passage through the narrow lumen of the uterine tube. Cytoplasmic factors within the blastomeres regulate cleavage, which occurs without net growth (Fig. 6.6) so as blastomere cell numbers increase, the cells become progressively smaller.

Initially, the cleavage divisions are synchronous and each cell or blastomere is identical, but then they start to divide at an independent rate. As synchrony is lost, the pattern of regular doubling of cell number is also lost. In human and mouse embryos, until the 8-cell stage, each of the cells is totipotent (i.e. is able to generate all cell lineages in the embryo/fetus and extraembryonic tissues). Experiments on mouse embryos have demonstrated that each of the cells has the capability of independently developing into an embryo. Cells from different origins at the same point of development can also be combined to form a mosaic or a chimera. In human IVF, a single blastomere can be removed from the blastocyst at this stage for genetic testing using the technique of PGD without prejudicing the outcome for the embryo if it is transferred to the uterus, since the remaining cells are all totipotent (see Chapter 7).

After the 8-cell stage, the cells change morphologically so some of the cells at the outer edge of the embryo become flatter. At ~day 4, as it reaches the uterine cavity, the embryo is a mass of cells known as the 'morula' (from the Latin word for mulberry). The dividing ball of cells enters a phase called 'compaction'. The inner cells are sealed off by outer cells, which adhere tightly in a sphere, developing a polarity and communicating via gap junctions. A fluid-filled cavity (blastocoele) forms between the inner and outer cell layers; the embryo is now known as a blastocyst. By the 64-cell stage, the cells of the

conceptus are irreversibly differentiated on the pathway to becoming embryonic (tissues that form the embryo) or extraembryonic tissue (tissues that form the placenta and membranes, etc.). Differentiation into a particular cell type seems to be related to positional information of the cells and the separation of cellular components into different daughter cells during cell division (environmental and divisional asymmetry), which induces particular genes to be expressed. Cells of the blastocyst initially differentiate into two distinct cell lines. Most of the outer layer of cells forms the trophoblast, which will develop into the placenta, chorion and extraembryonic tissue. Most of the cells of the inner cell mass will develop into the embryo, umbilical cord and the amnion (Fig. 6.7). At this stage, cells of the inner cell mass are capable of giving rise to all cells of the fetus and therefore the adult (but not to the placenta or extraembryonic tissues). These are embryonic stem cells (ESC) and are referred to as pluripotent.

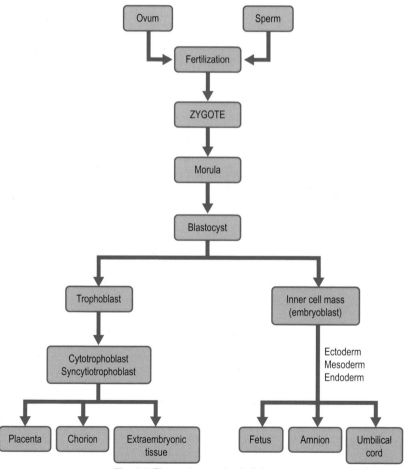

Fig. 6.7 The pathway of cell division.

PARENTAL IMPRINTING

Both maternal and paternal chromosomes are required for normal zygote formation and development but genes from both chromosomes are not always expressed. This is described as genomic imprinting and is due to gamete-specific patterns of DNA modification such as methylation. This means that, although each pair of chromosomes carries the same genes (with possibly different sequences), this information can be expressed differently depending on whether it originates from the maternal chromosome from the oocyte or from the paternal chromosome from the sperm (see Chapter 7). In genomic imprinting, methyl groups are attached to cytosine bases at specific locations in DNA during male and female gametogenesis. These epigenetic marks are therefore 'inherited' by the offspring so that a gene from one parent can be expressed, whereas the other parent's gene is imprinted and inactive. In the germ cells but not the somatic cells of the developing embryo, however, all imprinting is lost due to widespread demethylation before new imprints are established later in embryo development. Paternal gene expression favours development of the placenta and inhibits development of the embryo. Maternal imprinting seems to switch off some of the genes involved in placental development. Normally, the paternal copy of the X chromosome is preferentially activated in cells derived from the trophoblast. Conversely, in the inner cell mass, either the paternal or the maternal X chromosome is randomly inactivated (see Chapter 7). X chromosome inactivation occurs in all cells of human females, a process referred to as dosage compensation and is irreversible, except in oogonia. The inactivated X chromosome is referred to as a Barr body and most or all of its genes will never be expressed. Parental genetic imprinting is lost (reordered) on formation of new gametes, which have new patterns of parental imprinting established on the formation of new chromosome sets. It is thought that most imprinted genes are associated with placental tissue and so affect growth and development.

In mouse embryo cells, removal and replacement of one of the pronuclei with another of the opposite sex (so both pronuclei are of the same sex) results in abnormal development. If both the pronuclei are female (gynogenotes), early embryo development appears normal but placental development is impaired. If both pronuclei are male (androgenotes), placental development appears normal but embryonic development is extremely stunted. In both cases, very few androgenotes or gynogenotes survive until mid-gestation. Hydatidiform mole development in humans occurs as a result of diandric diploids, that is, when two sperm fertilize an oocyte and the maternal chromosome complement does not participate in development. The result is extreme overdevelopment of the placental tissues and extreme underdevelopment of the embryonic tissues. This situation could also arise from the fertilization of an oocyte with a diploid sperm. Digynic triploids (i.e. two maternal and one paternal chromosome sets) can occur if the polar body is retained.

Human oocytes can be induced to undergo spontaneous cleavage in the absence of fertilization by a sperm and develop into parthenotes (parthenogenesis). Early stages of cleavage, therefore, seem to be maternally imprinted. However, mouse parthenogenic oocytes arrest after the first cleavage divisions, at the time the embryonic genes would be expressed. It is thought that there is an increased risk of low birthweight in otherwise healthy infants born after assisted reproductive technologies (see p. 155), which may be partially related to different conditions very early in life affecting the imprinting of genes involved in fetal growth. Kaguya, a parthenogenic ('virgin birth') mouse that survived to adulthood, was produced by Kono et al. (2004) from an oocyte manipulated in vitro to have two haploid sets of maternal chromosomes together with expression of Igf2 and H19 genes by genetically engineering eggs to produce the growth factor, IGF-2, which is normally expressed from the paternal copy of chromosome 11. The method was very problematic and only two of 457 reconstructed eggs developed; there is a consensus that cloning of humans would be extremely difficult, of little merit and be likely to have major risks for maternal health and offspring development, as well as ethical issues.

TWINS

Throughout history, twinning has fascinated civilizations. The incidence of sets of twins in England was about 15.3 per 1000 live births in 2010 (Smith et al., 2014), an increase over previous years, which was seen in many countries because of the increased use of assisted reproductive technologies (ART) and an increase in maternal age at conception (note that the rate of triplet births is decreasing with changes in the numbers of embryos used in ART). The incidence of twins has stabilized in the USA in the 2004–2010 period at ~32 per 1000 live births, although figures vary markedly globally, with the highest birth rate of dizygotic twins in parts of Africa reaching 45 per 1000 live births. Monozygotic (identical) twin births occur globally at a similar rate of ~3.5 per 1000 live births. The ratio of monozygotic to dizygotic twins varies markedly from country to country and is affected by season, ethnic origin, parity and maternal age. Dizygotic twins arise from multiple ovulation and two fertilized oocytes implanting and developing; they have separate placentas and membranes (although sometimes these are fused). Monozygotic or identical twins are derived from one fertilized oocyte; the single zygote or embryo divides and then splits into two. Although it is possible that a 2-celled embryo could split resulting in twins, most twins result from the subdivision of the inner cell mass at the blastocyst stage (Fig. 6.8). About 75% of

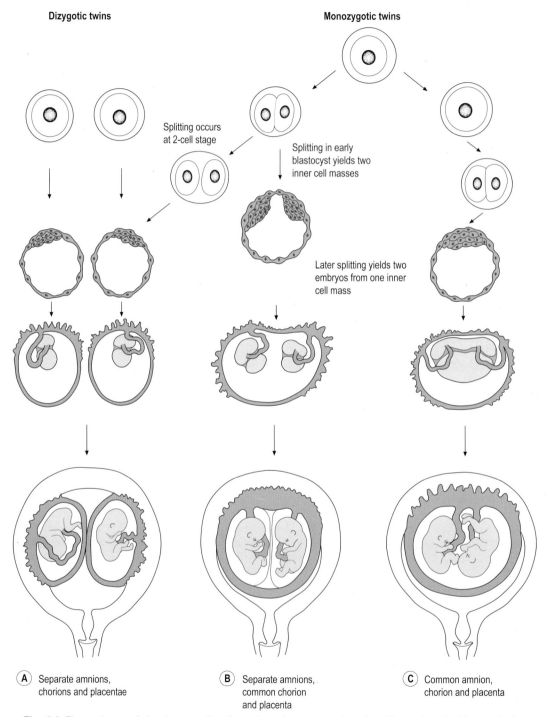

Dizygotic twins

Monozygotic twins

Splitting occurs at 2-cell stage

Splitting in early blastocyst yields two inner cell masses

Later splitting yields two embryos from one inner cell mass

(A) Separate amnions, chorions and placentae

(B) Separate amnions, common chorion and placenta

(C) Common amnion, chorion and placenta

Fig. 6.8 The pathway of development for dizygotic and monozygotic twins. (Reproduced with permission from Larsen, 1993.)

monozygotic twins share one placenta; the remainder have separate placentas and membranes. Twin pregnancies have a higher rate of obstetric complications, including fetal death, miscarriage and preterm labour, compared with singleton pregnancies. Very rarely, superfecundation results from the fertilization of two ova at different times during the same menstrual cycle resulting in fraternal twins with different biological fathers.

IMPLANTATION

The blastocyst may remain free-floating in the uterine cavity until implantation at day 7. The blastocyst accumulates fluid and expands. This, together with the digestion and thinning of the zona pellucida by uterine enzymes, results in shedding of the zona pellucida, described as 'hatching', at about 6–7 days postfertilization. The disappearance of the zona pellucida allows the cells of the blastocyst to come into contact with the epithelial lining of the uterus. The blastocyst consists of at least 100 cells, but some programmed cell death (apoptosis) has already occurred even at this very early stage of the lifecycle. In most blastocysts, there is a degree of degeneration of some trophoblast cells and some cells of the inner cell mass. After hatching, growth is no longer physically restricted and the blastocyst grows in mass as well as cell number. Embedding or nidation of the blastocyst normally occurs in the upper region of the uterus (the fundal region). The blastocyst implants at the embryonic pole, where the inner cell mass lies. The inner cell mass forms the embryonic disc (see Chapter 9).

The outer cells of the blastocyst secrete proteolytic enzymes and collagenase, which break down and destroy some of the cells of the endometrial surface, forming a depression in which the blastocyst lies. Implantation in humans is a very invasive process. Uterine muscle activity is low at this time because secretion of progesterone is high. Once implantation has occurred, the lining of the uterus closes over the blastocyst and the pregnancy is established within the endometrium. The trophoblast cells absorb nourishment from the decidua and secrete human chorionic gonadotrophin (hCG), which stimulates growth and secretory activity of the corpus luteum to produce steroid hormones that support continued growth of the decidua. Critical amounts of hCG are required for blastocyst survival.

MATERNAL RECOGNITION OF THE PREGNANCY

Successful implantation requires 'crosstalk' (reciprocated two-way communication between mother and embryo). The menstrual cycle, under the control of ovarian steroids, induces the biochemical, physiological and morphological changes, which prepare the uterus for blastocyst implantation. Many signals are involved in the crucial role of maintaining the corpus luteum, regulating uterine vascular permeability and maternal immunosuppression. Not all of the signals have yet been identified. hCG is involved in maintaining the corpus luteum and its essential endocrine role. hCG is luteotrophic, binding to the LH receptors and stimulating a progressive rise in progesterone and oestrogen secretion. Levels of hCG are abnormally low if implantation is inadequate, if trophoblast cell division is insufficient, if implantation is ectopic or if growth of the corpus luteum is deficient. Secretion of hCG from the trophoblast is regulated by trophoblastic gonadotrophin-releasing hormone (GnRH). hCG also binds to the embryonic trophoblast cells and affects the differentiation of cytotrophoblast into the syncytiotrophoblast (see Chapter 8). Before it becomes receptive, the uterus expresses high levels of the endogenous cannabinoid, anandamide. The concentrations of anandamide fall as receptivity increases, leading to the suggestion that the lower birthweight, which is associated with maternal cannabis (marijuana) use occurs because this balance is perturbed; tetrahydrocannabinol (THC) also crosses the placenta and affects neurodevelopment (Gunn et al., 2016).

Implantation and the three stages of apposition, adhesion (attachment) and penetration (invasion) require the endometrium to change and to become responsive. The endometrial stroma is modified (see Chapter 8); vascular permeability increases, and the endometrial cells become hypertrophied and produce prolactin. The processes that induce these changes are known as decidualization and the changed endometrium is called the decidua. The initial changes begin in the luteal phase of the menstrual cycle. The uterine glands become more tortuous, the spiral arteries develop and the endometrium becomes thicker and oedematous. Uterine secretions increase and intercellular spaces develop. The decidua forms a physical barrier to invasive trophoblast cell migration and generates cellular signals that promote trophoblast attachment. The decidualized endometrial cells also produce insulin-like growth factor binding protein 1 (IGFBP-1), which modulates interactions at the maternal–fetal interface and is involved in regulating growth.

Effectively, a nidation or implantation window, related to changes in the endometrial epithelium, occurs at about day 20–23 of the cycle (6–8 days after ovulation). The timing of the endometrial changes is mediated by preovulatory increase in 17β-oestriol and subsequent luteal progesterone secretion and has to synchronize with the time the fertilized ovum enters the uterus. Problems with coincident timing may explain infertility or impaired fertility. During this receptive period, tiny hair-like microvilli protruding from the endometrial cells transiently fuse into single, smooth, flower-like apical membrane protrusions called pinopodes or uterodomes. The pinopodes form a week after ovulation and are present for only 2 days before regressing. They absorb fluid and molecules from the uterine lumen, which tends to decrease the size of the uterine cavity and to increase the chance of apposition between the embryo and the endometrium. The transient absence of cilia may also prevent the blastocyst being swept away from the site of implantation. Progesterone stimulates pinopode formation, as well as increased uterine secretions, increased blood flow and oedema.

The microenvironment of the reproductive tract is influenced by the secretion of maternal proteins, which may then be further modified by proteins secreted by the developing embryo. Embryo-derived platelet-activating factor (ED-PAF) influences vasodilation and oedema of the decidua. It increases vascular permeability, induces thrombocytopenia, regulates prostaglandin synthesis and activates platelets. Prostaglandins are also involved in regulating decidual factors. Other substances thought to be involved in maternal–conceptus cross-talk include chemokines and cytokines (such as interleukins, interferons and tumour necrosis factor), inhibin and other growth factors (see Chapter 4), adhesion molecules (such as integrins), angiogenic and apoptotic factors, leptin and vitamin D. The expression of these proteins, peptides and steroids can act as markers of uterine receptivity. The uterine immune system plays an important role in implantation and trophoblastic growth and development; 30–40% of decidual cells are immune cells, predominantly uterine natural killer (uNK) cells (see Chapter 10).

CAUSES OF INFERTILITY

The average monthly fecundity rate of humans is about 20%; humans are not as fertile as other mammalian species. Infertility is usually defined as the failure to conceive a clinical pregnancy within 12 months of regular unprotected sexual intercourse. About 10–15% of couples have difficulties conceiving. Strictly speaking, infertility is a failure to produce gametes capable of fertilization and thus, conception never happens (by natural means). In practice, the term infertility is used for failure to continue a pregnancy to term (so there is no 'take home' baby). Subfertility is reduced fertility with a prolonged period of unwanted nonconception; it may require treatment. Some female infertility is due to primary ovarian failure (independent of hypothalamic and pituitary defects) or premature ovarian failure; these probably have genetic components but these have not been clearly identified. Women who experience prolonged hypovolaemic shock resulting from major haemorrhage (sometimes associated with surgery or a previous pregnancy) can develop anterior

pituitary necrosis, which can result in Sheehan's syndrome resulting in a loss of pituitary follicle-stimulating hormone (FSH) and LH secretion so that menopause begins abruptly and fertility is lost. About one-third of female infertility is related to tubal or peritoneal factors. This includes damage resulting in obstruction, narrowing or kinking of the uterine tubes, often related to pelvic inflammatory disease (PID) or sometimes scarring (adhesions) secondary to pelvic or tubal surgery. PID is also associated with irreversible damage and loss of the ciliated cells lining the uterine tubes, and thus the inability to transport the fertilized embryo to the uterus. Persistent tubal damage increases with each episode of infection or trauma. Previous ectopic pregnancy, prior abdominal surgery, especially if it caused peritubal adhesions, endometriosis, hydrosalpinx (where the uterine tube is blocked and filled with fluid), sepsis following abortion, appendicitis associated with rupture, uterine fibroids and tubal sterilization (ligation) can also affect tube patency and function. Female fertility can also be curtailed by failure to ovulate or to produce or respond to hormones during the menstrual cycle. Polycystic ovary syndrome (PCOS) is a relatively common cause of impaired fertility. Ageing affects the likelihood of ovulation within the menstrual cycle; it is thought that many women overestimate the length of their reproductive life. Unexpected premature menopause results in early infertility.

Male factor infertility is the underlying defect in one-third to a half of infertile couples. Oligoasthenoteratozoospermia (OAT: low number, poor motility, abnormal shape) is the most common cause. Other possible factors include azoospermia (zero sperm), the presence of anti-sperm antibodies or defects in the mechanisms by which the sperm interacts with the zona pellucida or oocyte membrane or failure of sperm-evoked oocyte activation. Most of these sperm-associated subfertility problems have been very effectively bypassed by the availability of ICSI for IVF. Although male reproductive functions do not cease abruptly, as with female menopause, paternal age has marked effects on sperm parameters and semen quality, hormone levels, libido and erectile function (Mazur and Lipshultz, 2018). Damage to the cells and tissues involved in spermatogenesis such as that caused by trauma or infection (like mumps or malaria) can affect sperm production. Defects of the genital tract (usually obstruction), antibodies or problems with ejaculation usually due to RE or impotence are the more common causes of male infertility. Recent data also suggest that the DNA methylation patterns in paternal sperm change significantly with paternal ageing and may have consequences for health outcomes in the offspring (Jenkins et al., 2018).

There are some factors that can affect fertility in both men and women. These include genetic factors such as Robertsonian translocations (see Chapter 7), where one of the parents has a chromosomal rearrangement, which means that their own genetic constitution is fine but they have an increased risk that their gametes are unbalanced and could potentially produce a nonviable embryo. Chromosomal abnormalities, especially where the number of sex chromosomes is abnormal, are associated with infertility. Endocrine abnormalities, particularly if they affect the hypothalamic pituitary axis such as pituitary tumours (e.g. prolactinaemia), Kallmann syndrome (a form of hypogonadotropic hypogonadism) and hypopituitarism, can affect fertility. Some metabolic/endocrine disorders such as diabetes, liver, kidney, thyroid and adrenal diseases also have effects on reproduction. Generally, untreated endocrine disorders are associated with infertility and treatment restores fertility. Sexually transmitted diseases, extremes of body weight in either partner, and advancing age can also affect fertility. Environmental factors such as virus infections, toxins, pesticides, solvents, pollutants (including cigarette smoke), alcohol and recreational drugs are all associated with reduced fertility (measured as a longer time to conception and/or increased risk of miscarriage). Some medical treatments, particularly those used to treat cancer, such as chemotherapy and radiation therapy for testicular cancers, can permanently affect fertility. Cryopreservation of gametes may be an option to preserve fertile gametes for subsequent IVF. Damage to sperm and possibly to sperm stem cells can result in male infertility, whereas damage to sperm DNA can result in genetic defects in the offspring, which result in miscarriage or postnatal defects. Conception should be avoided around the time of treatment and problems can be avoided completely by donation and storage of sperm for future use (sperm banking) before treatment is begun. Finally, there is also a significant probability that either both partners have fertility problems or that there is no explanation for failure of conception.

ASSISTED REPRODUCTIVE TECHNOLOGY (ART OR ARTIFICIAL FERTILIZATION)

Infertility is medically defined at the point when it is appropriate to offer intervention: when conception has not occurred after 12 months of unprotected intercourse in couples wishing to start a family or after 6 months if the woman is over 35 years old. Subfertility is thought to affect ~15–20% of couples. However, this figure depends on how subfertility is defined, as couples may also experience delays in achieving second and subsequent pregnancies. In practice, infertility cannot be cured but subfertility may be treated; medical intervention attempts to optimize conditions that will aid conception. The study of infertility is a relatively new field, open to new research, though research in humans is complicated by ethical considerations. It involves not just biological aspects of fertility but also social and psychological aspects. Many couples

---

BOX 6.3 Commonly Used Assisted Reproduction Procedures

- *In vitro* fertilization and embryo transfer (IVF+ET)
- Gamete intrafallopian transfer (GIFT)
- Zygote intrafallopian transfer (ZIFT)
- Intracytoplasmic sperm injection (ICSI)
- Donor insemination (DI)
- Intrauterine insemination (IUI)

---

seeking fertility treatment will not succeed. In the UK, fertility treatment is regulated by the Human Fertilisation and Embryology Act 2008 (see Box 9.3) and monitored by the Human Fertilisation and Embryology Authority (HFEA).

If gametes are available, either from the couple themselves or from a donor, assisted conception techniques can be used. Laboratory techniques can be used to prepare the gametes and bring them together in the laboratory to enhance fertilization (Box 6.3). Such techniques can be utilized in situations where there is damage to the uterine tubes (the site of normal fertilization), severe endometriosis, which may alter the uterine environment, male factor infertility (reduced number, motility or fertilizing ability of sperm) or coital dysfunction. ART is also used to treat unexplained infertility where they will test the fertilizing ability of the sperm, or where PGD is advisable to ensure that only embryos that do not carry the inherited genetic disorder carried by parents are delivered to the uterus.

Methods of selecting the gametes used for IVF are extremely important, especially when legal, ethical or religious reasons mean that destruction of supernumerary embryos has to be avoided. There may also be an association between a lower level of ovarian stimulation and better oocyte and embryo quality (Ubaldi and Rienzi, 2008). An oocyte is considered normal when, after the removal of the cumulus cells, which are also examined, it has a round clear zona pellucida, a small perivitelline space enclosing a single whole first polar body and cytoplasm, which appears pale, moderately granular and without inclusions. However, oocytes with morphological abnormalities can still be fertilized by ICSI, although abnormally shaped oocytes and giant oocytes are not associated with good outcomes. A large perivitelline space may be due to oocyte overmaturity. Similarly, sperm morphology can also be assessed; when strict selection criteria are applied, the success rate of ICSI is improved; a technique known as intracytoplasmic morphologically selected sperm injection (IMSI; Shalom-Paz et al., 2015). The criteria are based on the morphology of the sperm acrosome, midpiece, mitochondria, tail and nucleus but IMSI is expensive and time-consuming and so is not used routinely.

In Vitro Fertilization

IVF is now a routine procedure for certain types of infertility. It is often more efficient to treat infertility than investigate the causes first. Although IVF has given amazing opportunities to otherwise infertile couples to conceive, with more than 6 million babies born through IVF in the 40 years since the first successful birth of Louise Brown (Steptoe and Edwards, 1978), there are concerns that the technologies used traverse natural barriers, which normally prevent the transmission of genetic defects. There are a number of stages in a cycle of IVF treatment (Box 6.4). The couple may have more than one cause of infertility. IVF can also be used with oocyte donation, for instance, where the woman has ovarian dysfunction (such as premature menopause or Turner syndrome) or has a high risk of transmitting an inherited disorder as *in vitro* culture of the embryo permits preimplantation diagnosis (see Chapter 7). Ovarian stimulation is used to increase the number of mature oocytes that will be harvested, as some are likely to fail to be fertilized. The method is based on suppressing the natural menstrual cycle by inhibiting the LH surge with a GnRH agonist and then stimulating follicular development with hMG (human menopausal gonadotrophin, which contains FSH and LH), a technique called 'superovulation'. Ultrasound techniques can be used for both follicular assessment and the retrieval of oocytes. When several follicles have grown to a particular size (17–18 mm), ovulation is induced with human chorionic gonadotrophin. The oocytes are collected at a preovulatory stage so they are not truly mature. Ovarian hyperstimulation syndrome (OHSS) is a significant complication of fertility treatment involving ovarian stimulation (Nastri et al., 2010); it can cause ovarian enlargement, which may result in abdominal distension, increased vascular permeability, intravascular dehydration and the consequences of raised cytokine production such as thrombosis. Progesterone or hCG is necessary to support the luteal phase. The collected oocytes are then cultured.

BOX 6.4   Stages in an IVF Cycle

- Patient selection
- Ovarian stimulation
- Oocyte retrieval
- Semen preparation
- Possible cryopreservation of gametes (variable success rates)
- Insemination
- Assessment of fertilization
- Embryo cleavage
- Embryo transfer to uterus
- Cryopreservation of excess embryos
- Detection of pregnancy

BOX 6.5   Naegele's Rule

This rule was devised by Dr. Franz Karl Naegele who was a German obstetrician in the 19th century.

The rule estimates the expected date of delivery (EDD) from the first day of the woman's last menstrual period (LMP) by adding 1 year, subtracting 3 months and adding 7 days to that date. This approximates to the average normal human pregnancy, which lasts 40 weeks (280 days) from the LMP, or 38 weeks (266 days) from the date of fertilization.

Alternatively, 9 months and 7 days can be added.

Example:

LMP = 8 May 2019

+1 year = 8 May 2020

−3 months = 8 February 2020

+7 days = 15 February 2020.

Many women have either a longer or a shorter menstrual cycle. If this is the case, ovulation nearly always happens 14 days before the next menstrual period is due – it is usually the first part of the menstrual cycle (follicular phase) that varies. Therefore, short cycles, for instance of 26 days, the date estimated by Naegele's rule needs to have 2 more days added and long cycles, for instance of 32 days, the estimated date will be 4 days earlier than the date estimated by Naegele's rule.

It is estimated that only around 5% of babies arrive on their due date. Normal term is considered from the completion of the 37th week of pregnancy up until the completion of the 42nd week of pregnancy (usually written as T+14), so using Naegele's rule, a pregnancy would normally have a duration of between 266 and 294 days. After the 41st week, the term 'postmature' is used; current practice is to recommend induction of labour once 42 weeks have been completed (for singleton pregnancies), if maternal and fetal health are satisfactory. About 15% of babies will be born prematurely (before the completion of the 37th week).

The semen is prepared by separating the motile sperm from the seminal fluid and allowing them to capacitate in an artificial 'capacitating medium'. The capacitated sperm are introduced to the oocyte within a few hours of oocyte retrieval. The oocyte is enclosed by the cumulus cells of the corona radiata, which can be removed by the enzyme hyaluronidase to improve sperm access. The presence of the first polar body shows that the oocyte is at the metaphase II stage (see Fig. 7.11, p. 174) and ready to be fertilized.

At ~18 h after insemination, the oocytes are denuded by mechanical removal of the cumulus cells. If fertilization has occurred, two distinct pronuclei, and usually two polar bodies, will be observable under a microscope. At 24 h later, embryonic cleavage is evident and the quality of the embryo can be assessed morphologically for its potential to continue developing by the number of anucleate fragments and the evenness of the cells. Embryos with fragmented or uneven cells rarely continue developing. At around the 8-cell stage where embryonic cells are still totipotent, a blastomere can be removed for PGD (Handyside, 2018). Two or three embryos are then selected for transfer to the uterus about 48 h after the 2-cell stage; morphological scoring systems are used to assess embryo quality and potential viability. The zona pellucida tends to harden in culture and has to be eroded mechanically or by acid digestion to aid hatching prior to the transfer. Multiple births are common with IVF, although nowadays only two oocytes are implanted into older women, as the success rate is higher in younger women and the protocols try to avoid multiple gestation to increase the wellbeing of the infants. Successful implantation relies on both embryo quality and endometrial receptivity. Excess embryos can be cryopreserved using controlled freezing and storage in liquid nitrogen ($-196°C$) for later use (as can early embryos). Increased hCG levels 10–12 days after fertilization confirm pregnancy is established; levels of hCG usually double every 1.3 days.

In IVF treatment, injections of hCG can be given to prepare the follicles for ovulation following ovarian stimulation as it mimics the action of LH closely (see Chapter 3). Once the follicles have matured, the oocytes can be harvested. The administration of GnRH agonists in the luteal stage of the menstrual cycle has been shown to increase the implantation success of IVF and ICSI treatments (Razieh et al., 2009).

Intracytoplasmic Sperm Injection

ICSI has become the method of choice in couples where normal conception is prevented by severe male factor infertility and is now the most commonly used method of IVF. The use of ICSI now accounts for more than half of all IVF treatments worldwide, with significant differences between countries. Of the 68,000 IVF treatment cycles resulting in 20,000 births in the UK in 2016, 36% were via ICSI, down from a peak of 42% in 2011 (HFEA, 2018). In contrast, in regions such as Latin America and the Middle East, ICSI is used in 85–100% of IVF cases. In severe male factor infertility, the sperm are unable to fertilize the oocyte. In ICSI, a single noncapacitated, acrosome-intact sperm is gently aspirated into a glass micropipette, viewed using a microscope, and microinjected directly into the oocyte cytoplasm. The advantage of this method is that it is successful even with very severe sperm dysfunction. Sperm do not need to be motile and can even be harvested from the epididymis by microepididymal sperm aspiration (MESA) or percutaneous epididymal sperm aspiration (PESA). The success rates of ICSI are similar to IVF, but much higher when male-factor infertility exists.

Unlike conventional IVF, when sperm are to be used for ICSI capacitation is not included in their preparation, since interaction with the ZP and the oocyte plasma membrane will be bypassed by microinjection of a single sperm directly into the oocyte cytoplasm. Concerns have been raised about possible damage to the gametes during ICSI since hydrolytic enzymes from the sperm acrosome are released into the cytoplasm of the oocyte and the risk of mechanical damage to the oocyte, for example to the meiotic spindle that could potentially lead to aneuploidy. Also, ICSI bypasses almost all of the natural selection mechanisms that challenge the sperm in a normal conception. Thus, although ICSI works well in humans, particularly for male-factor infertility, success rates for live births from ICSI are lower than for conventional IVF, for reasons that are uncertain.

ICSI is also successful in animal species such as mice, but less so in species such as hamsters, which have large acrosomes (Yamauchi et al., 2002). There has been some discussion in the scientific literature about why ICSI in humans is less successful than conventional IVF, and also whether ICSI is associated with increased developmental defects (Esteves et al., 2018), although the evidence for the latter is inconclusive. Insufficient attention, perhaps, has been paid to the fact that introduction of the powerful acrosomal digestive enzymes directly into the oocyte cytoplasm might severely impact cell function at the very beginning of life, with potentially lifelong consequences. Early suggestions that this might be the case (Morozumi and Yanagimachi, 2005) and that acrosomal digestive enzymes should be removed prior to ICSI (Morozumi et al., 2006) have largely been ignored for human ICSI.

It is important to monitor the health of children born following assisted conception procedures. For example, the fertility of male offspring resulting from ICSI using a sperm which was incapable of normal fertilization, may well be affected; however, very little research in this area has been reported. Also, male offspring born following ICSI from fathers with Y chromosome deletions may inherit the same deletion. There are also increased incidences of *de novo* sex chromosome aberrations, inheritance of cystic fibrosis mutations and Y microdeletions. Over 1% of births in the UK and the USA are now due to ART, which also accounts for >30% of twin births. There is an increased complication rate in infants conceived through IVF, though some of this is probably due to the increased frequency of multiple births. However, singleton IVF infants are also more likely to be of lower birthweight and have birth defects. There is also an increased risk with IVF of rare epigenetic disorders, including Beckwith–Weidemann syndrome, Angelman syndrome, Russell–Silver syndrome and Prader–Willi syndrome, which are due to defects in genetic imprinting (see p. 189) (Cortessis et al., 2018). This appears to be related to postfertilization events such as embryo culture conditions used in

IVF or cryopreservation but the absolute number of children with these very rare disorders is very small.

Cryopreservation of oocytes, sperm or early embryos is an essential part of IVF. Cryopreservation provides the opportunity for sperm or spare oocytes and embryos to be stored for use in subsequent rounds of IVF. It can also be used to store early embryos that are surplus to requirements to be donated to other couples who are infertile, or carry a genetic disease but would find antenatal diagnosis and termination of an abnormal pregnancy to be unacceptable. The two cryopreservation techniques that are currently used are slow-freezing and vitrification, both of which minimize intracellular ice crystal formation which is essential to tissue viability. The use of frozen rather than fresh embryos for donation is becoming more common and in some countries is now used in most embryo transfers. Embryo donation has many ethical, legal and psychosocial implications. There is an increasing trend for patients facing intensive chemotherapy and other procedures to request gamete retrieval and cryopreservation; a more ethically complex area is requests for gamete retrieval from men who are terminally ill, dead, near-dead (for instance, in a persistent vegetative state) or brain-dead.

Case study 6.2 is an example of a couple preparing for pregnancy after IVF.

CASE STUDY 6.2

Elizabeth is a 42-year-old primipara who has been married for 20 years to Thomas. They had never used contraception. After initial investigations at a subfertility clinic, they were told that Thomas had a very low sperm count and that the sperm present were morphologically abnormal and displayed little motility. After eight rounds of IVF, Elizabeth and Thomas were offered ICSI and as a result, a pregnancy occurred.

- Should the advice that the midwife gives to Elizabeth and Thomas be any different to that given to a fertile couple?
- What kinds of anxieties and concerns would Elizabeth and Thomas have and how might these be addressed?
- Are there any more serious risks and complications for a developing fetus conceived by ICSI?

KEY POINTS

- The male gamete (sperm) is one of the smallest human cells and is motile, whereas the female gamete (oocyte) is one of the largest human cells and is immotile.
- Fertilization is the union of the sperm and the oocyte, resulting in a diploid zygote.
- Coitus requires circulatory and neuronal activity resulting in erection of the penis by increasing blood volume. Sexual arousal causes analogous physiological changes in the female.
- Assisted reproduction technologies and sex selection are widely practised in the agricultural livestock industries from where the technologies were derived for their application to humans. Gender selection in humans is practised using several approaches but sperm or embryo gender selection is ethically challenging and not widely used.
- In order to fertilize the oocyte, sperm undergo a series of changes: (1) development in the testes; (2) maturation in the epididymis; (3) capacitation in the female reproductive tract and changes in the sperm surface, which accompany the acrosome reaction. These alter the sperm plasma membrane, tail movement and metabolism to enable them to fertilize the oocyte.
- The acrosome reaction, and release of enzymes, results in digestion of a pathway through the follicular cells and zona pellucida. Interaction between the sperm and the zona pellucida and the oocyte membrane is mediated by species-specific receptors.

- Fusion of the gametes results in release of cortical granules and the zona reaction, and the shedding of Juno from the oocyte membrane both of which are blocks to polyspermy. Fusion also triggers metabolic changes, completion of the oocyte meiotic division, extrusion of the second polar body, DNA replication and initiation of the first mitotic division.
- The embryo or zygote undergoes cell cleavage as it is moved towards the uterus.
- As the number of cells increases, the embryo is described as a morula. The inner and outer cells undergo compaction and differentiate.
- The blastocyst has an outer layer of trophoblast cells (the future placenta) and an inner cell mass (the future embryo). After approximately 2 days in uterine fluids, the accumulation of fluid by the blastocyst causes the embryo to 'hatch' out of the zona pellucida.
- The trophoblast cells secrete hCG, which promotes the survival and further growth of the corpus luteum.
- Maternal recognition of the pregnancy allows embryonic development and uterine receptiveness to be coordinated.
- Implantation occurs about 7 days after fertilization.
- Assisted fertility techniques have been developed for couples who are subfertile.

APPLICATION TO PRACTICE

Primarily, the midwife is not involved with the treatment of subfertility and infertility. However, with the advance of technology, there are an increasing number of conceptions and successful pregnancies that result from fertility treatment.

An understanding of the complexities and interventions required to achieve conception is essential in order for the midwife to support women and partners. A knowledge of fertilization is also required in the understanding of contraceptive techniques.

ANNOTATED FURTHER READING

Balen AH: *Infertility in practice*, ed 4, Oxford, 2014, CRC Press.

A comprehensive textbook, based on the author's clinical experience of assisted reproductive techniques, which provides an up-to-date guide to the aetiology, assessment and management of human infertility including ethical issues and emerging techniques.

Carlson BM: *Human embryology and developmental biology*, ed 6, Edinburgh, 2018, Elsevier.

A recently updated and well-illustrated textbook, which covers the molecular basis of development, cellular aspects, developmental anatomy and the progression of development. Includes recent research findings, case studies, timeline information, review questions, clinical vignettes and useful end-of-chapter summaries. The textbook is packaged with an eBook that provides access to figures, text and animations.

Christianson MS, Bellver J: Innovations in assisted reproductive technologies: impact on contemporary donor egg practice and future advances, *Fertil Steril* 110:994–1002, 2018.

A good summary of the progression of assisted reproductive technologies since the 1980s, which identifies currently developing techniques and areas of innovation.

Fishel S: First in vitro fertilization baby – this is how it happened, *Fertil Steril* 110:5–11, 2018.

A fascinating account of the history of research into infertility and human embryology and the personal histories of Bob Edwards, Patrick Steptoe and Jean Purdy. It includes an interesting summary of some of the ethical issues and concerns about the work.

Human Fertilisation Embryology Authority (HFEA): *Fertility treatment 2014–2016 – Trends and figures*, London, 2018, HFEA.

A report of key information and statistics about the number and types of fertility treatment carried out in the UK including number of treatment cycles and birth measures. Note that HFEA regularly update material on their website: www.hfea.gov.uk.

Johnson MH: *Essential reproduction*, ed 8, Oxford, 2018, Wiley-Blackwell.

An integrated and well-organized research-based textbook, recently updated, that explores comparative reproductive physiology of mammals, including anatomy, physiology, endocrinology, genetics and behavioural studies.

Katkin E: *Conceivability: what I learned exploring the frontiers of fertility*, London, 2018, Simon & Schuster.

A personal and practical account, written by a lawyer, of fertility issues, of the science of conception and different approaches to infertility in countries across the world.

Ozyigit A, Ozyigit S: *The IVF guide: what you need to know about fertility, infertility and available treatment options*, London, 2018, Universal.

A concise but comprehensive guide, written for prospective parents and medical students, to in vitro fertilization and the current technologies used in reproductive medicine.

Simpson LL: What you need to know when managing twins: 10 key facts, *Obstet Gynecol Clin North Am* 42:225–239, 2015.

A concise overview of the management of twin pregnancy including dating, determination of chorionicity, possible abnormalities and best practice in monitoring twin pregnancies.

REFERENCES

Adashi EY, Cohen IG: Preventing mitochondrial diseases – embryo-sparing donor-independent options, *Trends Mol Med* 24:449–456, 2018.

Aitken RJ, Nixon B: Sperm capacitation – a distant landscape glimpsed but unexplored, *Mol Hum Reprod* 19:785–793, 2013.

Austad SN: The human prenatal sex ratio: a major surprise, *Proc Natl Acad Sci USA* 112:4839–4840, 2015.

Barroso G, Valdespin C, Vega E, et al.: Developmental sperm contributions: fertilization and beyond, *Fertil Steril* 92:835–848, 2009.

Bianchi E, Wright GJ: Sperm meets egg: the genetics of mammalian fertilization, *Annu Rev Genet* 50:93–111, 2016.

Bianchi E, Wright GJ: Izumo meets Juno, *Cell Cycle* 13:2019–2020, 2014.

Bianchi E, Doe B, Goulding D, Wright GJ: Juno is the egg Izumo receptor and is essential for mammalian fertilization, *Nature* 508:483–487, 2014.

Brenker C, Goodwin N, Weyand, et al.: The CatSper channel: a polymodal chemosensor in human sperm, *EMBO J* 31:1654–1665, 2012.

Brooker CG: *Human structure and function*, ed 2, St Louis, 1998, Mosby, p 477.

Chakravarty S, Kadunganattil S, Bansal P, et al.: Relevance of glycosylation of human zona pellucida glycoproteins for their binding to capacitated human spermatozoa and subsequent induction of acrosomal exocytosis, *Mol Reprod Dev* 75:75–88, 2005.

Cortessis VK, Azadian M, Buxbaum J, et al.: Comprehensive meta-analysis reveals association between multiple imprinting disorders and conception by assisted reproductive technology, *J Assist Reprod Genet* 35:943–952, 2018.

Cox LJ, Larman MG, Saunders CM, et al.: Sperm phospholipase C-zeta from humans and cynomolgus monkeys triggers Ca^{2+}

oscillations, activation and development of mouse oocytes, *Reproduction* 124:611–623, 2002.

Dixson AF: *Sexual selection and the origins of human mating systems*, Oxford, 2009, OUP.

Edwards RG, Bavister BD, Steptoe PC: Early stages of fertilization in vitro of human oocytes matured in vitro, *Nature* 221:632–635, 1969.

Esteves SC, Roque M, Bedoschi G, et al.: Intracytoplasmic sperm injection for male infertility and consequences for offspring, *Nat Rev Urol* 15:535–562, 2018.

Gunn JK, Rosales CB, Center KE, et al.: Prenatal exposure to cannabis and maternal and child health outcomes: a systematic review and meta-analysis, *BMJ Open* 6:e009986, 2016.

Gupta SK: The human egg's zona pellucida, *Curr Top Dev Biol* 130:379–411, 2018.

Handyside AH: 'Designer babies' almost thirty years on, *Reproduction* 156:F75–F79, 2018.

Hauzman EE, Papp Z: Conception without the development of a human being, *J Perinat Med* 36:175–177, 2008.

Heytens E, Parrington J, Coward K, et al.: Reduced amounts and abnormal forms of phospholipase C zeta (PLCzeta) in spermatozoa from infertile men, *Hum Reprod* 24:2417–2428, 2009.

Holt WV, Fazeli A: Do sperm possess a molecular passport? Mechanistic insights into sperm selection in the female reproductive tract, *Mol Hum Reprod* 21:491–501, 2015.

Human Fertilisation Embryology Authority (HFEA): *Fertility treatment 2014–2016 – Trends and figures*, London, 2018, HFEA.

Inoue N, Ikawa M, Isotani A, et al.: The immunoglobulin superfamily protein Izumo is required for sperm to fuse with eggs, *Nature* 434:234–238, 2005.

James WH: Evidence that mammalian sex ratios at birth are partially controlled by parental hormone levels around the time of conception, *J Endocrinol* 198:3–15, 2008.

Jenkins TG, Aston KI, Carrell DT: Sperm epigenetics and aging, *Transl Androl Urol* 7(Suppl 3):S328–S335, 2018.

Karabinus DS, Marazzo DP, Stem HJ: The effectiveness of flow cytometric sorting of human sperm (MicroSort®) for influencing a child's sex, *Reprod Biol Endocrinol* 12:106, 2014.

Kono T, Obata Y, Wu Q, et al.: Birth of parthenogenetic mice that can develop to adulthood, *Nature* 428:860–864, 2004.

Koopman WJH, Willems PHGM, Smeitink JAM, et al.: Monogenic mitochondrial disorders, *N Engl J Med* 366:1132–1141, 2012.

Kouidrat Y, Pizzol D, Cosco T, et al.: High prevalence of erectile dysfunction in diabetes: a systematic review and meta-analysis of 145 studies, *Diabet Med* 34:1185–1192, 2017.

Larsen WJ: *Human embryology*, ed 2, New York, 1993, Churchill Livingstone, p 481.

Levin RJ: *The human sexual response cycle, the textbook of clinical sexual medicine*, New York, 2017, Springer, pp 39–51.

Lewis Z, Price TA, Wedell N: Sperm competition, immunity, selfish genes and cancer, *Cell Mol Life Sci* 65:3241–3254, 2008.

Mazur DJ, Lipshultz LI: Infertility in the aging male, *Curr Urol Rep* 19:54, 2018.

Morozumi K, Yanagimachi R: Incorporation of the acrosome into the oocyte during intracytoplasmic sperm injection could be potentially hazardous to embryo development, *Proc Natl Acad Sci USA* 102(40):14209–14214, 2005.

Morozumi K, Shikano T, Miyazaki S, et al.: Simultaneous removal of sperm plasma membrane and acrosome before intracytoplasmic sperm injection improves oocyte activation/embryonic development, *Proc Natl Acad Sci USA* 103(47):17662–17666, 2006.

Nastri CO, Ferriani RA, Rocha IA, et al.: Ovarian hyperstimulation syndrome: pathophysiology and prevention, *J Assist Reprod Genet* 27:121–128, 2010.

Nomikos M, Kashir J, Swann K, et al.: Sperm PLCζ: From structure to Ca2+ oscillations, egg activation and therapeutic potential, *FEBS Letters* 587:3609–3616, 2013.

Orzack SH, Stubblefield JW, Akmaev VR, et al.: The human sex ratio from conception to birth, *Proc Natl Acad Sci USA* 112:2102–2111, 2015.

Quilter M, Hodges L, von Hurst P, et al.: Male sexual function in New Zealand: a population-based cross-sectional survey of the prevalence of erectile dysfunction in men aged 40–70 years, *J Sex Med* 14:928–936, 2017.

Razieh DF, Maryam AR, Nasim T: Beneficial effect of luteal-phase gonadotropin-releasing hormone agonist administration on implantation rate after intracytoplasmic sperm injection, *Taiwan J Obstet Gynecol* 48(3):245–248, 2009.

Shalom-Paz E, Anabusi S, Michaeli M: Can intra cytoplasmatic morphologically selected sperm injection IMSI technique improve outcome in patients with repeated IVF-ICSI failure? A comparative study, *Gynecol Endocrinol* 31(3):247–251, 2015.

Smith SM, Garic A, Berres ME, Flentke GR: Genomic factors that shape craniofacial outcome and neural crest vulnerability in FASD, *Front Genet* 5:224, 2014.

Steptoe PC, Edwards RG: Birth after the reimplantation of a human embryo, *Lancet* 2:366, 1978.

Suarez SS: Mammalian sperm interactions with the female reproductive tract, *Cell Tissue Res* 363:185–194, 2016.

Swann K, Lai FA: The sperm phospholipase C-ζ and Ca2+ signaling at fertilization in mammals, *Biochem Soc Trans* 44:267–272, 2016.

Sykes B: *The seven daughters of Eve*, London, 2001, Corgi Books.

Ubaldi F, Rienzi L: Morphological selection of gametes, *Placenta* 29(Suppl B):115–212, 2008.

Wallace DC: Mitochondrial DNA mutations in disease and aging, *Environ Mol Mutagen* 51:440–450, 2010.

Webster A, Schuh M: Mechanisms of aneuploidy in human eggs, *Trends Cell Biol* 27:55–68, 2017.

Wilcox AJ, Weinberg CR, Baird DD: Timing of sexual intercourse in relation to ovulation –effects on the probability of conception, survival of the pregnancy, and sex of the baby, *New Engl J Med* 333:1517–1521, 1995.

Williams AC, Ford CL: The role of glucose in supporting motility and capacitation in human spermatozoa, *J Androl* 22:680–695, 2001.

Yafi FA, Jenkins L, Albersen M, et al.: Erectile dysfunction, *Nat Rev Dis Primers* 2:16003, 2016.

Yamauchi Y, Yanagimachi R, Horiuchi T: Full term development of golden hamster oocytes following intracytoplasmic sperm head injection, *Biol Reprod* 67(2):534–539, 2002.

Overview of Human Genetics and Genetic Disorders

LEARNING OBJECTIVES

- To describe the organization of DNA and the packaging of genes in the chromosome and how they are expressed.
- To describe the general characteristics of dominant, recessive and X-linked genetic traits.
- To interpret a pedigree chart and explain simple genetic predictions.

- To discuss the principles of genetic screening and preimplantation genetic diagnosis.
- To relate current genetic research to midwifery practice.
- To discuss evolutionary influences upon human reproduction.

INTRODUCTION

Genetics is the science of genes, heredity and the variation of organisms. Although genetics is a component of virtually all areas of biology, it tends to be reductionist in nature. Life is the result of the genetic codes that all living things carry in almost all of their cells. The mechanisms that govern the manner in which genetic information is duplicated, altered, transferred and expressed provide a wealth of information about the biochemical processes of all living organisms. The advent of molecular biology has meant that many problems considered formidable until very recently may now be understood and resolved. Molecular biology has added new dimensions to understanding the origin of the human species, to creating new drugs and gene therapy and to sequencing of entire genomes of a variety of species, including disease-causing microorganisms, plants, insects and animals including humans.

CHAPTER CASE STUDY

Zara is informed by her midwife about the options available for routine antenatal screening. Zara wants to minimize the risk to her unborn child and asks the midwife for non-invasive prenatal testing (NIPT) (see p. 191).

- What information and training would the midwife need to be able to inform Zara about this type of antenatal screening?

Zara has a family history of Duchenne Muscular Dystrophy (an X-linked trait); it has been confirmed that she is a carrier (and has a 1:4 risk of having an affected male child).

- Would this warrant sex determination via NIPT to establish the presence of a Y chromosome?
- Would there be any benefit if Zara's partner James underwent genetic screening as well?

As part of the routine antenatal care Zara is receiving from her midwife at her local maternity unit, she is offered a 20-week anomaly ultrasound as part of the screening policy of the local maternity services. Zara is initially concerned because one of her friends had undergone amniocentesis after her ultrasound scan revealed cardiac, brain and limb abnormalities. Zara felt that this could be avoided if she opted for NIPT. Subsequently, Zara has NIPT, and is informed that her fetus is female and no genetic abnormalities were detected.

Zara's scan appears to be normal and the baby appears to be growing well but Zara is still concerned and wishes to discuss what further tests are available that would reassure her further.

- How would you, as Zara's midwife, reassure and counsel her and James through this difficult period?
- Are there any other situations, routinely managed in pregnancy, that may have risks that could be significantly reduced with the application of NIPT?

Within living organisms, the genetic information is usually carried in chromosomes where organization of the DNA provides a gene or 'blueprint' (genotype) directing protein synthesis and thus the expression of the genes into physical characteristics (phenotype). Characteristics are passed from one generation to the next in the form of genes. In sexually reproducing species, the genes are shuffled and repackaged into the gametes. Variations between genes affect survival so the individuals with the best-adapted characteristics to cope with environmental conditions have an advantage. This differential survival is described as natural selection.

Although DNA codes for the genes, not all the genes are expressed in any one cell or any one time. The phenotype is determined by which genes are expressed (turned on) and which are not. Epigenetics is the term used to describe the modifications to DNA which controls which genes are expressed. The modifications affect the transcription of DNA (the outcome) without changing the underlying DNA sequence. As well as the functions of the genes being identified as part of the determination of the DNA sequence (human genome), thousands of small noncoding RNAs have roles in mRNA stability, protein translation, protein modification and changes in the germline. All eukaryotic organisms have both nuclear DNA and mitochondrial DNA (mtDNA) (outside the nucleus), which is thought to be due to a serendipitous event in evolution, whereby the genomes of ancestral bacteria were engulfed and incorporated into eukaryotic cells as mitochondria. The bacterial origin of mitochondria is supported by observed similarities in the mode of mitochondrial replication by binary fission, genetic similarities between the mitochondrial genomes of some eukaryotic species and bacterial genomes and similar types of protein in the mitochondrial membrane and cell membranes of bacteria.

The study of genetics focuses on inherited characteristics, particularly those that are considered abnormal, how these arise and their effects on the individual. Genetics is a predictive science and its rules are based upon the application of statistics and probability. Evolutionary effects on genetics may determine the penetration of recessive genetic disorders such as cystic fibrosis into gene pools. The impact of genetics upon preimplantation diagnosis and antenatal screening to predict the probability of fetal abnormalities is of particular relevance for midwives.

A BRIEF HISTORY OF GENETICS

Historically, humans unknowingly but successfully applied genetics to the breeding and domestication of animals and plants. However, the first systematic study of genetic interactions is associated with the breeding experiments of Gregor Mendel, an Austrian monk, in the 1860s. Mendel established inheritance patterns of certain traits in pea plants and demonstrated that application of statistics to inheritance could be very useful. Subsequently, more complex forms of inheritance have been identified.

Mendel correctly identified the concept of genes long before the structures of DNA and chromosomes were understood. He proposed that 'particles of inheritance' were transmitted from one generation to the next and defined a concept that he described as an allele. The term 'allele' is now used to describe a specific variant or alternative form of a particular gene occupying a given locus (position) on a chromosome.

The term 'eugenics' was coined by Francis Galton (a cousin of Charles Darwin) who advocated that application of Darwinian theories and selective breeding could improve the quality of entire human populations, particularly with respect to talent and intelligence. In the late 19th century, eugenics societies formed in various parts of the world sought to promote such practices as marriage restriction, sterilization and custodial commitment of those thought to have unwanted characteristics and to positively encourage reproduction in those individuals perceived as the best and brightest. The popularity of the eugenics movement was already waning when the infamous eugenics programmes of Nazi Germany were revealed at the end of World War II.

Darwin's 'survival of the fittest' theory promoted the concept of natural selection and how environmental conditions determine survival and reproduction of organisms with particular traits. If environmental conditions do not vary much, these traits continue to be adaptive and become more common within the population.

Neo-Darwinism (or 'modern evolutionary synthesis') extends the scope of Darwin's ideas of natural selection by including modern genetic knowledge about DNA and concepts such as speciation, kin selection and altruism. It advocates that survival of a species is not necessarily by the fittest but by those that are most likely to reproduce successfully. This is reflected in the work of William Hamilton, popularized by Richard Dawkins over 40 years ago in his best-selling book *The Selfish Gene*, who asserted that the gene, rather than the organism or species, is the true unit of reproduction and the primary driver and beneficiary of evolution. The genes were described as 'selfish' because in order to replicate and be successful, they use organisms that contain them solely as vehicles to ensure survival (Dawkins, 2016). Obviously, reproduction is vital to ensure that the genes survive.

This gene-centred view of evolution portrays organisms solely as mechanical methods of survival to pass genes on to as many offspring as possible. However, there are a number of arguments against this view. Organisms are not perfectly adapted. It could be argued that some genes, which are not advantageous, have not been obliterated because other linked genes are advantageous and effectively protect them.

The other important point is that species not only interact with their environment but also positively alter their environment to optimize survival. The selfish gene hypothesis also accounts for how genes that seem to be harmful can evolve by natural selection.

The environment interacts with genes (the nature/nurture debate) and has a tremendous influence on how they are expressed, affecting susceptibility and resistance to disease. Genes may act in competition with each other, which may explain certain pathophysiological conditions and their aetiology. Some organisms may use their genes to alter the phenotype of another animal to increase their chances of survival. Co-evolution explains how the change of one organism can be linked to the change in a related organism. Each organism exerts selective pressure on the adaptation and evolution of the other. Examples include how angiosperm (flowering trees) and primates evolved, the existence of mitochondria (see Chapter 1) in eukaryotic cells and co-evolution of parasites with the acquired immunity of their hosts. Epigenetics and genetic imprinting (see p. 250) explain how gene expression can be affected by the environment.

Fred Sanger developed the methodology, now known as the 'Sanger Method', for sequencing DNA, in 1977. This ground-breaking method, which allowed long stretches of DNA to be accurately and rapidly sequenced, led to him being awarded his second Nobel prize in chemistry. This method was used for the Human Genome Project (HGP), 'the largest single undertaking in the history of biological science', which was established as a multinational cooperative research project in 1990 to map the common human nucleotide sequence of more than 3 billion DNA bases in some reference human genomes (the DNA of a few anonymous donors). It was hoped that identification of the 20,000–25,000 genes in the human genome would accelerate progress to diagnosing, treating and ultimately preventing diseases as well as answer questions about evolution. As individuals (except for identical twins) have unique genomes, the project involved determining the sequence of many versions of each gene. The international project was completed in 2003 and revealed that there are about 22,300 genes in humans, which code for proteins (Pertea and Salzberg, 2010). The mapping of the genome allows a framework for looking at differences in DNA sequences in individuals so variations in DNA sequence associated with diseases could be identified. The HGP has been supported by remarkable technological progress in bioinformatics, statistics and biotechnology. The HGP has also raised some complex ethical, legal and social implications, such as gene patenting.

The current medical and genetic technology has created ethical dilemmas associated with screening, detection and termination of abnormal fetuses. Current research in genetics (Box 7.1) can also be applied to population studies, such as tracing the origins of human migration movements,

---

> **BOX 7.1   Areas of Genetic Research**
>
> - Screening for fetal abnormality
> - Genetic counselling for parents with a family history of genetic disorders
> - Identification of fetal sex in the early (indifferent) embryological phase
> - Cloning of whole organisms
> - Gene manipulation not only to eradicate disease but also to improve existing disease states
> - Treatment by gene manipulation in animals to produce human proteins, hormones and so on
> - Genetic modification
> - Identification of individuals by genetic 'fingerprinting'

---

and to genealogy. Forensic genetics, though traditionally focused towards profiling human DNA in criminal investigations such as identifying the source of miniscule biological samples or identifying a body, is now being used for much wider applications. Examples include identifying animals involved in attacks, trafficking of protected species, identification of food contaminants and food-borne diseases and investigation of bioterrorism (Arenas et al., 2017). Post-conflict situations often require the search, recovery and identification of people who have gone missing (or 'been disappeared'); some of the best-known examples include tracing the real families of the adopted children of the Argentinian 'Los Desaparecidos' ('The Disappeared'). Another interesting application of genetic tracking is the research into the migration of the ancestral Polynesian population from South China through the Pacific to Aotearoa, New Zealand, in the second millennium AD (Anderson et al., 2015). There are also ethical concerns about how knowledge of the human genome might be used to discriminate against people, for instance, if it was known that their genes significantly increased the risk of disease it might affect employment or insurance premiums.

As genetics has developed, new scientific fields have been identified. Genomics refers to all aspects of molecular biology involved with identifying the structure and function of the genomes and their evolution and mapping. Genome editing or engineering encompasses modification of the genome of a living organism by inserting, deleting, modifying or replacing its DNA at specific locations of the gene by using specifically created nucleases known as molecular scissors.

A major advance in the field of genome manipulation arrived with the application of CRISPR (Clustered Randomly InterSpaced Palindromic Repeats) technology to human cells. CRISPR-Cas9 genome editing is based upon the methods used by bacteria to remember and defend against viral and bacteriophage infection; the bacterial 'immune system'. CRISPR techniques are able to target specific sequences of DNA in cells so that Cas9 can break the DNA at that point and inactivate the gene or, alternatively, using modified versions of Cas9, activate expression of the gene instead. These techniques allow researchers to study the gene's function and edit the gene in live cells by designing a guide RNA (gRNA), to precisely target specific nucleic acid sequences, such as those that result in diseases (Pandey et al., 2017). CRISPR technology also forms the basis for new diagnostic tools to identify genes and DNA sequences that are present in diseases of unknown cause. CRISPR will provide the technology to correct mutations in the human genome to treat genetic disease, as well as providing new and powerful diagnostic tools. Concerns have been expressed about ensuring both safety and efficacy in CRISPR use in humans as a diagnostic tool (Pan and Kraschel, 2018).

GENES AND CHROMOSOMES

Genes are the units of inheritance. Each gene is a length of DNA on a chromosome that contains the coded information to direct the synthesis of a specific protein chain. The differences between organisms are related to different proteins being synthesized (expressed) that have different structures and functions. Effectively, the genes act as a blueprint, or instruction manual, for the total development of the organism and how it will function and change during its lifetime (Box 7.2). Chromosomes are packages of DNA in the nucleus, on which the genes are linearly arranged. Chromosomes have two arms: a shorter 'p' arm and a longer 'q' arm, with a centromere between them. Chromosomes are important in cell replication and the passing of the genetic message from one generation to the next. DNA exists as an unstructured mass of threads in the nucleus. It consists of about 3 billion base pairs per cell nucleus, which if it could be stretched out, would be ~2 metres long. However, when the cell is undergoing division, the DNA becomes organized and compacted into chromosomes, which can be visualized by microscopy (see Chapter 1). This chromosomal organization allows biologists to identify genes and localize them to a particular chromosome to follow their pattern of inheritance. Each cell has the same genetic information in its nucleus as the original zygote (fertilized ovum) and all of the cells derived from it. Different cells behave in different ways because they express different subsets of genes to yield their characteristic set of proteins.

THE STRUCTURE OF DNA AND RNA

Watson, Crick, Franklin and Wilkins elucidated the biochemical structure of DNA, which was published in their seminal paper in 1953. Their description of the helical structure revealed how the molecule was able to replicate itself and thus explained the cellular mechanism of reproduction. DNA is composed of two strands of sugar phosphate molecules with pairs of bases that hold the chains together in a double helical structure (Fig. 7.1). The strands of DNA are made up of repeating units called 'nucleotides'. The DNA nucleotide has three components: a deoxyribose sugar, a phosphate group and a base. There are four types of bases: thymine and cytosine, which have single-ring structures, and adenine and guanine, which have double-ring structures. DNA exists as a double-stranded molecule wound into a helix. The strands are kept together by hydrogen bonding between the bases. The bases are of different sizes and have a different potential number of hydrogen bonds so they always pair in the same ways. Adenine (A) and thymine (T) pair with two hydrogen bonds: cytosine (C) and guanine (G) pair with three. This means that the sequence of the bases is complementary; the sequence of bases on one strand can be deduced from the sequence on the other strand.

DNA REPLICATION AND CELL DIVISION

The arrangement of base pairs of the two strands is like the rungs of a ladder or the teeth of a zip. When DNA replicates, the strands unwind and the hydrogen bonds, which hold the base pairs together, separate (unzip). Each strand acts as a template for the synthesis of another new strand of complementary DNA bases to form from nucleotides that enter the nucleus through the nuclear pores (Fig. 7.2). Two new DNA double helices are formed, each with one strand of 'old' DNA and a newly synthesized strand. Thus, the replication is described as semiconservative. Replication occurs as part of mitosis or cell division. Replication of DNA means that the chromosomes have double their nuclear material in

---

BOX 7.2   Genetics as a Language

Genetics can be considered as a language based on the DNA molecule. Linguistic development and evolution have a number of similarities. Studies looking at the origins of a particular word and how it has evolved to be slightly different in different languages are similar to the changes in genes. Genetic mutations are analogous to new words being introduced into the language (such as 'email').

- Language = genetics
- Vocabulary = genes
- Grammar = rules about the arrangement of information
- Literature = the instructions to make a human
- Alphabet = four bases of DNA
- Word = codon (three 'letter' code for an amino acid)

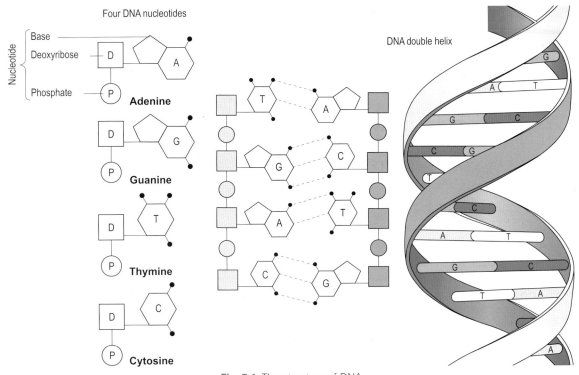

Fig. 7.1 The structure of DNA.

preparation for dividing into two separate cells. Therefore, the chromosome is formed of two identical chromatids.

Mitosis

The replication of the entire human genome is achieved through the process of mitosis, which is part of the cell cycle (Fig. 7.3). Cellular replication results in growth of tissues through hyperplasia (an increase in the number of cells); each cell has the identical genetic message (DNA content) to its parent cell. Mitotic rates are different for different types of cells. Cells that divide rapidly (have a high mitotic index) include skin and gut epithelial cells, spermatogonia and tumour cells. With increased age, the mitotic rate slows down so skin renewal, for instance, takes longer and the appearance of the skin is more aged. Drugs used to treat cancers also inhibit mitosis so their side-effects are mostly clearly manifested in normal cells with high mitotic rates, causing problems with nutrient absorption and decreasing male fertility. Many cells, such as brain, heart and liver cells, have an extremely slow rate of mitosis and do not regenerate or heal well after injury. Mitosis is a continuous process but for ease of description is traditionally described in distinct phases: prophase, metaphase, anaphase and telophase (Fig. 7.4). Interphase is the name given to the gap between mitotic divisions.

THE GENETIC MESSAGE

The structure of DNA allows both ease of replication and duplication of the genetic message prior to cell division, and is also a method of directing protein synthesis and ultimate cell function. The DNA message is interpreted as a specific protein product. The genes in the DNA strand contain exons, regions that will be translated to proteins, interspersed with introns, regions not transcribed into proteins. Proteins are synthesized at the ribosomes of the cell, whereas the encoded information, in the form of DNA, remains within the nucleus. The information is carried from DNA to the site of protein synthesis by the second type of nucleic acid, RNA. Whereas DNA is a double strand, RNA exists as a single strand of sugar phosphate units, and has ribose sugar units (instead of deoxyribose) and similar complementary base molecules to those found in DNA, except that uracil instead of thymine pairs with adenine. RNA also exists as different forms with different functions. Initially a gene is transcribed as nuclear (or 'pre-messenger') RNA (nRNA). This primary transcript, nRNA, synthesized by DNA transcription, is modified to form mRNA. It is messenger RNA (mRNA) that carries the message from the nucleus to the ribosome, as a complementary strand of mRNA is formed using a stretch of

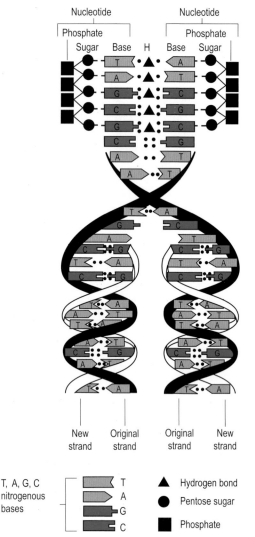

Fig. 7.2 DNA replication. (Reproduced with permission from Brooker, 1998.)

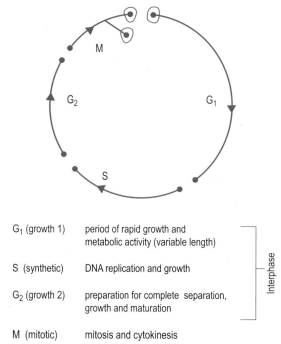

G₁ (growth 1)	period of rapid growth and metabolic activity (variable length)
S (synthetic)	DNA replication and growth
G₂ (growth 2)	preparation for complete separation, growth and maturation
M (mitotic)	mitosis and cytokinesis

Fig. 7.3 The phases of the cell cycle and cell content. (Reproduced with permission from Brooker, 1998.)

genes, which is why the HGP identified far fewer genes than was originally anticipated.

The DNA contains genes but only specific genes will be expressed in any particular cell at any particular time. Gene expression describes the means by which information from a gene drives the synthesis of a functional gene product, which is usually a protein. Molecular biology techniques have allowed in-depth investigation of the function of single genes. There are several ways in which gene expression can be regulated. These include controlling which particular genes are transcribed, selective processing of the transcribed DNA to control which RNA become cytoplasmic mRNA, selective translation of mRNA and post-translational modification of the proteins produced from mRNA.

Transcription

The process starts with the DNA strands separating like a zip pulling open in the middle. This is the reverse process to the way it coils when condensing into chromosomes (Fig. 7.5). Only one strand of DNA, the coding or 'sense' strand, is used as the template; the other is described as noncoding or 'non-sense'. The mRNA chain is built by DNA-dependent RNA polymerase enzymes as the bases pair with the DNA template. This is called 'transcription' (Fig. 7.6).

unwound DNA as a template. mRNA is shorter than nRNA because nRNA contains the introns that are spliced out (removed) as the nRNA moves from the nucleus, where it is made, to the cytoplasm where it is translated to produce an amino acid chain that will form the protein. Splicing allows genes to form different proteins because the exons can be spliced in different patterns with each pattern generating a specific protein. The process of splicing is carried out by small nuclear RNAs (snRNA or U-RNA) called 'spliceosomes'. The process where one gene can code for multiple proteins ('splice variants') means that there are about three times as many possible proteins as there are

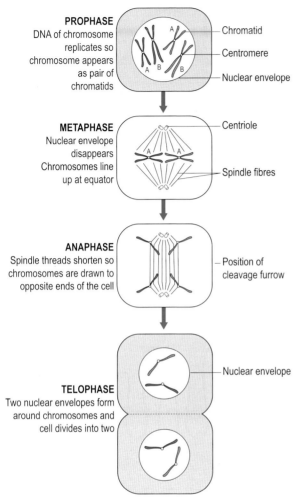

PROPHASE
DNA of chromosome replicates so chromosome appears as pair of chromatids

— Chromatid
— Centromere
— Nuclear envelope

METAPHASE
Nuclear envelope disappears
Chromosomes line up at equator

— Centriole
— Spindle fibres

ANAPHASE
Spindle threads shorten so chromosomes are drawn to opposite ends of the cell

— Position of cleavage furrow

TELOPHASE
Two nuclear envelopes form around chromosomes and cell divides into two

— Nuclear envelope

Fig. 7.4 The stages of mitosis.

The whole gene is transcribed but not all of it is used, so the primary transcription product mRNA is modified (cut and spliced) into functional mRNA (Fig. 7.7). The parts of the mRNA that are removed have been copied from parts of the gene called introns and those that are retained come from the parts of the DNA known as exons. It is estimated that only about 2–5% of the total genome (genetic code or DNA) is composed of exons and actually codes for protein synthesis. Some of the DNA modulates genetic expression, switching the process of protein synthesis on and off; these control genes are referred to as operator, regulator and inducer genes. Introns form the majority of the DNA sequence and do not appear to be involved in coding for protein synthesis, although they may allow different proteins to be formed from the same length of DNA. Much of

the genome (~98%) may be composed of redundant genes that are no longer activated and involved in the synthesis of proteins. These unused stretches of DNA can be used to compare tissue samples for DNA fingerprinting.

Single nucleotide polymorphisms or SNPs (pronounced 'snips') are DNA sequence variations that occur when a single nucleotide in the genome is altered, often with the substitution of cytosine with thymine. Variations that occur in at least 1% of the population are considered to be SNPs. There are >1.4 million SNPs in the human genome, occurring approximately every 100–300 bases and accounting for up to 90% of all human genetic variation. These variations in the human genome alter how individuals respond to disease, infection, drugs and so on. SNPs are valuable because they do not change much from generation to generation and can be targeted for biomedical research and development of drugs.

The term 'genome' refers to a complete DNA sequence of one set of chromosomes of an organism. As such, it does not describe the genetic polymorphism (diversity) of a species. To understand how variations in DNA cause particular traits or diseases requires comparison between individual genomes.

Protein Synthesis

When transcription and post-transcription modification are complete, the finished functional mRNA strand detaches from the DNA and leaves the nucleus, via a nuclear pore, to go to the ribosomes. Ribosomes are structures formed of two subunits made of protein and another type of RNA, ribosomal RNA (rRNA). mRNA attaches to ribosomes and the sequence of bases of the mRNA is decoded to direct the synthesis of a protein. This step is called 'translation' (Fig. 7.8). The mRNA sequence is 'read' three bases at a time. A particular sequence of three bases is called a codon; each codon prescribes that a specific amino acid is incorporated into the final amino acid chain of the overall protein structure. There are 20 amino acids; however, as a three-base genetic code allows the potential of $4 \times 4 \times 4 = 64$ permutations, most amino acids are coded for by more than one codon (Fig. 7.9).

Another form of RNA in the cytoplasm, called transfer RNA (tRNA), carries amino acids to the ribosome to be incorporated into the protein chain. There are different types of tRNA, each one with a specific binding site for a particular amino acid at one end and an 'anticodon', which recognizes the codon on the mRNA at the other end. The first amino acid of a new protein is always methionine. The next amino acid joins to the carboxyl group of methionine with a peptide bond. Successive amino acids join, forming a chain of amino acids until a 'stop' codon on mRNA signals the end of the protein chain. The sequence of amino

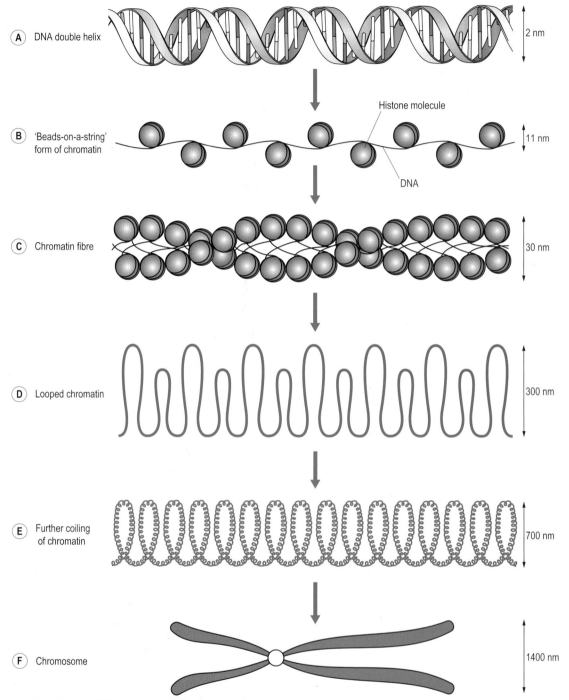

Fig. 7.5 (A–F) The stages of DNA packaging; in order for transcription to take place, the chromosomes must be uncoiled and 'unzipped' in the reverse process to that shown. (Adapted with permission from Goodwin, 1997.)

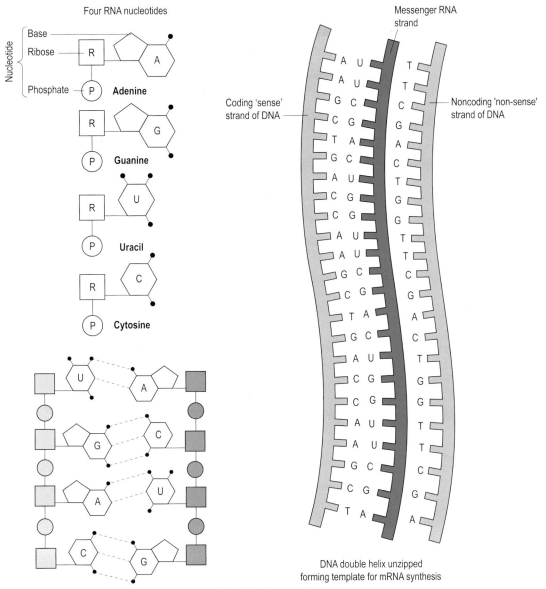

Fig. 7.6 Transcription.

acids determines the primary structure of the protein. The further configuration of the protein is determined by the interactions between different amino acids on the chain, which change the protein shape into a 'folded' structure; the final shape (configuration) of the protein determines its function. Hence, the sequence of bases of the gene, or region of DNA, determines the sequence of amino acids, which in turn prescribes the structure and therefore the function of the protein.

MUTATION

The copying of DNA has to be accurate. If mistakes are introduced into a region of DNA that is expressed as a protein (i.e. into an exon), the altered sequence of amino acids can change the structure of the protein. This permanent and transmissible change in base sequence of DNA is described as a mutation. Some mutations can lead to death of a cell or cause cancer. They are considered to

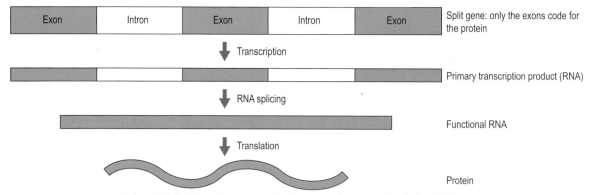

| Exon | Intron | Exon | Intron | Exon | Split gene: only the exons code for the protein |

↓ Transcription

Primary transcription product (RNA)

↓ RNA splicing

Functional RNA

↓ Translation

Protein

Fig. 7.7 Splicing. (Reproduced with permission from Goodwin, 1997.)

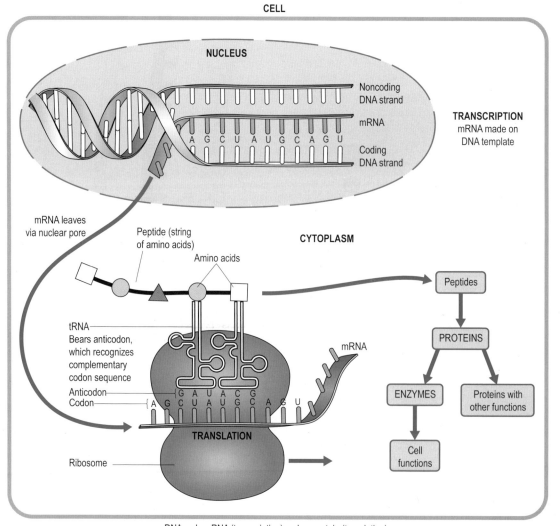

DNA makes RNA (transcription) makes protein (translation)

Fig. 7.8 The stages of protein synthesis translation.

First letter	Second letter				Third letter
	U	**C**	**A**	**G**	
U	UUU ⎤ Phe UUC ⎦ UUA ⎤ Leu UUG ⎦	UCU ⎤ UCC ⎦ Ser UCA ⎤ UCG ⎦	UAU ⎤ Tyr UAC ⎦ UAA stop UAG stop	UGU ⎤ Cys UGC ⎦ UGA stop UGG Trp	U C A G
C	CUU ⎤ CUC ⎦ Leu CUA ⎤ CUG ⎦	CCU ⎤ CCC ⎦ Pro CCA ⎤ CCG ⎦	CAU ⎤ His CAC ⎦ CAA ⎤ Gln CAG ⎦	CGU ⎤ CGC ⎦ Arg CGA ⎤ CGG ⎦	U C A G
A	AUU ⎤ Ileu AUC ⎦ AUA ⎤ Met AUG ⎦	ACU ⎤ ACC ⎦ Thr ACA ⎤ ACG ⎦	AAU ⎤ Asn AAC ⎦ AAA ⎤ Lys AAG ⎦	AGU ⎤ Ser AGC ⎦ AGA ⎤ Arg AGG ⎦	U C A G
G	GUU ⎤ GUC ⎦ Val GUA ⎤ GUG ⎦	GCU ⎤ GCC ⎦ Ala GCA ⎤ GCG ⎦	GAU ⎤ Asp GAC ⎦ GAA ⎤ Glu GAG ⎦	GGU ⎤ GGC ⎦ Gly GGA ⎤ GGG ⎦	U C A G

The abbreviated names of amino acids are:

Ala = alanine   **Gln** = glutamine   **Leu** = leucine   **Ser** = serine
Arg = arginine   **Glu** = glutamic   **Lys** = lysine   **Thr** = threonine
Asn = aspargine   **Gly** = glycine   **Met** = methionine   **Trp** = tryptophan
Asp = aspartic acid   **His** = histidine   **Phe** = phenylalanine   **Tyr** = tyrosine
Cys = cysteine   **Ileu** = isoleucine   **Pro** = proline   **Val** = valine

Fig. 7.9 Codons and the amino acids they code for. (Reproduced with permission from the Open University, 1988.)

be the driving force of evolution; favourable mutations tend to accumulate and less favourable ones tend to be removed by natural selection. It is estimated that mutations occur every 30 min in each person but a mutation in a functional gene only occurs once in five generations. A mutation can be described as 'descent with modification'. DNA has regions of 'hotspots' where the mutation rate can be up to 100 times more frequent than normal. New gene mutations are associated with increasing paternal age (>35 years); it is suggested that new gene mutations are exclusively inherited from the father and occur during spermatogenesis. Dominant mutations seem to arise predominantly in the male germline and may be induced by free radical damage (Aitken, 2017). Although the testes contain antioxidant enzymes and free radical scavengers and function at a relatively low oxygen tension, spermatogenesis is fuelled by an extremely high rate of mitosis and there are high rates of mitochondrial oxygen consumption by the cells involved. This means free radical production is high. Furthermore, the sperm themselves have poor intracellular antioxidant defence mechanisms to scavenge free radicals generated from metabolism so they are extremely vulnerable to free radical damage. The spontaneous mutation rate is about four times higher in sperm than in oocytes (Aitken, 2017). Other factors are also associated with the high mutagenesis rate. A high annual income, which is a surrogate marker of a healthy lifestyle, is inversely correlated with mutation rates (Linschooten et al., 2013). Paternal smoking in the 6 months prior to conception and father's age are positively correlated with mutation rate and increased incidence of diseases in the children.

In mitosis, there are accumulated errors in copying the genetic message. Each chromosome has telomere, a specialized length of DNA at its end, which gets shorter with each successive division. The telomere is made up of repeated nucleotide sequences (TTAGGG) associated with shelterin proteins that protect the ends of chromosomes from being misrecognized as DNA breaks in need of repair. Telomeres, therefore, protect the ends of chromosomes from damage and maintain chromosome stability. The process of DNA replication prior to cell division is unable to copy the ends of chromosomes, referred to as the 'end replication problem', so that in most cell types the telomeres shorten with each cell division with no effect on the neighbouring genes. Eventually, critically shortened telomeres will trigger replicative senescence so that each cell type has a finite number of cell divisions, the so-called 'Hayflick limit' named after Leonard Hayflick who first described this built-in 'counter' of cell divisions. The sequence of TTAGGG is repeated about 2,500 times (15,000 base pairs) in human telomeres and 50–100 base pairs are lost with each successive cell division due to a combination of the 'end replication problem' and oxidative stress. Interestingly, expression of the telomere-maintaining enzyme telomerase is a common feature of tumorigenesis, allowing tumour cells to become immortalized, avoiding the Hayflick limit with unlimited replicative potential.

A base pair may be spontaneously replaced by a different base pair (a 'point mutation') thus altering the codon and ultimately the amino acid sequence. Age, environmental pressure, radiation and chemicals increase mutation rate. One notable example is haemophilia, the sex-linked genetic condition that afflicted male members of the European Royal Family for several generations. The spontaneous mutation for changed haemoglobin structure may have occurred in one of the gametes that formed the zygote that became Queen Victoria. This type of mutation is referred to as a substitution. Mutations may arise as an insertion or deletion of a nucleotide into or from the DNA strand; these 'frame-shift' mutations cause a shift in the 'reading frame' after which all codons and the resulting amino acids in the protein are different, grossly affecting the gene product. Mutations may also occur by the complete insertion of new codons or by the deletion of a complete codon, thus altering protein structure by inserting or deleting a single amino acid in the protein sequence. The effects of these mutations can be complicated if codons are duplicated and repeated one after the other, for example in the polyglutamine and polyarginine expansions that cause Huntington disease and fragile X syndrome, respectively.

Many mutations occur in the noncoding areas of DNA, so protein structure and function are not affected by the change; these mutations are described as 'silent' as they appear to have no effect. If the mutation results in a different codon that codes for the same amino acid as the original, there will also be no effect. However, a different base, or a missing base, will cause a change in the final sequence of amino acids of the protein, which may have serious effects on protein folding, structure and function. An example is sickle cell anaemia (Box 7.3; Fig. 7.10).

BOX 7.3   Sickle Cell Anaemia

Most haemoglobin (Hb) in adults is HbA, which has two α-peptide chains and two β-peptide chains forming the haemoglobin molecule. Sickle cell anaemia is an example of a single point mutation where the substitution of one base changes the codon and results in the substitution of one amino acid (Fig. 7.10). Uracil replaces adenine so, instead of glutamic acid, valine is inserted in the protein chain at position 6. Valine has a different charge to glutamic acid so the protein folds differently. The result is that the protein structure of the β-chain of haemoglobin is changed, which affects the molecular shape and oxygen-binding properties. The red blood cells distort into a characteristic rigid sickle shape, particularly at low oxygen tension. Sickle cell anaemia is inherited as an autosomal recessive condition; the affected person has two mutant haemoglobin S genes, one inherited from each parent. The parents are heterozygotes (usually HbA/HbS) and are thus clinically normal but are carriers of the sickle cell gene. Homozygotes (HbS/HbS) have chronic haemolytic anaemia and are prone to vaso-occlusive 'sickling' crises (where the abnormally shaped red blood cells block capillaries because they are not elastic and restrict blood flow to an organ). The red blood cells are recognized as abnormal by the macrophages of the spleen and other organs which break them down. A sickled red blood cell has a lifespan of about 10–20 days compared with about 90–120 days of healthy red blood cells; synthesis of new red blood cells by the bone marrow cannot match the rate of their destruction, which results in anaemia.

MEIOSIS

The basic characteristics of meiosis – two cell divisions without intervening DNA replication, halving the chromosome complement of the resulting cells – are conserved in evolution. Each species has a characteristic number of chromosomes; humans have 46 chromosomes, arranged as 23 pairs. One chromosome of each pair is maternally derived (from the ovum); the other is paternally derived (from the sperm). (The members of each pair are said to be homologous; see below). Human gametes contain only 23 chromosomes, which is half the normal number of chromosomes in other human cells. This reduction from the diploid number of chromosomes (46) to the haploid number (23) is accomplished by meiosis. Meiosis is the process whereby a diploid parent cell produces four haploid daughter cells, resulting in gametes, or sex cells, that are not identical to their parent cells. These gametes are haploid and during meiosis the

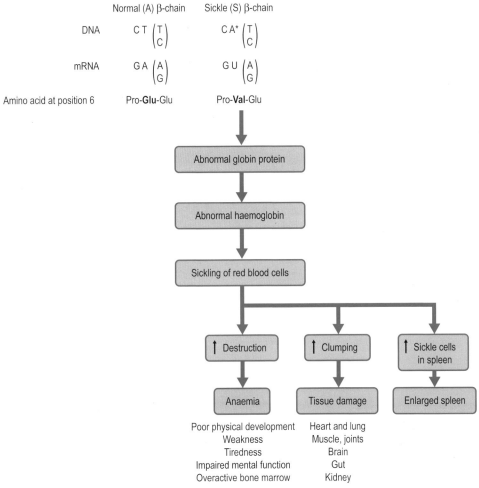

Fig. 7.10 The sickle cell mutation and its effects.

genetic instructions are randomly assorted, thus generating unique combinations. Meiosis is also described as 'reduction division' because the number of chromosomes is reduced from 46 (i.e. 23 pairs) to 23. It occurs in two successive divisions (meiosis I and II), each of which can be divided into steps (Fig. 7.11). Meiosis II is very similar to mitosis.

In anaphase I, there is random segregation of each member of the chromosome pairs with a maternal and a paternal chromosome randomly going to a particular end of the cell. This would theoretically generate 2^{23} (i.e. 8,388,608) different possibilities of gamete combination. However, the exchange of genetic material ('crossing over') between each pair of chromosomes adds far more variation. Meiosis allows the genomes of the parents to be combined to form an individual whose genome is related to their parents and siblings but is unique.

Mammalian oogenesis begins meiotic development during fetal development but arrests in meiosis I and does not complete meiosis I until ovulation; the second division is only completed if the egg is fertilized. Oogenesis, therefore, requires several stop-and-start signals and, in humans, may last for several decades. The longer an oocyte is immobilized at prophase I, the greater is the chance of failure of separation of the homologous chromosomes (nondisjunction). Often genetic abnormalities arise as extra genetic material is incorporated into the genome. If an extra chromosome is inserted, the condition is referred to as trisomy (Table 7.1). Most combinations of trisomy are not viable, but there is no reason to believe that certain chromosomes are more susceptible to failed disjunction. Those trisomies observed are probably those that are compatible with fetal survival, although they may cause congenital abnormalities

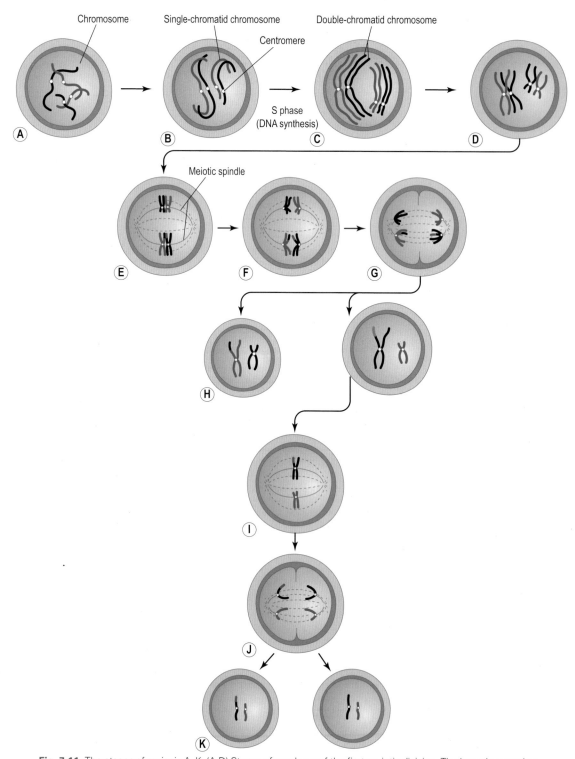

Fig. 7.11 The stages of meiosis A–K. (A-D) Stages of prophase of the first meiotic division. The homologous chromosomes approach each other and pair; each member of the pair consists of two chromatids. A single crossover is shown in one pair of chromosomes, resulting in the interchange of chromatid segments. (E) Metaphase. The two members of each pair become oriented on the meiotic spindle. (F) Anaphase. (G) Telophase. The chromosomes migrate to opposite poles. (H) Distribution of parental chromosome pairs at the end of the first meiotic division. (I-K) Second meiotic division which is similar to mitosis except the cells are haploid. (Reproduced from Moore KL, Persaud TVN, Torchia MG: *The developing human: clinically oriented embryology*, 11 ed, Elsevier 2020, Fig. 2.2.)

TABLE 7.1 Examples of Chromosome Disorders

Disorder	Example	Incidence	Outcome	Notes
Polyploidy	Triploidy 69 chromosomes (69,XXX, 69,XXY, 69,XYY)	Occurs in 2% of conceptions but early spontaneous abortion is normal	Lethal	Usually arises from fertilization of oocyte by two sperm or from a diploid gamete. 69,XXY is most common. Polyploid cells occur normally in the bone marrow and liver as a stage of cell division
Trisomy	Trisomy 13/T13	1/5000 live births	Patau syndrome	Usually due to nondisjunction of chromosomes or chromatids at anaphase. Trisomy increases with increased maternal age and is sometimes associated with radiation or viral infection. There may be a familial tendency
	Trisomy 18/T18	1/3000 live births	Edward syndrome	Maternal age effect. Incidence at conception much higher – most affected fetuses abort spontaneously. More female fetuses seem to survive
	Trisomy 21/T21	1/700–1000 live births	Down syndrome	Incidence at conception is higher. Maternal age effect; the extra chromosome is maternal in 85% cases. The most serious complications are intellectual disability and congenital heart problems
	47,XXY	1/1000 male births	Klinefelter syndrome	Trisomies involving sex chromosomes usually result in a less serious outcome. Condition is usually diagnosed during investigations for infertility
	47,XYY	1/1000 male births		Often asymptomatic, some effects on IQ. Only XX and XY offspring observed
Monosomy	Monosomy X (45,X)	1/5000 female births, much higher at conception	Turner syndrome	Due to nondisjunction in either parent; 80% of affected females have maternal X so it is the paternal chromosome that is missing

Continued

TABLE 7.1   Examples of Chromosome Disorders—cont'd

Disorder	Example	Incidence	Outcome	Notes
Deletion and ring chromosome	Wolf–Hirschhorn syndrome (partial deletion of short arm of chromosome 4); Cri du chat syndrome (partial deletion of short arm of chromosome 5)	Incidence of deletions and/or duplications is 1/2000 births	Chromosome imbalance of autosomes is usually associated with intellectual disability and multiple dysmorphic features	A deletion is the loss of part of chromosome. A ring chromosome is due to deletions in both arms of a chromosome and the fusion of the proximal sticky ends. Microdeletions are deletions that can just be detected by light microscopy
Duplication				Duplication is where there are two copies of a segment of chromosome. This is more common and less harmful than deletions
Inversion			The carriers of balanced inversions and translocations are healthy because the cells have all the genetic material but gamete formation is affected so there is a high rate of miscarriage and malformation	A segment of the chromosome is inverted through 180° between breaks. Usually does not cause clinical problems but unbalanced gametes may result
Translocation	Reciprocal			Translocations involve transfer of chromosomal material between chromosomes. Two chromosomes are broken and repaired abnormally or there is recombination between nonhomologous chromosomes at meiosis. Reciprocal translocations involve transfer of material between two chromosomes
	Robertsonian (centric fusion)			Robertsonian translocation involves transfer of material, which leaves a large chromosome, and a fragment of a chromosome, which is unable to replicate; most common centric fusion translocations are 13/14 and 14/21. Balanced carriers have 45 chromosomes and are healthy. Gametogenesis is affected

or affect neonatal survival. Sometimes extra chromosomal material may become attached to a chromosome, making it abnormally long. Rarely, triploidy occurs where the chromosomes of the zygote are in triplicate rather than the normal duplicate complement. This condition is not compatible with embryo survival but is sometimes found in products of a failed conception (early miscarriage) and is associated with a high incidence of hydatidiform mole (see Chapter 6). Imperfect disjunction also causes conditions where the genome is lacking part or a whole chromosome. For example, there is only one X chromosome present in Turner syndrome (see Chapter 5) and Wolf–Hirschhorn syndrome is caused by a microdeletion (loss of a small amount of chromosomal DNA) from the short arm of chromosomes 4.

AUTOSOMES AND SEX CHROMOSOMES

Each gene has a specific location on a specific chromosome, which is referred to as a locus (plural: loci). Each chromosome may have 1000–2000 different genes, each with its own location and function. The visualization of the chromosomes from a cell is described as a karyotype (Box 7.4) (see Case study 7.1). Of the 23 pairs of chromosomes that constitute the human genome, 22 pairs of chromosomes can be seen in both sexes; these are referred to as the autosomes and contain the autosomal genes. The 23rd pair of chromosomes comprises the sex chromosomes; these are homologous within the female (i.e. XX) but in the male the XY arrangement consists of a pair of nonhomologous chromosomes.

CASE STUDY 7.1

Surya presents herself to a midwife at 8 weeks' gestation demanding that she needs to know the sex of her baby because if it is female she would rather have a termination than proceed with the pregnancy.
- What should the midwife do in this situation?
- Are there any circumstances when fetal sex determination is justified?

BOX 7.4 Karyotyping

Karyotyping is the method of counting and visualizing the chromosomes. Pictomicrographs of the stained chromosomes, arrested in the metaphase stage of mitosis, are arranged in a standard format in which they are ordered by their characteristics such as their size and the position of their centromeres. For a fetal karyotype, a sample of amniotic fluid is removed. The cells are centrifuged to concentrate the fetal cells. The supernatant can also be used diagnostically for biochemical tests such as investigation of enzyme deficiencies, protein defects and gene alterations. Alternatively, cells may be taken from the chorionic villus. A karyotype of adult cells is usually derived from a sample of venous blood, where the anuclear red blood cells are haemolysed and the washed remaining cells are, therefore, white blood cells containing nuclei.

The fetal cells or white blood cells are grown in tissue culture. The time taken for this depends on the number of cells in the original sample. Contamination of the sample can interfere with the success of the method. Colchicine, a chemical poison, is added to the culture medium to prevent spindle formation. Thus, mitosis in all cells is halted at the metaphase stage when the chromosomes are maximally contracted and well defined as paired chromatids (in the typical X-shaped appearance). The cells, all halted at the same stage, can be separated from the culture medium. Exposure of the cells to hypotonic saline causes the nucleus to swell so the chromosomes spread out. The cells are then fixed and stained. Visualization of the karyotype is done by computer-aided photographic techniques. The chromosomes are ordered according to size with the homologous autosomes being paired together. The chromosomes of pair number 1 are the longest and those of pair number 22 are the shortest. The position of the centromere is also used to sort the chromosomes into order. Stains that bind preferentially to some areas of the chromosome, producing a distinct pattern of bands, can be used to identify the chromosomes. Karyotypes can be used to identify gross abnormalities such as additional or missing chromosomes and missing or duplicated parts of chromosomes. However, a normal karyotype does not reveal the presence of abnormal genes at specific loci. In order to identify such genes, the chromosomes are stained, which produce a pattern or banding enabling an abnormal gene or a marker gene to be identified. A marker gene is a gene that is often found in close proximity to an abnormal gene; the closer the marker gene to the abnormal gene, the higher is the association.

Occasionally, results from karyotyping may be confounded by mosaicism. Mosaicism, a different number of chromosomes in different populations of cells may occur for instance where the chorionic (placental) tissue has a different number of chromosomes to the fetus.

Sex Chromosomes

The sex chromosomes provide the mechanism for the determination of sex and the differentiation into male morphology, which is usually dependent on the inheritance of a Y chromosome (see Chapter 5). As well as sex determination and identity, other genetic traits can be inherited on the sex chromosomes.

It is thought that the sex chromosomes originated from a pair of autosomes (see Chapter 5) during the evolution of sex determination (Graves, 2018). The X and Y chromosomes are very different in size and sequence compared with the other 22 pairs of autosomes. The human X chromosome has been described as 'smart and sexy' because it has a disproportionate allocation of genes identified to be involved in reproduction and intelligence and the Y chromosome has been described as a 'wimpy' degenerate copy of the X chromosome with few active genes (Graves, 2018). The Y chromosome is very small in comparison to the X chromosome and is completely different from the X chromosomes except at its tips. These identical regions at the tips, known as the pseudoautosomal regions, contain most of the Y chromosome genes involved in control of growth and allow the pairing of the X and Y chromosome and crossing over during cell division. The X chromosome is ~5% of the total length of a single set of chromosomes and bears ~3000–4000 genes, many of which are conserved (identical to those of other placental mammals). The Y chromosome contains only ~45–50 genes, many of which appear to be nonfunctional; others are involved with male differentiation and spermatogenesis, implantation and promoting placental growth. The Y chromosome is one of the fastest evolving components of the human genome. It is suggested that the Y chromosome is particularly vulnerable to mutations and gene deletions because it cannot retrieve lost genetic information by homologous recombination and that, over the past 300 million years, it has already lost most of its original 1500 genes and continues to deteriorate. Indeed, Graves (2018) suggested that if the present rate of decay continued (losing about five genes per million years), the genes of the Y chromosome would disappear in a few million years. This has already happened in some East European rodents such as the mole vole, which has lost the Y chromosome and all of its genes from the genome and expresses new sex-determining genes. An alternative view is that the Y chromosome, rather than approaching oblivion, has evolved extremely effective mechanisms to survive indefinitely as an efficient carrier of male-specific genes, rationalized by evolutionary selection (Griffin and Ellis, 2018). Without meiotic crossing-over in meiosis, it is protected from genetic decay. The palindromic sequences ensure efficient self-recombination. Furthermore, the Y chromosome has not lost any genes since the ancestral paths of humans and chimpanzees diverged about 6 million years ago.

Alleles

Each pair of autosomes is homologous; this means that their gene arrangements, although not necessarily the specific gene at each locus, are identical. So, although the genes at a specific locus code for a specific physiological feature, these features in themselves may vary. For example, the genes at a particular locus may code for eye colour, but this could be blue eye colour on the chromosome inherited from one parent and brown eye colour on the chromosome inherited from the other parent. (However, note that eye colour is due to both pigmentation of the iris and light scattering properties and so is actually a trait affected by more than one gene). Genes that code for the same physical feature but produce variations in that feature are called alleles.

If the genes are identical alleles, then the structure and coding of the pair are referred to as being homozygous. If the genes are differing alleles, then the pair is referred to as being heterozygous. If one copy of a gene is required for a trait to be expressed (i.e. for the feature to be 'visible' in the resultant individual), the gene is described as being dominant. If two copies are required, the gene is described as being recessive. Autosomal traits (genetic instructions carried on the autosomes) can be expressed as either dominant or recessive traits. Simple inheritance of these traits can be predicted diagrammatically (see Figs 7.12 and 7.16).

PREDICTION OF GENETIC OUTCOMES

Genetic predictions forecast the chance of an ovum carrying a specific combination of genes being fertilized by a sperm carrying a specific combination of genes. The convention is to show the dominant gene as a capital letter. The genetic potential is described as the genotype; how it is expressed is called the 'phenotype'. Combination diagrams and Punnett squares give the same results, and are used to predict the chance (probability) of a particular outcome or phenotype (Figs 7.12 and 7.13).

The genetic rules that dictate eye colour often follow the traditional form of dominant and recessive interaction (Box 7.5). However, it is important to realize that, like so many other physiological states, expressed characteristics may be the outcome of multifactorial genes where more than one gene is involved. The environment may also influence the expression of genes. For instance, inheriting genes for tall stature does not necessarily mean the child will be tall. In the absence of appropriate nutrition at critical times of growth, the genetic potential may not be realized.

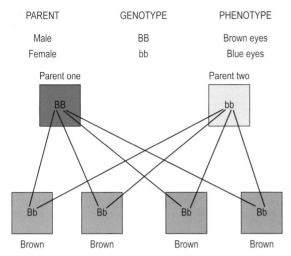

PARENT	GENOTYPE	PHENOTYPE
Male	BB	Brown eyes
Female	bb	Blue eyes

Fig. 7.12 Combination diagram illustrating the genetic outcomes of crossing a homozygous male with brown eyes (carrying two dominant genes for brown eye colour, BB) and a homozygous female with blue eyes (carrying two recessive genes for blue eye colour, bb). All the offspring will be heterozygous, carrying one recessive gene and one dominant gene. All the children will have the phenotype of brown eye colouration.

		Parent one Gametes	
		B	**B**
Parent two Gametes	b	**Bb**	**Bb**
	b	**Bb**	**Bb**

Fig. 7.13 Punnett square.

BOX 7.5 Selected Examples of Recessive and Dominant Traits

Autosomal trait	Recessive trait
Brown eye colour	Blue or grey eye colour
Curly hair	Straight hair
Dark brown hair	All other colours
Near or far sight	Normal vision
Normal skin pigment	Albinism
Normal hearing	Deafness
Migraine headaches	Normal
A or B antigen (A, B or AB blood group)	No A or B antigen (O blood group)
Rhesus antigen (Rh+ blood group)	No Rhesus antigen (Rh– blood group)

CHARACTERISTICS OF DIFFERENT TYPES OF INHERITANCE

Autosomal Dominant Inheritance

The trait is expressed by a gene on an autosome and is expressed provided that at least one chromosome has the dominant gene. Each person expressing the trait usually has a parent with the trait (Fig. 7.14 shows a pedigree chart for a pattern of autosomal dominant inheritance; the symbols used in these charts are shown in Box 7.6). This means that a particular characteristic or disorder can be traced through several generations if it has little effect on survival. However, a trait occurring in a new generation may be the result of polygamic behaviour (illegitimacy) or a fresh mutation. Autosomal dominant traits also tend to be extremely variable in expression so they may be undetectable and appear to 'skip' a generation. For instance, polydactyly (an extra digit) may be manifest as a tiny pedicle, rather than an extra finger. Autosomal dominant disorders are often caused by defects in structural proteins.

If an affected person mates with an unaffected person, the chances of any child being affected are one in two (i.e. 50%). Some autosomal diseases or traits do not affect the predicted 50% of offspring. These are described as having incomplete penetrance. Conversely, a highly penetrant gene is expressed regardless of environmental and other factors.

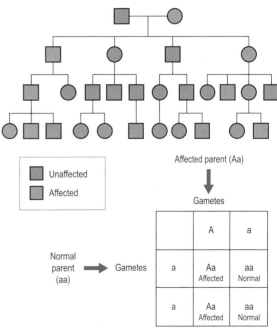

Fig. 7.14 Inheritance of a dominant trait.

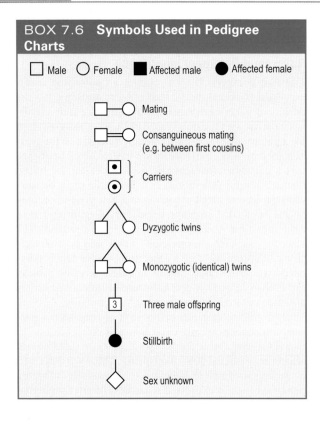

BOX 7.6 Symbols Used in Pedigree Charts

☐ Male   ○ Female   ■ Affected male   ● Affected female

☐—○ Mating

☐═○ Consanguineous mating (e.g. between first cousins)

⊡ ⊙ Carriers

☐△○ Dyzygotic twins

☐△○ Monozygotic (identical) twins

☐ 3 Three male offspring

● Stillbirth

◇ Sex unknown

TABLE 7.2 Examples of Autosomal Dominant Diseases

Trait	Incidence
Familial hypercholesterolaemia	1/500 births
von Willebrand disease	1/20–30,000
Huntington disease	1/18,000
Achondroplasia	1/26,000

	A	a
A	AA	Aa
a	Aa	aa

Expected outcome might be 25% chance of child with normal height, but AA is lethal lung deformity so observed outcome is 2:1 chance of achondroplasia: normal height.

Fig. 7.15 Inheritance of achondroplasia.

offspring of parents of normal height). Achondroplasia is the result of a mutation in the fibroblast growth factor receptor, which is normally inhibited but the mutated form leads to shortened bones. Humans exhibit selective rather than random mating, often being attracted to partners of similar height, intelligence and other physical attributes. In consequence, individuals with achondroplasia partner each other with a higher frequency than expected by chance. If two people with achondroplasia mate, there would seem to be a theoretical one in four chance of a child having normal stature (Fig. 7.15). However, homozygosity (two genes for achondroplasia) results in the fetus having lethal respiratory problems, which are incompatible with survival. Hence the actual ratio of newborn children is one in three. (Arguably, achondroplasia could be viewed as a recessively inherited respiratory condition that confers dwarfism on the heterozygote.)

Autosomal Recessive Inheritance

As with autosomal dominant inheritance, this type of inheritance can affect both sexes equally. However, the recessive trait is expressed only if the defective gene is present on both alleles, which means it has been inherited from both parents. If the parents are heterozygotes, each carrying one recessive gene for the trait and one normal dominant gene, they express the dominant gene and are described as 'carriers' of the recessive gene. In some conditions, the carriers

In the UK, the most common dominantly inherited traits are Huntington disease and achondroplasia (Table 7.2). Huntington disease, a degenerative neuropsychiatric disorder initially characterized by dystonia (spasmodic movements of the body and limbs) and ultimately dementia, is usually not expressed until the third or fourth decade when the person affected is likely to have already reproduced. The age at onset and progression of the disease is linked to the number of polyglutamine sequence repeats in huntingtin, the disease-causing protein. The codon for glutamine is CAG and the more CAG (cytosine-adenosine-guanine) repeats there are in the gene that codes for the abnormal huntingtin protein, the more severe the disease and the earlier its onset. Diagnosis via identification of the huntingtin gene (*IT15*) can occur before the expression of symptoms, which raises several ethical issues such as the age of the individual being tested and whether an individual has the right to know whether their parent is affected if the parent does not wish to know.

Another complication occurs in the case of inherited achondroplasia (dwarfism) (note that 80% of cases of achondroplasia are caused by new mutations in the

TABLE 7.3 **Examples of Recessively Inherited Diseases**	
Trait	**Carrier Frequency**
β-Thalassaemia	One in six Cypriots
Cystic fibrosis	1 in 25 Northern Europeans
Phenylketonuria	1 in 10,000 Europeans
Sickle cell anaemia	Varies among Mediterranean, Middle Eastern and Afro-Caribbean races
Tay–Sachs disease	1 in 30 Ashkenazi Jews

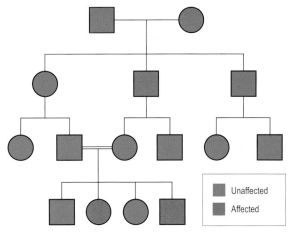

Cystic fibrosis

Carrier rate = $\frac{1}{25}$ **(Cc)**   Chance of two parents being carriers = $\frac{1}{25}$ x $\frac{1}{25}$ = $\frac{1}{625}$

	C	c
C	CC Normal	Cc Carrier
c	Cc Carrier	cc Affected

Live birth rate approximately $\frac{1}{25}$ x $\frac{1}{25}$ x $\frac{1}{4}$ = $\frac{1}{2500}$

Fig. 7.16 Inheritance of cystic fibrosis, a recessive trait.

Legend: Unaffected / Affected

may exhibit mild signs of a disease or have an unusual level of certain biochemical markers that can be measured in genetic testing.

Most inherited enzyme disorders are recessive. Another characteristic of recessive disorders is that they show a variation in birth frequency among different populations (Table 7.3). It is suggested that the reason some recessively inherited disorders reach such a high incidence within a population is because advantages are conferred on the heterozygotes. For example, it is recognized that carriers of the gene for sickle haemoglobin (see Box 7.3), namely HbS or C, have a resistance to *Plasmodium falciparum*, the parasite that causes the most dangerous form of malaria (but not to other types). Obviously, such an advantage will selectively increase the number of people within the population who carry the gene. The incidence of malaria and the inheritance of other forms of altered haemoglobin, such as β-thalassaemia, can be mapped to the same parts of the world.

In the Caucasian population, the most common autosomal recessive condition is cystic fibrosis. The carrier rate within the population is about 1 in 25 people. This means that there is a 1 in 25 chance that any person might be heterozygous for (i.e. carry) the cystic fibrosis gene. The chance, therefore, of two carriers mating is 1 in 625 (25 × 25) (Fig. 7.16). If two heterozygous parents have children, there is a one in four chance that any child will be affected and a one in two chance that any child will be a carrier of the gene themselves. The live-birth rate of children with cystic fibrosis is about 1 in 2500 (625 × 4). Because of the relatively high incidence of the disease, parents who already have an affected child or those whose family history has a strong incidence of the disease will be offered genetic counselling. Carriers of the cystic fibrosis gene appear to have resistance to gastrointestinal conditions, tuberculosis

and cholera, and to have increased fertility. Cystic fibrosis is a condition that has the potential to be treated by gene therapy (Box 7.7).

Sex-linked Inheritance

The sex chromosomes not only determine the sex of the embryo but also have other structural genes. Female and male genetic endowments are different. Very few genes appear to be carried on the Y chromosomes so sex-linked inheritance usually relates to X-linked inheritance. Most genes carried on the X chromosome are recessive. The effects of a recessive X-linked gene are usually masked in the female by the presence of the paired normal gene upon the other X chromosome. However, should such a woman carry an abnormal gene, she may pass it on to her sons. Males inherit only one of the paired X chromosomes; therefore, if they acquire the abnormal gene on the X chromosome the disease will automatically be manifest because the Y chromosome lacks the corresponding allele of the

BOX 7.7   Advances in Gene Therapy

Recent advances in gene therapy have led to techniques to insert normal genes into human cells and tissues which express abnormal genes. Gene therapy aims to supplement a defective allele with a functional allele and focuses on single-gene defects such as cystic fibrosis, muscular dystrophy, sickle cell anaemia and haemophilia. This is achieved by using a modified virus that acts as a vehicle by which the normal gene is carried into and thus incorporated into the genome. The altered virus is unable to replicate and so causes no harm to the recipient. In treatment of cystic fibrosis, the cells of the nasal passages and lining of the lungs are exposed to the virus in the form of an inhaled spray. So far, all human gene therapy has targeted at somatic (body) cells; germline engineering (altering stem cells or gametes) remains controversial.

TABLE 7.4   Examples of Sex-linked Recessive Disorders

Trait	UK Frequency/ 10,000 Males
Red–green colour blindness	800
Haemophilia A (factor VIII)	2
Haemophilia B (factor IX)	0.3
Duchenne muscular dystrophy	3
Fragile X syndrome	5

other X chromosome that is found in the female. Also, if a female inherits two abnormal genes, one on each X chromosome, the condition is usually incompatible with life and the embryo is lost at a relatively early stage. X-linked recessive disorders therefore affect many more males than females. Very few sex-linked abnormalities are inherited as dominant traits which affect would both male and female offspring. One example is vitamin D-resistant rickets.

Most sex-linked diseases (Table 7.4) involve a female carrier partnered with a trait-free man (Fig. 7.17). There is a one in two chance that any male offspring will inherit and express the disorder and a one in two chance that any female offspring will carry the trait. An affected man cannot pass the disorder to his sons because they will receive a Y chromosome only, but all of his daughters will be carriers of the disease.

Only males have the genes from the Y chromosome, which is small and contains very little active genetic coding. However, it does contain the SRY (sex-determining region of the Y chromosome) gene, which when activated, directs male embryonic development (see Chapter 5). The male, however, still requires the presence of an X chromosome as this contains many genes that are vital for normal development to occur.

The female inherits two X chromosomes but evidence suggests that only one of the chromosomes is activated within the cell. On examination of the cell nucleus, one chromosome is always contracted, forming a characteristic Barr body at the outskirts of the nucleus. The number of Barr bodies is one of the tests used in determining the sex of a baby born with ambiguous genitalia. The contracted Barr body chromosome was assumed to be inert, but a small number of genes appear to remain active and expressed.

Although the second X chromosome in females is inactivated, this is usually incomplete so a proportion (perhaps 15%) of X-linked genes will be expressed at higher and variable levels in women. As X chromosome inactivation is random, some female cells will express the paternal X chromosome, whereas the others will express the maternal X chromosome so women are genetic mosaics with respect to X-linked gene expression.

There are examples of mosaic phenotypes where a heterozygous woman has a mix of dominant and recessive expression. For instance, in X-linked ectodermal dysplasia, affected males have smooth skin with no sweat glands. Female carriers may have patches of normal skin interspersed with patches of dysplastic skin. Similarly, females who are heterozygous for ocular albinism may have a mosaic pattern of pigmentation in their irises. There also seems to be some form of dosage compensation, as the inheritance of two X chromosomes does not result in twice the amount of proteins coded for by genes on the X chromosome. The explanation is that, early in embryonic development, a process called X-inactivation or 'Lyonization' occurs in which one of the X chromosomes is permanently inactivated (Box 7.8 and Fig. 7.18). As random chromosomes are selected for inactivation, different regions of the adult body have different chromosomes inactivated.

The three main types of inheritance are summarized in Box 7.9.

Other Types of Inheritance

Blood groups A and B are inherited as co-dominant genes, whereas the gene for blood group O is recessive (Fig. 7.19; Box 7.10). Some disorders are inherited via the mitochondria. The mitochondria of the zygote and subsequent cells are exclusively derived from the oocyte (see Chapter 6); therefore, no paternal mitochondria are passed on to the next generation. Disorders of mitochondrial metabolism are passed from mother to child but never from father to child. The unique matrilineal transmission of mtDNA has been particularly useful for the study of population genetics

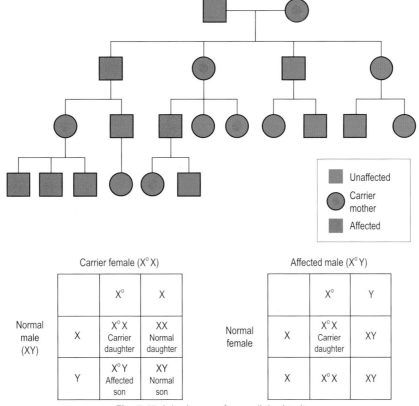

Fig. 7.17 Inheritance of a sex-linked trait.

BOX 7.8   X-inactivation or Lyonization

X chromosome inactivation or Lyonization (named after Dr. Mary Lyon who first proposed the hypothesis in 1961) occurs at approximately 15 days into the gestation (Huynh and Lee, 2005). In humans, the cell mass of the embryo at around this stage is approximately 5000 cells (Fig. 7.18). The female embryo randomly inactivates all but one X chromosome on each cell; once inactivated, all the cells descending from each parent cell retain their pattern of either paternal or maternal inactivation. In some animals, such as marsupials, it is always the paternally derived X chromosome that is deactivated but in mammals it appears that either one of the pair is inactivated. Random inactivation would predict that 50% of female cells would have an active paternal X and 50% have an active maternal X; however, skewed patterns of inactivation can arise, which means that the X chromosomes from one parent may be predominantly inactivated so the X chromosomes from the other parent will then be expressed. This could lead to the dominant proportion of expressed X chromosomes carrying a disorder that can be expressed. The inactivated chromosome appears as a sex chromatin body (Barr body) and is identified as it always divides late in mitosis. However, not all the chromosomes are totally inactivated: the pseudoautosomal region of the short arm and other loci remains active to prevent the manifestation of Turner syndrome in all normal genotypical women.

---

and evolutionary biology. This has been particularly useful in determining family lineage, such as the notable case of grand Duchess Anastasia, the Russian princess who was the youngest daughter of Tsar Nicholas II. The Russian royal family was murdered by the Bolshevik secret police in 1918

but persistent rumours suggested that Anastasia may have escaped as her grave was not found. DNA analysis showed that the mtDNA of members of the present Royal Family was different to that of the person who claimed to be Anastasia and subsequently the remains of all four of the children of

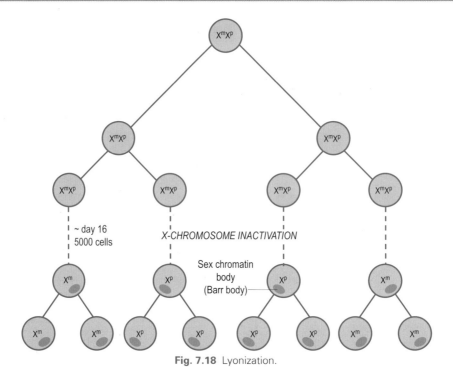

Fig. 7.18 Lyonization.

BOX 7.9 Characteristics of Different Types of Inheritance

Autosomal Dominant Inheritance
- Effects are manifest in heterozygotes
- Affected person + person: half of offspring are affected
- Unaffected persons do not transmit condition
- Fresh mutation may produce abnormal genes
- An affected person usually has an affected parent
- Traits are often variably expressed and may not be penetrant (an individual can have the mutant gene but have a normal phenotype)
- Often structural, receptor or carrier proteins are affected and clinical effects tend to be less severe than those due to recessively inherited traits

Autosomal Recessive Inheritance
- Effects are manifest in homozygotes
- Affected person receives genes from both parents
- Heterozygote = 'carrier'
- Heterozygote parents
  - One in four chance that offspring will be affected
  - One in two chance that offspring will be carriers
  - One in four chance that offspring will be unaffected

- Variation in birth frequency
- Recessive traits usually result in enzyme defects

Sex-linked Inheritance
- Sex chromosomes carry genes and determine sex
- Sex-linked = X-linked
- Most conditions are rare
- Genes involved are usually recessive
- Female carrier
  - One in two chance that male offspring will be affected
  - One in two chance that female offspring will also be carriers
- Affected male
  - All sons will be normal
  - All daughters will be carriers

PHENOTYPES OF PARENTS		PHENOTYPES OF OFFSPRING POSSIBLE	IMPOSSIBLE
A	A	A, O	B. AB
A	B	A, B, AB, O	none
A	AB	A, B, AB	O
A	O	A, O	B, AB
B	B	B, O	A, AB
B	AB	A, B, AB	O
B	O	B, O	A, AB
AB	AB	A, B, AB	O
AB	O	A, B	AB, O
O	O	O	A, B, AB

Antigens A and B are inherited as dominant traits, whereas O is inherited as a recessive trait

Fig. 7.19 Inheritance of ABO blood groups.

BOX 7.10   Erythrocyte Surface Antigens: Blood Group Classifications

The reason for the evolution of differing blood groups in humans remains a mystery except that at some point during evolutionary history they may have been advantageous to ensure overall survival of the population. Other animals do not have the same number or type of blood groups. The more common human blood cell antigens give rise to the blood groups A, B, AB and O (Table 7.5).

Other surface antigens commonly found in practice are Duffy, Rhesus D, C, E and Kell. The presence of other antigens explains why, even with closely matched blood, recipients can react to the blood of the donor. The Rhesus antigen, which is present in ~85% of the population, has implications for fetal survival (see Chapter 10).

BOX 7.11   Incidence of Chromosomal Abnormalities

- Incidence of major chromosomal abnormality
  - About 1 in 200 live births
  - About 1 in 20 perinatal deaths (stillbirths and early neonatal deaths)
  - About 1 in 2 early spontaneous abortions
- About 1 in 100 births: single-gene (unifactorial) disorder
- About 1 in 50 births: + major congenital abnormality

Nicholas II were identified (Rogaev et al., 2009). Determining patterns of inheritance can be complicated, however, where different genes resulting in different inherited disorders apparently cause the same effect, such as blindness.

The presence of 23 pairs of normal chromosomes indicates a normal karyotype (see Box 7.4).

CHROMOSOMAL ABNORMALITIES

Changes within the genetic message, for instance those due to mutation, may involve large parts of the chromosome (Box 7.11). If the changes can be seen by light microscopy such as a marked structural abnormality or an atypical number of chromosomes, they are termed 'gross aberrations' and can be detected from an examination of the karyotype. Chromosomal abnormalities can be classified as numerical or structural, affecting either the autosomes or the sex chromosomes. These types of abnormality are easier than a single-gene abnormality to detect.

Numerical Abnormalities

The loss or gain of one or more chromosomes is described as aneuploidy (wrong number of chromosomes), whereas cells with the correct number of chromosomes are euploidic. It is estimated that 10–25% of all human fetuses are aneuploidal, predominantly due to nondisjunction in maternal meiosis, although trisomy 18 most often results from nondisjunction in meiosis II. Aneuploidy appears to occur more frequently in humans than in other species, possibly because of deliberate or occupational exposure to environmental factors such as tobacco smoke, alcohol, oral contraception use, radiation exposure and industrial chemicals, which is probably one of the reasons for a high rate of miscarriage in humans.

Aneuploidy is usually due to nondisjunction in the formation of the gametes resulting in a zygote that does not have 46 chromosomes. Monosomy describes the loss of a complete chromosome and trisomy describes the addition of a single chromosome, as in Down syndrome (trisomy 21 or T21 caused by an additional copy of chromosome 21) (see Table 7.1). Monosomy and triploidy (an extra complete set of 23 chromosomes) are usually lethal. Most autosomal trisomies are also lethal except those involving chromosomes 13, 18 or 21 but these, and the sex chromosome trisomies, are the main causes of intellectual and developmental disabilities. It is interesting to note that chromosomes 13, 18 and 21 carry the fewest genes. Abnormal numbers of sex chromosomes have a less serious effect on development; for instance, a missing sex chromosome can result in a Turner syndrome monosomy (45,X0).

Female meiotic recombination seems prone to errors. It is estimated that 10% of human pregnancies are aneuploidic related to segregation errors of maternal origin, increasing to over 50% at the end of the reproductive lifespan, whereas segregation errors in the sperm account for far fewer cases of aneuploidy. Although it is possible that paternally

TABLE 7.5   **ABO Blood Groups**

Blood Type	A	B	AB	O
Antigen on RBC (agglutinogen)	A	B	A + B	None (universal donor)
Antibody in plasma (agglutinin)	b	a	None (universal recipient)	a + b
Can donate to:	A and AB	B and AB	AB	All
Can receive from:	A and O	B and O	All	O
Distribution in UK (%)	42	9	3	46
Genotype	AA, AO	BB, BO	AB	OO
Phenotype	A	B	AB	O

derived aneuploidies are preferentially eliminated or culled (resulting in spermocyte death), it is more likely that more recombination errors occur in maternal meiosis and/or that the mechanisms for detecting and correcting or eliminating them are less stringent (such as mutations and recombination failure in the oocyte evading cellular checkpoints). It is proposed that the most likely reason for nondisjunction in the oocyte is age-related deterioration of the meiotic spindle (related to advanced maternal age) and the motor proteins that move chromosomes along it.

Down Syndrome

Down syndrome is the most common chromosomal anomaly at birth affecting about one in 700–1000 live births (depending on the screening protocols and pregnancy termination policies in different countries). The conception rate is much higher but it is associated with a high incidence of spontaneous abortion and stillbirth. Either the ovum or the sperm carries the extra chromosome 21. Although nondisjunction is usually associated with older maternal age, there is evidence to suggest that older men, perhaps because of a lower incidence of coitus, also have an increased rate of nondisjunction in their sperm formation. The relationship between maternal age and the genetic quality of the oocyte is more complex. The maternal age curve for trisomy incidence in naturally occurring pregnancies is J-shaped (Nagaoka et al., 2012); at the youngest maternal ages there is also a slight increase in the incidence of Down syndrome with a much more marked increase in the 10-year period preceding menopause. This suggests there are multiple mechanisms involved in human aneuploidy. It has been proposed that there may be an evolutionary advantage of increased aneuploidy in human females, possibly because aneuploidy usually results in failure of implantation or pregnancy thus increasing the interpregnancy spacing and preserving maternal resources, which enhances the likely survival of live-born offspring (Wang et al., 2017).

Affected children with trisomy 21 have typical stigmata of Down syndrome (Box 7.12). Their life expectancy tends

BOX 7.12   **Down Syndrome (Trisomy 21): Clinical Features**

- Slanting palpebral fissure, almond-shaped eyes
- A roundish head and flat facial profile
- Small nose and chin, protruding tongue
- Low-set ears
- Simian crease (single palmar crease) in 50% of cases
- Folds of redundant skin around neck
- Clinodactyly (inwardly curved little/5th finger) in about 50% of cases
- Extra space between first/big and second toes
- Usually have mild/moderate intellectual disability (IQ 35–69)
- Slower growth rate and short adult height
- Hearing and vision problems
- Congenital heart malformations occur in 40% of cases
- Prone to presenile dementia in fifth decade

to be shorter because of increased susceptibility to infection, congenital heart disease, testicular cancer and leukaemias. Individuals with Down syndrome have increased oxidative damage to neurons, which results in accumulation of excess amyloid β-peptide and characteristics of accelerated brain ageing, such as amyloid plaques and neurofibrillary tangles, similar to that in Alzheimer's disease. (The gene for the amyloid precursor protein is located on chromosome 21.)

Over half of the conceptions with trisomy 21 fail, suggesting that the extra copy of chromosome 21 interferes with intrauterine development. Although males with Down syndrome are infertile, females with Down syndrome can reproduce but have lower rates of fertility; theoretically, half the ova will have an extra copy of chromosome 21 but the effects on uterine development mean that the live-birth rate does not correlate with the conception rate.

About 2–4% of babies with Down syndrome have 46, rather than 47, chromosomes. The extra chromosomal material from a chromosome 21 is attached to another

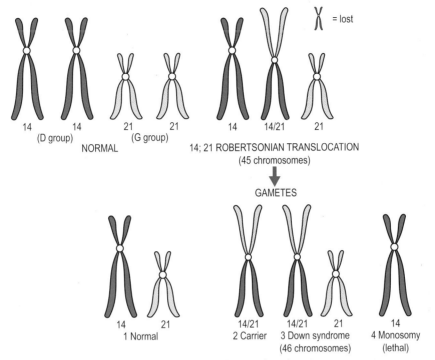

X = lost

14   14   21   21   14   14/21   21
(D group)   (G group)

NORMAL   14; 21 ROBERTSONIAN TRANSLOCATION
                              (45 chromosomes)

GAMETES

14   21   14/21   14/21   21   14
1 Normal   2 Carrier   3 Down syndrome   4 Monosomy
                                   (46 chromosomes)   (lethal)

Fig. 7.20 Robertsonian translocation.

chromosome (Robertsonian or balanced translocation; see Table 7.1). Usually, one of the parents is a carrier of Down syndrome and has the translocation in a balanced form; 45 chromosomes with the extra copy of chromosome 21 attached to another chromosome (Fig. 7.20). This means that the translocation carrier is not directly affected but will produce a proportion of gametes with an unbalanced complement of chromosomes. There is frequently an associated history of recurrent spontaneous abortion due to lethal arrangements of chromosomes in the gametes. In some cases of Down syndrome, the condition is mosaic with some normal cells (46 chromosomes) and some with trisomy 21 (47 chromosomes); the intellectual development and prognosis of these individuals is closer to normal.

In the UK, a screening test (for trisomies 21, 18 and 13) is offered to women in their first trimester, between 10 and 14 weeks of pregnancy, at the same time as the pregnancy dating scan; the 'combined test' is a nuchal translucency (NT) measurement during the scan plus measurement of serum free β-hCG and pregnancy-associated plasma protein A (PAPP-A) in maternal blood. This detects about 90% of affected pregnancies (trisomy 21, 18 or 13) with a false-positive rate of about 5%. For women who present late (between 14^{+2} and 20 weeks) or where a NT measurement was not possible, the 'quadruple test' to screen for

CASE STUDY 7.2

Josie is 48 years old and has four children between 14 and 24 years of age. She attends the midwives' clinic in a state of shock as her doctor has just informed her she is 8 weeks' pregnant.

- What advice would the midwife give Josie in relation to antenatal screening?

  Josie attends her local maternity unit at 12 weeks' gestation for a nuchal translucency scan and is given an estimated risk of a one in six possibility of a Down syndrome baby.

- What further investigations could be offered to Josie and how can the midwife best support her during this period of investigation?

trisomy 21 is offered in the second trimester; this measures serum free β-hCG, α-fetoprotein, unconjugated oestriol and inhibin A. The screening tests in conjunction with maternal age indicate risk. If the risk is high, the woman will be offered diagnostic testing: chorionic villus sampling (CVS; between weeks 11 and 14) or amniocentesis (from 15 weeks) and a mid-gestation ultrasound scan.

Case study 7.2 looks at a woman's concerns related to screening for Down syndrome.

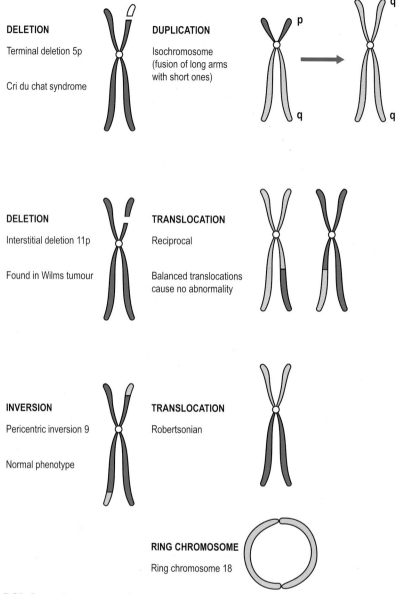

Fig. 7.21 Gross chromosome aberrations: deletions, inversion, duplication and translocations.

Structural Abnormalities

Autosomal Abnormalities

Structural chromosomal abnormalities include translocations, where material is exchanged between chromosomes, inversions, where a segment of the chromosome is rotated through 180°, and deletions, where segments of chromosomes are lost (Fig. 7.21). Cri du chat syndrome, which is rare, is associated with a partial deletion of the short arm

of chromosome 5. The chromosome 5 with the deletions is usually of paternal origin. Deletions at the ends of chromosomes can leave the affected chromosomes with fragile sites that adhere to each other, forming ring chromosomes that are unstable during cell division. In inversions, a parent may have the correct amount of chromosomal material and therefore no clinical problem, but the chromosomes align inappropriately in meiosis so gamete formation is affected. Many chromosomal disorders affect fertility.

BOX 7.13 Fragile X Syndrome

Fragile X syndrome is one of the commonest causes of intellectual disability in males. It is inherited as an X-linked trait, affecting 1 in 1000 male babies. The fragile site on the X chromosome is on the long arm. Affected males often have a large head, prominent chin and ears and may develop large testes at puberty. A significant proportion of carrier women have intellectual disability.

BOX 7.14 Epigenetic Control of Growth

Insulin-like growth factor 2 (IGF2) is encoded by the IGF2 gene which is imprinted. A fetus inherits two copies of the IGF2 gene, one from each parent. Usually, the paternal copy is expressed and the maternal gene is silenced. If the maternal gene is expressed as well as the paternal gene, the fetus has Beckwith–Wiedemann syndrome, which results in a high birthweight and other markers of overgrowth such as macroglossia (enlarged tongue) and an increased risk of childhood cancer. If both the maternal and paternal genes are silenced, the result is Silver–Russell (or Russell–Silver) syndrome, which is due to fetal undergrowth. Both conditions are rare but they occur with increased frequency in offspring derived from ICSI (see Chapter 6) suggesting the manipulation of gametes and embryos may affect imprinting.

Sex Chromosome Abnormalities

Sex chromosome anomalies are relatively common but produce fewer adverse effects than autosomal anomalies. Generally, the greater the number of extra sex chromosomes, the higher is the degree of intellectual disability. Many sex chromosome anomalies also affect reproductive performance (see Chapter 5).

An example of an X chromosome abnormality is fragile X syndrome (Box 7.13).

EPIGENETICS AND IMPRINTING

Epigenetic modifications to the genome produce heritable changes in gene expression, which do not involve a change in sequence of bases in the DNA. Thus, the phenotype of the offspring is changed because bases in DNA are modified in some way without their sequence being altered. Epigenetics is the basis of genetic imprinting (see below). The expression of genes can be switched on or off by DNA methylation (the addition of a methyl group to a cytosine residue of DNA), by phosphorylation or by modification of the DNA-associated histone proteins. During embryonic development, for example, imprinting switches off the expression of key genes so that only the gene from one of the parents is expressed as the functional protein. This additional mechanism of regulation of gene expression has created challenges in animal cloning experiments and in human ovarian tissue cryopreservation.

Imprinted genes cluster in particular parts of the genome, which are rich in CpG nucleotides (where a cytosine nucleotide is next to a guanine nucleotide linked by a phosphate group – CpG denotes Cytosine–phosphate–Guanine). CpG dinucleotides do not occur as often as predicted suggesting that they are vulnerable to mutation. The regions of the DNA strand, which have a high prevalence of CpG nucleotides are called 'CpG islands'. CpG islands often occur at the beginning of a gene. Most of the cytosine nucleotides in CpG islands are methylated. Methylation usually switches off – 'silences' – the gene. Histone modification of the DNA strand affects whether transcription factors can access the DNA to direct the transfer (transcription) of genetic material to RNA. There are about 22,300 genes in the human genome of which several hundred are thought to be imprinted, predominantly affecting growth (including function of the placenta) and development including brain development (Keverne, 2010) (Box 7.14).

Some genes are expressed when inherited from one parent but are not expressed when inherited from the other parent. This is genetic imprinting, the suppression or silencing of certain alleles on the chromosomes depending on their parental origin. Following fertilization, some genes are only expressed if they were inherited from the mother (the paternal gene being imprinted and therefore silenced), whereas others are expressed only if they were inherited from the father with the maternal gene being imprinted. Expression of some imprinted genes is spatially and temporally regulated and may only be active for a limited window during development.

Imprinted genes result in monoallelic gene expression and a number of diseases have been linked to defects in the normal imprinting process. The importance of genetic imprinting can be clearly seen in situations where imprinted genes are either inactivated or deleted on the normally active allele. The diseases Präder–Willi syndrome (PWS) and Angelman syndrome (AS) result, respectively, from a paternal (PWS) or a maternal (AS) deletion of the same region of chromosome 15 and since the alleles derived from the other parent are silenced by being imprinted, the genes are not expressed and their proteins are absent. In PWS, genes are deleted from the paternal chromosome 15, which are also imprinted on the maternal allele. In AS, the same region of chromosome 15 as that affected in PWS is deleted on the female allele and imprinted on the allele derived from the male.

Paternally imprinted genes tend to enhance fetal growth, whereas maternally expressed genes tend to constrict growth (see p. 256 for discussion of the 'conflict hypothesis'). Much of the research has been carried out in mice but in most genes, the imprinting status is conserved between species. Mouse genome manipulation demonstrates that androgenote mice, which have only paternal DNA, have a poor embryonic development and gynogenote mice, which have only maternal DNA, have poor placental development. In the mouse placenta, the paternal X chromosome is imprinted so that only the maternal genes are expressed and the paternal genes are silenced (Keverne, 2009). It is suggested that this may be important in avoiding a maternal immune rejection response to allogeneic fetal proteins that could be encoded by the paternal X chromosome (see Chapter 10). Gene expression in the brain is complex probably affecting behaviour, cognition and personality. In the preoptic area of the mouse brain, there is a high incidence of genes that are parentally imprinted; this area of the brain is a testosterone-dependent sexually dimorphic region, which is important for male sexual behaviour and maternal care (Gregg et al., 2010).

The appropriate establishment and maintenance of the epigenetic imprints are essential for normal growth and development. Aberrant gene expressions due to imprinting problems are called 'epimutations'. These can occur during imprint erasure, when the primordial germ cells migrate to the gonadal ridges in embryonic development (see Chapter 9), during imprint establishment when gametogenesis occurs or during imprint maintenance, throughout the life of the organism. The paternal genome is actively demethylated within a few hours of fertilization, whereas the maternal genome is demethylated passively during the first few cleavages of the embryo in a species-dependent manner. This pattern of demethylation, which erases most imprinted genes from the parents in the preimplantation stage, spares some imprinted genes, which are then maintained throughout development. Assisted reproductive techniques (ART) are associated with an increased risk of epigenetic disturbance, which is more likely when gametes are manipulated (affecting imprint establishment) or when the preimplantation embryo is manipulated (affecting imprint maintenance). As the first ART involving invasive manipulation of gametes and embryo are fairly recent events, it is not yet clear whether there will be any long-term epigenetic-medicated repercussions, the so-called 'ART ticking time bomb' (Grace and Sinclair, 2009).

GENETIC SCREENING

The detection of abnormal genetic conditions, such as cystic fibrosis (Case study 7.3), has been the focus of much

CASE STUDY 7.3

Tania has a brother who was diagnosed as having cystic fibrosis some years ago. Tania has been identified as being a carrier. Tania presents herself at the midwives' clinic with an unplanned pregnancy at 8 weeks' gestation. Her partner, Paul, has no family history of cystic fibrosis.

- What reassurance and advice can the midwife give to Tania?
- What referrals should the midwife make and how should this be explained to Tania?

ongoing research. There are three particular areas in which genetic investigation can be used to assess risk factors and confirm diagnosis of genetic disorder: parental screening, preimplantation screening and antenatal assessment.

Parental Screening

Individuals from families with a known prevalent genetic disorder may be tested to confirm whether they carry the abnormal gene. The findings form the basis of genetic counselling in which both the risks of passing on the abnormal gene and the possible consequences for a child are discussed. Frequently, this follows the delivery of an affected baby, especially if there is no family history. The condition may have arisen by spontaneous mutation and so the chances of it reoccurring in subsequent pregnancies may be much smaller than if the parents were carriers of the defective gene.

Preimplantation Genetic Diagnosis and Preimplantation Genetic Screening

Preimplantation genetic diagnosis (PGD) is a technique that allows diagnosis of genetic and chromosomal disorders in an embryo before pregnancy is established. It was developed as a test for couples carrying genetic disorders who were at risk of having a child with the disorder such as identifying and selecting female embryos from parents at risk of having a child with an X-linked recessive disorder if they had a son (Chen et al., 2018). However, the technique is also now used extensively in preimplantation genetic screening for optimizing IVF outcome in couples who do not carry a genetic disorder because chromosomal aberrations occur at high frequency in all embryos and can be detected before implantation thus reducing the otherwise inevitable implantation failure and early pregnancy loss thus increasing pregnancy rate in women who have poor IVF success rates. *In vitro* fertilization techniques (see Chapter 6) allow genetic analysis on polar bodies extracted from the oocyte before fertilization (first polar body)

BOX 7.15 Molecular Detection of Abnormal Genes

Molecular genetics studies human variations and mutations at the level of the gene and is important for understanding and identifying genetic diseases. Application of molecular genetic methods allows DNA diagnosis from very small amounts of tissue.

Fluorescent *In Situ* Hybridization

This involves the use of a genetic probe, which attaches to the target gene that it is designed to detect. The probe has a fluorescent label and so the abnormal gene can be visualized. Fluorescent in situ hybridization is used to identify microdeletions, aneuploidy and translocations.

Polymerase Chain Reaction

A small fragment of DNA is selectively amplified (at least a million times) by enzymatic procedures to produce large quantities of the relevant restriction fragments. These fragments can then be visualized by electrophoresis through an agarose gel, which is stained with a fluorescent dye. Polymerase chain reaction (PCR) is used to identify single-gene disorders such as fragile X syndrome, Huntington disease and muscular dystrophy. PCR can be used for any condition for which gene sequencing, and therefore the information required to design primers for selective amplification, is available.

and/or after fertilization (second polar body). Testing at the polar body stage is carried out in some countries where the legal regulation of testing of embryos is more rigorous; the integrity of the embryo is not affected by this approach. Genetic testing is usually carried out on a single cell from a day 3 cleavage-stage embryo or on trophoblast cells from the blastocyst at day 5 or 6. These techniques thus allow selection of normal disease-free embryos for subsequent implantation. PGD and preimplantation genetic screening (PGS) utilize molecular techniques such as fluorescent *in situ* hybridization, DNA analysis and quantitative polymerase chain reaction (qPCR; see Box 7.15), next generation sequencing (NGS) and array comparative genomic hybridization (aCGH) to detect single-gene disorders, such as thalassaemia or cystic fibrosis, or to screen for structural or numerical chromosome disorders. PGD offers an alternative to prenatal diagnosis and selective termination of an affected pregnancy, which may be important for couples who cannot contemplate termination of a pregnancy. The identification and selection of euploid embryos also has a positive effect on the clinical outcome of assisted

reproductive technologies (see Chapter 6) as chromosomal abnormalities are one of the major causes of spontaneous abortion and implantation failure. The use of PGS in IVF embryos is not without controversy. Initially results from nonrandomized studies were published about the increased pregnancy rate, decreased rate of miscarriage and trisomies. But in 2007, the 'Mastenbroek controversy' study reported that PGS reduced the rates of pregnancies and live births in women of advanced maternal age who had received IVF treatment (Mastenbroek et al., 2007). There are also concerns about the consequences of removal of embryonic cells and some paradoxical case reports of normal babies being born after the embryos were diagnosed with aneuploidy but implanted because there were no apparently euploid embryos available (Chen et al., 2018).

Antenatal Assessment

It is common throughout the UK for the screening for certain genetic disorders to be offered to all women. The tests predict the mathematical probability of a pregnancy being affected. If a test results in a high risk of abnormality, a diagnostic procedure such as chorionic villi sampling or amniocentesis may be offered. The aim is to detect chromosomal and anatomical abnormalities. 'Soft markers' are nonspecific and often transient or ethnic-specific findings of minor structural variants that can be detected by ultrasound (Ebrashy et al., 2016). These are considered of being of limited significance unless there are other markers that predict the probability of risk. Clinical tests include first trimester NT ultrasound, second trimester maternal serum screening and second semester ultrasound for anatomical survey. Methods of prenatal screening have to be adapted for women with multiple gestation. This is particularly important as the incidence of multiple gestation increases (Bender and Dugoff, 2018). Offspring of multiple gestation are at increased risk of abnormality but interpretation of the test results presents additional challenges. In women, who conceive after egg donation, it is the age of the ovum donor that is important.

First Trimester Nuchal Translucency Ultrasound

The first trimester ultrasound evaluates the fetus and uterus. At around 12 weeks' gestation, the nuchal fat pad at the back of the fetus's neck can be measured using ultrasound assessment. NT indicates the risk of cardiovascular anomalies. The NT measurement increases with crown–rump length so the findings combined with maternal age and fetal size (crown–rump length) indicate a higher or lower risk of the fetus having Down syndrome. The detection rate is about 83%. If the NT measurement is higher than normal, but the karyotype is normal, the fetus may be checked later for other physiological conditions such as cardiac abnormalities. The NT test is a screening test rather than a diagnostic test; there are other conditions besides trisomy 21 (Down syndrome) which cause abnormal results. The NT test can identify increased risk of trisomy 21 and other chromosomal abnormalities such as trisomy 18, trisomy 13, Turner syndrome, triploidy and other defects and genetic abnormalities.

Two aspects can be measured: the NT (between 11 and 14 weeks' gestation) and the thickness of the nuchal fold between 16 and 24 weeks' gestation. If either are increased, there is an increased risk of a genetic or physical abnormality being present. It is important not to confuse the two measurements. The change in NT may be related to oedema due to cardiac conditions, or failure of the neck lymphatic structures to develop at the right time, or both. Each case has to be assessed on an individual basis taking into consideration the maternal age and fetal size (crown–rump length), although generally measurements <1.9 mm are probably normal, whereas those >3 mm are probably abnormal. In the first trimester, the accepted method for noninvasive screening for trisomy 21 is to consider a combination of maternal age, free β-hCG and pregnancy associated plasma protein A in maternal serum and the fetal NT results. If these markers are combined, the detection rate is about 90% with a false-positive rate of 5%. Other markers of abnormalities that are assessed include the hypoplasticity of the nasal bone (indicating an absent nasal bone, more common in trisomy), echogenic intracardiac focus (indicating mineralization of myocardium or papillary muscle and possible regurgitation of the tricuspid valve, more common in trisomy 21) and echogenic bowel (which is seen as the bowel appearing as bright as bone). Some of these additional observations and others such as dilation of the renal pelvis (pyelectasis) and a single umbilical artery are classified as soft markers. The first trimester ultrasound can also accurately date the age of the fetus.

Second Trimester Maternal Serum Screening Tests

The risk of trisomy 21 can also be estimated by a combination of noninvasive blood tests, such as the levels of hCG (human chorionic gonadotrophin, which is usually raised in singleton trisomy 21 pregnancies), AFP (alpha/α-fetoprotein, which is usually low in a trisomy 21 pregnancy), β-hCG, unconjugated oestriol and inhibin-A at around 16 weeks in combination with maternal age (Table 7.6). These tests have various formats and are often referred to as double, triple or Bart's, and quadruple test, etc. Trisomy becomes more common with an increase in maternal age and is linked to an increasing failure of the division of the oocyte to be completed normally. The results from the biochemical indicators are combined with the maternal age risk and compared with normal values, adjusted for gestational age, to establish the likelihood ratio (probability or risk) of the pregnancy being affected. The second trimester is considered to be a particularly important time for antenatal screening.

Combined and Integrated Tests

Combined testing refers to combining the results of blood tests and ultrasound scans before the completion of the 14th week of pregnancy usually to predict risk of Down

TABLE 7.6	Combination Test Screening for Chromosomal Abnormalities			
Indicator	**Source**	**Rationale**	**Considerations**	
Alpha fetoprotein (AFP)	Amniotic fluid and maternal serum (MSAFP – levels ~1000 times less than amniotic fluid)	MSAFP levels are reduced in pregnancies affected by trisomy 21 and other trisomies. AFP leaks from exposed capillaries into amniotic fluid in fetuses with neural tube defect and some other malformations	The results are interpreted using appropriate standards for ethnic background: MSAFP is lower in Asian women and higher in black women. Levels are reduced in mothers with insulin-dependent diabetes	
Human chorionic gonadotrophin (hCG)	Maternal serum	Values are higher in trisomy 21 and lower in trisomy 18	Free β-subunit is measured	
Unconjugated oestriol (E3)	Maternal serum	Values are lower in trisomy 21		
Pregnancy-associated plasma protein A (PAPP-A)	Maternal serum	Values are lower in trisomy 21	PAPP-A increases with gestation. PAPP-A measurement may be used in first trimester screening	

syndrome; this is more sensitive than using blood tests and ultrasound examination in isolation. Integrated testing involves two blood tests, one in the first trimester (ideally between 10 and 12 weeks) followed by another blood test in the second trimester (ideally between 15 and 20 weeks). The results of the tests are evaluated using sophisticated risk evaluation software.

Ultrasound

All pregnant women in the UK are currently offered an anomaly ultrasound scan at approximately 20 weeks' gestation. The scan entails the detailed examination of the gross anatomical structures, such as internal organs, head, limbs and spine, and assessment of fetal growth. Many physical abnormalities, such as cardiac defects and limb length, are markers which may indicate the presence of a genetic abnormality. The more abnormal the ultrasound findings, the higher the risk of fetal aneuploidy. Abnormalities include structural malformations, increased nuchal thickness, short ear length, short femur or humerus, an extra vessel in the umbilical cord, a wide space between the toes and increased bowel echogenicity. This has led to the development of ultrasound scoring systems to identify fetuses at risk and support to the suggestion that ultrasound alone may be an alternative method of detecting genetic abnormalities in women who are reluctant to undergo amniocentesis.

Amniocentesis and Chorionic Villus Sampling

Diagnosis of the above disorders can usually only be confirmed with more invasive procedures such as CVS and amniocentesis (withdrawal of amniotic fluid) (Fig. 7.22). Both of these procedures enable the karyotype of the fetus to be examined, enabling fetal sexing, the identification of a trisomy or the presence of markers indicating the presence of abnormal alleles. Other invasive techniques are fetoscopy and cordiocentesis (fetal blood sampling) and biopsy. These procedures carry a slightly increased risk of procedure-related loss; however, the spontaneous abortion rate is higher in pregnancies with chromosomal abnormalities.

The fetal cells in the amniotic fluid or villus sample are grown in culture to produce enough cells for testing. The time taken for a result depends on the number of cells in the original sample and their growth rate, which can be affected by contamination with blood or maternal cells. The cell sample is greater in CVS so results are usually quicker; the other advantage of CVS is that is carried out earlier at 10–12 weeks' gestation. CVS is usually used to confirm the suspicion of trisomy 21 but is can identify many other chromosomal abnormalities. Occasionally, results can be complicated by chromosomal mosaicism where an individual has a combination of two or more cell lines, each with different chromosome numbers, derived from one zygote. For example, 1% of people with trisomy 21

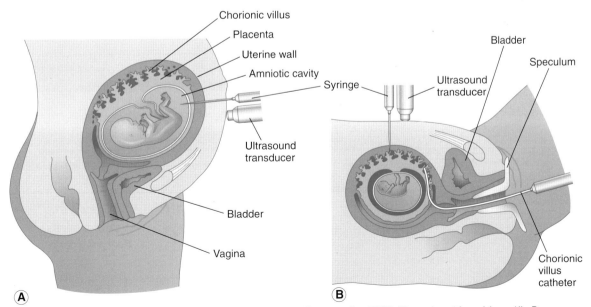

Fig. 7.22 (A) Amniocentesis; (B) transvaginal chorionic villus sampling (CVS). (Reproduced from Moore KL, Persaud TVN, Torchia MG: *The developing human: clinically oriented embryology*, 11 ed, Elsevier 2020, Fig. 6.13.)

are mosaics with both trisomic cells and normal cells; the clinical outcome is much better in these cases but if the abnormal cells are in the gonads there may be a high risk of producing abnormal gametes.

Amniocentesis and CVS are both invasive methods of prenatal diagnosis with inherent risks for the pregnancy. Alternative less-invasive methods of obtaining fetal cells and nucleic acids (DNA and RNA) are being studied because they are not associated with the same increased risk of miscarriage. The placenta is not a totally impermeable barrier. Some fetal cells transfer to the maternal circulation (see microchimerism, p. 286); there is approximately one fetal cell per millilitre of maternal blood. These intact fetal cells can be separated from maternal cells by flow cytometry (automated cell sorting equipment) as the cells have different morphological characteristics. Developments in molecular biology mean that PCR amplification assays (see p. 191) can be used for prenatal screening and genetic diagnosis. The discovery that cell-free fetal DNA and RNA (nucleic acids probably derived from invading fetal cells which are released during apoptosis of the trophoblast during placental development) can also be extracted from the maternal blood in the first trimester is the basis of non-invasive prenatal testing (NIPT aka the "SAFE" test) which is a relatively new procedure offered in the UK from 2018 (Mackie et al., 2017). NIPT was originally used for accurate determination of fetal sex (by

identifying the presence of Y chromosomal material in maternal blood) from 9 weeks gestational age which is much earlier than determination of fetal sex by ultrasound. It is also used to detect blood NI group incompatibility, aneuploidy and single-gene disorders such as Huntingdon disease, cystic fibrosis, thalassemias and leukaemia (Hudecova and Chiu, 2017). If NIPT results indicate a increased probability of abnormalities, definitive diagnosis by less safe invasive tests is offered. NIPT means fewer amniocentesis tests are carried out. Where the technique is applied to the detection of genetic diseases, such as cystic fibrosis, caused by a single gene variant, the result is definitive and does not require confirmation by an invasive test; this is known as non-invasive prenatal diagnosis (NIPD). Table 7.7 summarizes the prenatal diagnostic procedures and Box 7.15 describes the techniques for molecular detection of abnormal genes.

EVOLUTION

Evolution is the study of genetic variation within populations and how this variation allows populations to evolve in response to changes within the environment in which they live. The variation of genes within a defined population is referred to as the gene pool. Charles Darwin's famous book *On the Origin of the Species by Means of Natural Selection, or the Preservation of Favoured Faces in the Struggle for Life* (commonly known as

TABLE 7.7 Prenatal Diagnostic Procedures

Procedure	Gestation at Which Test is Performed (Weeks)	Conditions Screened for or Diagnosed
Noninvasive techniques		
NT measurement by ultrasound scan	12	Screen for trisomic conditions and other abnormalities
AFP test	16	Screen for neural tube defects
Triple/double/Bart's/combined test	16	Screen for trisomies
Ultrasound scan	20	Diagnosis of gross physical defects
Noninvasive prenatal testing (NIPT)	9–10	Screen for trisomies and other aneuploidies, diagnosis of fetal sex (if risk of X-linked conditions) and some single gene disorders
Invasive techniques		
CVS	10–12	Diagnosis of chromosomal abnormality
Amniocentesis	16	Diagnosis of chromosomal abnormality
Fetoscopy		Diagnosis of chromosomal abnormality
Cordocentesis (removal of fetal blood from the umbilical cord)		Diagnosis of metabolic disorders
		Assessment of antibody status in haemolytic disease
		Detection of fetal infection
Organ biopsy (liver, skin, etc.)		Metabolic disorders
		Hereditary disorders

The Origin of the Species) (1859) presented the argument that all organisms descended from a common ancestor and advocated natural selection as the mechanism of evolution. The mechanism of evolution is still contested, particularly how other mechanisms such as random genetic drift have contributed to evolution and the effects of gradual accumulation of small genetic changes rather than fewer large ones.

As described earlier in this chapter, many disease processes have their aetiology in the physical expression (phenotype) of an abnormal gene (genotype). They are normally recessive, so the effects of the abnormal gene are masked by the presence of a normal gene. The physical effects of recessive genes are only seen when there are two recessive genes present in the genome, for instance, in cystic fibrosis (see also Case study 7.4, which looks at the Rhesus-negative blood type). Some abnormal genes may be partially expressed or modified by the presence of a normal gene. Many heterozygous, partially expressed genetic conditions may, in the right environment, impart a beneficial effect on the individual. An example is the sickle cell trait HbA/HbS or HbA/HbC (see Box 7.3). If one recessive gene is present, the anaemia condition may be expressed in a minor form. Whilst this can cause problems for individuals in periods of stress and physiological change, such as pregnancy, the symptoms are usually not life-threatening; on the contrary, in the malaria zones of the world the sickle cell trait is beneficial to heterozygotes as it affords some protection from the malaria parasite. This is because entry of the parasite into the red blood cell causes the cell to die before the parasite has time to reproduce. In the major form of the disease when the individual inherits two abnormal genes, one from each parent, the haemoglobin configuration is abnormal. The erythrocytes are sickle-shaped and fragile which leads to severe complications of blood cell lysis and coagulation. Hence, although the homozygous form has implications for the survival of the affected individual, the abnormal gene is maintained within the gene pool because its partial form confers advantage in the gene pool of the population by increasing resistance to falciparum malaria. The absence of the Duffy surface antigen, which is usually present on the erythrocyte cell membrane, also affords protection against malaria as the malarial parasite attaches itself to this particular antigen to enable it to enter the cell.

CASE STUDY 7.4

Jane is a 30-year-old woman expecting her second baby. Her first baby was born 3 years ago in rural Africa. She has now returned to this country at 36 weeks' gestation. The blood group results from her first antenatal visit show that Jane's blood group type is O, Rhesus-negative.

- What are the implications of this?
- If it is known that her partner has the same blood group, what are the risks of the pregnancy being affected?
- If Jane's first baby was Rhesus-positive, what risk is there to the current fetus and how does it depend on its own blood group?
- If a baby is affected by haemolytic disease of the newborn, what clinical symptoms are likely to be evident and how can they be treated?
- If the first baby had been born in England, how would Jane have been treated?

The environment is ever changing and so the process of evolution as a result continues to facilitate adaptation to such changes. The process of evolution itself may then complicate our own understanding of human physiological processes. More than one regulatory system may develop at different times within our evolutionary progression. Different prevailing environmental conditions would thus influence the evolution of changes within the regulation mechanisms to match the change within the environment. Human physiological processes can be described as being in two evolutionary states that are either progressing or declining. Our reproductive physiology may still be influenced by processes that evolved to cope with the Pleistocene environment, in which it is believed that the genus *Homo* first evolved, even though these may now be in a state of evolutionary decline. In contrast, it is believed that our physiological processes may be responding to 'younger' evolutionary influences and therefore be in a state of evolutionary progression. Depending on the external (exogenous) and internal (endogenous) conditions present, the response to either of these evolutionary types may still be initiated.

KEY POINTS

- Genetics is a reductionist science that uses mathematical probability to predict the risk of inheriting certain characteristics, usually of medical relevance. Techniques such as combination diagrams and Punnett squares can be used to predict the probability of inheriting single-gene traits.

- DNA is the 'blueprint' of the organism, which is organized into chromosomes within the cell nuclei. A gene is a unit of a chromosome, or length of DNA, that codes for a particular instruction. Humans have 23 pairs of chromosomes: 22 pairs of autosomes and a pair of sex chromosomes (XX in females and XY in males).

- The structure of DNA facilitates its semiconservative replication prior to cell division, thus each cell of an organism has the same DNA.
- Mitosis is normal cell division producing daughter diploid cells with 23 pairs (i.e. 46) of chromosomes. Meiosis is a specific cell division in gamete formation that results in the number of chromosomes being reduced to 23 (the haploid number).
- DNA controls protein synthesis by acting as a template for the formation of mRNA (transcription); mRNA induces protein synthesis by directing the incorporation of amino acids into the protein (translation).
- There are accumulated errors in replicating DNA, which may manifest as mutations causing proteins with abnormal structure and function to be formed.

- A trait that is dominantly inherited is expressed if the individual has at least one copy of the gene, whereas a recessively inherited trait is expressed only if the individual inherits the gene from both parents. Sex-linked traits affect males more than females, who may be carriers.
- Chromosomal abnormalities may be numerical or structural and have serious clinical implications for those affected.
- Detection of fetal abnormalities is a routine part of antenatal care, which has developed screening programmes to assess risk and tests to confirm diagnosis.

APPLICATION TO PRACTICE

It is important to realize that the genetic diversity of a population drives the process of evolution and adaptation to changes in the external environment.

Many genes are labelled as abnormal but they may be essential variants that may at least contribute to the survival of the population as a whole.

The focus of antenatal screening of the fetus is based upon the detection of risk of abnormal karyotypes using tests that are noninvasive such as ultrasound scanning and the measurement of fetal DNA and other biomarkers in maternal blood. Diagnostic testing to confirm the abnormal karyotype is through invasive tests, such as CVS and amniocentesis, which carry a small increased risk of miscarriage. In many situations, the conditions being screened for have a genetic cause. Knowledge of this is essential for the midwife to be able to understand and explain what the tests actually involve and what the results may indicate.

Midwives have an increasing role in the care of women suffering from pregnancy loss for whatever reasons, so an in-depth knowledge of fetal abnormalities is essential in providing care for the women.

Preimplantation genetic diagnosis can be performed on early embryos following IVF before implantation. This means that some genetic conditions can be identified as part of the embryo selection procedures so that only nonaffected embryos are replaced into the uterine cavity. This does not, however, guarantee a healthy infant and couples undergoing this technique may have high anxiety levels.

ANNOTATED FURTHER READING

Dawkins R: *The extended phenotype: the long reach of the gene*, Oxford, 2016, OUP.
A follow-up book to the Selfish Gene, which extends the concept that the gene is the unit of selection; a well-written and controversial book by an author known for his communication skills.

Department of Health: *NHS fetal anomaly screening programme handbook*, London, 2018, DoH.
This booklet, written for health professionals, gives in-depth details of the principles, background and current methods used in the UK for antenatal screening.

Edwards L, Hui L: First and second trimester screening for fetal structural anomalies, *Semin Fetal Neonatal Med* 23:102–111, 2018.
A comprehensive review of current and emerging methods to detect fetal anomalies, which summarizes the principles, detections rates and limitations of the methods.

Ennis C: *Introducing epigenetics; a graphic guide*, London, 2017, Icon Books.
A slim and succinct book about genetics, cell biology and epigenetics written by a journalist with a background in science and research expertise in cancer and genetics.

Frati P, Fineschi V, Di SM, et al.: Preimplantation and prenatal diagnosis, wrongful birth and wrongful life: a global view of bioethical and legal controversies, *Hum Reprod Update* 23:338–357, 2017.
A review of the technologies used in preimplantation and prenatal diagnoses and the ethical dilemmas raised by these tests.

Hartl DL: *Essential genetics and genomics*, ed 7, Burlington, 2018, Jones and Bartlett.
A popular and well-illustrated textbook, suitable for beginners, which clearly explains genetic concepts from the principles of hereditary and genetic analysis to molecular genetics.

National Collaborating Centre for Women's and Children's Health: *Antenatal care: routine care for the healthy pregnant woman*, 2008. London. NICE (latest update 2019).

This guidance details the current recommendations and methods for routine antenatal screening in the UK.

Read A, Donnai D: *New clinical genetics*, Oxford, 2015, Scion Publishing.

A case-based textbook, targeted at medical students and clinicians, which describes genetic mechanisms, diseases, diagnosis and the application of new technologies and diagnostic tools.

Russell PJ: *iGenetics: a Mendelian approach*, ed 3, New York, 2013, Pearson.

A modern approach to genetics, which covers fundamentals of genetics using an experimental enquiry-solving approach includes experimental data from research studies, critical thinking skills, problems and worked examples and comments on applications in 'focus on genetics' boxes.

Rutherford A: *A brief history of everyone who ever lived: the stories in our genes*, London, 2016, Weidenfeld & Nicolson.

An interesting and unique history of what makes us humans as a species.

Ryan F: *The mysterious world of the human genome*, London, 2015, William Collins.

A summary of the human genome project and its implications, which considers how genetic issues affect health and public policy; includes chapters on the potential cure of genetic diseases, the use of DNA in forensic science and paternity testing, and mapping the movements of humans from their African birthplace.

Shearer WT, Lubin BH, Cairo MS, Notarangelo LD: Cord blood banking for potential future transplantation, *Pediatrics* 140, 2017.

A fascinating review of the sources and uses of stem cells, the value of cord blood banks and processes for quality control and accreditation, which generates some useful information to discuss with parents.

Tobias ST, Connor JM, Ferguson-Smith MA: *Essential medical genetics*, ed 6, Oxford, 2013, Wiley-Blackwell (updated).

An updated and well-written text that introduces the basic principles and clinical applications of genetics with a focus on the molecular mechanisms involved in genetic disorders and diseases. Also covers the genetics of common diseases and cancer, prenatal screening and gene therapy.

Turnpenny PD, Ellard S: *Emery's elements of medical genetics*, ed 15, New York, 2017, Elsevier.

A comprehensive classic textbook, which is divided into three parts. Section A focuses on the scientific basis of human genetics and covers genetic principles, risk prediction and factors influencing inheritance. Section B covers medical aspects of genetics including genetic diseases, genetic factors in diseases and genomics. Section C deals with clinical applications, including genetic counselling, ethical issues, screening and diagnosis.

REFERENCES

Aitken RJ: DNA damage in human spermatozoa; important contributor to mutagenesis in the offspring, *Transl Androl Urol* 6:S761–S764, 2017.

Anderson A, Binney J, Harris A: *Tangata whenua: a history*, Wellington, 2015, Bridget Williams Books.

Arenas M, Pereira F, Oliveira M, et al.: Forensic genetics and genomics: much more than just a human affair, *PLOS Genetics* 13:e1006960, 2017.

Bender W, Dugoff L: Screening for aneuploidy in multiple gestations: the challenges and options, *Obstet Gynecol Clin North Am* 45:41–53, 2018.

Brooker CG: *Human structure and function*, ed 2, St Louis, 1998, Mosby. pp 8, 20, 514.

Chen HF, Chen SU, Ma GC, et al.: Preimplantation genetic diagnosis and screening: current status and future challenges, *J Formos Med Assoc* 117:94–100, 2018.

Darwin C: *On the origin of the species by means of natural selection*, London, 1859, John Murray.

Dawkins R: *The selfish gene: 40th Anniversary edition*, ed 4, Oxford, 2016, OUP.

Ebrashy A, Kurjak A, Adra A, et al.: Controversial ultrasound findings in mid trimester pregnancy. Evidence based approach, *J Perinat Med* 44:131–137, 2016.

Goodwin B: *Health and development: conception to birth*, Milton Keynes, 1997, Open University.

Grace KS, Sinclair KD: Assisted reproductive technology, epigenetics, and long-term health: a developmental time bomb still ticking, *Semin Reprod Med* 27:409–416, 2009.

Graves JAM: Weird animals, sex, and genome evolution, *Annu Rev Anim Biosci* 6:1–22, 2018.

Gregg C, Zhang J, Butler JE, et al.: Sex-specific parent-of-origin allelic expression in the mouse brain, *Science* 329:682–685, 2010.

Griffin DK, Ellis PJI: The human Y-chromosome: evolutionary directions and implications for the future of 'maleness'. In Palermo GD, Sills ES, editors: *Intracytoplasmic sperm injection*, Bloomberg, 2018, Springer International Publishing AG, pp 183–192.

Hudecova I, Chiu RW: Non-invasive prenatal diagnosis of thalassemias using maternal plasma cell free DNA, *Best Pract Res Clin Obstet Gynaecol* 39:63–73, 2017.

Huynh KD, Lee JT: X-chromosome inactivation: a hypothesis linking ontogeny and phylogeny, *Nat Rev Genet* 6:410–418, 2005.

Keverne B: Monoallelic gene expression and mammalian evolution, *Bioessays* 31:1318–1326, 2009.

Keverne EB: Neuroscience: a mine of imprinted genes, *Nature* 466:823–824, 2010.

Linschooten JO, Verhofstad N, Gutzkow K, et al.: Paternal lifestyle as a potential source of germline mutations transmitted to offspring, *FASEB J* 27:2873–2879, 2013.

Mackie FL, Hemming K, Allen S, et al.: The accuracy of cell-free fetal DNA-based non-invasive prenatal testing in singleton pregnancies: a systematic review and bivariate meta-analysis, *BJOG* 124:32–46, 2017.

Mastenbroek S, Twisk M, van Echten-Arends J, et al.: In vitro fertilization with preimplantation genetic screening, *New Engl J Med* 357:9–17, 2007.

Nagaoka SI, Hassold TJ, Hunt PA: Human aneuploidy: mechanisms and new insights into an age-old problem, *Nat Rev Genet* 13:493–504, 2012.

Open University: *DNA: molecular aspects of genetics.* Unit 24 in the Science foundation course (S102), Milton Keynes, 1988, OU, pp 14, 36.

Pan A, Kraschel KL: CRISPR diagnostics: underappreciated uses in perinatology, *Semin Perinatol* 42:525–530, 2018.

Pandey VK, Tripathi A, Bhushan R: Application of CRISPRCas9 genome editing in genetic disorders, *J Genet Syndr Gene Ther* 8:321–330, 2017.

Pertea M, Salzberg SL: Between a chicken and a grape: estimating the number of human genes, *Genome Biol* 11:206, 2010.

Rogaev EI, Grigorenko AP, Moliaka YK, et al.: Genomic identification in the historical case of the Nicholas II royal family, *Proc Natl Acad Sci USA* 106:5258, 2009.

Wang S, Hassold T, Hunt P, et al.: Inefficient crossover maturation underlies elevated aneuploidy in human female meiosis, *Cell* 168:977–989, 2017.

8

The Placenta

- To describe the development of the placenta, membranes and umbilical cord.
- To describe the structure of the placenta, membranes and umbilical cord and recognize common structural variants.
- To identify the roles of the placenta.
- To describe the formation and role of amniotic fluid.
- To discuss how abnormal placental development might affect fetal development including intrauterine

growth restriction and other outcomes of the pregnancy.
- To describe methods for monitoring placental function and wellbeing.
- To outline the development of the placenta in twin pregnancies.
- To discuss the role of the placenta in delivery of nutrients and how this can affect fetal growth and later risk of chronic disease.

INTRODUCTION

The development of the placenta is critical for fetal survival because of the importance of the placenta in maternal–fetal transfer. It transfers nutrients to the fetus and establishes stable surroundings for fetal development, buffering the fetus from maternal and environmental stressors. The placenta has a range of functional activities (Table 8.1), including synthesizing and secreting hormones, providing immune support, transporting a range of nutrients, gas exchanges, waste and heat removal and detoxification of xenobiotic substances. The placenta flourishes in an immunologically foreign environment and has an important role in the immunological acceptance of the fetal allograft (see Chapter 10). The structure of the placenta means that, although optimal diffusion gradients are established, maternal and fetal blood never actually mix. The placenta has an extraordinary ability to undergo structural and functional adaptations that limit the effect of adverse situations such as hypoxia (a state of inappropriately 'low' oxygen), nutrient deficiency and exposure to drugs and toxins. Placental blood flow requires synchronous development of the maternally derived uteroplacental circulation and the fetoplacental vasculature. Compromised development of either component is associated with adverse outcomes of pregnancy such as preeclampsia and fetal growth restriction (FGR) and effects on both maternal health and fetal/infant wellbeing.

CHAPTER CASE STUDY

At Zara's 20-week scan, the ultrasonographer documented in her report that the placenta was situated on the anterior wall of the uterus with the majority of the placental body situated in the middle and lower pole of the uterine body with the lateral edge of the placenta ~2 cm from the internal cervical os.

- What are the possible complications that could arise from this situation?
- How do you think the midwife should discuss these possible complications with Zara and how they could be recognized?
- Why is it common for women with this situation to have vaginal bleeding around 34 weeks of pregnancy?
- Are there any conditions or factors related to low lying placentas and, if so, how can these be managed?

The placenta and the chorion (outer membrane) are derived from the trophoblast layer of blastocyst cells (see Fig. 6.6, p. 149). Other extraembryonic tissues develop from the inner cell mass. These include the amnion (inner membrane) and amniotic fluid, the yolk sac, the allantois

TABLE 8.1   Summary of Placental Functions

Function	Placental Role
Respiration	Maternal oxyhaemoglobin dissociates in the intervillous spaces. O_2 diffuses through the walls of the villi where it binds to fetal haemoglobin forming fetal oxyhaemoglobin. Transfer is increased by the higher affinity of fetal haemoglobin for O_2. The lower CO_2 level facilitates transfer of CO_2 in the reverse direction in pregnancy
Nutrition	Active transport of glucose, iron and some vitamins and passive transport of other nutrients. The placenta can metabolize proteins, fats and carbohydrates into simple molecules. Fats cross the placenta less easily so the fat-soluble vitamins (A, D, E and K) cross slowly. The placenta stores glycogen, which can be converted to glucose when required
Excretion	Waste products of metabolism, CO_2 and heat cross from the fetus to the mother
Protection	The placenta acts as a barrier against most bacteria (such as cocci and bacilli). However, smaller microorganisms (such as the syphilis bacterium) and viruses (including rubella, varicella-zoster, cytomegalovirus, coxsackie and HIV) can cross the villi. The placenta transfers IgG antibodies and Rhesus antibodies to the fetus. Drugs including teratogens, anaesthetics and carbon monoxide (from smoking) can cross the placenta. The placenta also expresses enzymes involved in detoxification
Endocrine role	Initially, the trophoblast produces hCG, which maintains the corpus luteum and its production of steroid hormones. From the 3rd month onwards, oestrogen and progesterone are produced in large quantities by the placenta. hPL is produced from the syncytiotrophoblast. The placenta also produces a broad range of other hormones including corticosteroids, ACTH, TSH, IGFs, prolactin, relaxin, endothelin and prostaglandins
Immunological role	The trophoblast has unique immunological properties, such as nonclassical HLA-G and HLA-E expression, that protect the conceptus from immune rejection
Provision of stem cells	The placental tissue, including Wharton's jelly and cord blood, is a potential source of stem cells, which may have therapeutic potential

(a largely vestigial structure in humans) and the extraembryonic mesoderm. The umbilical cord and the blood vessels of the placenta are derived from the extraembryonic mesoderm.

The human placenta is haemochorial (Box 8.1), which means that maternal blood comes into contact with the placental trophoblast cells; this type of organization is also seen in chimpanzees and gorillas and in rats and mice. The uteroplacental unit is a dynamic interface where the fetal and maternal components cooperate to establish conditions that promote the growth and development of the fetus. The placenta as seen at delivery is just the fetal component or chorionic plate. The maternal component or basal plate is the placental bed, which underlies the fetal component and the uteroplacental circulation that vascularizes the placental bed. Between the chorionic and basal plates are the intervillous spaces where the maternal–fetal exchange occurs. Conversion of the maternal spiral arteries, by the trophoblast tissue, to dilated and flaccid vessels is an essential step for successful pregnancy. Abnormal placental function is strongly associated with fetal complications, but study of

BOX 8.1   Types of Placental Organization and Nutrition

Placentas are classified depending on how the maternal and fetal blood supplies are organized.

- Haemochorial: the chorion (placental tissue) is in direct contact with maternal blood (e.g. human, rodent); remodelling of the uterine vasculature is essential for success of the pregnancy.
- Endotheliochorial: the endometrium of the maternal blood vessels is in contact with the chorion (e.g. dogs, cats).
- Epitheliochorial: a more primitive structure in which the maternal epithelium of the uterus is in contact with the chorion (e.g. cows, pigs).

the human placenta, particularly the maternal component, is not easy. Placentation in the human and other great apes is unique, which means that observations from other species can be applied to humans only with caution.

Placental reserve needs to exceed fetal requirements (otherwise the fetus could be compromised under conditions of hypoxia or compromised nutrient supply). 'Placental efficiency' is a concept defined as birthweight (grams of fetus) produced per gram of placenta developed at any stage of gestation or as the placental:fetal or birthweight:placental weight ratio (BWPW) (Salavati et al., 2018). Placental weight and size are rather crude proxies for placental function and efficiency. Placental:fetal weight ratio decreases and efficiency increases during gestation, particularly in the last week. Both maternal and fetal signals can affect the phenotype of the placenta and how it grows. Fetal growth predicts later onset of adult disease (see Chapter 9) and as fetal growth is largely determined by the placental control of nutrient flow, placental growth and development are crucial in programming of later health (Thornburg et al., 2016).

Placental efficiency is affected by the surface area for exchange, the thickness of the barriers between fetal and maternal circulations and the arrangement of the fetal and maternal blood vessels ('vascular architecture'). It is the latter variable that appears to account for species differences in placental efficiency. The most efficient human placentas are those which are small in diameter and thin; it is thought that these small placentas must functionally adapt to increase nutrient transporter expression and become more efficient. Placental efficiency is enhanced by an increase in both the number of carrier proteins involved in the transport of substances across the placenta and the placental perfusion. The mechanisms by which the placenta responds to external cues appear to involve insulin-like growth factors (IGFs), which regulate placental nutrient allocation for fetal growth (Sferruzzi-Perri and Camm, 2016). It is also suggested that placental shape may be important in predicting later risk of disease (Thornburg et al., 2016). Most placentas are oval rather than round; the length (long axis) is ~2.5 cm greater than the width (short axis). The regulators of the growth of the axes are not known but there are relationships between the dimensions and disease outcomes and lifespan, which have been identified from birth cohort studies.

UTERINE RECEPTIVITY

Successful implantation requires synchronous development of the human embryo and the endometrium so the embryo is implantation competent and the endometrium is receptive to implantation. The first phase of the development of uterine receptivity is regulated by the steroid hormones produced by the follicular cells. Initially oestrogen drives the renewal and proliferative growth of the endometrial lining following menstruation. Postovulation,

progesterone from the corpus luteum causes the endometrium to differentiate into a secretory tissue; the glands and blood vessels proliferate and entwine and the connective tissue becomes oedematous. Progesterone also stimulates the development of microvilli to increase the apical surface area of the columnar epithelial cells of the endometrium. Smooth muscle myosin also increases and the stromal (connective tissue) cells proliferate.

Decidualization promotes changes in the endometrium that make it receptive to implantation. After ovulation in the human (and other closely related primate species: 'higher primates'), spontaneous decidualization of the endometrium occurs. This involves angiogenesis (so blood flow increases), natural killer (NK) cells infiltrating into the endometrium, and the endometrial stromal cells thickening and accumulating lipid and glycogen; these differentiated cells are now called decidual cells. In most placental mammals, decidualization of the endometrium is fetus-induced rather than hormone-induced so it only occurs after successful fertilization. It has been suggested that spontaneous decidualization is an adaptation in mammals with invasive haemochorial placentation (Emera et al., 2012) possibly as a protective mechanism or to provide a mechanism for embryo selection. In species, like humans, with spontaneous decidualization, postovulatory progesterone is the main signal. If fertilization does not occur and progesterone levels drop, then menstruation results. In those species with hormone-induced spontaneous decidualization, progesterone withdrawal leads to apoptosis of the endometrial stroma cells (see Chapter 4).

Synchronous development and communication between the maternal endometrium and the embryonic tissue are required for successful establishment of pregnancy. The signals involved in the exquisitely sensitive dialogue between the embryo and the endometrium include human chorionic gonadotrophin (hCG), interleukin-1 and insulin-like growth factor 2 (IGF-2) (see Chapter 4). Whereas mammalian embryos have intrinsic invasive potential and can initiate implantation-type reactions in many different tissues, the endometrium is receptive to implantation for a limited duration known as the implantation or nidation window (Aplin and Ruane, 2017).

Implantation occurs in the receptive or mid-secretory phase of the menstrual cycle, about 7 days after fertilization. The cells of the endometrial epithelium have cells that are both ciliated and have microvilli (Aplin and Ruane, 2017). During the implantation window, microvilli on the surface of these uterine endometrial cells become less prolific and shorter and fuse together to form single flower-like projections from the cells called pinopods (or pinopodes) or uterodomes. These smooth bleb-like protrusions form under the influence of progesterone (during the mid-luteal phase) only in the preferred sites of embryo–endometrial interaction and thus act as markers of uterine receptivity The pinopods are only present for 2–3 days during which implantation must occur; if blastocyst competency does not coincide with the endometrium being receptive, then implantation is defective and fails (Davidson and Coward, 2016). The interaction between the endometrium and the developing trophoblast is facilitated by a number of cytokines, metalloproteinases, surface integrins and growth factors, including IGFs and their binding proteins, which create a specific microenvironment, which modulates trophoblast function. Perhaps surprisingly, the uterine environment is proinflammatory; signals such as prostaglandin E2 (PGE$_2$) and a proinflammatory profile of cytokines such as interleukin 6 (IL-6) and tumour necrosis factor (TNF) are essential (Griffith et al., 2017). If a woman takes nonsteroidal anti-inflammatory drugs (NSAIDs, e.g. aspirin or ibuprofen) during this time and the inflammatory reaction is suppressed, the risk of implantation failure is increased. After implantation, the endometrium changes to an anti-inflammatory state, which prevents fetal rejection (see Chapter 10).

It is evident that implantation is a rather inefficient process in the human; the probability of natural conception per menstrual cycle (defined as fecundity) is only about 30% and over 75% of failed pregnancies are thought to be due to implantation defects (Cha et al., 2012). Defective implantation, if it results in pregnancy at all, is associated with a poor outcome. Repeated implantation failure (RIF) refers to failure of good quality embryos to implant following several *in vitro* fertilization (IVF) cycles; it is thought that nonreceptive endometrium is a significant factor (Simon and Laufer, 2012).

Implantation

Implantation is the consequence of a well-organized sequence of events involving synchronized crosstalk between the receptive endometrium and a functional and implantation-competent blastocyst (Aplin and Ruane, 2017). Implantation in the receptive phase is classically described as occurring in three stages: apposition, adhesion and invasion. Implantation cannot occur during the preceptive (preparatory) phase (first 7 days after ovulation) or in the refractory nonreceptive phase after the implantation window, when the uterine environment becomes hostile to the blastocyst surviving.

The trophoblastic cells overlying the inner cell mass are known as the polar trophoblast; it is these cells that initiate the adhesion and implantation processes. The blastocyst enters the uterus about 4 days after fertilization. It probably floats freely in the uterus for up to 72 h before hatching out of the protective zona pellucida and coming into

contact with the endometrium (Evans et al., 2016). The blastocyst rolls freely over the endometrium until it reaches a receptive area. This process is thought to be mediated by signals such as selectins, which are expressed on the surface of the polar trophoblast cells of the newly hatched blastocyst (Feng et al., 2017). The blastocyst then orientates itself so that the embryonic pole of the blastocyst implants into the maternal endometrium first. The interaction of the trophoblast cells overlying the inner cell mass modulates gene expression to promote these cells becoming invasive when they contact the maternal endometrium (Aplin and Ruane, 2017). Inappropriate implantation of the blastocyst, so there is reduced contact between the polar trophoblast and the uterine endothelium, is associated with abnormalities of umbilical cord insertion, growth of the placenta and fetus and even failure of pregnancy. The endometrium produces MUC1, a mucin glycoprotein, which prevents the blastocyst adhering to areas of the endometrium with poor chances of implantation. The optimally receptive areas of the endometrium secrete a cascade of signals, including chemokines and growth factors, which attract the blastocyst to the pinopodes. The apposition of the blastocyst to the endometrium further triggers the production of adhesion molecules, such as integrins and cadherins, which firmly anchor the blastocyst to the endometrial pinopodes (Fig. 8.1). This process is enhanced because the endometrial surface expresses receptors for selectins. The tethering of the blastocyst to the endometrium stimulates

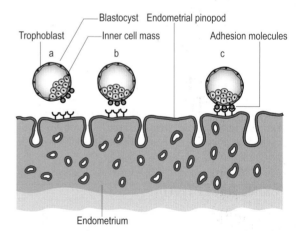

Fig. 8.1 The sequence of implantation: (a) the blastocyst comes close to the endometrial pinopods and the trophoblast overlying the embryonic pole expresses selectins; (b) the trophoblast selectins are recognized by the selectin receptors on the endometrium, which (c) triggers the production of adhesion molecules. (Reproduced with permission from Achache and Revel, 2006.)

the polar trophoblastic cells to undergo rapid mitosis and proliferate as the invasion of the uterine wall commences. Implantation may be affected by conditions such as maternal antiphospholipid syndrome where maternal autoimmune antiphospholipid antibodies cause implantation to be dysregulated; there is a high incidence of pregnancy loss associated with this condition (Salmon et al., 2017) (Case study 8.1).

CASE STUDY 8.1

Trudy is a 36-year-old, para 1, gravida 11. She attends the midwives clinic at 6 weeks' gestation, very distressed as this was not a planned pregnancy. Trudy informs the midwife that her last baby was born at 32 weeks' gestation, very small for dates and that Trudy had also developed fulminating preeclampsia, which was the main reason for the early delivery. Three days after this delivery, Trudy developed severe difficulty in breathing, which was diagnosed as a pulmonary embolism. Trudy then informs the midwife that all her other pregnancies had been spontaneous miscarriages at around 10 weeks' gestation.

The midwife reviews Trudy's postobstetric notes and discovers that Trudy has antiphospholipid syndrome and that at her last delivery, it was documented that the placenta was small and infarcted. As a result of this, the midwife immediately refers Trudy to attend a consultant clinic as an emergency.

- Why did the midwife refer Trudy to the consultant as an emergency?
- What treatment would be offered to Trudy and how will the pregnancy be managed?
- What is the significance of the placental infarcts and what was the most likely cause?

DIFFERENTIATION INTO CYTOTROPHOBLAST AND SYNCYTIOTROPHOBLAST

There are two distinct cell layers in the blastocyst (see Chapter 6): the inner cell mass, which is surrounded by an outer sphere of a single layer of mononucleated trophoblast cells. The trophoblast is the first cell type of the embryonic tissue to differentiate; this outer layer rapidly proliferates and develops into the placental tissue and fetal membranes.

The trophoblast differentiates into two layers: the outer syncytiotrophoblast and the inner cytotrophoblastic layer. Some of the proliferative cytotrophoblast cells fuse together to form a multinucleated syncytium (a united mass of fused cellular material): the syncytiotrophoblast (Fig. 8.2). This outermost layer of the placenta has little proliferative and transcriptional activity; the maintenance and growth of the syncytiotrophoblast throughout gestation is almost entirely dependent on the incorporation of cytotrophoblast cells into the layer. Apoptosis (programmed cell death) of trophoblast tissue increases throughout pregnancy as a normal part of trophoblast turnover and syncytiotrophoblast formation. The nuclei of the cells newly incorporated into the syncytiotrophoblast are initially similar to the nuclei of the cytotrophoblast cells but then undergo morphological changes; the chromatin condenses so the nuclei become smaller and denser eventually resembling late apoptotic nuclei. Some of these nuclei aggregate and are packaged into syncytial (or syncytiotrophoblastic) knots, which are shed from the apical surface of the syncytiotrophoblast into the maternal circulation. In a normal pregnancy, these syncytial knots are consistently present and increase with gestational age so they can be observed to assess placental maturity. Excessive knot formation (Tenney-Parker change) is associated with placental pathology and possibly preeclampsia. Syncytial knots can be identified in maternal blood in the uterine veins but are destroyed in the maternal pulmonary vessels as they pass through the pulmonary circulation. In hypertensive disorders of pregnancy such as preeclampsia, syncytiotrophoblast renewal is overactive; there is an increase in apoptosis often complicated by aponecrosis. The syncytial knots of preeclamptic pregnancies are more prominent and are smaller so they can survive the maternal pulmonary vasculature and trigger a maternal systemic inflammatory response including an activated endothelium and increase in proinflammatory markers (Kovo et al., 2017). In addition, the placenta may communicate with and modulate maternal physiology by releasing extracellular vesicles containing proteins, lipids and nucleic acids into the maternal circulation (Adam et al., 2017).

The surface of the syncytiotrophoblast is covered with microvilli, which increase the surface area. The syncytiotrophoblast expresses transporters, enzymes and receptors on its surface. It also produces hCG and human placental lactogen (hPL), which are crucial to the maintenance of the pregnancy. hCG enhances differentiation of cytotrophoblasts into the syncytiotrophoblast. Electron microscopy reveals the syncytiotrophoblast to be a mass of cytoplasm containing remnants of the original cell membranes before fusion, evenly dispersed nuclei and a few intermediate cells. This syncytial organization of cells is unusual; other than the trophoblast and osteoclasts, multinucleated cells are usually only seen in some tumour cells and in inflammatory giant cells, a fused mass of various cells such as

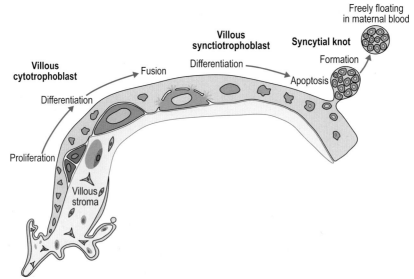

Fig. 8.2 The differentiation of villous cytotrophoblast into villous syncytiotrophoblast and the shedding of syncytial knots into maternal blood. (Reproduced from Huppertz, 2008.)

macrophages and other cells, which arise in response to an infection (McNally and Anderson, 2011). A range of tumour cells also secrete hCG, which can be detected in urine (Cole, 2017). hCG can be used clinically as a tumour marker; usually the tumours produce hCG at much lower concentrations than those characteristic of trophoblast cells and affect individuals late in life, so hCG is a fairly specific and sensitive biomarker of pregnancy.

The cytotrophoblasts, which form the inner layer of placental cells, are large clear discrete cuboidal cells each with a single nucleus and a few organelles enclosed in a well-defined cell membrane. These cells have marked mitotic activity and DNA synthesis. The outer syncytiotrophoblast layer increases in volume throughout the 2nd week as cells detach from the proliferating layer of cytotrophoblast and fuse with the mass of the syncytiotrophoblast. The syncytiotrophoblast has an invasive phenotype, secreting enzymes that attack the endometrium and hormones, which sustain the pregnancy. Projections from the syncytiotrophoblast penetrate between the maternal endometrial cells and into the underlying connective tissue. Syncytiotrophoblast invasion is aggressive; between 6 and 9 days postfertilization the embryo becomes completely implanted into the endometrial stroma. The hydrolytic enzymes produced cause breakdown of the extracellular matrix between the cells of the endometrium thus eroding a pathway. The syncytiotrophoblast is also involved in absorption of nutrients secreted by the uterine glands in the first trimester of pregnancy (histiotrophic nutrition).

The surface of the syncytiotrophoblast has tiny processes extending from it that penetrate between the endometrial cells, pulling the conceptus into the uterine wall. As implantation progresses, the expanding syncytiotrophoblast rapidly envelops and surrounds the entire blastocyst. The endometrial epithelium regenerates over the site of implantation, forming the decidua capsularis (Fig. 8.3). By 9 days, the embryo is completely embedded within the endometrial wall with the syncytiotrophoblast forming a complete mantle around the entire conceptus so it is the only embryonic tissue in direct contact with the maternal tissue; this is important in protecting the embryo from rejection. The syncytiotrophoblast is thicker and better developed over the embryonic pole of the blastocyst. Implantation is complete by about 10–12 days after fertilization. A plug of a cellular material called the coagulation plug or operculum seals the small hole at the point of implantation (Fig. 8.4).

In the 1st week of development, as the free-floating embryo (conceptus) moves towards the uterine cavity propelled by the ciliary movement and peristaltic muscular contractions of the uterine tube, the cells can obtain nutrients from secretions of the uterine tubes and endometrium and eliminate waste products by simple diffusion. As the developing syncytiotrophoblast expands after implantation, it erodes the maternal tissue that it encounters such as capillaries, superficial veins and endometrial or uterine glands (Burton et al., 2016), so that maternal red blood cells and secretions from the endometrial glands enter small

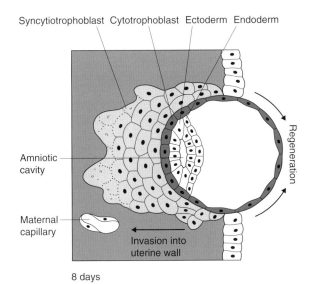

Syncytiotrophoblast Cytotrophoblast Ectoderm Endoderm

Regeneration

Amniotic cavity

Maternal capillary

Invasion into uterine wall

8 days

Fig. 8.3 Regeneration of endometrium over the site of implantation.

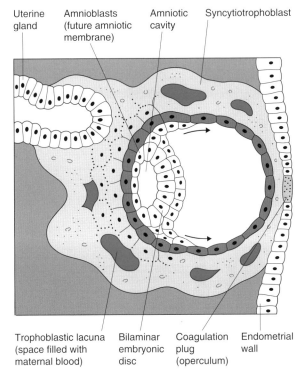

Uterine gland   Amnioblasts (future amniotic membrane)   Amniotic cavity   Syncytiotrophoblast

Trophoblastic lacuna (space filled with maternal blood)   Bilaminar embryonic disc   Coagulation plug (operculum)   Endometrial wall

Fig. 8.4 Implantation of blastocyst into the endometrial wall at 9 days postfertilization.

spaces (lacunae; see below) within the mass of syncytiotrophoblast tissue. The endometrial glands secrete a fluid that contains glucose, lactate, pyruvate, maternal proteins,

lipids, amino acids as well as signalling molecules and powerful mitogenic growth factors (Burton and Jauniaux, 2017). The uterine fluid is phagocytosed by the outer layer of blastocyst cells and subsequently by the syncytiotrophoblast and provides the nutritional substrates for embryonic and placental development for most of the first trimester (Burton et al., 2016). Nutrition provided by the secretions of the uterine glands is described as 'histiotrophic' nutrition; these secretions are sometimes described as 'uterine milk'. The secretions are rich in carbohydrate, lipid and growth factors; they are secreted through openings in the basal plate to the intervillous spaces and are taken up by syncytiotrophoblast tissue (Burton and Jauniaux, 2018). By the end of the first trimester, there is a transition to haemotrophic nutrition from the uteroplacental circulation, which provides a system in which the maternal and fetal circulations come into close contact to facilitate transfer of substances from one system to the other.

The fluid-filled trophoblastic lacunae (literally 'little lakes') within the syncytiotrophoblast coalesce to form larger lacunae, which are the precursors of the intervillous spaces. As maternal blood vessels are progressively invaded, the lacunae fill with maternal blood. Maternal capillaries near the syncytiotrophoblast expand to form maternal sinusoids, which rapidly anastomose with the trophoblastic lacunae. As this development continues, the lacunae become separated by columns of syncytiotrophoblast, or trabeculae, which effectively form a framework on which the intervillus develops. The trabecular columns project radially from the blastocyst. The cytotrophoblast at the core of the columns proliferates locally to form extensions, which grow into the columns of syncytiotrophoblast. The growth of these protrusions is induced by the newly formed extraembryonic mesoderm (Fig. 8.5). The result is the primary stem villus, an outgrowth of cytotrophoblast covered by syncytiotrophoblast, which penetrates into the blood-filled lacuna (Fig. 8.6).

EXTRAVILLOUS CYTOTROPHOBLAST AND REMODELLING OF THE UTERINE VESSELS

Cytotrophoblast Migration and Invasion

The cytotrophoblast layer has several distinct roles: (1) it acts as proliferative progenitor or stem cell layer to generate and construct the developing syncytiotrophoblast, which covers the villi like a glove (Burton et al., 2016); (2) it forms the proliferative column cytotrophoblast of the anchoring villi; (3) it detaches from the cell columns and migrates into the maternal stroma to form interstitial cytotrophoblasts; and (4) it forms invasive extravillous or endovascular trophoblast cells, which migrate through the connective

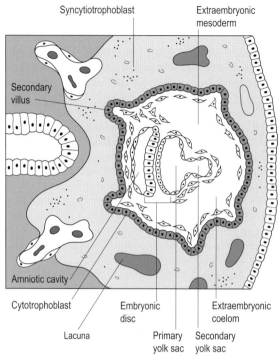

Fig. 8.5 Formation of extraembryonic mesoderm.

tissue of the uterus seeking maternal spiral arteries, which they will remodel and then replace the maternal endothelial cells (Maltepe and Fisher, 2015). From about 12 days postfertilization, these cells invade the maternal capillaries and spiral arteries of the decidua. The extravillous cytotrophoblast cells initially plug the lumen of the maternal vessels that have been invaded; the maternal endothelial cells of the maternal blood vessels are replaced by the extravillous cytotrophoblast cells. The extravillous cytotrophoblast cells interact with uterine NK cells of the maternal immune system, promoting release of cytokines and proteases cause de-differentiation and loss of the smooth muscle cells of the artery walls.

Plugging of the lumen of the invaded maternal blood vessels prevents bleeding and is achieved by day 14, which coincides with the expected date of the next menstrual period. If the maternal vessels are not plugged adequately during implantation and early development, then vaginal bleeding may occur, which is associated with an increased risk of spontaneous miscarriage. Subchorionic haematomas can be seen on ultrasound investigation; they are associated with an increased risk of premature rupture of the membranes and risk of preterm delivery possibly because the clot of blood releases free iron, which causes oxidative stress (OS) (Burton and Jauniaux, 2017). The

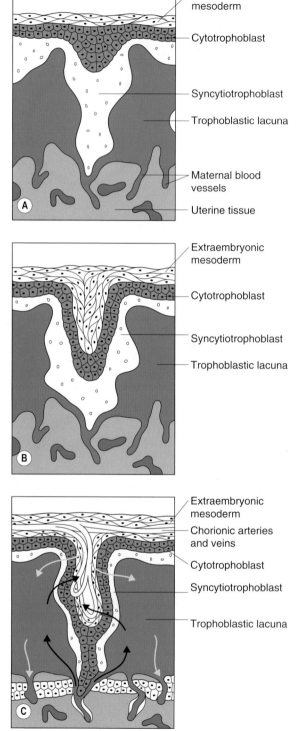

Fig. 8.6 The stem villus: (A) primary (11–13 days); (B) secondary (16 days); (C) tertiary (21 days).

plugs prevent flow of maternal blood into the intervillous space in early pregnancy but allow a slow seepage of plasma through a network of tiny intercellular clefts (Maltepe and Fisher, 2015) so the lacunar spaces enclosed by the syncytiotrophoblast initially contain exudate from maternal vessels and secretions from uterine glands rather than blood. The developing placenta forms an effective barrier between the mother and developing embryo that persists for the first trimester after which the trophoblastic plugs are dislodged and maternal blood flow to the intervillous space is established (Maltepe and Fisher, 2015), causing a rise in intraplacental oxygen concentration. It is at this time that peak hCG secretion occurs. The plugging of the vessels means that normal first trimester development occurs in a relatively hypoxic environment. When the vessels are unplugged towards the end of the first trimester, maternal blood comes into contact with the syncytiotrophoblast covering the chorionic villi so the environment becomes normoxic with higher intrauterine oxygen levels because the haemochorial placenta is established. From this time, placental nutrients are provided by haemotrophic nutrition from the maternal blood supply in the intervillous space via diffusion across the syncytiotrophoblast.

The increasing oxygen level and concomitant OS also stimulate cytotrophoblast proliferation and differentiation and the increased expression of antioxidant enzymes. Doppler ultrasound shows there is no intervillous blood flow in normal pregnancies before this period and oxygen electrodes have demonstrated that an oxygen gradient exists across the placenta and decidua. Where maternal–placental blood flow is observed in the first trimester, it is often associated with nonviable pregnancies (Soares et al., 2017) The advantage of development in a hypoxic environment is that the developing embryo is particularly vulnerable to damaging reactive oxygen species (ROS) during the sensitive period of organogenesis and the first trimester placenta has limited antioxidant capacity; thus, limiting fetal exposure to oxygen may be protective. However, ROS are also used as signalling molecules controlling gene expression in development. Hence, the redox environment of early development has to be tightly regulated (Timme-Laragy et al., 2017) otherwise normal development is disrupted leading to structural and functional changes. Congenital abnormalities caused by recreational drugs, such as cocaine and alcohol, abnormal maternal metabolism affecting the first trimester, such as uncontrolled type 1 diabetes and a hyperglycaemic environment, and prescribed medications, such as thalidomide and drugs for epilepsy, have their effect by disrupting the delicate balance between ROS and antioxidant defence mechanisms.

The differentiation of trophoblast cells is influenced by the local oxygen levels. In the maternal decidua, oxygen levels are about 8–10% whereas in the placenta in the first trimester, they are about 3–5% (Parks, 2017). This appropriate low level of oxygenation early in the first trimester is physiological (and should not be considered hypoxic) and promotes trophoblast proliferation, whereas higher levels of oxygenation at this time inhibits proliferation and induces migration. When the trophoblastic plugs are removed and maternal blood enters the intervillous space at the end of the first trimester, oxygen levels in the placenta are raised to maternal levels or slightly higher. Hypoxia in the second and third trimesters can damage the placenta and compromise fetal wellbeing and growth (Parks, 2017). Fetal hypoxia is caused by three distinct classes of problem: preplacental factors associated with inadequate oxygenation of the maternal blood due, for instance, to high altitude or maternal anaemia; uteroplacental factors usually because maternal blood flow is obstructed; and postplacental hypoxia, which paradoxically is associated with normoxic (or hyperoxic) conditions. In this scenario, the fetal vessels have a high resistance to blood flow so fetal blood flow is decreased and less oxygen is extracted from the maternal blood. This leads to higher oxygen levels in the placental tissue, which inhibit villus branching; oxidative damage due to hypoxia-reperfusion also occurs.

In most other mammalian species, organogenesis is complete and embryonic development is advanced before placental attachment. In human development, implantation is highly invasive so the precocious conceptus is embedded in the uterine wall even before the primitive streak is evident (Wamaitha and Niakan, 2018). Hence, it is thought to be much more sensitive to OS, an imbalance between production of free radicals and antioxidant defences. OS is common in normal pregnancy but is tightly regulated. Excessive OS leads to excessive consumption of antioxidants so levels decline; this is associated with damage to DNA, lipids and proteins and premature placental ageing and compromised function (Torres-Cuevas et al., 2017). Embryonic and placental cells are particularly vulnerable to OS because they undergo extensive DNA replication and cell division. The syncytiotrophoblast is exposed to the highest concentration of oxygen as it is closest to the maternal blood and has low levels of antioxidant enzymes. Pregnancy complications such as maternal diabetes generate more oxidative free radicals, thus more OS, and are associated with a higher incidence of miscarriage, preterm delivery, vasculopathy, fetal structural defects and growth restriction, which is thought to be due to OS (Cuffe et al., 2017).

Spiral Artery Conversion

From early gestation onwards, villus growth and considerable remodelling of the placenta occur, including remarkable changes in the maternal blood vessels underlying the

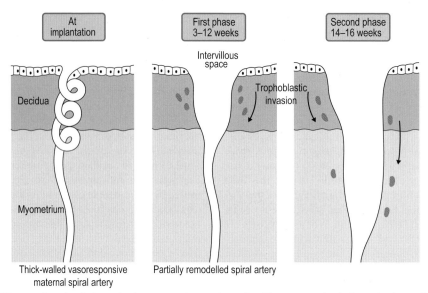

Fig. 8.7 Conversion of spiral arteries into uteroplacental arteries. The maternal spiral arteries have thick muscular walls and are responsive to vasoactive substances. They are remodelled by the trophoblastic cells in two waves, ultimately forming nonresponsive dilated vessels. Where remodelling is inadequate, a proportion of the vessels retain the structure of preimplantation or partially remodelled vasoresponsive vessels.

fetal placenta ensuring that they are capable of delivering large volumes of blood to the placental intervillous spaces at an appropriate rate and pressure to protect but provide for the delicate fetal villi. The fetal placental villi are perfused by the low-pressure developing fetal circulation and are immersed in maternal blood, which normally circulates at a much higher pressure and velocity; this model is sometimes described as being like a mop (the placental villus) in a bucket (intervillous space) of maternal blood (Moffett and Loke, 2006). Failure of the spiral arteries to be remodelled appropriately is associated with a number of common complications of pregnancy including preeclampsia, FGR, recurrent first and second trimester losses, spontaneous preterm labour and premature rupture of the membranes (Burton and Jauniaux, 2018). In the early weeks, while the lacunae are forming, a subset of the cytotrophoblastic cells (described as extravillous trophoblast or EVT) move from the tips of the anchoring villi to colonize the decidua and myometrium of the placental bed. It is this invasion of extravillous cytotrophoblast cells into the maternal blood vessels that promotes maternal recognition of the fetus and the subsequent production of blocking antibodies (see Chapter 10), which are important for the viability of the pregnancy. The extravillous cytotrophoblast cells are involved in physiologically remodelling of the maternal spiral arteries. The smooth muscle of the tightly coiled spiral arteries is destroyed and replaced by fibrinoid produced

by the invading EVT. The removal of the smooth muscle converts the thick-walled muscular spiral artery into a wide-mouthed funnel-shaped uteroplacental vessel with a diameter 5–10× greater than the original spiral artery (Parks, 2017) and thus low impedance to blood flow (Fig. 8.7). The remodelled blood vessel is no longer vasoresponsive to maternal or fetal signals. Another subset of ET form transient endovascular plugs to occlude the lumen of the spiral artery (see above); these disintegrate about week 12 of development when the maternal blood is able to pass into the intervillous space.

After an apparent rest phase of a couple of weeks (weeks 14–16), there is a resurgence of the EVT migration and spiral artery remodelling continues in the second trimester. This phase of remodelling is faster and the remodelling extends to parts of the spiral arteries, which are deeper in the myometrium; the sphincters in the myometrial segments of the spiral arteries are also destroyed, which also facilitates maternal blood flow to the intervillous space (Parks, 2017). The remodelling changes the blood flowing into the intervillous space from a high-speed intermittent jet to a gentle but generous flow, which allows better mixing and is less likely to promote fibrin deposition. Insufficient remodelling of the spiral arteries is associated with failure of the fetus to reach its genetic growth potential (FGR or intrauterine growth restriction [IUGR]) and preeclampsia (Box 8.2).

BOX 8.2 Preeclampsia

Preeclampsia is a placental condition; it can occur in the absence of a fetus in a molar pregnancy. One of the most convincing theories about the aetiology of preeclampsia and the associated condition of IUGR (which can occur independently or with preeclampsia) is that they are due to placental malperfusion secondary to deficient spiral artery conversion (Burton and Jauniaux, 2018). In normal pregnancies, all spiral arteries in the placental bed are invaded by cytotrophoblast cells. In preeclampsia, it seems that only a proportion of the maternal vessels are invaded and that a significant number of vessels show complete absence of physiological changes. The second wave of arterial invasion may be the stage that is most compromised owing to the endovascular trophoblast failing to reach the intramyometrial portion of the vessels. This means that the spiral arteries are not completely transformed to uteroplacental vessels. Maternal uteroplacental blood flow is therefore restricted, which results in placental abnormalities and fetal complications such as IUGR. The effect is compounded by the persistence of vasoresponsiveness of the spiral arteries, which retain the ability to constrict and limit placental perfusion, like the spiral arteries of a nonpregnant uterus (see Chapter 4). Impaired placental perfusion increases the risk of ischaemia–reperfusion type insult, which leads to the generation of reactive oxygen species (oxidative stress). Oxidative stress results in increased generation of oxygen free radicals, which lead to the formation of lipid peroxides that alter cell membranes. The incorporation of cholesterol, oxidized free fatty acids and LDLs into membranes is increased, which leads to a biological cascade of leukocyte activation, platelet adhesion and aggregation and the release of vasoconstrictive agents (Burton and Jauniaux, 2017). Acute atherotic changes can lead to the development of intimal plaques, which can project into the vessel lumen and restrict blood flow. In addition, endoplasmic reticulum (ER) stress is also triggered by ischaemia–perfusion and hypoxia. ER stress can lead to inhibition of protein synthesis and reduced expression of amino acid transporters (thus affecting growth) as well as activating apoptosis. There are serious maternal complications of preeclampsia, which have been attributed to a putative and as-yet unidentified placentally derived 'factor X', which is released into the maternal circulation; possible candidates include proinflammatory cytokines from the syncytiotrophoblast, products of placental oxidative stress, antiangiogenic factors and trophoblastic apoptotic debris such as syncytiotrophoblast microfragments all of which could contribute to activation of maternal endothelial cells and cause the peripheral syndrome of preeclampsia (Fig. 8.8).

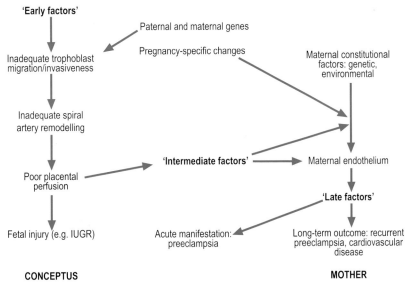

Fig. 8.8 Interactions between the conceptus and the mother in the development of preeclampsia. (Reproduced with permission from Lala and Chakraborty, 2003.)

Maternal spiral arteries maintaining a high vasculature resistance because of incomplete or failed remodelling are predisposed to hypoperfusion, hypoxia, reperfusion injury, OS, and occlusion by coagulation.

The remodelled vessels passively dilate and accommodate a greatly increased blood flow (~30% of maternal cardiac output) but they are not responsive to vasoactive agents. The effect of this interaction between the trophoblastic cells and the maternal blood vessels is that a low-pressure, high-conductance vascular system is established, which provides an adequate maternal blood flow to the placenta and thus a plentiful provision of oxygen and nutrients to the fetus. The maternal uteroplacental circulatory system is mostly complete by mid-gestation. In contrast, the fetal villus tree continues to branch and develop throughout the pregnancy, ensuring that the capacity of the placenta matches the growth of the fetus.

As the maternal cardiac output increases by about 40% (see Chapter 11), the net effect is to increase the uterine blood flow by about 15-fold from about 45 mL/min to over 750 mL/min at term (James et al., 2017). Evaluation of placental blood flow using different types of Doppler ultrasound methods, contrast-enhanced ultrasound (CEU) and magnetic resonance imaging (MRI) techniques provides insights into placental vascularization and the implications for both mother and fetus (Mourier et al., 2017). Doppler ultrasound is noninvasive, low-cost and widely available. It is used to assess blood flow in arteries and veins as the ultrasound waves are reflected by the moving red blood cells. Flow in the uterine arteries gives a picture of the maternal vascular effects of the invading placenta, predicting possible preeclampsia and IUGR. Umbilical artery Doppler ultrasound assesses the fetal circulation and identifies placental vascular resistance, which indicates IUGR and effects of placental deficiency. Before pregnancy and in the first trimester, the uterine arterial waveform, observed in Doppler ultrasound assessment of the blood flow in uterine artery, usually has low end-diastolic flow velocity and early dicrotic notch during diastole. The Doppler assessment visualizes the uteroplacental circulation noninvasively by using high-frequency sound. The normal uterine artery waveform has a characteristic shape, which changes as the blood vessels are remodelled and their resistance to blood flow falls. These changes start about 4 weeks after implantation and are particularly dramatic in the second trimester. By 18–20 weeks' gestation, successful trophoblastic invasion alters the waveform to one showing a high diastolic flow velocity and loss of the dicrotic notch. If the dicrotic notch and low end-diastolic velocity persist, this indicates that the uterus still has high resistance to blood flow, which is predictive of IUGR and

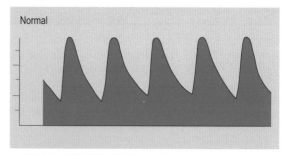

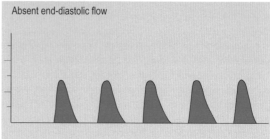

Fig. 8.9 Doppler ultrasound waveforms showing diastolic flow and dicrotic notch. (Reproduced with permission from Miller and Hanretty, 1998.)

severe preeclampsia (Fig. 8.9). Three-dimensional (3D) power Doppler angiography is a relatively new and safe method, which scans the region of interest (part of the placenta) and generates a 3D reconstruction. It is able to quantify vascularization in the small vessels of the placenta and identify women at risk of preeclampsia in the second and third trimesters (Mourier et al., 2017). CEU uses gas-filled, liquid-encapsulated microbubbles, which are injected into the maternal circulation; it is used for research but not routinely in clinical environments until its safety is confirmed. MRI techniques can be used to investigate tissue deeper than ultrasound can penetrate. MRI scans are usually avoided in pregnancy unless there is a life-threatening condition because there are concerns about the effects of the high level of magnetic radiation on the fetus.

A number of pathologies including placental infarction or abruption, preeclampsia and recurrent pregnancy loss are associated with defects due to maternal malperfusion of the placental vascular bed (Parks, 2017). Some placental lesions have been associated with nutrient deficiencies, maternal smoking and OS but the cause of most lesions is never determined (Redline, 2015).

Placental pathologies may be due to defective trophoblast function and/or impaired maternal decidualization. There are gender differences in placental development and structural and functional responses to maternal diet

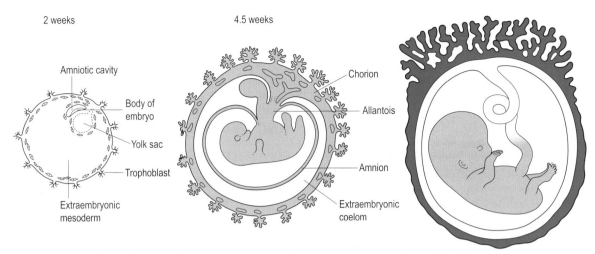

Fig. 8.10 Early villus formation occurs in a sphere-like organization around the whole of the enlarging conceptus; eventually most of the villi will degenerate leaving only the ovoid development of the fetal placenta.

and stress, and exposure to environmental chemicals (Rosenfeld, 2015). For instance, in response to poorer maternal nutrition in Saudi Arabia, it appears that the placentas of male babies were heavier but smaller in every dimension except thickness (Alwasel et al., 2014). This suggested that the male placentas had compensated by increasing the depth of the spiral artery invasion. The placentas of female infants appeared to have a greater surface area suggesting more effective regional specialization possibly due to more extensive spiral artery recruitment. There are also gender-specific differences in placental size, and responses to maternal nutrient deprivation, and its relationship to later hypertension (van Abeelen et al., 2011).

The placenta-related disorders of pregnancy, such as miscarriage, preeclampsia and placenta accreta, are almost unique to humans. Placenta accreta, a type of abnormal placental attachment, was first described in the 20th century and occurs more commonly in women who have previously had a caesarean section, uterine curettage, or endometritis (inflammation of the endometrium). It is suggested that these situations are associated with myometrial defects, uterine scarring and abnormal decidualization, which promotes excessive vascular remodelling in subsequent pregnancies increasing the risk of placenta accreta (Jauniaux et al., 2018).

VASCULARIZATION OF THE PLACENTAL VILLI

Fetal blood cells are derived from angioblasts that aggregate to form cell clusters called blood islands in the extraembryonic mesoderm surrounding the yolk sac (see Chapter 9). The blood vessels that perfuse the placenta also develop in the extraembryonic mesoderm. In the 3rd week postfertilization, the extraembryonic mesoderm associated with the cytotrophoblast penetrates into the core of the primary stem villi transforming them into secondary stem villi. This mesoderm develops into the blood vessels and connective tissue of the villi. It forms at the same time as the embryonic vasculature with which it will eventually connect. Haemangioblasts (precursors of blood cells) appear and capillaries form. The haemangioblasts are multipotent cells that form both the haematopoietic stem cells, which will go on to generate all cellular components of blood, and the endothelial cells that line all blood vessels. Under experimental conditions, it has been demonstrated that a single haematopoietic stem cell can re-form an animal's entire blood system (Krause et al., 2001). This extraordinary regenerative capacity is harnessed clinically in bone marrow transplantation therapy.

The linking of the blood vessels of the villi with the vessels of the embryo results in a circulating blood system so the villi begin to be perfused by the fetal circulation by ~28 days after fertilization. The fetal red blood cells containing embryonic haemoglobin allow oxygen transfer at low partial pressures of oxygen and low pH. The villi containing differentiated blood vessels are described as tertiary stem villi. By the end of the 4th week after fertilization, these chorionic villi cover the entire blastocyst surface forming a spherical shell of villi projecting outwards into the maternal tissue (Fig. 8.10). It is possible to remove a sample of the developing placental villi from this shell for genetic testing (Box 8.3). The placental membrane now permits diffusion of gases, nutrients and waste materials. (It is not appropriate to describe the placenta as a 'barrier' as very few substances cannot cross the placental tissue). Until about 20 weeks' gestation, there are four layers of the placental membrane: the endothelium lining the fetal capillaries of the villus, the connective tissue in the villus core, a layer of cytotrophoblast cells and a maternal-facing layer of syncytiotrophoblast (Fig. 8.11). From mid-gestation, most of the cytotrophoblast layer of many villi disappears and

the placental barrier becomes very thin and attenuated. The syncytiotrophoblast comes into direct contact with the endothelium of fetal capillaries to form a vasculosyncytial placental membrane, which means the maternal and fetal blood may only be about 2–4 μm apart.

DEVELOPMENT OF THE DISCOID PLACENTA AND CHORIONIC MEMBRANE

From the 4th week to the 16th week, the villus growth over the entire surface of the blastocyst is remodelled. About two-thirds of villi orientated towards the uterine cavity degenerate and regress, leaving behind an area that develops into the typical placental structure and shape seen at delivery. The regression creates an area of mechanical weakness because the spiral arteries are unplugged and bleeding may occur between the developing fetal membranes and the underlying decidua basalis at the end of the first trimester; this may result in threatened miscarriage, which is the most common complication of this stage of pregnancy (Burton and Jauniaux, 2017). As the embryo starts to enlarge, the uterine wall where it has implanted starts to protrude into the uterine cavity (Fig. 8.12). The protruding portion of the embryo is covered by the decidua capsularis, a thin layer or capsule of endometrium. The layer of decidua under the embryonic pole of the embryo is the decidua basalis, which forms the maternal part of the placenta. The remaining areas of the decidua are described as the decidua parietalis.

In the 3rd month, as the fetus enlarges and grows to fill the uterus, the thin rim of decidua capsularis covering the bulge gradually thins and attenuates so the chorion comes into contact with the decidua parietalis of the opposite wall of the uterus. Before the trophoblastic shell comes into contact with the uterine wall on the opposite side, trophoblasts and other cells of fetal origin reach the uterine cavity and can be collected by flushing or aspiration (Fiddler, 2014). This is a potential technique for minimally invasive prenatal diagnosis from week 5 or 6 until weeks 13–15.

BOX 8.3   Chorionic Villus Sampling

In the chorionic villus sampling (CVS) procedure, 20–40 mg of placental tissue can be obtained from a villus for genetic diagnosis of trisomy 21, for example, or of a single-gene defects such as cystic fibrosis or β-thalassaemia. After 10 weeks' gestation, the tissue can be extracted transabdominally by needle aspiration or transcervically using curved biopsy forceps. The collected trophoblast cells, which divide very rapidly, can be cultured for 24 h and then the chromosome number can be determined (see Chapter 7). Because of the problems associated with mosaicism (see Chapter 7), a more accurate determination of chromosome number and structure is obtained by using fibroblast cells taken from the vascular core of the villus. These cells grow more slowly so they have to be cultured for 2 weeks before being stained and examined (which means the results of the test take longer). As fibroblast cells are derived from the mesoderm, they originate from the inner cell mass and are embryonic rather than the trophoblast-derived cells from the outer layers of the villus. Placental mosaicism is associated with increased fetal loss and IUGR. There is a 1–2% procedure-related loss in CVS, although it should be remembered that the procedure is being performed because there is already a concern about the pregnancy. Pregnancies associated with genetic abnormality have a much higher risk of spontaneous failure.

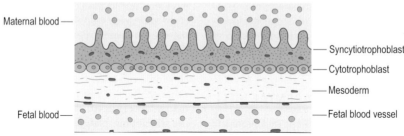

Fig. 8.11 Exchange of substances across the placenta occurs across a barrier consisting of four layers of tissue: syncytiotrophoblast, cytotrophoblast, mesoderm and fetal blood vessel wall. (Reproduced with permission from Miller and Hanretty, 1998.)

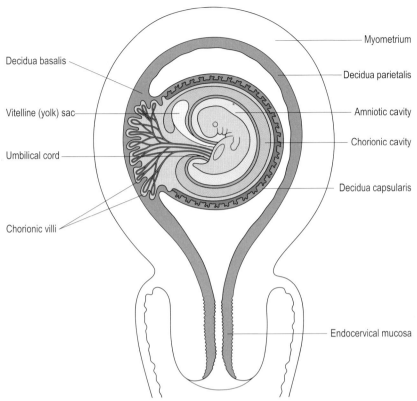

Fig. 8.12 Protrusion of the developing conceptus into the uterine cavity and formation of the decidua capsularis.

Visualizing the size of the chorionic, or embryonic, sac by ultrasound can be used to determine the gestational age of the embryo because its growth between weeks 5 and 10 is very fast and characteristic. This is particularly important where the woman is uncertain about the date of her last menstrual period.

The uterine cavity is obliterated by 12 weeks' gestation. The enlarging blastocyst compresses the trophoblastic layer of villi, distal to the entry pole, which limits blood (and therefore nutrient) supply to the villi in this region of the decidua capsularis. The underlying villi cannot continue to grow and slowly degenerate and regress so by the 5th month this region becomes devoid of villi and smoother. This avascular and flattened surface of the decidua capsularis and atrophied chorion form the chorion laeve, the utero-placental membrane, which is also known as the chorionic membrane or bald or smooth chorion. Effectively, the chorion is extraplacental trophoblast with similar immunological properties; it may also be an important source of hCG, particularly in early pregnancy. The portion of the trophoblastic tissue associated with the decidua basalis implants

further and receives a plentiful supply of nutrients so these villi continue to grow well. This area of the chorion, therefore, retains villi that proliferate and progressively arborize (take on a tree-like branched appearance) forming the chorion frondosum (*frondosus* is Latin for leaf), which ultimately develops into the definitive discoid fetal placenta. The placenta is a union between the chorion frondosum derived from the fertilized ovum and the decidua basalis (basal plate) formed from the maternal uterine wall. It is anatomically complete by the end of the first trimester but continues to grow throughout the pregnancy.

DEVELOPMENT OF THE AMNION (INNER MEMBRANE)

The amniotic cavity first appears at about day 7. The primitive ectoderm cells enclosing the cavity become flattened forming amnioblasts, cells that become the fetal-facing (innermost) amniotic membrane. These cells secrete amniotic fluid, thus the embryo is enclosed in the fluid-filled amniotic sac. The outer surface of the amnioblast cell layer becomes covered with mesoderm. As the embryo and amniotic sac expand, the amnion comes into contact with the chorion. The chorionic cells are lined with mesoderm cells on the inner side. When the amnion and chorion meet, the two layers of mesoderm loosely fuse forming the amniochorionic membrane. The fetal membranes protect the fetus and secrete factors into the amniotic fluid, which affects amniotic fluid activity and also can influence the maternal uterine physiology. An important aspect of examining the placenta and membranes is to ensure that both membranes are present following birth. The amnion and chorion should be easily separated; the chorion is attached to the edge of the placenta, whereas the amnion can be separated from the surface of the placenta with attachment around the base of the cord.

Amniotic Fluid

Amniotic fluid has an important role in protecting the fetus, cushioning it from external impact and stresses to prevent fetal injury. It also allows the embryo to float freely, which facilitates symmetrical fetal growth and movement, preventing fetal parts from adhering together or to the amnion, allows practice breathing and swallowing exercises and increases placental surface area. Amniotic fluid has bacteriostatic and growth-promoting properties; it is important in maintaining a constant body temperature and is also involved in maintaining amnion integrity, suppressing myometrial contractions and maintaining cervical length and consistency (Loukogeorgakis and De Coppi, 2017).

Initially, amnioblasts (cells of the amnion) actively secrete amniotic fluid into the developing amniotic sac, then the fluid is derived from maternal tissue by diffusion across the fetal membranes and decidua parietalis. In the first half of gestation, before skin keratinization takes place, fluid and electrolytes diffuse freely through the fetal skin (Moore et al., 2015) so the composition of the amniotic fluid at this time is similar to that of fetal tissue fluid. After 20 weeks, the skin becomes keratinized and transudation from maternal and fetal blood vessels contributes less to the amniotic fluid. From 11 weeks, fetal urine contributes to the amniotic fluid. Fetal gastrointestinal and lung secretions are also important. Fetal swallowing and exchange across the amnion mean that turnover of fluid is rapid, particularly close to term; the water content is exchanged every 3 h. By term, lung fluid may contribute about 100 mL per day, respiratory secretions about 300–400 mL and fetal urine 500 mL per day. The fetus may swallow up to 0.5–1 L of fluid per day; the extra water crosses the gut, enters the fetal circulation and can then cross the placenta. By term, the normal volume of amniotic fluid is 500–1000 mL; assessment of amniotic fluid volume is used to monitor fetal

wellbeing. Polyhydramnios is an excess amount of fluid (over 2000 mL), which is usually associated with multiple pregnancies, fetal swallowing problems such as oesophageal atresia (blockage of the gut) and serious defects of the nervous system. A low volume of amniotic fluid (<500 mL) is classified as oligohydramnios, a condition often associated with impaired fetal renal function or placental insufficiency. Premature rupture of the fetal membranes can also cause oligohydramnios. Complications of oligohydramnios are associated with compression of the fetus (which might affect development of the lungs, limbs of face) or compression of the umbilical cord.

Amniotic fluid provides a useful tool to monitor fetal development and wellbeing. A small amount of amniotic fluid (20–30 mL) can be removed in amniocentesis for testing. Amniotic fluid is an aqueous solution in which fetal cells, such as desquamated skin cells, are suspended. It contains maternal and fetal proteins, carbohydrate, fat, hormones, enzymes and pigments. The fetal cells suspended in the amniotic fluid can be used for genetic testing (see Chapter 7). If the fetus has a neural tube defect (see Chapter 9), concentrations of α-fetoprotein (AFP, derived from spinal fluid) in the amniotic fluid are very high. Levels of AFP are low in Down syndrome (trisomy 21) and are measured as part of the triple screen test (see Chapter 7). Components of amniotic fluid are also used to predict preterm labour, premature cervical effacement, fetal infection and fetal lung maturity (see Chapter 15). Amniotic stem cells from the amniotic fluid and fetal membranes have potential therapeutic applications for tissue engineering and regenerative medicine such as repair of defective tissues and treatment of congenital and inflammatory diseases (Loukogeorgakis and De Coppi, 2017). As they are pluripotent embryonic stem cells, they have higher capacity for proliferation and differentiation than adult stem cells so there is interest in harvesting and culturing them (to expand the tissue mass) and storing them in tissue banks.

GROWTH AND MATURATION OF THE PLACENTAL VILLI

The placental villi continue to grow for most of the pregnancy. There is a widely held belief that the placenta ages during the pregnancy and that at term it is declining into functional senescence. Instead, the continuous morphological changes should be viewed as an increase in functional efficiency rather than ageing. Thus, in early pregnancy, the placenta is a highly invasive and proliferative tissue and in later pregnancy, although its growth rate slows down, it continues to mature and increase in efficiency. Placental efficiency is favoured by the attenuated maternal–fetal barrier and reduced diffusion distance rather than by an increase in weight. Although the rate of placental growth does decline in the later part of gestation, this decrease in growth rate is not irreversible or inevitable. If the maternal environment becomes unfavourable, for instance because of maternal anaemia or increased altitude, fresh villus growth will ensue and the placenta will expand its surface area and continue branching past term. In all placentas, total placental DNA levels continue to increase linearly beyond the 40th week of gestation reflecting continued growth.

Growth of the placenta (see Fig. 8.6, p. 206) can be divided into three stages. Earlier in pregnancy, the trabeculae develop side-branches of syncytiotrophoblast protrusions (syncytial spouts), which may be filled with a core of cytotrophoblast. These primary (or stem) villi protrude into the intervillous spaces. Later on, more lateral branches develop, increasing the total surface area for exchange, and the layers forming the placental barrier become more refined. In the 9th week, the tertiary stem villi lengthen to form mesenchymal villi as extraembryonic mesodermal cells penetrate the cytotrophoblast; the presence of this mesenchymal core transforms the villi into secondary or mesenchymal villi. Haematopoietic stem or progenitor cells develop within the mesoderm of the secondary villi forming the first placental blood cells and endothelial cells. Maternal and embryonic vascular systems do not connect; their development is similar and coordinated but independent and separate. The formation of placental blood vessels and cells transforms the villi into tertiary villi. The placental vascular network involves vasculogenesis, angiogenesis and remodelling of the spiral arteries. Vasculogenesis is the formation of the first blood vessels from cells differentiated from the mesenchymal stem cells and angiogenesis is the development of new blood vessel networks by branching and elongation of existing vessels (Pereira et al., 2015). Vasculogenesis starts about 3 weeks after fertilization; there is a gradual transition to angiogenesis, which markedly accelerates from mid-gestation (Li et al., 2018). The resulting vascular bed is about 12–15 m^2 with a total length (if all vessels were laid end to end) of about 550 km. The processes of blood vessel development are controlled by various growth factors, including the vascular endothelial growth factor (VEGF) family, fibroblast growth factors (FGFs) and angiopoietins (Li et al., 2018). Placental vascular development is influenced by the balance of ROS, which are involved in cellular signalling pathways (Pereira et al., 2015).

By the 16th week, the terminal extensions of the tertiary stem villi reach their maximum length. At this stage, the villi are described as immature intermediate villi. The cells of the cytotrophoblast layer become more dispersed within the villi creating gaps in the cytotrophoblast layer of the villus wall. Near the end of the second trimester, the tertiary stem villi form numerous side-branches and are described as mature intermediate villi. The earliest mature intermediate villi finish forming by about week 32 and then begin to produce small nodule-like secondary branches characteristic of the terminal villi. This is the final structure of the placental villus tree. The terminal villi are not formed by active outgrowth of the syncytiotrophoblast but by coiled and folded villus capillaries that bulge against the villus wall and expand by unfurling. Two types of chorionic villi can be identified: anchoring (or stem) villi, which attach the placenta to the decidua basalis, and the more numerous shorter branch villi, which extend only into the intervillous space and have a solely nutritive role.

The blood-filled intervillous space, into which the villi project, is formed from the trophoblastic lacunae that grow and coalesce. Therefore, the intervillous space is lined on both sides with syncytiotrophoblast. The maternal face of the placenta is the basal plate, which consists of syncytiotrophoblast lining plus a supporting layer of decidua basalis. The fetal side is formed of the layers of the chorionic plate.

The functional unit within the placenta is the placentome (or placental lobe), a villus tree arising from the chorionic plate within the intervillous space, which is perfused by a spiral artery. There are about 50–100 such units within the placenta. The terminal villi have low vascular resistance so provide a high fetoplacental flow; they are the major sites of nutrient and gaseous exchange in late gestation. The progressive development and branching of the placental tree structure is important for fetal growth and development. For instance, in IUGR pregnancies requiring elective preterm delivery, there are fewer terminal villi, which seem to have an abnormal extravillous cytotrophoblast structure.

On the basal (maternal) surface, the placenta is subdivided into cotyledons (lobes) by wedge-like placental septa, which appear in the 3rd month. The placental (decidual) septa grow into the intervillous space from the maternal side of the placenta, separating the villi into 10–40 cotyledons. Each cotyledon has two or more anchoring villi and many branch villi. The placental septae do not fuse with the chorionic plate, so maternal blood can flow freely from one cotyledon to another. This means that the villi are bathed in a lake of maternal blood that is constantly exchanging; this organization of placental perfusion is described as haemochorial. Haemochorial placentation is efficient because the syncytiotrophoblast is in contact with maternal blood optimizing maternal–fetal transport of gases, nutrients, water and ions. The syncytiotrophoblast can also endocytose the immunoglobulin IgG. In addition, hormones produced by the fetoplacental unit can easily access the maternal circulation. There are, however, some costs to the haemochorial arrangement; bleeding may be extensive at parturition and cells can be transferred between mother and fetus, for instance, resulting in microchimerisms (see Chapter 10) or erythroblastosis fetalis (haemolytic disease of the newborn due to Rhesus incompatibility).

PLACENTAL BLOOD FLOW

The fetal blood reaches the placental blood system via the two umbilical arteries that spiral around the umbilical vein (Fig. 8.13). On reaching the chorion, the vessels usually each supply half of the placenta. The arteries (which are vessels carrying blood away from the fetal heart carrying deoxygenated blood) divide repeatedly to form a branching network of smaller arteries and capillaries running through the intervillous space. The fetal blood flow through the placenta is about 500 mL/min, propelled by the fetal heart. Smooth muscle fibres contracting in the villi may help to pump blood back from the placenta to the fetus.

The maternal blood enters the intervillous space via about 100-150 of the remodelled spiral arteries. There is a pressure gradient from the maternal arteries to the intervillous space to the maternal endometrial veins from which the blood returns to the maternal circulation. Most organs have a progressive decrease in arterial diameter as the blood nears its target tissue. In the uteroplacental vessels, the remodelled spiral arteries increase in diameter as the vessels approach the intervillous space. Therefore, the intervillous space is a low-pressure system; the blood gently flows through and washes over the fetal placental tissue. The placenta has little resistance to maternal blood flow and a high vascular conductance so there is little fall in pressure across the intervillous space. The main determinant of the rate of maternal blood flow is the vascular resistance in the myometrial arteries. Myometrial contractions can decrease or stop afferent blood flow to the intervillous space. This effect is probably due to the compression or occlusion of the veins draining this space. During a contraction, the space distends so the fetus is not totally deprived of oxygen.

IUGR and 'Placental Insufficiency'

Poor placental function is implicated in a range of pregnancy-related disorders, such as fetal hypoxia, IUGR (Box 8.4) and preeclampsia, many of which predispose to low birthweight and/or preterm delivery, which are the

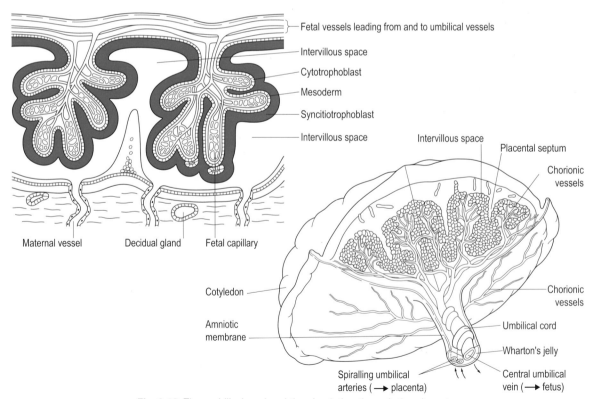

Fig. 8.13 The umbilical cord and the circulation through the placenta.

BOX 8.4 Intrauterine Growth Restriction (IUGR)

IUGR (also known as fetal growth restriction, FGR) increases the risk of disability or death for the fetus and neonate in the perinatal period and predisposes the individual born following IUGR to later adult disease (see Chapter 12). Although there is no internationally agreed definition for IUGR, it is usually defined as small for gestation age (SGA) and as a birthweight below a certain percentile (10th, 5th or 3rd percentile). It may be further qualified as also including a longitudinal decrease in the growth of the abdominal circumference, increased fetal head:abdomen circumference ratio or oligohydramnios. Risk factors for IUGR include acquired blood borne infections (such as malaria, rubella and cytomegalovirus), pre-existing maternal disease (cardiovascular, endocrine, autoimmune), aneuploidies, metabolic factors and placental disorders including abnormal placental position. However, for most infants with evidence of IUGR, there is no known cause; idiopathic IUGR is often described as 'placental insufficiency'. In IUGR, there are marked reductions in the placental delivery of amino acids to the fetus, which is reflected in decreased deposition of tissue. This is probably due to both blood flow and arteriovenous differences in nutrient concentrations being compromised as well as reduced activity in the placental amino acid transport systems. Placental transport of glucose in IUGR seems no different to a normal placenta but the placental expression of the lipoprotein receptors and lipoprotein lipases involved in transfer of maternal fatty acids is altered. In IUGR, there also appears to be increased placental permeability and increased placental oxygen utilization. Where there is IUGR with a normal umbilical blood flow, amino acid and LC-PUFA concentrations are significantly reduced and nonesterified fatty acids levels are increased. However, when umbilical blood flow is also impaired in severe IUGR, fetal blood flow to the brain, liver and heart is altered leading to the fetus becoming hypoxic and lactacidaemic with subsequent effects on the fetal growth trajectory. Associated with these changes, the fetus adapts to nutrient intake not meeting demand by increasing protein catabolism, reducing metabolic rate and making endocrine adaptations; these adaptation mechanisms are not without cost and may have lifelong health consequence (see Chapter 12). The most serious complications of IUGR occur in fetuses weighing <500 g. One approach to correcting IUGR might be placental gene therapy, particularly as growth factors (such as insulin growth factors, placental growth factor and VEGF) are all implicated in failure of trophoblast remodelling of the uterine spiral arteries, which appears to be the underlying abnormality in both IUGR and preeclampsia. Although development of such treatment is theoretical at the moment, it does raise interesting ethical questions about whether the patient in such a scenario is the woman or her fetus and whether gene therapy could be justified if it was safe and effective, where there was reasonable certainty that the fetus would suffer irreversible and substantial harm without the intervention and where the risk to the mother was negligible.

---

leading causes of prenatal morbidity and mortality. Often the terms 'placental insufficiency' or 'uteroplacental vascular insufficiency' are used to describe suboptimal placental function. However, despite the importance of identifying and assessing placental insufficiency, these terms are not precisely defined (Hunt et al., 2016).

A proportion of those babies with a low birthweight (<2.5 kg) may have failed to achieve their growth potential because placental transfer of oxygen and nutrients was inadequate. Like all essential organs, the placenta has a considerable physiological reserve. It has been estimated that the placenta could lose 30–40% of its villi (and therefore surface area) without affecting its function. The placentas of growth-restricted fetuses may exhibit pathological changes such as reduced syncytiotrophoblast area and volume, reduced vascularization of the villi, increased placental apoptosis and/or increased thickness of the exchange barrier (Burton and Jauniaux, 2018).

Placental insufficiency is more likely to be due to inadequate maternal uteroplacental blood flow and reduced uteroplacental perfusion, primarily due to the failure of trophoblastic invasion and impaired remodelling of the spiral arteries into low resistance vessels in the early stages of pregnancy (Burton and Jauniaux, 2018). There are several consequences of the incomplete conversion of the spiral arteries: (1) the maternal blood will flow into the intervillous space at a higher velocity and in a pulsatile fashion, which means that the villus tree is less likely to be perfused evenly, there is less time for exchange and mechanical damage to the delicate placental villi can result in shedding of placental fragments and release of procoagulants (Roberts, 2014); (2) some vascular smooth muscle is likely to be retained, predisposing to intermittent placental perfusion due to spontaneous vasoconstriction of the spiral arteries; (3) higher shear forces result in an increased risk of atherosclerosis including the accumulation of foam calls and occlusion of the lumen of the artery; and (4) malperfusion causes ischaemia-reperfusion injury, which results in OS and the release of proinflammatory cytokines and apoptosis.

In addition to the impaired uteroplacental blood flow, which is characteristic of IUGR, there is also impaired placental transfer of nutrients (Dimasuay et al., 2016), possibly because the placenta responds to decreased blood flow or hypoxia by down-regulating key placental transporters, particularly amino acid and lipid transporters. Maternal levels of insulin-like growth factor I (IGF-I) and leptin are also decreased in IUGR pregnancies.

Case study 8.2 describes a case of a small baby.

CASE STUDY 8.2

Polly was diagnosed as carrying a small-for-dates baby. She spontaneously delivered Thomas at 39 weeks, and although he weighed only 2.4 kg, he appeared healthy and vigorous. The midwife noted that the third stage appeared complete but failed to identify that the placenta appeared relatively large.

- Do you think that there is any need to weigh placentas and to compare the placental and fetal birthweights?
- Are there any situations where the weight and condition of the placenta may be used as a possible indicator for disease states in later life?

Fetoplacental Blood Flow

Blood leaving the right atrium is diverted into the ductus arteriosus, into the aorta and down to the lower body (see Chapter 15). At term, about 40–50% of the fetal cardiac output goes to the placenta via the umbilical arteries. Blood flow from the aorta to the umbilical arteries is high because the resistance to flow in these vessels is low compared with the systemic circulation of the lower body. The vessels of the fetoplacental circulation lack autonomic innervation but a variety of substances can affect the smooth muscle of the stem villus arteries. Of particular interest are paracrine agents, which have a local effect on the fetoplacental circulation. Both prostacyclin and nitric oxide (NO), which have vasodilatory and anticoagulant effects, are produced by the vessel endothelium and their production is compromised by stress. It is thought that flow-mediated release of NO may have an important role in maintaining the high flow and low resistance uteroplacental vasculature of healthy pregnancies. Endogenous production of NO is upregulated in pregnancy. As NO is derived from oxidation of the amino acid L-arginine, dietary interventions

aimed at enhancing NO bioavailability, for instance by providing L-arginine supplements or promoting dietary sources (such as beetroot and green leafy vegetables), have been investigated as possible ways to improve uteroplacental vascular function and increase fetal growth (Cottrell et al., 2017). Studies carried out so far are interesting but not conclusive.

Optimal placental exchange requires adequate vascularization of the placental bed by the maternal arteries matched by circulation of fetal blood to the placenta. The fetus does not appear to have a mechanism to increase umbilical flow in response to hypoxia or volume depletion. It has limited ability to increase cardiac output. Therefore, the fetus adapts to hypoxia or decreased nutrient availability by decreasing oxygen consumption and growth rate. It is advantageous to be a smaller infant in a nutrient-restricted postnatal environment. The cardiac output is redistributed to the heart, brain and adrenal glands at the expense of the flow to the body and gut. Hypoxia and acidosis cause cerebral vasodilatation and constriction of the pulmonary and femoral vessels. Blood flow to the liver is high when oxygen and nutrients are plentiful but the hepatic circulation is bypassed to a greater extent if placental exchange is compromised.

It is hypothesized that perfusion of the placental vessels is controlled to match the maternal perfusion of the uteroplacental vessel in a similar way to the perfusion–ventilation matching in the neonatal or adult pulmonary system (see Chapter 1). If an area of the placenta is underperfused by the maternal blood flow, hypoxia ensues. The endothelium of the placental vessels responds by vasoconstriction (by decreasing NO synthesis and increasing endothelin-1 production), so that fetoplacental blood flow is diverted to a better-perfused villus tree.

PLACENTAL TRANSPORT MECHANISMS

Many substances are transported from the maternal blood in the intervillous space to the fetal blood in the capillaries of the villi and vice versa. The transfer of substances across the placenta occurs in both directions, to and from the fetus. By term, most exchange occurs in the terminal villi, which have a high surface area and small diffusion distance, perhaps of only a few microns in some areas. The surface area of the placenta is estimated to be 5 m² at 28 weeks, increasing to about 12–15 m² from the terminal villi at term (Burton and Fowden, 2015). The precise mechanisms of placental transport for many substances are still to be characterized. Transport mechanisms include simple diffusion and transporter-mediated mechanisms and exocytosis/endocytosis. The effectiveness of the transport mechanism depends on the morphological characteristics of the placenta (like surface area and barrier thickness) and on the abundance and distribution of specific transporters. Simple and facilitated diffusion depends on the concentration gradient, the placental permeability the surface area and the thickness of the interhemal membrane; however, passive diffusion alone is not likely to be adequate for fetal requirements for nutrients.

Lipophilic substances (which are soluble in lipid such as respiratory gases and lipophilic drugs) are permeable through cell membranes so their transport depends on the concentration gradient and the relative rates of maternal and fetal blood flow. Because the placenta provides a large surface area, the transfer of respiratory gases depends on the materno–fetal concentration difference, which depends on the flow rates of the uterine and umbilical circulations (Burton et al., 2016). This exchange is described as 'flow-limited' because it depends on the refreshment and depletion of the blood on each side of the exchange membrane: the maternal reservoir pool in the intervillous spaces and the fetal recipient pool in the blood vessels of the placental villi. Changes in either maternal or fetal blood flow rates will affect the transport of respiratory gases and lipophilic substances.

Diffusion of hydrophilic substances (soluble in aqueous solutions but poorly soluble in lipid bilayers) is relatively slow and limited by the diffusion distance (placenta thickness) and the surface area of the membranes of the placental barrier. This exchange is described as 'diffusion-limited' (Burton et al., 2016). To some extent, the placenta can adapt to stressors such as high altitude or maternal smoking by increasing its surface area, reducing the thickness of the diffusion barrier or by increasing uterine artery blood flow (Browne et al., 2015).

The fetal capillary endothelium may limit transport of large proteins (such as albumin, IgG and AFP). Transport studies of the syncytiotrophoblast suggest that there may be water-filled channels or pores in the human placenta, which allow solutes of 1350–5200 Daltons (Da) through (Burton and Fowden, 2015). These channels remain speculative as they have not yet been visualized but they would explain the observation that large proteins can diffuse across the human placenta. In addition, small defects in the syncytiotrophoblast occur in all human placentas (Burton and Fowden, 2015). These defects lead to fibrin plaques being deposited; it is suggested that the plaques might offer a route across the placenta for hydrophilic molecules, maternal immune cells, pathogens and large proteins such as AFP.

There are specific transport proteins on the placental plasma membrane involved in the efficient transfer of metabolically important substances, particularly molecules, which are charged or hydrophilic such as glucose, amino acids and fatty acids and micronutrients such as iron, folate and copper. These transport proteins are channels, carriers or active transporters.

Glucose is the most important nutrient for the fetus, which is dependent on maternal supply as there is no de novo gluconeogenesis during fetal life (Luscher et al., 2017). Glucose demands of the fetus are high; 80% of fetal energy is derived from the oxidation of maternal glucose and glucose utilization rates are estimated to average about 5 mg/kg per min (Blackburn, 2018), which is markedly higher than adults at 2–3 mg/kg per min. In FGR, the placenta may produce lactate and ketone bodies as alternative energy substrates, which the fetal can use to produce ATP and glycogen.

Glucose transport is predominantly carried out by facilitative diffusion the glucose transporters GLUT1 and GLUT3. The GLUT transporters are membrane proteins that transport glucose and other hexoses down a concentration gradient much faster than is possible by simple diffusion. Glucose transport by GLUT1 is concentration dependent, bidirectional and independent of insulin. GLUT1 expression is higher on the maternal side of the syncytiotrophoblast, which favours mother-to-fetus transfer and protects against glucose being transported from the fetus during maternal hypoglycaemia. GLUT1 expression is downregulated by hyperglycaemia so fetal development is partially protected if there is maternal hyperglycaemia. A significant proportion of the glucose taken up by the placenta is used by the placenta for its own metabolic requirements, which are high.

Compared with GLUT1, GLUT3 provides the minor contribution to glucose transport to the developing fetus but may be important during periods of maternal hypo- or hyperglycaemia. It is expressed on the apical but not the basal side of the syncytiotrophoblast and has a higher affinity (lower K_m) for glucose for supply to the fetus when maternal plasma glucose levels are low. Fetal glucose levels are usually slightly lower than maternal levels, which they usually reflect. The difference between fetal and maternal glucose levels increases with the severity of IUGR.

Some substances, such as certain amino acids and calcium, are transported by active (energy-dependent) transport against their electrochemical gradients. Amino acid transport by the placenta has a significant effect on the fetal growth rate; amino acids are required for fetal protein synthesis, as precursors for other metabolic requirements and are also metabolized to produce ATP. There are several amino acid transporters in the uterine and placental tissues, which transport particular groups of amino acids depending on the structure of their side-chain, e.g. neutral, cationic or aromatic. Functionally, amino acids can be considered in three categories: (1) accumulative (system A) transporters, which are expressed on both the apical and basal placental surfaces and generate a pool of amino acids within the trophoblast tissue; (2) exchange transporters, which exchange an amino acid in the pool for a different one; and (3) facultative transporters, which control the export of amino acids across the basal membrane (Burton et al., 2016).

Maternal signals such as steroid hormones, insulin and IGFs, and adipokines from adipose tissue affect placental amino acid transport. When maternal anabolic pathways are dominant, amino acid transfer is stimulated and when maternal catabolic pathways are dominant, amino acid transfer is reduced (Vaughan et al., 2017). This adaptation promotes maternal survival and long-term reproductive success when food is restricted. Placental transfer of amino acids is reduced in IUGR in preeclampsia probably because fewer transporters are expressed and their function is downregulated (Luscher et al., 2017), so the maximum rate of transfer is reduced. Amino acid levels are usually higher in the fetus than in the mother as expected with active transport systems but, when the fetus is growth-restricted, maternal amino acid levels are not as low as in normal pregnancies.

Fatty acids, particularly the long-chain polyunsaturated fatty acids (LC-PUFA), are important for synthesis of phospholipids and cell membranes, and growth and development of the brain and nervous system; they may also be oxidized as fuel. The fetus is dependent on placental transfer of free fatty acids, since intact triglycerides cannot cross the placenta. There are also binding sites for lipoproteins on both the apical and basal aspects of the syncytiotrophoblast, which may be particularly important in the transport of maternal cholesterol to the fetus.

The syncytiotrophoblast expresses lipases, which hydrolyse maternal triglyceride to free fatty acids. These can then be transported across the placental tissue by different types of fatty acid transport proteins. Some of these are specific for medium to long chain fatty acids and others preferentially transfer LC-PUFA (Lewis et al., 2018).

The placental nucleoside transporters enable the fetus to meet its high demands for nucleosides to synthesize nucleotides; transport of nucleosides is decreased by ethanol, nicotine and caffeine. There are additional mechanisms for the transport of some very large molecules such as receptor-mediated pinocytosis for IgG (see Chapter 10). There is a net flux of water to the fetus via osmosis, mostly across the placenta.

Steroid hormones cross the placenta but peptide hormones seem to be poorly transferred. Gas transfer occurs by diffusion and is limited by blood flow. As well as oxygen and carbon dioxide, the placenta permits diffusion of other gases such as carbon monoxide and inhalation anaesthetics. The placenta itself has a high rate of oxygen consumption; much of this oxygen is used for oxidative phosphorylation of glucose. The consequent production of ATP is used mainly for placental synthesis of peptide and steroid hormones and for transport of nutrients.

The placenta has a protective function and, although it is not an efficient barrier, it limits transfer of some xenobiotic substances to the fetus. The placenta expresses cytochrome P450 enzymes so, like the liver, it can metabolize and detoxify a number of drugs. There are also export pumps in the syncytiotrophoblast, which reduce placental transfer of potentially toxic substances. However, some bacteria such as *Treponema pallidum* (which causes syphilis) and protozoa such as *Toxoplasma gondii* (which causes toxoplasmosis), two infectious conditions that can occur during pregnancy, and a number of viruses (including HIV, cytomegalovirus, rubella, polio and varicella) can readily cross the placenta and infect the fetus.

The placenta acts as a nutrient sensor and regulates nutrient transfer depending on the ability of the maternal circulation to supply the nutrients. Furthermore, the placenta has its own nutrient demands; it extracts a fixed proportion of maternal nutrients (70% of the glucose and 40% of the oxygen) (Johnson, 2018) and can also take nutrients, such as amino acids, from the fetal circulation for its own nutrient needs. This means the fetus is vulnerable to nutrient deprivation as it is restricted to the surplus nutrients that remain after placental demands are met. Even minor placental dysfunction can restrict nutrient transfer and blood flow to the fetus while maintaining the high level of placental nutrition. Similarly, placental oxygen uptake also seems to remain constant even when there are acute reductions in uterine oxygen supply, so it is the fetal level of oxygenation, which is compromised in such conditions. If uterine perfusion is reduced, delivery of glucose and amino acids to the fetus can be compromised. Such a reduction in substrate availability can affect growth and metabolism of the fetus. The fetal compensatory responses include down-regulation of the insulin and IGF-1 axis and hepatic glucose metabolism. This results in glycogenolysis and endogenous protein breakdown, which increase fetal glucose and amino acid levels but potentially compromise growth. Endocrine responses include hypothyroidism, bone demineralization and upregulation of the adrenocortical axis. An increase in fetal red blood cell mass may not only exacerbate placental dysfunction but also result in increased risk of thrombocytopenia, increased blood viscosity and platelet aggregation.

PLACENTAL HORMONE PRODUCTION

Placental hormones have a role in adjusting maternal physiology to provide the optimal environment for fetal development (see Chapter 11); however, roles for all of the placental products have not yet been elucidated. Concentrations of placental protein hormones, such as hCG and hPL, are higher in the maternal blood than in the fetus because the placenta conjugates hormones entering the fetal compartment or otherwise limits the transfer of the hormones (Johnson, 2018). Conversely, levels of steroid hormones are about 10 times higher in the fetal circulation. Emerging evidence suggests that the placenta may exhibit circadian rhythms in hormone secretion (Valenzuela et al., 2015) and express the clock genes required for mammalian circadian functions. Factors that alter the normal pattern of circadian rhythm such as shiftwork are associated with an increased risk of poorer outcomes of pregnancy, such as preterm delivery, IUGR and preeclampsia. The human placenta also synthesizes melatonin, a hormone produced by the pineal gland postpartum, which regulates sleep–wake (night–day) cycles and circadian rhythms. Hormonal concentrations also change in response to environmental challenges such as changes in maternal blood flow, compromised maternal diet and hypoxia, probably in response to changed gene expression. In the fetal compartment, environmental conditions that favour fetal growth increase concentrations of anabolic hormones such as thyroxine, insulin and IGF-1 and decrease concentrations of catabolic hormones such as catecholamines and cortisol; growth hormone has little effect on fetal growth since fetal growth hormone receptors are not expressed until late in pregnancy (Malcomson and Nagy, 2015).

The placenta has a broad endocrine capacity and extraordinary biosynthetic diversity, producing many hormones that are the products of other endocrine organs after birth, both steroid and peptide/protein hormones. The placenta synthesizes hypothalamic releasing hormones (such as gonadotrophin-releasing hormone (GnRH) and corticotrophin-releasing hormone [CRH]), pituitary hormones (such as oxytocin, antidiuretic hormone and adrenocorticotrophic hormone [ACTH]), hormones that regulate metabolism (such as leptin and ghrelin), vasoactive peptides, neurohormones and cytokines (such as activin A, inhibins and IGFs) (Johnson, 2018). Some of these hormones affect both maternal and fetal physiology; others appear to act predominantly within the placenta. Some of the placental forms of hormones are distinctly different to those produced by the other maternal endocrine glands.

The syncytiotrophoblast is probably the source of most placental products including hormones, growth factors and cytokines, although the cytotrophoblast may also produce hCG, hPL, inhibin, relaxin and placental releasing hormones. The major steroids produced are progesterone and oestrogens (oestriol). The production of oestrogens

requires both maternal and fetal precursors, so monitoring maternal oestrogen levels during pregnancy is a useful indicator of fetal wellbeing. Cholesterol from maternal low-density lipoproteins (LDL) is the usual precursor for steroid hormone production. Oestriol synthesis requires 16α-hydroxydehydroandrosterone sulphate derived from the fetal liver and adrenal gland. Most of the steroid hormones produced also enter the maternal circulation and also affect her physiology (see Chapter 11). The placenta also produces neuropeptides (although it has no nerves), which may regulate placental steroid and peptide hormone production, leptin, growth factors and cytokines; it is suggested that the expression of placental neuropeptides may be involved in regulating the duration of gestation (Vitale et al., 2016).

hCG and Steroids

Embryo development requires progesterone to maintain uterine quiescence. Initially hCG from the trophoblast rescues the corpus luteum from atresia, thus maintaining the production of oestrogen (oestradiol and oestrone) and progesterone from the corpus luteum. Release of hCG from the trophoblast is detectable about 7 days after fertilization; however, concentrations of hCG and luteal steroid hormones are not directly correlated. The corpus luteum becomes redundant at about 7–9 weeks after fertilization when steroid hormone production is taken over by the placenta (and the corpus luteum markedly regresses from about week 10). This change in site of production is described as the luteoplacental (or luteal-placental) shift. It is thought that delayed or inadequate steroid hormone production by the placenta is likely to result in miscarriage or unsuccessful assisted reproduction (Schindler et al., 2015); low progesterone concentrations after 7 weeks are correlated with increased likelihood of pregnancy failure. Iatrogenic low progesterone levels can result from the use of GnRH analogues to synchronize follicular development and ovulation when pregnancy has resulted from IVF. Low progesterone levels are also associated with polycystic ovary syndrome and endocrine problems. Progestational agents such as hCG or progestogens can be used to provide transient hormonal support in women with a history of recurrent miscarriage. hCG is the first hormonal signal from the embryo; hCG mRNA is transcribed from the 8-cell stage of embryonic development (see Chapter 9) before implantation has started (Makrigiannakis et al., 2017). It can be detected in maternal serum and urine once implantation has occurred about 9–10 days postfertilization when secretions from the trophoblast enter the maternal blood vessels. hCG is composed of 2 subunits; the α-subunit is common to all glycoprotein hormones such as luteinizing hormone (LH), follicle-stimulating hormone (FSH) and thyroid-stimulating hormone (TSH). Dissociated α- and β-subunits of hCG, as well as the intact dimer (the complete hCG molecule formed of two subunits), are measurable in pregnancy. hCG exists in three different isoforms: 'regular' hCG produced from the syncytiotrophoblast cells, sulphated (hCG-S) produced by the pituitary gland and hyperglycosylated (hCG-H), which has additional branching oligosaccharide side-chains, produced from the cytotrophoblast (Nwabuobi et al., 2017). The hyperglycosylated form is the dominant form produced early in pregnancy when invasive trophoblastic activity is high and from choriocarcinomas (Evans, 2016). Altered levels of hCG-H are associated with pregnancy complications such as inadequate placentation in preeclampsia and IUGR and excessive invasive cytotrophoblasts in Down syndrome (Evans, 2016). hCG-H promotes trophoblastic invasion, cytotrophoblast differentiation and proliferation and migration of EVTs (Makrigiannakis et al., 2017). It is also important in the preparation of the endometrium for implantation; decidualization during and prior to the implantation window is mediated by hCG-H. The role of hCG, particularly hCG-H, in maintaining hormone production by the corpus luteum is clearly established; however, peak production of hCG occurs after the function of the corpus luteum has already started to decline, suggesting other roles for the hormone.

hCG contributes to maternal tolerance of the embryo; it affects T-cell modulation and adjusts the Th-1/Th-2 balance (see Chapter 10), regulates macrophage migration and inflammation and regulates uterine NK cell proliferation (Makrigiannakis et al., 2017). It may also be involved with fetal testosterone production and male sexual differentiation (see Chapter 5). Because of the structural similarity between hCG and LH, hCG is used in ART for controlled ovarian stimulation (see p. 157) because it reduces the risk of ovarian hyperstimulation syndrome. However, although both LH and hCG can bind to LH receptors of the corpus luteum, the effect is not identical. The structural differences in the beta subunit mean that the pharmacokinetics are different and hCG has a significantly longer half-life than LH (Klement and Shulman, 2017).

The risk of breast cancer is decreased by a first childbirth before the age of 24 years (Rao, 2017). Studies in animal models and on human breast cancer cell lines suggest hCG might be responsible for this protective effect; further research in this field may lead to hCG as a possible clinical therapy for breast cancer prevention (Schuler-Toprak et al., 2017). The observations that hCG promotes myometrial quiescence (Nwabuobi et al., 2017) have led to clinical studies to investigate whether it could suppress the premature myometrial contractions that lead to preterm birth (Rao, 2016). The beta subunit of hCG is measured in urine by immunoassay in standard pregnancy tests. hCG-H is a biomarker of early pregnancy and is probably a better predictor of a viable pregnancy than regular hCG because failing pregnancies produce minimal hCG-H (Nwabuobi et al., 2017). Commonly found endocrine disrupting chemicals (EDC), such as bisphenol A (BPA) used in the manufacture of plastics and parabens used as preservatives in cosmetics, might interfere with the production of hCG and negatively affect fetal development (Paulesu et al., 2018).

Human Placental Lactogen

hPL (also known as human chorionic somatomammotropin, hCS) is also a product of the syncytiotrophoblast; it is structurally and functionally similar to human growth hormone and prolactin. Levels of hPL increase throughout gestation and correlate well with placental syncytiotrophoblast mass so it used to be used to clinically evaluate placental function before other more modern and reliable tests became available. By term, 1–3 g of hPL is produced per day (equivalent to 5–7 mg/mL in maternal blood). hPL affects maternal metabolism, erythropoietin activity, fetal growth, mammary gland development and ovarian function; it induces insulin resistance, decreases maternal glucose utilization and promotes carbohydrate intolerance (see p. 328). It increases lipolysis so free fatty acid levels increase; the fatty acids are preferentially metabolized by the mother so glucose and ketones are spared for fetal metabolism. Lower hPL levels are associated with preeclampsia, aborting molar pregnancy (hydatidiform mole), choriocarcinoma and placental insufficiency. Higher than normal hPL levels are associated with multiple pregnancies, placental tumours, intact molar pregnancy, diabetes and Rhesus incompatibility.

Placental Growth Hormone

PGH is synthesized by the syncytiotrophoblast; it is also known as growth hormone 2 (GH2) or growth hormone variant (GH-V). PGH is structurally similar to hPL and pituitary growth hormone. It has high somatogenic (growth) activity and low lactogenic activity, binding to the GH and prolactin receptors. PGH gradually replaces pituitary growth hormone in the maternal circulation and becomes the predominant form in pregnancy (Velegrakis et al., 2017). Levels of PGH increase throughout pregnancy to replace pituitary growth hormone, which has a pulsatile secretory pattern. PGH is important in facilitating maternal metabolic adaptation to pregnancy; it stimulates lipolysis, glycogenolysis and anabolic pathways to regulate the amount of glucose and amino acids available for placental extraction from the maternal circulation. PGH is regulated by levels of glucose and insulin in maternal plasma. The effects of PGH (and hPL) are mediated by maternal IGF-1; levels of PGH correlate with the birthweight of newborns. However, women who give birth to large for gestational age (LGA) infants tend to have lower levels of PGH in early pregnancy (Ringholm et al., 2015). PGH may be a useful marker of pregnancy pathologies (Liao et al., 2018). Levels of PGH in amniotic fluid or maternal serum may be useful indictors of an increased risk of Down syndrome and other trisomies, maternal diabetes, IUGR, preeclampsia and LGA.

THE ALLANTOIS AND YOLK SAC

The allantois and yolk sac (or umbilical vesicle) are semi-vestigial fetal membrane structures that may have a more important role in other species, such as birds and reptiles, where the yolk sac is important in nutrition of the maternally isolated eggs and the allantois has a respiratory and excretory role. The allantois forms from a pocket of the hindgut embedded within the umbilical cord, which is incorporated into the developing urinary system. Blood cells develop in the wall of the allantois during weeks 3–5 and its blood vessels become the vessels of the umbilical cord, which forms in the region of the body stalk and is covered by the developing amnion. The embryonic structures and the right umbilical vein disappear, leaving two arteries and one vein. The yolk sac develops on the ventral side of the embryonic disc and is important in nutrition of the embryo while the uteroplacental circulation is forming. The primordial germ cells (see Chapter 5) and the blood islands develop in the tissue of the yolk sac. The yolk sac becomes thin and elongated and is incorporated into the umbilical cord and primitive gut. Its role in haematopoiesis is taken over by the liver in the 6th week of development and the duct becomes obliterated. The remnant of the yolk sac remains between the chorion and amnion; it may be seen as a calcified yellow nodule ~4 mm long when the fetal membranes are examined after delivery.

THE PLACENTA AT TERM

The mature placenta is usually an oval/round disc with a diameter of ~18–22 cm and 2–3 cm thick in the middle, petering out towards the edges. At the placental margins, the basal and chorionic surfaces of the placenta unite to form the fetal chorionic membrane. On average, a placenta weighs about one-sixth of the weight of the fetus, about 470–500 g. The amniotic membrane is smooth so the fetal aspect of the placenta, the chorionic plate, appears shiny and grey. The amnion is a single layer of epithelial cells and avascular connective tissue, which is weakly attached and can be easily removed from the delivered placenta. The basal plate is the maternal surface of the placenta, which appears grooved and lobed with a dull red colouration. This basal surface is a mixture of EVTs, maternal decidua cells and immune cells such as macrophages and uterine natural killer (uNK) cells, extracellular matrix, fibrinoid and blood clots. The chorionic membrane retains the ridged appearance owing to the regression of the early villi. The umbilical cord is usually inserted slightly eccentrically into the chorionic plate. The umbilical cord gets progressively longer with the duration of the pregnancy as fetal activity and traction on the cord increases its length. At term, the umbilical cord is normally between 50 and 60 cm long. If the cord is abnormally short, it can cause bleeding problems. If it is long (>70 cm), it may prolapse through the cervix or entangle with the fetus, possibly forming knots that could obstruct fetal circulation during delivery, potentially causing fetal distress and death.

Examination of the cord including its length is used clinically as a marker of undetected intrauterine events such as unexplained fetal death (Gayatri et al., 2017); although it is not clear whether cord length is long because of traction associated with entanglement or whether entanglements occur because the cord is long. There may be a genetic component to abnormally long cords. Long cords are more likely associated with increased parity, maternal size (height and BMI) and diabetes, large placenta and birthweight and male sex (Linde et al., 2018). For a normal vaginal delivery, a cord length of at least 32 cm is thought to be necessary to avoid fetal distress, cord tearing and possible abruption. Very short cords are associated with poor fetal movement (such as in oligohydramnios) and prenatal exposure to alcohol and drugs such as cocaine; short cords have been associated with compromised neurological development. Short cords are more likely to be associated with female sex, small placenta and anomalous cord insertion (Linde et al., 2018). The risks of fetal malformation, placental complications and poor outcome of pregnancy are higher with short cords. Most umbilical cords are twisted; usually the twists are counterclockwise 'left twists' every few centimetres. Cords without any twists are often associated with single umbilical artery (SUA) and an increased risk of perinatal mortality. Excessive twisting, which can compromise blood flow, is also associated with fetal morbidity and mortality. True knots in the umbilical cord occur in about 0.3–1% of births and are associated with an increased risk of perinatal death (Mehta et al., 2017). The vessels of the cord, two arteries carrying blood from the fetus and one vein carrying blood to the fetus, are embedded in Wharton's jelly. This jelly is a connective tissue, similar to the vitreous humor of the eye, that protects the vessels of the cord. Wharton's jelly responds to temperature changes at delivery and contributes to physiological clamping of the vessels in the umbilical cord (see Chapter 13). It is also a source of adult-type stem cells, which may have therapeutic potential.

EXAMINATION OF THE PLACENTA

Examination of the placenta, fetal membranes and umbilical cord at delivery is an important responsibility of the attendant midwives. Most placentas and most babies are normal. A quick visual inspection of the maternal and fetal surfaces can pick up the occasional abnormal specimen; unusual odour, which could indicate a bacterial infection; and substantial amounts of fresh clot could indicate premature placental separation. Cord length and diameter are assessed and the distance of insertion to the nearest placental margin. The cord is checked for vessel number, true knots, twisting, discolouration, congestion and thrombosis. There are usually two arteries and the persisting left umbilical vein. A single umbilical artery (SUA) occurs in about 1% of births, and 4–11% of twin pregnancies; it is more common for the left umbilical artery to be missing (Iqbal and Raiz, 2015). SUA is associated with IUGR, preterm labour, SGA infants and an increased frequency of fetal and chromosomal abnormalities, particularly of the renal, respiratory and cardiovascular systems (Luo et al., 2017); however, it is normal for the arteries to fuse together just above the fetal surface. Sometimes more vessels are present because the right umbilical vein has not regressed. Although an abnormality in the number of vessels is associated with congenital abnormalities, it is not clear whether the wrong number of vessels is a cause or a result of the abnormality. About 20% of infants with SUA will have other major congenital abnormalities; the remainder are often slightly small and have an increased risk of perinatal and paediatric mortality. Macrosomic babies of diabetic mothers tend to have thicker and oedematous cords, whereas thin delicate cords are associated with IUGR. The cord can be inserted into the placental bed in different ways. Insertion of the cord is usually approximately central but may be lateral. Abnormal insertion of the cord can create problems at delivery (Table 8.2). If the cord is ruptured, it indicates that there may have been some fetal blood loss during labour. The chorionic plate opacity and colour including the amount of fibrin and thrombosis in the subchorionic region can also be assessed.

The type of membrane insertion and their completeness are assessed. The membranes are easier to examine if the placenta is held up by the cord. Usually, the two membranes hang down in a neat uniform way. The placenta is continuous with the chorion but the amnion should be able to be separated from the chorion up to the base of the cord. If the membranes are ragged and torn, some parts of the membrane may be retained in the uterus, which can impede uterine involution and staunching of blood loss. Meconium can discolour the membranes in late gestation; fresh meconium may also be present.

A healthy placenta is normally rounded and uniform but shape is quite variable. Unusual shapes may be a result of uterine cavity abnormalities. Placental weight is usually between 350 and 750 g; excessively light or heavy placentas are associated with pathological conditions. An excessively large or oedematous (soft) placenta is associated with maternal diabetes, hydrops or cardiac abnormalities. Maternal diabetes tends to result in placentas with a deep red colour, rather than the usual maroon. The placenta is also examined for abnormal numbers of lobes (Table 8.2) or missing areas of the maternal surface, which could indicate that a lobe has been retained, potentially causing serious postpartum bleeding and prevention of milk let down (lactation) due to continued placental progesterone secretion. Depending on whether twins are monozygotic or dizygotic, the placenta may be shared or regions fused (Box 8.5). The maternal surface is examined for completeness, adherent blood clot, lesions (such as infarcts and thrombi) and degree of calcification. Cysts are common on the surface and are associated with fibrin deposition but are usually not significant. True placental infarcts are also common, they tend to be small (<1 cm) and located at the placental margins. Haemorrhages on the maternal surface are usually due to premature separation and are more common with hypertensive disorders, ascending infection, smoking and cocaine use.

Sometimes a dense raised white rim may be observed on the periphery of the fetal placental bed; this is called a 'circumvallate placenta'. It is thought to be caused by deep implantation of the placenta into the maternal decidua and subsequent partial separation of the placental from the uterine wall. This results in the folding back of the membrane towards the chorionic surface. The rim is a double fold of fetal membranes with degenerated decidua and fibrin between them. The clinical significance of the condition is uncertain but it may be a risk factor for antenatal haemorrhage and/or severe intermittent uterine contractions. It is more common in multigravidae and in women who have previously had a circumvallate placenta.

In some cultures and also in Westernized societies, women may wish to consume their placenta following delivery (placentophagy). This is normal practice in most mammalian species and is protective in that it removes the evidence of a recent birth and presence of vulnerable newborn. Placentophagy may be promoted as a 'traditional medicine' to prevent postnatal depression and fatigue, to increase milk supply, for health or nutritional benefits and/or to speed recovery (Farr et al., 2018).

Case study 8.3 describes an example of placental abnormality revealed by inspection.

TABLE 8.2   Placental Abnormalities

Condition	Description and Cause
Abruptio placentae	Separation of normally situated placenta from site of implantation after 24th week of gestation but before delivery of the fetus. More common in women with high parity and history of obstetric problems. May cause uterine tenderness and tetany, and variable bleeding. Complications may include disseminated intravascular coagulation (DIC), postpartum haemorrhage (PPH) and shock. It is essential to avoid vaginal examination until placenta previa has been excluded
Placenta previa	Abnormally implanted placenta, positioned partially or totally (over the os) in the lower segment, which obstructs normal delivery. More common in multigravidae, particularly those of high parity and with multiple pregnancy. Usually causes painless vaginal bleeding. Factors that cause damage and scarring of the endometrium increase risk. Possibly due to deficient decidua in fundus at implantation. The placenta is likely to be large and may have succenturiate lobes (see below)
Abnormal insertion of cord	Vasa previa is a rare condition that may occur with velamentous insertion of cord where some of the umbilical vessels cross the internal os. Velamentous insertion occurs in 1% of singleton pregnancies. The cord is attached to the membranes outside the placental boundary and blood vessels, unprotected by Wharton's jelly, and is at risk from compression and tearing
Abnormal conformation of placenta	Placentation may be extrachorial, where the surface area of the chorionic plate is less than the basal (maternal) area. A circumarginate placenta has a flat ring at the transition from placenta to chorion. A circumvallate placenta has a raised rolled ring at the transition and is associated with increased incidence of growth restriction
Succenturiate (accessory) lobes	Variations in shape and number of lobes do not normally affect the outcome of the pregnancy. The placenta may have accessory lobes or be completely bilobed. This may cause problems in determining whether the placenta has been completely expelled at delivery
Hydatidiform mole and choriocarcinoma	Abnormal placental development where the embryo is absent or nonviable. Related to abnormal fertilization and survival of paternal chromosomes only. Hydatidiform mole is a noninvasive usually benign chorionic development and choriocarcinoma is a malignant and invasive tumour derived from trophoblast tissue, possibly from a hydatidiform mole. The villi are not vascularized in either case (as extraembryonic mesoderm is derived from the inner cell mass). Pregnancy-related tumours such as hydatidiform mole and choriocarcinoma are classified as gestational trophoblastic disease (GTD)
Abnormal adherence of chorionic villi	In placenta accreta, the villi adhere to the uterine wall, which has an abnormal decidual layer due to excessive invasion. In placenta percreta, the villi penetrate right through the myometrium to the perimetrium. The placenta fails to separate properly in the third stage of labour and maternal haemorrhage is likely

BOX 8.5   The Placenta in Multiple Pregnancies

Dizygotic (nonidentical) twins and monozygotic (identical) twins resulting from early splitting of the blastocyst prior to implantation can have separate placentas and membranes. However, if the two blastocysts implant in close proximity, the placentas and chorion may fuse. If monozygotic twins arise from division of the inner cell mass, they usually have separate amnions but share the placenta and chorion. The vascular systems within the placenta may remain separate but can fuse. If the vascular systems fuse within the placenta, twin-to-twin transfusion syndrome (TTTS) may occur where the twins have an unequal blood supply. This condition, which occurs in 10–15% of monozygotic twins (thus affecting 1 in 400 pregnancies; 1 in 1600 babies) with a shared placenta, can threaten the survival of both twins because the donor twin is anaemic and the recipient twin is polycythaemic and prone to cardiac hypertrophy and heart failure. Modern treatments have increased the survival of twins but the survivors are at increased risk of brain injury and neurodevelopment consequences.

CASE STUDY 8.3

Following what appeared to be a normal delivery, the midwife inspected the placenta and membranes. She discovered a hole in the membranes that had blood vessels leading to it, radiating out from the main body of the placenta.

- What do you think the midwife concluded from these findings?
- What care and observation will the woman require?
- How will this be explained to the woman and what information might she require?

KEY POINTS

- The placenta orchestrates pregnancy. It controls physiological changes in the mother and nurtures the fetus.
- It derives largely from the trophoblast layer of the embryo, which differentiates into two layers: the cytotrophoblast and the syncytiotrophoblast.
- The cytotrophoblast undergoes rapid mitosis and the syncytiotrophoblast aggressively digests and invades the maternal endometrial wall.
- Fragments of maternal blood vessels are engulfed forming lacunae and a framework for villi development.
- Extravillous cytotrophoblast invades the maternal circulation resulting in remodelling of the spiral arteries.
- Extraembryonic mesoderm, originating from the inner cell mass, invades the core of the villi and establishes the vasculature of the villi.

- The villi continue to grow and remodel throughout the pregnancy; the barrier to diffusion is reduced as fetal requirements increase.
- The placenta has specific transport mechanisms and a range of endocrine activities. It also has an important immunological role.
- Amniotic fluid, produced by the amniotic membrane, cushions and protects the fetus. It is also important in the development of the respiratory and urinary systems.
- Inadequate maternal uteroplacental blood flow, described as placental insufficiency, is associated with the aetiology of preeclampsia and IUGR.
- Examination of the placenta is important in detecting any abnormality or retention of placental tissue.

APPLICATION TO PRACTICE

The placenta has an important physiological role in supporting and maintaining pregnancy. Dysfunction of the placenta and its development results in abnormal conditions observed in pregnancy, which may affect the health of the mother and baby before and after birth.

Knowledge of the gross anatomy and the variants in the placental structure is essential in the postnatal examination of the placenta and membranes.

ANNOTATED FURTHER READING

Armaly Z, Jadaon JE, Jabbour A, Abassi ZA: Preeclampsia: novel mechanisms and potential therapeutic approaches, *Front Physiol* 9:973, 2018.

This is an overview of the pathogenesis of preeclampsia focusing on endothelial injury. Preeclampsia is still a 'medical mystery', but the identification of biomarkers has significant relevance for the identification of possible therapeutic options.

Benirschke K, Burton GJ, Baergen RN: *Pathology of the human placenta*, ed 6, New York, 2012, Springer (soft cover edition 2016).

This comprehensive and heavily illustrated reference text, which covers the structure of the placenta at birth, types of placenta, early development and cellular details, remains the authoritative textbook in the field. The latest edition includes recent research, artificial reproductive technologies and legal aspects.

Burton GJ, Jauniaux E: Pathophysiology of placental-derived fetal growth restriction, *Am J Obstet Gynecol* 218:S745–S761, 2018.

An excellent and well-illustrated description of normal and abnormal placental development, which presents the evidence that deficient remodelling of the uterine spiral arteries in early pregnancy is the primary cause of placental-related IUGR.

Burton GJ, Jauniaux E: The cytotrophoblastic shell and complications of pregnancy, *Placenta* 60:134–139, 2017.

Another well-written review, by two of the best-known experts in placental development, which describes the formation of the cytotrophoblastic shell and presents convincing arguments that impaired development is associated with growth restriction, early-onset preeclampsia, spontaneous miscarriage, preterm rupture of the membranes and premature onset of labour.

Carter AM, Enders AC, Pijnenborg R: The role of invasive trophoblast in implantation and placentation of primates, *Philos Trans R Soc Lond B Biol Sci* 370:20140070, 2015.

A review of the evolution of invasive placentation in primates; some interesting comparisons of the implantation and development of placentas of different primates.

Djaafri F, Stirnemann J, Mediouni I, et al.: Twin-twin transfusion syndrome – what we have learned from clinical trials, *Semin Fetal Neonatal Med* 22:367–375, 2017.

A good explanation of the aetiology of TTTS, how it is assessed and currently treated with a review of clinical trials, their short- and long-term outcomes and issues about the ongoing management of TTTS.

Khong TY, Mooney EE, Nikkels PGJ, et al.: *Pathology of the placenta: a practical guide*, New York, 2019, Springer International Publishing.

An extensive resource about the pathology of the human singleton placenta, which covers nomenclature, definitions and clinical aspects.

Li Y, Lorca RA, Su EJ: Molecular and cellular underpinnings of normal and abnormal human placental blood flows, *J Mol Endocrinol* 60:R9–R22, 2018.

An excellent and well-written description of placental blood flow and the molecular and cellular mechanisms involved in its contribution in the uteroplacental compartment and how they can be impaired in the development of clinical phenotypes.

Maltepe E, Fisher SJ: Placenta: the forgotten organ, *Annu Rev Cell Dev Biol* 31:523–552, 2015.

An in-depth review of placental development, transport and metabolism, which provides details about signalling pathways involved. Finishes with a brief commentary about the development of artificial placentas and extra corporal membrane oxygenation (ECMO) to promote survival of extremely premature infants.

Moser G, Windsperger K, Pollheimer J, et al.: Human trophoblast invasion: new and unexpected routes and functions, *Histochem Cell Biol* 150:361–370, 2018.

An excellent description of the remodelling of the spiral arteries and how they connect to the intervillous spaces of the placenta; good links to pathological conditions.

Nakayama M: Significance of pathological examination of the placenta, with a focus on intrauterine infection and fetal growth restriction, *J Obstet Gynaecol Res* 43:1522–1535, 2017.

A practical step-by-step guide to how to prepare a placenta for examination, the approaches to examination, interpretation of the findings and clinical implications; excellent links to IUGR, chorioamnionitis and other placental pathologies.

Robillard PY, Dekker G, Chaouat G, et al.: Historical evolution of ideas on eclampsia/preeclampsia: a proposed optimistic view of preeclampsia, *J Reprod Immunol* 123:72–77, 2017.

A review of the history of theories about preeclampsia and the current state of understanding.

Sultana Z, Maiti K, Aitken J, et al.: Oxidative stress, placental ageing-related pathologies and adverse pregnancy outcomes, *Am J Reprod Immunol* 77, 2017.

A timely account of oxidative stress and its normal and beneficial roles as well as the recognition of it as key component of the pathogenesis of adverse outcomes of pregnancy.

REFERENCES

Achache H, Revel A: Endometrial receptivity markers, the journey to successful embryo implantation, *Hum Reprod Update* 12:731–746, 2006.

Adam S, Elfeky O, Kinhal V, et al.: Fetal-maternal communication via extracellular vesicles – implications for complications of pregnancies, *Placenta* 54:83–88, 2017.

Alwasel SH, Harrath AH, Aldahmash WM, et al.: Sex differences in regional specialisation across the placental surface, *Placenta* 35:365–369, 2014.

Aplin JD, Ruane PT: Embryo-epithelium interactions during implantation at a glance, *J Cell Sci* 130:15–22, 2017.

Blackburn ST: *Maternal, fetal, neonatal physiology: a clinical perspective*, ed 5, Philadelphia, 2018, Saunders.

Browne VA, Julian CG, Toledo-Jaldin L, et al.: Uterine artery blood flow, fetal hypoxia and fetal growth, *Philos Trans R Soc Lond B Biol Sci* 370:20140068, 2015.

Burton GJ, Fowden AL: The placenta: a multifaceted, transient organ, *Philos Trans R Soc Lond B Biol Sci* 370:20140066, 2015.

Burton GJ, Fowden AL, Thornburg KL: Placental origins of chronic disease, *Physiol Rev* 96:1509–1565, 2016.

Burton GJ, Jauniaux E: Pathophysiology of placental-derived fetal growth restriction, *Am J Obstet Gynecol* 218:S745–S761, 2018.

Burton GJ, Jauniaux E: The cytotrophoblastic shell and complications of pregnancy, *Placenta* 60:134–139, 2017.

Cha J, Sun X, Dey SK: Mechanisms of implantation: strategies for successful pregnancy, *Nat Med* 18:1754–1767, 2012.

Cole LA: Human chorionic gonadotropin (hCG) and hyperglycosylated hCG, seven semi-independent critical molecules, *J Mol Oncol Res* 1:22–44, 2017.

Cottrell E, Tropea T, Ormesher L, et al.: Dietary interventions for fetal growth restriction – therapeutic potential of dietary nitrate supplementation in pregnancy, *J Physiol* 595:5095–5102, 2017.

Cuffe JS, Xu ZC, Perkins AV: Biomarkers of oxidative stress in pregnancy complications, *Biomark Med* 11:295–306, 2017.

Davidson LM, Coward K: Molecular mechanisms of membrane interaction at implantation, *Birth Defects Res C Embryo Today* 108:19–32, 2016.

Dimasuay KG, Boeuf P, Powell TL, Jansson T: Placental responses to changes in the maternal environment determine fetal growth, *Front Physiol* 7:12, 2016.

Emera D, Romero R, Wagner G: The evolution of menstruation: a new model for genetic assimilation: explaining molecular origins of maternal responses to fetal invasiveness, *Bioessays* 34:26–35, 2012.

Evans J: Hyperglycosylated hCG: a unique human implantation and invasion factor, *Am J Reprod Immunol* 75:333–340, 2016.

Evans J, Salamonsen LA, Winship A, et al.: Fertile ground: human endometrial programming and lessons in health and disease, *Nat Rev Endocrinol* 12:654–667, 2016.

Farr A, Chervenak FA, McCullough LB, et al.: Human placentophagy: a review, *Am J Obstet Gynecol* 218, 401 e1–e11, 2018.

Feng Y, Ma X, Deng L, et al.: Role of selectins and their ligands in human implantation stage, *Glycobiology* 27:386–391, 2017.

Fiddler M: Fetal cell based prenatal diagnosis: perspectives on the present and future, *J Clin Med* 3:972–985, 2014.

Gayatri R, Crasta J, Thomas T, et al.: Structural analysis of the umbilical cord and its vessels in intrauterine growth restriction and pre-eclampsia, *J Fetal Med* 4:85–92, 2017.

Griffith OW, Chavan AR, Protopapas S, et al.: Embryo implantation evolved from an ancestral inflammatory attachment reaction, *Proc Natl Acad Sci USA* 114:E6566–E6575, 2017.

Hunt K, Kennedy SH, Vatish M: Definitions and reporting of placental insufficiency in biomedical journals: a review of the literature, *Eur J Obstet Gynecol Reprod Biol* 205:146–149, 2016.

Huppertz B: The anatomy of the normal placenta, *J Clin Pathol* 61:1296–1302, 2008.

Iqbal S, Raiz I: Isolated single umbilical artery in twin pregnancies and its adverse pregnancy outcomes – a case report and review of literature, *J Clin Diagn Res* 9:AD01–AD04, 2015.

James JL, Chamley LW, Clark AR: Feeding your baby in utero: how the uteroplacental circulation impacts pregnancy, *Physiology (Bethesda)* 32:234–245, 2017.

Jauniaux E, Collins S, Burton GJ: Placenta accreta spectrum: pathophysiology and evidence-based anatomy for prenatal ultrasound imaging, *Am J Obstet Gynecol* 218:75–87, 2018.

Johnson MH: *Essential reproduction*, ed 8, Oxford, 2018, Wiley-Blackwell.

Klement AH, Shulman A: hCG triggering in ART: an evolutionary concept, *Int J Mol Sci* 18, 2017.

Kovo M, Bar J, Schreiber L, Shargorodsky M: The relationship between hypertensive disorders in pregnancy and placental maternal and fetal vascular circulation, *J Am Soc Hypertens* 11:724–729, 2017.

Krause DS, Theise ND, Collector MI: Multi-organ, multi-lineage engraftment by a single bone marrow-derived stem cell, *Cell* 105:369–377, 2001.

Lala PK, Chakraborty C: Factors regulating trophoblast migration and invasiveness, *Placenta* 24(1):575–587, 2003.

Lewis RM, Childs CE, Calder PC: New perspectives on placental fatty acid transfer, *Prostaglandins Leukot Essent Fatty Acids* 138:24–29, 2018.

Li Y, Lorca RA, Su EJ: Molecular and cellular underpinnings of normal and abnormal human placental blood flows, *J Mol Endocrinol* 60:R9–R22, 2018.

Liao S, Vickers MH, Stanley JL, et al.: Human placental growth hormone variant in pathological pregnancies, *Endocrinology* 159:2186–2198, 2018.

Linde LE, Rasmussen S, Kessler J, Ebbing C: Extreme umbilical cord lengths, cord knot and entanglement: risk factors and risk of adverse outcomes, a population-based study, *PLoS One* 13:e0194814, 2018.

Loukogeorgakis SP, De Coppi P: Amniotic fluid stem cells: the known, the unknown, and potential regenerative medicine applications, *Stem Cells* 35:1663–1673, 2017.

Luo X, Zhai S, Shi N, et al.: The risk factors and neonatal outcomes of isolated single umbilical artery in singleton pregnancy: a meta-analysis, *Scientific Reports* 7:7396, 2017.

Luscher BP, Marini C, Joerger-Messerli MS, et al.: Placental glucose transporter (GLUT)-1 is down-regulated in preeclampsia, *Placenta* 55:94–99, 2017.

Makrigiannakis A, Vrekoussis T, Zoumakis E, et al.: The role of HCG in implantation: a mini-review of molecular and clinical evidence, *Int J Mol Sci* 18, 2017.

Malcomson RDG, Nagy A: The endocrine system. In Khong TY, Malcomson RDG, editors: *Keeling's fetal and neonatal pathology*, Heidelberg, 2015, Springer, pp 671–702.

Maltepe E, Fisher SJ: Placenta: the forgotten organ, *Annu Rev Cell Dev Biol* 31:523–552, 2015.

McNally AK, Anderson JM: Macrophage fusion and multinucleated giant cells of inflammation, *Adv Exp Med Biol* 713:97–111, 2011.

Mehta S, Singla A, Sinha S, Grover A: Long cord: a knotty affair, *J Clin Diagn Res* 11:QJ01, 2017.

Miller AWF, Hanretty KP: *Obstetrics illustrated*, ed 5, New York, 1998, Churchill Livingstone, pp 12, 99.

Moffett A, Loke C: Immunology of placentation in eutherian mammals, *Nat Rev Immunol* 6:584–594, 2006.

Moore KL, Persaud TVN, Torchia MG: *The developing human: clinically oriented embryology*, ed 10, Philadelphia, 2015, Saunders.

Mourier E, Tarrade A, Duan J, et al.: Non-invasive evaluation of placental blood flow: lessons from animal models, *Reproduction* 153:R85–R96, 2017.

Nwabuobi C, Arlier S, Schatz F, et al.: hCG: Biological functions and clinical applications, *Int J Mol Sci* 18, 2017.

Parks WT: Manifestations of hypoxia in the second and third trimester placenta, *Birth Defects Res* 109:1345–1357, 2017.

Paulesu L, Rao CV, Ietta F, et al.: hCG and its disruption by environmental contaminants during human pregnancy, *Int J Mol Sci* 19, 2018.

Pereira RD, De Long NE, Wang RC, et al.: Angiogenesis in the placenta: the role of reactive oxygen species signaling, *Biomed Res Int* 2015:814543, 2015.

Rao CV: Why are we waiting to start large scale clinical testing of human chorionic gonadotropin for the treatment of preterm births? *Reprod Sci* 23:830–837, 2016.

Rao CV: Protective effects of human chorionic gonadotropin against breast cancer: how can we use this information to prevent/treat the disease? *Reprod Sci* 24:1102–1110, 2017.

Redline RW: Classification of placental lesions, *Am J Obstet Gynecol* 213:S21–S28, 2015.

Ringholm L, Juul A, Pedersen-Bjergaard U, et al.: Lower levels of placental growth hormone in early pregnancy in women with type 1 diabetes and large for gestational age infants, *Growth Horm IGF Res* 25:312–315, 2015.

Roberts JM: Pathophysiology of ischemic placental disease, *Semin Perinatol* 38:139–145, 2014.

Rosenfeld CS: Sex-specific placental responses in fetal development, *Endocrinology* 156:3422–3434, 2015.

Salavati N, Gordijn SJ, Sovio U, et al.: Birth weight to placenta weight ratio and its relationship to ultrasonic measurements, maternal and neonatal morbidity: a prospective cohort study of nulliparous women, *Placenta* 63:45–52, 2018.

Salmon JE, Mineo C, Giles I, et al.: Mechanisms of antiphospho-lipid antibody-mediated pregnancy morbidity. In Erkan D, Lockshin MD, editors: *Antiphospholipid syndrome: current research highlights and clinical insights*, Cham, 2017, Springer International Publishing, pp 117–143.

Schindler AE, Carp H, Druckmann R, et al.: European Progestin Club Guidelines for prevention and treatment of threat-ened or recurrent (habitual) miscarriage with progestogens, *Gynecol Endocrinol* 31:447–449, 2015.

Schuler-Toprak S, Treeck O, Ortmann O: Human chorionic gonadotropin and breast cancer, *Int J Mol Sci* 18, 2017.

Sferruzzi-Perri AN, Camm EJ: The programming power of the placenta, *Front Physiol* 7:33, 2016.

Simon A, Laufer N: Assessment and treatment of repeated implantation failure (RIF), *J Assist Reprod Genet* 29:1227–1239, 2012.

Soares MJ, Iqbal K, Kozai K: Hypoxia and placental develop-ment, *Birth Defects Res* 109:1309–1329, 2017.

Thornburg KL, Kolahi K, Pierce M, et al.: Biological features of placental programming, *Placenta* 48(Suppl 1):S47–S53, 2016.

Timme-Laragy AR, Hahn ME, Hansen JM, et al.: Redox stress and signaling during vertebrate embryonic development: regulation and responses, *Semin Cell Dev Biol* 80:27–28, 2017.

Torres-Cuevas I, Parra-Llorca A, Sanchez-Illana A, et al.: Oxygen and oxidative stress in the perinatal period, *Redox Biol* 12:674–681, 2017.

Valenzuela FJ, Vera J, Venegas C, et al.: Circadian system and melatonin hormone: risk factors for complications during pregnancy, *Obstet Gynecol Int* 2015:825802, 2015.

van Abeelen AFM, de Rooij SR, Osmond C, et al.: The sex-specific effects of famine on the association between placental size and later hypertension, *Placenta* 32:694–698, 2011.

Vaughan OR, Rosario FJ, Powell TL, Jansson T: Regulation of placental amino acid transport and fetal growth, *Prog Mol Biol Transl Sci* 145:217–251, 2017.

Velegrakis A, Sfakiotaki M, Sifakis S: Human placental growth hormone in normal and abnormal fetal growth, *Biomed Rep* 7:115–122, 2017.

Vitale SG, Lagana AS, Rapisarda AM, et al.: Role of urocortin in pregnancy: An update and future perspectives, *World J Clin Cases* 4:165–171, 2016.

Wamaitha SE, Niakan KK: Human pregastrulation development, *Curr Top Dev Biol* 128:295–338, 2018.

9

Embryo Development and Fetal Growth

LEARNING OBJECTIVES

- To describe the formation of the bilaminar and trilaminar embryonic discs in weeks 2 and 3 of development.
- To outline the events involved in folding of the embryonic disc into the characteristic shape of the human embryo.
- To define key embryological terms: gastrulation, neurulation, primitive streak, somites and notochord.
- To outline events in embryonic development in the first 8 weeks.

- To describe developmental characteristics of the fetal organ systems.
- To discuss factors affecting fetal growth and the implications these have for future health.
- To relate the timing of development with sensitive periods and to appreciate the developmental factors limiting survival of a preterm baby.
- To outline how fetal abnormalities can result from abnormal embryonic development.

INTRODUCTION

Fetal age is timed from fertilization, whereas pregnancy is dated from the first day of the last normal menstrual period (gestational age). This means that the timing of the pregnancy is 2 weeks more than the true fetal age. The average length of pregnancy is 280 days (40 weeks) when the fetus is 266 days old (38 weeks). During the 9 months of pregnancy, the single cell of the zygote divides to produce 6 trillion cells of the mature fetus. On average, an adult cell is the product of about 47 cell divisions from the zygote, at least 40 of which occur before birth. The first 3 weeks of development are often described as the pre-embryonic period when the cells differentiate into germ layers from which all the organs and tissues develop. The sequence of events in this stage, albeit with a different time course, is similar in most multicellular animals, including *Drosophila* (fruit fly), nematodes, amphibians and birds as well as mammals. The embryonic stage, embryogenesis or organogenesis, lasts from fertilization to week 8 in the human. During this time, the organ systems are established and the embryo develops distinct human characteristics. The fetal stage, from week 9 to birth, is largely a period of growth, during which time the systems become more refined and mature as the fetus gains weight and prepares for birth. Understanding the key concepts of embryology and fetal development is important in monitoring the wellbeing of the fetus and developing appropriate healthcare programmes and interventions to promote better reproductive health outcomes. This field has important applications in prenatal diagnosis and treatments as well as prevention and management of infertility, subfertility and birth defects. Pregnant women are also obviously interested in knowing how their baby is developing and changing during the duration of the pregnancy. (Development in the 1st week after fertilization is described in Chapter 6.)

CHAPTER CASE STUDY

Zara's best friend, Aderyn attends the midwifery clinic for the first time when she is 6 weeks pregnant. This is her second pregnancy. Early in her first pregnancy last year, the fetus was discovered to have an extensive open lesion in the lumbosacral region of the spine. Sadly, this baby did not survive beyond birth.

Aderyn, prior to this pregnancy, had received prenatal care and advice (see Chapter 12) and had followed a pre-conceptual care plan in preparation for pregnancy.

- How should the midwife coordinate Aderyn's care early in this pregnancy?
- Who else should be involved in her care and what investigations and ongoing treatments will be required?

EMBRYONIC WEEK 2

By the end of the 1st week, the blastocyst has entered the uterine cavity, hatched out of the zona pellucida and started the process of implantation into the endometrial wall. Two types of cells are evident: the outer trophoblast (see Chapter 6) and the inner cell mass (also known as the embryoblast or pluriblast because the cells are pluripotent). The inner cell mass gives rise to all cell types and tissues of the embryo and also contributes towards some of the extraembryonic membranes. The undifferentiated cells from the blastocyst are embryonic stem cells (ESC), which are pluripotent (have the potential to give rise to all three embryonic germ layers) and have some potential therapeutic uses (Box 9.1). At about day 7 after fertilization, the cells of the inner cell mass start to proliferate and differentiate rapidly. The inner cell mass becomes flattened into an almost circular bilaminar embryonic disc with the cells forming two distinct layers (Fig. 9.1). The cells adjacent to the blastocyst (exocoelomic) cavity are small and appear distinctly cuboidal. These form the hypoblast or primitive endoderm layer, a transitory layer that will subsequently be replaced by the definitive endoderm (from the ectoderm), which then gives rise to the future gut and its derivatives. Cells from the hypoblast layer migrate forming a membrane called the exocoelomic or Heuser's membrane, which lines the cytotrophoblast so the blastocyst cavity is also enclosed. This is the cavity that will develop into the primitive (primary) yolk sac. The hypoblast also influences the development and position of the primitive streak and thus the embryonic axis of development.

BOX 9.1 Stem Cells

Stem cells are unspecialized cells that have the ability to self-renew and to differentiate into a number of cell types. This ability to produce a variety of differentiated cell types means that stem cells are a potential source of replacement cells that could be used to treat variety of diseases and repair damaged tissues. There are several categories of stem cells defined according to the variety of cells they are able to produce. Totipotent stem cells are able to produce all of the cells present in the fetus and adult together with those in the extraembryonic tissues such as placenta. Pluripotent cells are able to produce any cell in the body, multipotent cells can produce particular types of related cells, for example blood cells, whereas oligopotent (a few types of very similar cells) and unipotent (one cell type) have progressively more restricted lineages.

There are a number of sources of stem cells, which are usually classified as being embryonic (pluripotent) or adult (multipotent) stem cells. Embryonic stem cells (ESC) can be harvested from inner cell mass of the blastocyst (the trilaminar embryonic disc). Research using ESC is controversial because human ESC are taken from early embryos, which are destroyed. ESC can be obtained from a cloned embryo, which would make them genetically compatible with the recipient and therefore avoid the issue of immune rejection. A potentially important and recent advance is to 'persuade' differentiated cells to return to the undifferentiated stem cell state by expression of specific genes, a technique referred to as induced pluripotency (iPS). This also offers the advantage that somatic cells from an adult can be converted into stem cells and then be used to treat diseases in the same person, again, avoiding the problem of tissue immune rejection.

Adult stem cells are derived from progenitor cell populations such as bone marrow cells, which can be differentiated into liver, kidney, muscle and nerve cells as well as blood cells. Skin dermis cells can be transdifferentiated into many types of tissue including neurons, smooth muscle cells and fat cells. It is also possible that brain cells could be harvested from dead organ donors. A major concern of stem cell use is to control stem cell division and differentiation of the cells they produce to ensure that tissues are regenerated with the correct cell types but tumours do not grow.

Most adult stem cells are multipotent but some stem cells from the umbilical cord and cord blood cells are pluripotent. It is possible to reprogramme multipotent adult stem cells to become pluripotent. In some countries, parents are asked whether they would like to have their baby's cord blood cells frozen in case they can be used later in life to treat a disease. The blood is taken from the umbilical vein of the cleaned cord once the baby has been delivered; it is checked for infectious agents, tissue-typed and then stored in liquid nitrogen. Stem cells can be used either autologously (for the person they came from) or as an allogeneic treatment, where the donor and recipient are different individuals. The information given to new parents suggests a much wider use of the stem cells harvested from their baby's umbilical blood but many of these applications are currently at the research stage. To date, stem cells have been used in humans to treat leukaemia and restore eyesight using limbal stem cell therapy. The treatment of type 1 diabetes, spinal cord injuries, neurodegenerative and other diseases by stem cells is a very active area of research.

7 days

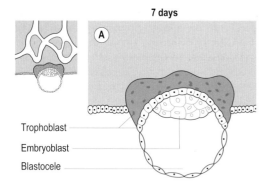

Trophoblast

Embryoblast

Blastocele

8 days

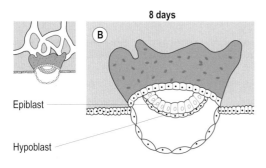

Epiblast

Hypoblast

9 days

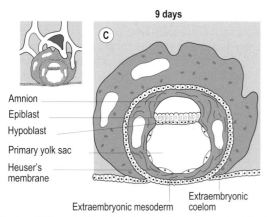

Amnion

Epiblast

Hypoblast

Primary yolk sac

Heuser's membrane

Extraembryonic mesoderm

Extraembryonic coelom

Fig. 9.1 Differentiation of the inner cell mass into the bilaminar disc: (A) 7 days; (B) 8 days; (C) 9 days. (Reproduced with permission from Fitzgerald and Fitzgerald, 1994.)

The thicker upper layer of cells of the blastocyst is formed of columnar epiblast cells, which will differentiate into the primitive ectodermal layer, which will subsequently form the embryo from the three primary germ layers. Some of the epiblast cells spread laterally to form the amnioblasts of

the amniotic membrane that encloses the amniotic cavity. The epiblast also gives rise to the extraembryonic mesoderm, which will go on to form parts of the chorion and the connecting stalk, the primordium of the umbilical cord.

There are two waves of endoderm cell remodelling of the blastocyst cavity, which form initially the primary yolk sac and then, at the beginning of the 5th week, the definitive (secondary) yolk sac (Fig. 9.2). The formation of the definitive yolk sac creates the chorionic cavity and the extraembryonic mesoderm, which gives rise to the vascular structures of the placenta (see Chapter 8). The definitive yolk sac synthesizes several proteins including alpha-fetoprotein (AFP). The bilaminar disc lies between two fluid-filled cavities: the amniotic cavity on the epiblast (ectoderm) side and the yolk sac cavity on the hypoblast (endoderm) side. (The primitive yolk sac will shrink away from the cytotrophoblast in the 4th week, creating the chorionic cavity with the extraembryonic coelom, which fills with fluid and becomes the largest cavity in the developing conceptus.)

At the end of the 2nd week, a region of endodermal cells starts to thicken and become columnar, forming the prechordal plate (Fig. 9.3). This marks the cranial region (head end) and is the site of the future mouth. At this site, the ectoderm is tightly fused to the endoderm. The prechordal plate is also important in influencing further development of the cranial structures including the eyes and the forebrain (Box 9.2).

By the 2nd week, according to the embryologist's 'rule of twos', the following have taken place:

- two germ layers have formed: the hypoblast and the epiblast
- two trophoblastic layers have formed: cytotrophoblast and syncytiotrophoblast
- two waves of remodelling have occurred: that of the blastocyst into the primary and then the definitive yolk sac
- two novel cavities have formed: the amniotic cavity and the chorionic cavity
- two layers have formed from the extraembryonic mesoderm
- prechordal plate develops indicating the site of the mouth.

EMBRYONIC WEEK 3

At this stage, when the woman may first realize she is pregnant (the week following the first missed menstrual period or she may have had a positive pregnancy test), embryo development is rapid. Three significant embryonic events occur: the primitive streak appears, the notochord develops and three germ layers differentiate forming the trilaminar disc. A line of epiblast cells, starting from the caudal region (tail end) at the other side from the prechordal plate, undergoes very rapid cell proliferation, forming the primitive streak in the midline (see Fig. 9.3). The primitive streak is a morphological sign of gastrulation on the dorsal surface of the embryonic disc. At its cranial (head) end, the primitive streak forms the primitive node. A groove is formed in the primitive streak and a small depression or pit forms in the primitive node. These are formed because some of the epiblast cells rearrange in a coordinated fashion and invaginate (move inwards) to the centre of the embryonic disc, which is known as a gastrula at this stage.

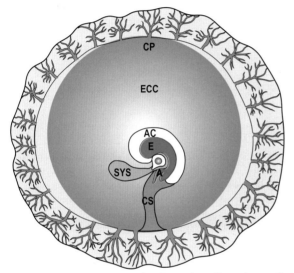

Fig. 9.2 First-trimester gestational sac about 3 weeks postfertilization, showing chorionic plate (CP) surrounding entire sac, extraembryonic coelom (ECC), amniotic cavity (AC) and embryo (E) with its secondary yolk sac (SYS) providing nutrients. (Reproduced with permission from Jauniaux et al., 2003.)

During gastrulation, the movement of cells causes the bilaminar embryonic disc to be converted into a trilaminar embryonic disc consisting of three germ layers (ectoderm, mesoderm and endoderm), which give rise to specific tissues of the body (Fig. 9.4). The middle layer is the mesoderm (loosely arranged spindle-shaped cells), from which connective tissue, smooth and skeletal muscle, the cardiovascular system and blood cells, the cartilage, bone and tendons of the skeleton and the reproductive and endocrine systems develop (Fig. 9.5). The ectoderm (columnar cells) will develop into the epidermis, central and peripheral nervous systems, the retina, parts of the ear, neural crest cells and some of the connective tissue of the head. Therefore, the ectoderm, which will give rise to the skin, is in contact with amniotic fluid in the amniotic cavity from very early on in embryonic development. The endoderm (cuboidal cells) gives rise to the epithelial linings of the gut and respiratory systems including the accessory organs of the gut and some glandular structures such as the pancreas and liver. The three germ layers interact, controlled by signalling molecules that induce cellular interactions and cause structural alterations and more complex interactions resulting in cellular differentiation.

The endodermal prechordal plate is fused to the ectoderm forming the oropharyngeal membrane (future mouth). Below the primitive streak, there is another area of fusion between the ectoderm and endoderm; this is the cloacal membrane (the future anus). Rare birth complications such as imperforate anus may arise from abnormal development of the cloacal membrane.

During gastrulation, some mesoderm cells migrate towards the prechordal plate forming a cord of adhesive cells (notogenesis) (Fig. 9.6). This cord is the notochordal process, which subsequently develops a lumen to form the notochord canal. The notochord evolves into a flexible rod-like tube that gives the trilaminar disc a

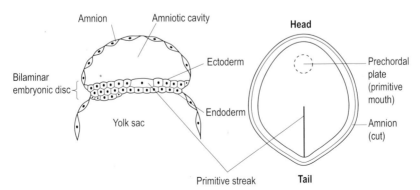

Fig. 9.3 Formation of the prechordal plate (future mouth) and primitive streak on the bilaminar and trilaminar embryonic discs.

BOX 9.2 Totipotency and Pluripotency

The zygote and cells from only the first few cell divisions of the blastocyst are termed 'totipotent', which means that each cell has the ability to develop into all cells of the organism and form all the types of body tissue. At the fourth cleavage division after fertilization, when the 8-cell embryo divides to form 16 cells, totipotency is lost. Genetic screening can be carried out at the 8-cell stage by the technique of preimplantation genetic diagnosis by removing one of the eight cells before the fourth division for analysis. Since all cells at this stage are totipotent, the zygote will develop normally from the seven remaining cells. Also, if single cells are removed at this stage into separate zona pellucidae and allowed to implant, identical offspring will develop; this 'reproductive cloning' in humans is banned on ethical grounds.

Following the loss of totipotency, the embryonic cells differentiate into pluripotent stem cells. These pluripotent cells can form any of the three types of germ cell layer (endoderm, mesoderm or ectoderm) and are therefore capable of becoming any cell in the body but cannot form a unique individual because they cannot form extraembryonic mesoderm and placental tissue.

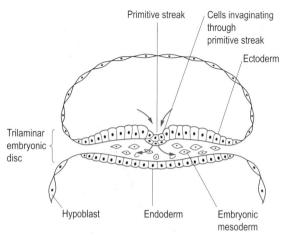

Fig. 9.4 The invagination of cells of the primitive streak between the ectodermal and endodermal layers creates a trilaminar embryonic disc. (Reproduced with permission from Fitzgerald and Fitzgerald, 1994.)

degree of rigidity and defines the central head–tail axis of the embryo. The notochord predominantly functions as a midline tissue running from head to tail that provides signals that direct the development of the surrounding tissue. If identical twins are going to develop, there are two parallel notochords. If there are two notochords that cross, conjoined (Siamese) twins result; the position where the notochords cross dictates where the twins will be conjoined, for example twins with cephalic joining have a higher crossover point of their notochords than twins who are joined at the hips (Ferrer-Vaquer and Hadjantonakis, 2013).

As well as defining the longitudinal axis of the embryo, the notochord initiates the development of the axial musculoskeletal structures (bones of head and spinal cord) and contributes to the intervertebral discs; the vertebral column forms around the notochord. Furthermore, the notochord induces neurulation and the formation of the neural plate and neural tube, which give rise to the primitive central nervous system (see below). The developing notochord induces the ectodermal layer overlying it to thicken and form a slipper-shaped neural plate, which will give rise to the central nervous system (brain and spinal cord) and the retina. During the 3rd week of embryonic

development, aggregates of mesoderm on either side of the notochord form pairs of bead-like blocks called 'somites', which direct the segmented structure of the body and induce the overlying ectoderm to form structures of the nervous system.

The formation of the primitive streak, the three germ layers, the prechordal plate and the notochord is described as gastrulation. Gastrulation marks the beginning of morphogenesis, the emergence and development of body form and structure. It begins with the appearance of the primitive streak at day 14. The primitive streak is considered to be an important concept in the bioethics of embryological research. Its presence defines the time when experimental manipulation of human embryos is legally obliged to stop under the terms of the UK Human Fertilisation and Embryology Act of 1990 (amended 2008; Box 9.3). Gastrulation is a very sensitive stage of embryogenesis; the cell populations are very vulnerable to teratogenic insult at the beginning of the 3rd week of development (Sadler, 2017). For instance, high levels of alcohol can kill cells in the craniofacial region of the embryonic disc affecting brain and face development (fetal alcohol syndrome). The primitive streak usually regresses and disappears. The very rare tumours of the neonate can be a result of remnants of primitive streak proliferating to form a sacrococcygeal teratoma (a tumour, usually nonmalignant, located at the base of the coccyx or tailbone). During the 3rd week of development, as well as gastrulation, the primitive nervous system and cardiovascular system begin to develop.

Box 9.4 is a summary of the events taking place in weeks 1–3.

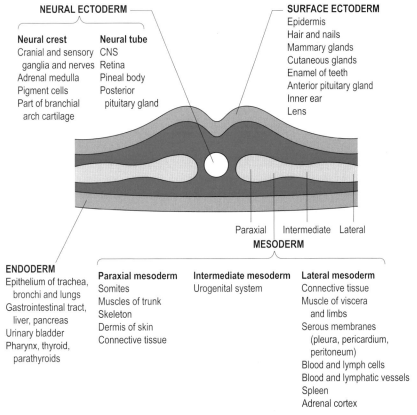

NEURAL ECTODERM

SURFACE ECTODERM
Epidermis
Hair and nails
Mammary glands
Cutaneous glands
Enamel of teeth
Anterior pituitary gland
Inner ear
Lens

Neural crest
Cranial and sensory
  ganglia and nerves
Adrenal medulla
Pigment cells
Part of branchial
  arch cartilage

Neural tube
CNS
Retina
Pineal body
Posterior
  pituitary gland

Paraxial   Intermediate   Lateral
MESODERM

ENDODERM
Epithelium of trachea,
  bronchi and lungs
Gastrointestinal tract,
  liver, pancreas
Urinary bladder
Pharynx, thyroid,
  parathyroids

Paraxial mesoderm
Somites
Muscles of trunk
Skeleton
Dermis of skin
Connective tissue

Intermediate mesoderm
Urogenital system

Lateral mesoderm
Connective tissue
Muscle of viscera
  and limbs
Serous membranes
  (pleura, pericardium,
  peritoneum)
Blood and lymph cells
Blood and lymphatic vessels
Spleen
Adrenal cortex

Fig. 9.5 The neural and surface ectoderm, the endoderm and the mesoderm will differentiate into future tissues of the body.

EMBRYONIC WEEKS 4–8: ORGANOGENESIS

During this period of embryonic development, the trilaminar disc folds into a C-shaped cylindrical embryo and all the major structures and organ systems are established. Folding is due to differential growth of parts of the embryonic disc. However, apart from the cardiovascular system, few of the systems are functioning at this stage. Organogenesis, the development of the organ systems, is a critical period during which the processes are susceptible to external influences that can cause disruption and subsequent serious congenital abnormalities. By the end of the 8th week, the embryo becomes known as the fetus and has a distinct human appearance (Fig. 9.7). Human growth and development can be crudely classified as three types:

- Growth: cell division
- Morphogenesis: development of form, shape, size and peculiar features of organ systems, etc. This is controlled by a choreographed sequence of precise and coordinated changes in the expression and regulation of specific genes and involves cells changing fate, size, shape, location and interactions with other cells
- Differentiation: maturation of cells forming tissues and organs capable of specialized function.

Growth is achieved by hyperplasia (cell division) and hypertrophy (increase in cell size). Initially the cells are pluripotent stem cells, which are similar and not differentiated or specialized into any particular cell type; they have the capability to follow different routes of development. Embryonic development is controlled by the genetic code but involves synchronized interaction of both genetic and environmental components, which control cell and tissue interactions, regulated cell proliferation and migration and apoptosis (Moore et al., 2015). The cells differentiate into one of the more than 200 different cell types found in the body, in two phases. Before differentiation occurs, there is a stage of determination during which the cell becomes restricted in its capability to develop along different pathways. As the cells differentiate fully, they develop specific morphological and functional characteristics of mature and complex specialized cells.

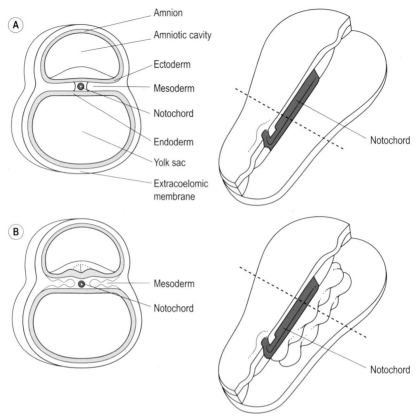

Fig. 9.6 Notochord formation: (A) 17 days and (B) 18 days. (Reproduced with permission from Goodwin, 1997.)

Differentiation is initiated and coordinated by the establishment of a signalling centre or polarizing region in a small bud of undifferentiated cells, for example, in the development of the vertebrate limb. This process by which cells influence the surrounding cells to develop in a specific way is known as induction. Induction involves the surrounding cells or cellular matrix ('inducers') to produce signals, which have an effect on the responding cells ('responders') via cell receptors. The signal may be a diffusible molecule such as a protein secreted by a cell. In the mammalian signalling pathway that controls development, the observation that mutations in the genes controlling differentiation resulted in the embryos developing spine-like projections led to the signalling molecules endearingly being named hedgehogs (Sonic hedgehog, Indian hedgehog and Desert hedgehog). As well as the signal being a diffusible molecule, which can travel from the inducing tissue to the reacting tissue, the signal may require contact with the extracellular matrix or to be translated into an intracellular signal.

Competence is the capacity to respond to the signal from an inducer, which requires the responding tissue to be activated by a competence factor. The inducing signal may be nonspecific but the reacting tissue can generate a specific response. The reacting tissue needs to express both the receptor for the signal and the intracellular components of the pathways, which result in the signal–receptor activation causing downstream effects. If any of the components are missing or are not expressed in a specific window of time, induction of the response will fail. These signal–response interactions often involve epithelial cells, which are usually joined together forming tubes or sheets, and mesenchyme cells, which are more dispersed. For instance, the epithelial cells forming the lining of the gut interact with the neighbouring mesenchyme cells to form the gut-associated organs such as the pancreas and liver and the epithelial tissue interacts with the limb mesenchyme cells to produce the initial limb buds. Continued signalling or 'crosstalk' between the different cell types allows differentiation to progress. The

BOX 9.3 Human Fertilisation and Embryology Act

This is an act of the UK parliament, which was originally passed into law in 1990 and reviewed in 2008 to take into account scientific and social change. It regulates all embryos created by processes outside the body including 'human-admixed' or hybrid embryos created from human and animal tissue for research purposes. The hybrid embryos usually have very little animal tissue (<1%) and are used to create stem cells. Other types of hybrid embryos are permitted including true chimeras, transgenic human embryos (with genetically modified DNA to include a few animal genes) and true hybrid embryos (for instance, as a result of a human egg being fertilized by an animal sperm. The hybrid embryonic tissue can be used to study genetic defects; it is only permitted to be kept in culture for a maximum of 14 days (and cannot be implanted into uterine tissue).

The Act bans sex selection for nonmedical reasons (it is permitted for medical reasons, usually that males will be affected by a serious disease such as an X-linked disorder, e.g. Duchenne muscular dystrophy). The Act established the provisions to recognize same-sex couples as legal parents of children conceived using donated tissue and considered the welfare of any child created; it replaced the term 'need for a father' to 'the need for supportive parenting' (which opponents of the Bill argued denigrated the role of the father). It also lifted the restrictions on the access to the data collected to facilitate follow-up research of infertility treatment. The act also considered preimplantation diagnosis and tissue typing to generate a 'saviour sibling' who is a tissue match for an older sibling with an untreatable genetic condition. Bone marrow cells or stem cells from the umbilical cord of the saviour sibling can be used to treat the older sibling. Further information including extensive explanatory notes can be found at: www.legislation.gov.uk

BOX 9.4 Summary of Pre-embryonic Period: Weeks 1–3

Week 1: Fertilization to Produce Zygote
- Cleavage of zygote while travelling in uterine tube
- Cell division without increase in mass to form the morula
- Fluid accumulation: hollow blastocyst formed
- 'Hatching' out of zona pellucida
- Blastocyst cells differentiate into trophoblast and inner cell mass
- Implantation in decidual wall

Week 2: Inner Cell Mass Forms Bilaminar Embryonic Disc of Hypoblast and Epiblast
- Trophoblast differentiates into dividing cytotrophoblast and invasive syncytiotrophoblast (see Chapter 8)
- Lateral movement of cells from epiblast layer encloses yolk sac, forming the extraembryonic mesoderm
- Prechordal plate (mouth) develops at caudal end
- Day 14: primitive streak develops

Week 3: Gastrulation
- Cells from primitive streak invaginate and migrate between the epiblast and the hypoblast forming the mesoderm
- Trilaminar disc of three germ layers: ectoderm (epiblast), mesoderm and ectoderm (hypoblast)
- Notochord forms, inducing development of the neural plate and giving rise to axis of development
- Somites become evident
- Neurulation begins

activate or inhibit gene expression. Juxtacrine factor signalling involves proteins on the surface of one cell or in the extracellular matrix interacting with the receptor on the surface of another cell or signals being transmitted from one cell to another via gap junctions. Differentiation can allow some plasticity. Branching morphogenesis is the formation of branched epithelial tubules, which is essential to the development of several tissues including the kidneys, lungs, breasts and salivary glands.

One of the cornerstones of embryology is the concept that cells of the three layers of the developing embryo migrate to the final destinations (Paluch et al., 2016). The migrating cells are polarized (i.e. have a front and back and a specific direction of movement, which is related to the intracellular cytoskeleton arrangement) to sense chemical signals and 'home' towards them by amoeboid (crawling) movement, which involves pushing out a leading edge of

crosstalk occurs by the cells producing growth and differentiation factors, which act at a paracrine (involving diffusible factors) or juxtacrine (involving nondiffusible factors) level.

Paracrine factors act by triggering a signalling transduction pathway in which a signalling molecule (or 'ligand') interacts with its receptor often triggering enzymatic activity in the receptor or receptor-interacting proteins, which then initiate a cascade of protein phosphorylation steps (see Chapter 3) that terminate with a transcription factor being activated. The transcription factor can then

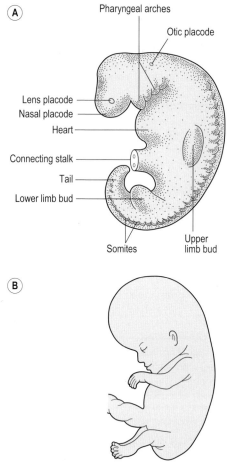

Fig. 9.7 (A) 4-week-old and (B) 8-week-old fetus. ((A) Reproduced with permission from Fitzgerald and Fitzgerald, 1994.)

the cell and pulling the trailing edge. In gastrulation, cell migration leads to the formation of the three layers of the trilaminar disc, which then migrate to target regions where they differentiate. For instance, the muscle precursor cells migrate from the somites to their targets in the limbs. Failure of cells to migrate at all or to the correct location is thought to result in abnormalities or to have life-threatening consequences. For instance, congenital defects in brain development leading to neurodevelopmental disorders, such as intellectual disability, schizophrenia, autism and epilepsy, are ascribed to abnormal neuronal positioning due to defective cell migration (Moffat et al., 2015). Collective cell migration also occurs in postnatal life and is central to other physiological processes such as effective immune responses and repair of injured tissues in the wound healing process (Scarpa and Mayor, 2016). Migration can also occur in pathological processes, including vascular disease and tumour metastasis, in which some tumour cells migrate to new sites where they form secondary tumours. Apoptosis or programmed cell death is another mechanism important in embryonic development. Apoptosis involves the cells effectively autodestructing in a precisely timed manner. For example, neurons in the developing brain or the embryo digits, which are initially fused until the tissue between them breaks down, separating them. However, if the latter process goes wrong, for example with mutations in bone morphogenic proteins (BMPs), separation may be incomplete so that animals are born with webbed fingers and toes (syndactyly). Embryogenesis also involves cell recognition and adhesion.

Folding

The disc-like arrangement of the germ layers is converted into a recognizable C-shaped vertebral embryo by folding in the 4th week of development. Folding is due to a differential rate in growth of the different parts of the embryo. The embryo is in a contained space so as it grows, it curves and ridges of tissues form. The embryonic disc grows rapidly particularly in the long axis, because of the growth of the brain and tail, so folding occurs at the cranial (head) and caudal (tail) ends of the disc. Although this is a momentous stage of development, relatively little is known about it. The yolk sac does not grow and, as the outer rim of the endoderm is attached to the yolk sac, the embryo becomes convex or 'C'-shaped. Folding occurs at the cephalic (head) and lateral regions on day 22 and at the caudal (tail) end of the embryo on day 23 (Fig. 9.8). Rapid growth of the spinal cord and somites causes the lateral folding. The cephalic, lateral and caudal edges of the embryonic disc are brought into apposition and the layers fuse along the midline, which transforms the endoderm into the gut tube. Initially the foregut and the hindgut fuse, leaving the midgut open to the yolk sac. The folds cause a constriction between the embryo and yolk sac. The yolk sac gives rise to the primitive gut. The amnion expands, enveloping the connecting stalk and neck of the yolk sac, forming the umbilical cord. Folding is precisely coordinated and is controlled. Failure at this point results in abdominal wall defects such as omphalocele and gastroschisis (failure of the gut to be fully enclosed within the abdominal wall).

The developmental pattern involves synchronized tissue communication, interaction and differing growth rates. Adjacent tissues induce changes in the movement and behaviour of neighbouring cells. These are well-controlled and dynamic events. Signals integrating genetic and environmental influences control cell proliferation, migration, autophagy and apoptosis (Agnello et al., 2015). The classification of regulated cell death is changing as our

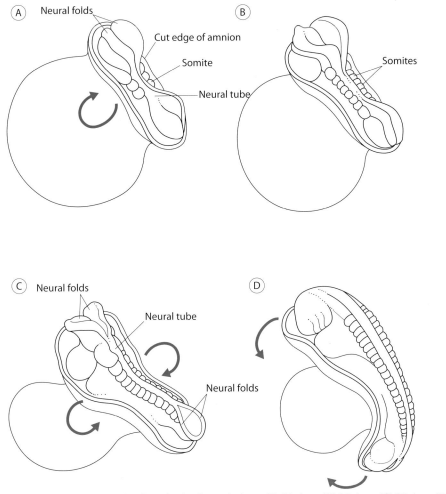

Fig. 9.8 Folding of the embryonic disc into the fetal morphology: (A) 21 days; (B) 22 days; (C) 23 days; (D) 25 days. (Reproduced with permission from Goodwin, 1997.)

understanding of the mechanisms involved improves. Simplistically, cell death can be classified into three types: type 1 (apoptosis); type 2 (autophagy); and type 3 (necrosis). Apoptosis is a form of programmed cell death where a cell is triggered to commit suicide either by the activation of death receptors on its plasma membrane (e.g. by cytotoxic T cells) or by the release of cytochrome c from the mitochondria. In response to signals due to cell stress (intrinsic pathway) or from other cells (extrinsic pathway), the cells undergo a series of characteristic changes such as plasma membrane blebbing, loss of the mitochondrial membrane potential, caspase activation, DNA fragmentation, flipping of phosphatidylserine from the inner to the outer leaflet of the cell membrane and the formation of apoptotic bodies. Dying cells retain their otherwise inflammatory content

and signal their demise to macrophages which then engulf and degrade them into harmless noninflammatory products. Apoptosis is an energy dependent process (requires ATP) and is involved in the removal of transient or unrequired structures, to alter tissues and to remove damaged cells.

Autophagy is a pathway by which cellular components and organelles are degraded and recycled so cell resources are conserved. Cell death will be induced by autophagy if the cell is badly damaged but cells will survive if the damage is repairable. Autophagy involves destruction by hydrolytic enzymes from lysosomes and can result in many cells being eliminated. It also protects cells from metabolic stress. During embryogenesis, both apoptosis and autophagy are important in the removal of extraneous cells and to control cell fate by restricting cell number and organizing morphogenesis and pattern formation; these two processes of cell death exhibit complex crosstalk pathways and cooperate to increase or limit cell death.

Although all cells have the same DNA in their nuclei, the pattern of gene expression will differ depending on the signals received giving rise to cell differentiation and the existence of >200 distinct cell types in humans. For example, a skin cell expresses the genes that control the behaviour of a skin cell because they are switched on by the signals skin cells receive. A liver cell has the same genes as the skin cell but expresses different genes. In addition to regulation of gene expression by myriad activators and repressors, epigenetic modification of DNA (see Chapter 7) can also control whether the gene is silenced or expressed.

The Organization of the Basic Body Plan

Techniques and concepts used to study molecular genetics (how the genetic code is expressed) in bacteria, yeast, *Caenorhabditis elegans* (*C. elegans*), *Drosophila*, sea urchin and mice can be applied to mammalian embryogenesis, including human development. The DNA in the nucleus codes for the basic body plan, which establishes the developmental pattern of the early embryo. The genes that control the basic body plan are evolutionarily highly conserved, i.e. the same in very diverse species. This region of about 180 base pairs of DNA, known as the 'homeobox', is found in the genes that regulate anatomical development (morphogenesis) of the embryo. The homeobox encodes a protein domain called the homeodomain, which can bind to DNA specifically. Homeobox genes encode transcription factors that switch on cascades of other genes, for instance all the ones needed to make a particular body part. Other morphogenic agents, signals and growth factors activate the homeobox genes. *Hox* genes are a particular subgroup of homeobox genes, which are found in a special gene cluster, the HOX cluster. *Hox* genes determine the patterning of the body axis. They direct the identity of particular body regions, determining where limbs and other body segments will develop in the fetus. Limb abnormalities such as polydactyly (extra digits) may result from abnormal *Hox* genes. There appears to be a series of three sequential steps in the conversion of the oval trilaminar embryonic disc into the cylindrical configuration with the endoderm on the inside, the ectoderm on the outside and the mesoderm in between (Fig. 9.9) (Carlson, 2018). These steps result in segmentation of the embryo. Gap genes subdivide the embryo into broad regional domains along the anterior–posterior axis. Pair-rule genes are involved in the formation of individual body segments

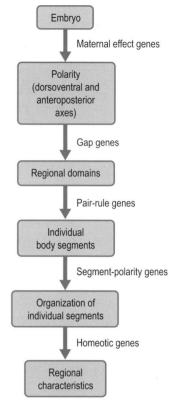

Fig. 9.9 Organization of the vertebrate body plan.

(mirror image of left and right) and segment-polarity genes control the anterior–posterior organization of each segment. As the embryo develops, the segmental plan becomes less evident; remnants can be seen in the arrangement of the backbone and ribs and abdominal muscles and in the organization of the spinal nerves.

Box 9.5 summarizes the events taking place during weeks 4–8.

NINTH WEEK TO BIRTH: FETAL PERIOD

During this period, the fetal body grows rapidly and the tissues and organs differentiate and mature (see below). The head growth rate becomes relatively slower so, by birth, the length of the head is about a quarter of the total length. Growth rate and the greatest straight or crown–rump length can be used to assess embryonic or fetal age (Box 9.6) and ultrasound examination can be used to examine developmental details and external characteristics of the embryo (Box 9.7). With neonatal expert care, a fetus can be viable and may survive birth from 22 weeks (see Chapter 13), although morbidity is higher with earlier age at birth.

BOX 9.5   Summary of Embryonic Period: Weeks 4–8

4th Week

- 4–12 somites are prominent
- Neural tube fusing but neuropores open at rostral (anterior) and caudal ends
- Folding produces characteristic C-shaped curved embryo
- Otic (auditory) pits present (primitive ear)
- Optic vesicles formed
- Upper limb buds appear (as small swellings), then lower limb buds
- Five pairs of pharyngeal (brachial) arches present (craniofacial rudiments: will form face, jaw, ear and neck)
- Beating heart prominent
- Forebrain prominent
- Attenuated tail
- Rudiments of organ systems established
- Rostral neuropore, then caudal neuropore, close
- Crown–rump length (CRL) 4–6 mm

5th Week

- Rapid brain development and head enlargement (cephalization)
- Facial prominences develop
- Upper limb buds become paddle-shaped
- Lower limb buds are flipper-like
- Mesonephric ridges denote position of mesonephric (interim) kidneys
- CRL 7–9 mm

6th Week

- Joints of upper limbs differentiate
- Digital rays (fingers) of upper limbs evident

- External ear canal and auricle (pinna) formed
- Retinal pigment formed so eye is obvious
- Head very large, projects over heart prominence
- Spontaneous movements and reflex responses to touch
- CRL 11–14 mm

7th Week

- Notches between digital rays partially separate future fingers and toes
- Liver prominent
- Rapidly growing intestines herniate out of small abdominal cavity into umbilical cord
- CRL 16–18 mm

8th Week

- Digits of hand start to separate (but still webbed)
- Notches visible between digital rays of feet
- Stubby tail disappears
- Purposeful limb movements occur
- Ossification begins in long bones of lower limbs
- Head still disproportionately large (about half of total embryo length)
- Eyelids closing
- Ears are characteristic shape but still low set
- External genitalia evident (but differences not distinct enough for sexual identification)
- CRL 27–31 mm

Box 9.8 is a summary of the changes during the fetal period.

DEVELOPMENT OF ORGAN SYSTEMS

The Central Nervous System

Neurulation is the formation of the neural plate and neural folds and the closure of these folds to form the neural tube, which is the precursor of the brain and spinal cord. The neural tube is completed by the end of the 4th week. The developing notochord induces the overlying ectoderm to thicken forming the neural plate, a raised slipper-like plate of neuroepithelial cells. This will give rise to the central nervous system (brain and spinal cord) and other structures such as the retina. In the middle of the 3rd week, the neural groove appears in the centre of the neural plate (Fig. 9.10). To each side of the groove are neural folds, which enlarge

BOX 9.6   Estimation of Embryonic/Fetal Age and Stage of Gestation

- Greatest length (GL) is used to measure embryos of about 3 weeks, which are straight
- CRL (crown–rump length) is equivalent to sitting height, and is used to measure older, curved embryos (though note growth rate is often slower before embryonic death)
- Size of the chorionic cavity
- Carnegie embryonic staging system uses external characteristics to estimate developmental stage
- Number of somites
- Fetal head measurements, such as biparietal diameter and head circumference
- Abdominal circumference
- Femur length and foot length

BOX 9.7 Ultrasound Examination

- Estimation of size and age of fetus (embryo)
- Detection of congenital abnormality
- Detection of antenatal soft markers (such as nuchal thickness, hypoplastic nasal bone, shortened fetal long bones, single umbilical artery) indicates increased risk of chromosomal and other abnormality
- Evaluation of growth rate
- Investigation of uterine abnormality or ectopic pregnancy
- Guidance for chorionic villus sampling

at the cranial end as the start of the developing brain. Marked development of the brain is a characteristic of embryonic development in primates; human brain growth exceeds that of other primate species. At the end of the 3rd week, the neural folds start to fuse forming the neural tube, which separates from the surface ectoderm. The neural crest cells, which detach from the lateral edges of the neural folds, give rise to the spinal ganglia and ganglia of the autonomic system as well as a number of other cell types (Box 9.9). The paraxial mesoderm, closest to the notochord and developing neural tube, differentiates to form prominent paired blocks of tissue, or somites. The first somites appear from day 20. There are about 30 pairs of somites by day 30

BOX 9.8 Summary of Changes in the Fetal Period

9–12 Weeks
- Growth in body length and limbs accelerates
- Ears are low set, eyes are fused
- Primary ossification centres develop in skeleton, notably skull and long bones
- Intestines return to abdominal cavity and body wall fuses
- Erythropoiesis (formation of red blood cells) decreases in liver and begins in spleen
- Urine formation begins
- Fetal swallowing of amniotic fluid

13–16 Weeks
- Rapid growth
- Coordinated limb movements (not felt by mother)
- Active ossification of skeleton
- Slow eye movements
- Ovaries differentiated and contain primordial follicles
- External genitalia recognizable
- Eyes and ears closer to normal positions

17–20 Weeks
- Growth slows down
- Limbs reach mature proportions
- Fetal movements felt by mother ('quickening')
- Skin covered with protective layer of vernix caseosa, held in position by lanugo (downy hair)
- Brown fat deposited

21–25 Weeks
- Fetus gains weight
- Skin wrinkled and translucent, appears red–pink

- Rapid eye movements begin
- Blink-startle responses to noise
- Surfactant secretion begins but respiratory system immature
- Fingernails are present
- May be viable if born prematurely

26–29 Weeks
- Lungs capable of breathing air
- Central nervous system can control breathing
- Eyes open
- Toenails visible
- Fat (3.5% body weight) deposited under skin so wrinkles smooth out
- Erythropoiesis moves from spleen to bone marrow

30–34 Weeks
- Pupillary light reflex
- Skin pink and smooth, limbs chubby
- White fat is about 8% of body weight
- From 32 weeks, survival is usual

35–38 Weeks
- Firm grasp
- Orientates towards light
- Circumference of head and abdomen are approximately equal
- White fat is about 16% of body weight, 14 g fat gained per day
- Skin appears bluish-pink
- Term fetus is about 3400 g, crown–rump length is about 360 mm

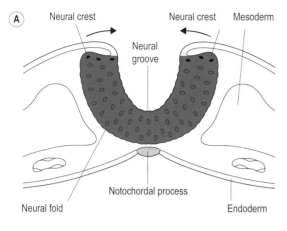

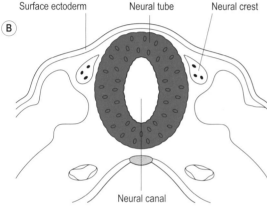

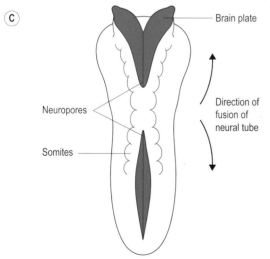

Fig. 9.10 The neural groove and neural tube fusion: (A) 21 days; (B) and (C) 23 days.

BOX 9.9 Tissues Arising from Cells of the Neural Crest

- Spinal ganglia
- Ganglia of the autonomic system
- Adrenal medulla
- Thyroid gland
- Glial cells
- Schwann cells
- Melanocytes (pigmented)
- Pharyngeal arch cartilage
- Odontoblasts (of teeth)
- Pupillary and ciliary muscles of eye
- Dermis and hypodermis of neck and face
- Meninges

---

increasing to a total of 44 pairs, but the cranial ones begin differentiation as new somites are added at the caudal end. The somites differentiate into sclerotomes, myotomes and dermatomes, which give rise to the axial skeletal bones, skeletal muscles and the dermis of the skin, respectively. The number of somites indicates the age of the embryo. The limbs carry with them the nerves from the somites from which they developed. The somatic pattern of development is important in understanding referred pain (see Chapter 13).

Neural tube defects (NTD) are one of the most common congenital abnormalities (see Chapter 12), resulting from the partial or complete failure of the neural tube to close during embryogenesis. Neurulation begins in the middle of the neural tube and proceeds cranially (towards the head) and caudally (towards the tail). Anencephaly (absent brain) results if the neural tube fails to close in the cranial region so the brain and spinal cord fail to develop properly and are fully exposed to the exterior; this condition is lethal and most cases are diagnosed by antenatal ultrasound scans and the pregnancies terminated. Failure of neurulation at the caudal end results in spina bifida. The extent to which spina bifida results in loss of neurological function depends on the severity of the lesion, the number of differing layers that have failed to fuse and the level of the lesion in the spinal cord. The most common site for spina bifida is the lumbosacral region, which suggests that close of the neural tube in this region is more susceptible to environmental and genetic influences. Neurulation is very sensitive to disturbances such as teratogenic drugs or lack of folate, which is required for DNA synthesis of the rapidly dividing cells (see Chapter 7).

Most neurons are formed between 10 and 18 weeks; this is therefore the critical window or period for brain development. Undernutrition or other insults in the first trimester may result in microcephaly (small cerebral cortex and cranial vault) because there is impaired neural stem cell proliferation and fewer neurons are produced. The head circumference is usually >2 or 3 standard deviations below the mean and because the face grows at a normal rate, the head has a characteristic shape. Congenital microcephaly is also associated with environmental factors such as cytomegalovirus, rubella (German measles), or varicella (chicken pox) virus infections and toxoplasmosis as well as genetic disorders such as trisomy 18 (Edward syndrome). Zika virus, which was declared a Public Health Emergency of International Concern by the WHO for a period in 2016, is transmitted by mosquitos and can cause microcephaly in the fetus, despite many pregnant women having mild symptoms (Merfeld et al., 2017). Microcephaly can also be due to degeneration of the brain and may develop after birth. Microcephaly can also be a genetic abnormality. Mutations of the gene for the abnormal spindle-like microcephaly-associated protein (*ASPM*) can cause microcephaly. The *ASPM* gene product is required for regulation of spindle assembly in mitosis of the neuroblasts (primitive nerve stem cells that produce neurons). It is thought that strong positive selection of the *APSM* gene was responsible for a significantly increased size of the cerebral cortex in primate evolution (Rosales-Reynoso et al., 2018). Although this appeared to be supported by the observation that a novel allele of the gene arose about the same time as contemporary human populations developed agriculture and cities and began to use written language, the relationship between *APSM* alleles and brain size and neuronal development has been questioned (Woodley et al., 2014). Microcephaly usually results in intellectual disability, abnormal head size and facial features, poor motor function, seizures and poor development of speech because of the absence of a normal sized cerebral cortex. Although intellectual disability can result from genetic abnormalities and exposure to teratogens such as viruses, the leading causes of intellectual disability are maternal alcohol and drug abuse causing disorders such as the fetal alcohol spectrum.

In later gestation, undernutrition affects the growth of the organs; however, the brain size seems to be protected by blood and nutrients being redistributed to the brain at the expense of other tissues. As brain size in humans is proportionately larger, the effects of protecting the brain size from undernutrition may be exaggerated compared with other species. However, this concept has been challenged because the human brain develops gradually and has a high energy requirement, and it has been suggested that its plasticity may make its development particularly vulnerable to even moderate undernutrition (Giussani, 2011). Glial cells (neuroglia) begin to develop at about 15 weeks. These are the groups of non-neuronal cells that support, protect and provide oxygen and nutrients to the neurons, maintain homeostasis and produce myelin; they include oligodendrocytes, microglia, astrocytes, ependymal cells, Schwann cells and satellite cells. Most of the glial cells originate from the neural crest cells and neural tube. In the second half of pregnancy, the glial cells hypertrophy and the axons and dendrites undergo marked growth in length. This rapid nervous system growth spurt continues until the second postnatal year and at a slower rate for at least the first decade, and is unique to humans who have an usually large brain for their body size (Sousa et al., 2017). The relatively slow development of the human brain, particularly in infancy and early childhood, has led to the worldwide public health policy emphasis on the 'first 1000 days' (conception until about 2 years) and '0–3' (years), as this period has a significant effect on the final function and structure of the brain (Cusick and Georgieff, 2016). This is the time when early brain development is most vulnerable to stress and inflammation, issues with social support and attachment, and whether optimal nutrition is available. The fetal response to impaired nutrition tends to 'spare' the brain at the cost of somatic growth, hence the asymmetric (disproportionate) growth patterns of babies born after intrauterine growth retardation (IUGR) where their heads seem disproportionately bigger. However, neither brain function nor neurology is perfectly protected; neuronal number tends to be reduced and myelination disturbed. The fetal (and infant) brain is more vulnerable to insults but has a higher level of plasticity so it can recover to some extent. The effects of nutritional deficiencies and stress have different outcomes depending on their timing, dose and duration because parts of the brain undergo development and growth in different critical windows (Lindsay et al., 2019). Brain development is also vulnerable to hypoxia; the fetus compensates for a lack of oxygen by decreasing oxygen consumption and redistributing blood flow to essential regions such as the brain (Giussani, 2016).

Human brain size, particularly brain:body ratio, is enormous compared with other primate species. Bite muscles of the jaw are very strong and enclose the skull in nonhuman primates. It is hypothesized that early humans (~2.4 million years ago) developed a single gene mutation that resulted in humans being unable to produce one of the main proteins (MYH16) usually present in primate jaw muscles (Stedman et al., 2004). The weaker jaw muscles relaxed their grip on the skull, allowing the human brain to grow and expand. Alternative explanations suggest that environmental changes forced humans to invent tools and develop manual dexterity, that natural selection favoured bigger brains because they permitted more complex and supportive societies or that evolution in an environmental niche where marine food provided a good source of long chain fatty acids allowed marked brain development (Wroe et al., 2010); this is known as the 'Aquatic Ape' theory. Impaired nutrition, particularly early in development, permanently affects brain size and cell number (assessed by head circumference estimated by ultrasound measurement); neurodevelopmental abnormalities occur at increased frequency in IUGR children.

Fetal sensory organs develop around the middle of gestation. At 24 weeks, the fetus will respond to noise and stimulation such as tapping on the maternal abdomen. As gestation progresses, the fetus exhibits increased sensitivity and responds to an increased range of sound frequencies. Babies are thought to enjoy being carried and cuddled because they can hear sounds of their mother's heart, breathing and digestive system, to which they became accustomed *in utero*. This is why kangaroo care has become popular where babies are bound close to the maternal or paternal chest by soft material such as a papoose or shawl.

Gastrointestinal System

The gut begins as a single tube running from mouth to anus. The mouth and anus are fused areas of endoderm and ectoderm (see above). The tube is therefore fixed at both ends so that when it grows it convolutes and loops (Fig. 9.11). Some parts of the tube dilate, such as the stomach and colon, and the gut rotates around other structures such as the developing liver. Between the 6th and 8th week of development, the proliferation of the epithelial cells lining the gut obliterates the lumen, which is then gradually recanalized. Early growth of the gut is extremely rapid so it extrudes into the amniotic cavity. If it is not withdrawn at about 10 weeks, the abdominal wall fails to close and the baby is born with exomphalos (omphalocele) or gastroschisis; some of the gut or abdominal organs remain outside the abdominal wall at birth. The incidence of gastroschisis is increasing; it is more common in infants born to young underweight mothers, and to those who smoke or drink. Gastroschisis can be detected by ultrasound and by raised AFP levels in amniotic fluid and maternal serum. Normal fusion of the lateral body folds occurs at the linea nigra, the abdominal line that becomes pigmented in pregnant women (see Chapter 11). Normal growth of the gut depends on fetal swallowing. A fetus swallows about one-third of the total volume of amniotic fluid per hour by the 16th week of development. Not only does amniotic fluid provide about 10% of the fetal protein requirements but it also seems to be associated with effective development of the gastrointestinal mucosa, liver and pancreas and promotion of growth.

The digestive enzymes are present from about 24–28 weeks, with the exception of lactase, which is expressed later in fetal life. Peristaltic coordination of the fetal gut is evident from the 14th week of development. By 34 weeks there is coordination of sucking, swallowing and peristalsis. As the gut matures, it produces mucus, which will

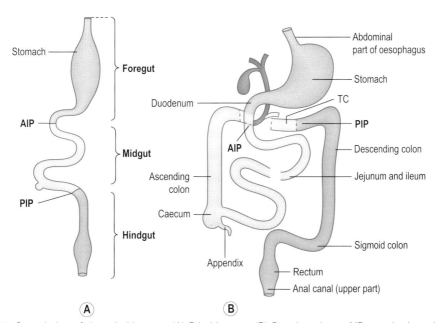

Fig. 9.11 Convolution of the primitive gut. (A) Primitive gut. (B) Developed gut. AIP, anterior intestinal portal; PIP, posterior intestinal portal; TC, transverse colon. (Reproduced from Singh V, *Textbook of clinical embryology* 2 ed, Elsevier 2017, Fig. 13.5.)

eventually be required to lubricate the passage of food and faeces during transit. The mucus accumulates in the fetal gut as meconium (a combination of mucus and products secreted by the liver). Adrenaline, produced in response to fetal distress, stimulates contractions of the gut and can lead to meconium-stained amniotic fluid. This is common in premature labour from 34 weeks and in postmature labour (over 42 weeks); meconium staining of the liquor is rare before 34 weeks but can been observed in maternal listeriosis infections. The assumption that the fetal gut is sterile until birth has recently been challenged (see Chapter 16). There is emerging evidence, from the identification of bacteria or bacterial products in the amniotic fluid, placenta, fetal membranes and meconium (Collado et al., 2016), that suggests the seeding of the gut microbiota (see Chapter 15) starts *in utero*. The source of these bacteria may be by bacterial translocation from the maternal circulation and/or from the vaginal tract (Stinson et al., 2017).

The pancreas, liver and gall bladder all originate from evaginations of the lining of the gut tube. The liver reaches metabolic maturity relatively late in gestation, storing glycogen in the last 9 weeks. Inadequate placental transfer of amino acids will affect tissues with high protein requirement such as liver, gut and skeletal muscle (Vaughan et al., 2017). The placenta is extremely metabolically active and extracts 40–60% of glucose and oxygen from the maternal circulation, some of which transfers from maternal to fetal circulation and then is re-extracted from the fetal circulation. In IUGR, the rate of placental extraction from the fetal circulation increases and can lead to loss of lean body mass from the fetus and wasting. There is a hierarchy: the fetus may become catabolic to nourish the placenta and both fetus and placenta may be compromised in attempting to sustain maternal requirements. As hepatic stores of glycogen and fat are mobilized in IUGR, the liver is the first organ affected as its glycogen is depleted so the head:abdomen ratio is an important indicator of IUGR (because the size of the liver makes a significant contribution to the abdominal circumference). The fetal liver has important roles in both the development of the immune system and as a source of fetal blood cells. Haematopoiesis is a major function of the liver during fetal life. The haematopoietic stem cells, from which blood cells develop, undergo a huge expansion in the fetal liver before they relocate to their final site in the bone marrow. Progenitor B-lymphocytes (see Chapter 10) develop in the fetal liver. The liver retains hepatic cells throughout life and is one of the few organs that can regenerate (to some degree) in postnatal life. The fetal liver is a potential source of stem cells for regenerative medicine related to therapy for liver and pancreas (Semeraro et al., 2013).

CASE STUDY 9.1

At 11 weeks' gestation, Julie has an ultrasound scan. She is asked to return for a further scan in 2 weeks as her unborn baby appears to have some gut tissue herniating into the umbilical cord. Julie seeks advice from her midwife.
- Is this normal?
- How might you reassure Julie that the ultrasonographer was just being cautious?
- If there were a pathological condition present, what two conditions are most likely?
- How would they be further investigated before Julie is advised upon the prognosis?
- What specific care and planning would be required to facilitate safe delivery and aftercare if an abdominal abnormality is diagnosed?

Case study 9.1 is an example of developmental abnormality of the gut.

The Face and Neck

The face is formed between weeks 5 and 12 from the pharyngeal apparatus, which is made up of the pharyngeal (brachial) arches, pouches, grooves and membranes derived from neural crest cells. The pharyngeal arches form the face, nasal cavity, mouth, larynx, pharynx and neck. The endoderm of the pouches forms the parathyroid glands, thymus, tonsils and middle ear. The thyroid gland begins as epithelial cell proliferation of the tongue, which descends towards the trachea. The nose grows downwards as a pillar of tissue (Fig. 9.12). Initially the nose is flat but by 14 weeks' gestation, facial development is completed and the nose, chin, lips and cheeks exhibit their characteristic shapes. The eyes, which are formed from a combination of nervous tissue and specialized ectoderm, are initially in a lateral position but move medially. The ears are initially low-set (note that low-set ears that persist are often an indicator (marker) of chromosomal abnormalities and syndromes). Below the nose, maxillary and mandibular processes extend to form the floor of the nose and the roof of the mouth. The upper lip is formed from processes that extend to meet centrally. Inadequate fusion of the maxillary processes causes congenital malformations of the mouth, such as cleft lip and/or palate. Palatal fusion is complete by the 11th week.

The Skeleton and Skull

The skeleton develops from the mesoderm layer and the neural crest. Most bones are formed initially from condensed mesenchyme tissue as cartilage, which then

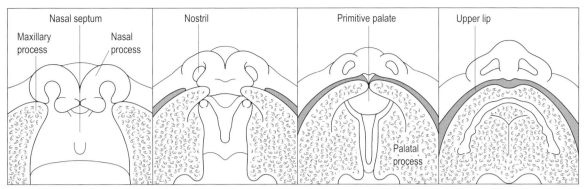

Fig. 9.12 Growth of the palate and nose between the 6th and 9th week. (Reproduced with permission from James and Stephenson, 1998.)

undergoes ossification. The ribs and vertebral column develop from the sclerotome components of the somites. The skull develops from mesenchymal tissue surrounding the brain. It is formed from the neurocranium, which protects the brain, and the viscerocranium, which forms the skeleton of the face. Each of these elements of the skull has membranous and cartilaginous components. Ossification is of the membrane rather than of cartilage and begins from the base of the skull.

The bones of the calvaria (cranial vault) have not completed development at birth. In the fetus, the flat bones of the calvaria are held together by soft fibrous sutures made of dense connective tissue, which allows some flexibility. The fetal head can mould to the shape of the maternal pelvis and distort as it passes through the birth canal. During delivery, the frontal bone becomes flatter, the occipital bone is drawn out and the parietal bones overlap (this is described as 'moulding'). The head usually returns to a normal shape a few days after delivery. Six large membranous fontanelles are formed where the sutures meet (see Chapter 13). The posterior fontanelles close at about 3 months after birth and the anterior ones close when the infant is about 18 months old. Raised intracranial pressure can be detected by palpating these fontanelles; a depression indicates dehydration. The fontanelles are useful landmarks in defining the fetal position in relation to the maternal pelvis during labour. Occipital anterior positions provide the optimal position to facilitate moulding. In suboptimal positioning, such as occipital posterior positions associated with deflexion of the head, abnormal moulding can be observed resulting in a dome-like appearance of the baby's head.

The fetal skull is relatively large compared with the skeleton. The newborn skull has relatively thin bones compared with those in later life. The face is relatively small and has a characteristic neonatal roundish shape because the jaws are small. The paranasal sinuses (which give the individual shape of the face and resonance of the voice) are virtually absent and the facial bones are underdeveloped. After birth, brain growth is rapid so the calvaria increase markedly during the first 2 years. The calvaria continue to grow until the child is about 16 years old; the skull bones then thicken and further growth is arrested. Apert syndrome, a genetic disorder, results from premature fusion of the fetal skull plates, which prevents the skull from growing normally and affects the shape of the face; diagnosis is confirmed by genetic testing and corrective surgery can be used to enlarge the calvaria.

The Muscles and Limbs

The first skeletal muscles to develop are the back muscles from the paired somites. Bone formation is closely associated with muscle growth and the nervous connections from the spinal cord. The muscle structures of the spine provide stability to the vertebral column. The limbs become evident initially as buds or bulges associated with particular somites in the 4th week of development. The limb buds are formed from migration of muscle cells from the myotomes. The cells form pairs of muscle masses. Adhesive cells form a compacted region between the two muscle masses, which differentiates into cartilage. Cartilage is stiff but flexible, whereas bone is stronger but more brittle and able to fracture. Ossification, the conversion to bone structure, begins from about 8 weeks but is still not complete by birth. This preponderance of cartilage in the skeleton aids flexibility at delivery. The arms are slightly ahead of the legs in development because the fetal circulatory system gives an advantage to the upper body (see Chapter 15). Bones and muscles closest to the body develop first so the humerus and femur develop before the distal regions of the limbs. The differential timing of development means that drugs such as thalidomide affect different limbs and parts of the limbs depending on time of exposure of the fetus to the teratogens (Box 9.10). By 41 days, the fingers and toes develop from paddle-like plates. As mentioned above, the sculpting of the digits is due to apoptosis of the tissue between the digital rays. A common minor congenital defect observed at birth is a failure of separation of the digits. By 9 weeks, the body skeleton is almost complete, although the skull bones are still forming. Development of the limbs and digits can be impaired by amniotic bands (derived from tears in the amnion possibly as a result of infection or toxic insult), which encircle and constrict parts of the fetus.

The Cardiovascular System

This is one of the first systems to develop; its function is important extremely early in development, unlike some of the other systems that do not have to achieve full function until after birth. This is because, as the embryo becomes larger, diffusion of oxygen and nutrients is no longer adequate. The heart starts beating at about 22 days after fertilization and blood flow starts shortly afterwards.

The primordial vascular system develops by vasculogenesis (new vessel formation from angioblasts) and later development is by angiogenesis (new vessels budding and branching off the existing vessels and remodelling). A few cells in the mesoderm of the yolk sac lose adherence and start to move, forming clusters called blood islands (Fig. 9.13). The haemocytoblasts (or haemangioblasts), the precursors of both blood cells and blood vessel endothelial cells, are nucleated and start to synthesize primitive forms of haemoglobin. The outer cells of the blood islands, angioblasts, develop characteristics of endothelial cells, the cells that line blood vessels. The blood islands fuse, forming vascular channels that eventually amalgamate to form a primitive vascular network with identifiable routes. Blood vessels form by vasculogenesis, where the vessels develop from blood islands, and by angiogenesis. The endothelial cells interact with pericytes, vascular smooth muscle cells, to form the vessel walls. The organization of the bloodflow across the yolk sac is similar to the geographical organization of river deltas where little streams meander and merge, following the route of least resistance.

Expansion and elastic resistance of the blood vessel walls, which become rhythmic generating a peristaltic pattern, propel the blood cells. Blood vessel differentiation and growth is orchestrated by a relatively restricted range of signals including cell adhesion molecules, morphogens, transcription factors and angiogenic growth factors and their receptors that regulate the differentiation of many cell types (Wigle and Eisenstat, 2015). It is thought that abnormal molecular regulation of blood vessel formation is the cause of capillary haemangiomas, the most

---

BOX 9.10　Thalidomide

Thalidomide was marketed in the 1950s as a nonaddictive sedative and antiemetic drug suitable for treating nausea and vomiting of pregnancy (morning sickness). The drug was distributed in 46 countries under different names and became one of the best-selling drugs worldwide with aggressive marketing as a completely safe drug (Vargesson, 2015). Congenital malformations of the limbs and ears rose in parallel with sales of the drug with a lag of 7–8 months. The drug was withdrawn from the UK in November 1961; 5850 infants were affected, of whom 40% died, leaving 3900 survivors (UK data). Worldwide, there were over 10,000 severe birth defects reported making this the greatest man-made medical disaster in history. Thalidomide disturbs cartilage formation and the establishment of the nerve connections to muscles. It is teratogenic 20–36 days after fertilization. Limb development begins at 24 days. Early exposure to thalidomide caused unique birth defects including absence of arms; later exposure successively affected development of ears, legs and thumbs. The damage to the embryo occurs during a short critical window between 20 and 36 days after fertilization, however before and after this period thalidomide is contraindicated in pregnancy. Absence of limbs is called 'amelia' and absence of long bones, so a hand or foot comes directly from the torso, is called 'phocomelia' ('seal limb'). Different species metabolize the drug differently; fetal development in the rodent test species (rats and mice) was not affected. Thalidomide and its analogues have effects on inflammation and blood vessel growth (angiogenesis). Today, thalidomide is used for treatment of a broad range of medical conditions including leprosy, inflammatory bowel disease, HIV, multiple myeloma and other cancers.

---

common tumours of the infant. Capillary haemangiomas are dense masses of capillary endothelial cells, which are usually associated with craniofacial structures and appear as a red raised mass of tissue. They are usually benign and self-limiting but occasionally they may proliferate or ulcerate and bleed, or they may persist as 'port-wine stains' or 'strawberry birthmarks'. Capillary haemangiomas may be present at birth or may develop in the first few months of life; about 10% of all babies have them and they are more common in female infants, in babies of Caucasian origin and those born prematurely.

The primitive heart develops from a horseshoe area of embryonic mesoderm, anterior to the prechordal plate. It forms two tubes, one on each side of the foregut, which fuse to form a single heart tube. The primitive atrium forms where the flow from the umbilical veins from the placenta joins with the blood vessels from the head, generating the greatest volume of blood. The swirling vortex of blood leaving the primitive atrium induces the development of the primitive ventricle, which becomes the main source of pumping activity. The characteristic shape of the heart is generated by the flow of blood cells within the vascular channels; this causes the heart tube to form an S-shaped loop that will eventually take on the configuration of the heart (Fig. 9.14). By 21-22 days after fertilization, the cells surrounding the heart have become differentiated as myocardial cells capable of eliciting an organized response, so the heart, which consists of four chambers in series, begins beating.

The development of the outer layers of the blood vessel walls is stimulated by blood flowing in the vessel. In areas where there is more turbulence, the vessel wall responds by developing more elasticity; the ratio of elastin and collagen is important in establishing the elasticity of the vessel walls (Flavahan, 2017). Therefore, the heart and arterial structures develop thicker and more elastic walls. The mature organization of the chambers of the heart is achieved by the ingrowth of the septa towards the central atrioventricular endocardial cushion in the centre and apoptosis of excess tissue (see Fig. 9.14). Abnormalities in the endocardial cushion development or excess apoptosis result in cardiac malformations including atrial and ventricular septal defects (known as a 'hole in the heart') and defects or transpositions of the great vessels. Abnormalities of the cardiovascular system are the more common human birth defect partly because they often allow normal fetal development and only become significant from birth, when oxygenation is dependent on pneumatic function of the lung and cardiopulmonary blood flow. Most cardiovascular abnormalities have multifactorial causes due

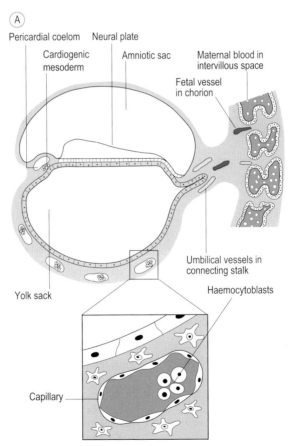

Fig. 9.13 Formation of the first blood vessels: (A) appearance of blood islands; (B) vessels at 24 days. ((A) Reproduced with permission from Fitzgerald and Fitzgerald, 1994; (B) reproduced with permission from Goodwin, 1997.)

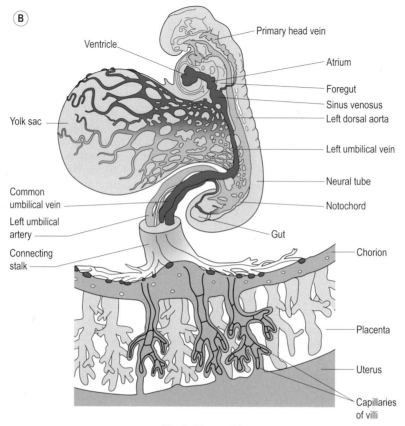

Fig. 9.13, cont'd

to the interaction of environmental and genetic factors including altered blood flow during embryonic development (Midgett et al., 2017). Cardiovascular teratogens include vitamin A, alcohol and some viruses; maternal gestational disorders such as hypertension and diabetes are also associated with an increased risk. Many chromosomal abnormalities and genetic syndromes cause heart malformations probably because so many different genes are involved in the complex embryonic development of the cardiovascular system.

The function and growth of the fetal heart depends on afterload. The fetal heart has small systolic reserve so if afterload is increased, for instance by placental insufficiency, the likely outcome is a growth-restricted baby with an enlarged heart (cardiomegaly) because of changes in the function of the cardiomyocytes and remodelling of the heart and major vessels (Miranda et al., 2017). If the fetus receives less than adequate nutrition or oxygenation during its development, then blood flow is diverted to the brain and heart. The decreased flow to the peripheral vessels

results in the development of less elastic tissue, which is the basis of the 'Barker hypothesis' or the Developmental Origins of Health and Disease (DOHaD), which suggests that intrauterine undernutrition causes compromised growth and development of organs during the critical window of fetal development leading to permanent changes that increase the risk of cardiovascular disease in adult life (Menendez-Castro et al., 2018). The risk of subsequent disease is accentuated if the nutrient supply after birth is more than adequate. The initial response to impaired nutrition is to increase placental growth in an attempt to increase nutrient transport; if this is not adequate, blood flow is diverted to the brain (and other essential organs such as heart, adrenal glands and placenta). Therefore, adults, who were small at birth, but with relatively large placentas, have an increased risk of developing hypertension because of structural alternations in blood vessels, such as lower vessel elasticity during fetal development (Fig. 9.15). It is suggested that compromised fetal nutrition leads to organs being formed with fewer cells, such as cardiomyocytes

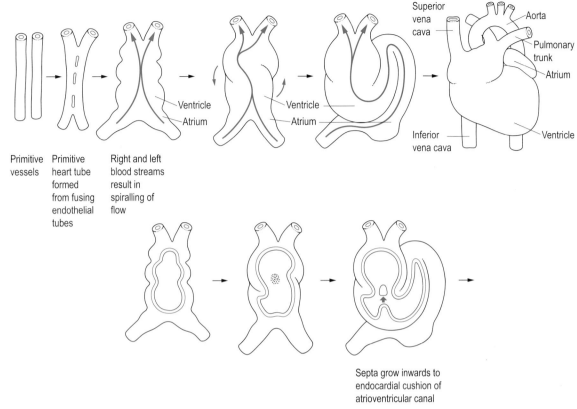

Fig. 9.14 Formation of the heart from bending of the cardiac tube (21–35 days) and formation of the heart chambers.

in the case of the heart, which leads eventually to early exhaustion of organ function and increased risk of chronic disease developing in adult life.

The Respiratory System

The trachea and major bronchi develop as out-pouches of the primitive alimentary tract. This development depends on interaction between the endodermal bud from the developing foregut and the splanchnic mesoderm it invades at about day 22. The bud bifurcates between day 26 and day 28. In the 5th week of development, three secondary buds develop on the right branch and two on the left; these are the main bronchi and primitive lobes of the lungs. There are four stages in the development of the respiratory system: the 'embryonic phase' from weeks 3 to 5; the 'pseudocanalicular phase' from 5 to 16 weeks; the 'canalicular phase' from 16 to 26 weeks; and the 'terminal sac phase' from 24 weeks until birth (Fig. 9.16). One of the most critical stages in development is the production of phospholipid-rich surfactant from the type II pneumocytes, allowing efficient inflation of the alveoli and gas exchange following birth, and therefore postnatal survival. Although the cells can be identified and production of surfactant begins at about weeks 20–22, production of surfactant increases significantly after 30 weeks when amounts become adequate for survival if the infant is born prematurely. Glucocorticoids are administered to more preterm infants in an attempt to increase surfactant production. The diaphragm starts to develop as the peritoneal membrane high in the neck and descends as the lungs and heart develop. This is the reason why diaphragmatic pain is often felt as referred pain in the shoulder. If the development of the diaphragm is incomplete, it results in a diaphragmatic hernia, which allows the abdominal contents to protrude into the chest cavity. In severe cases, the abdominal contents can restrict growth and development of the lungs (causing pulmonary hypoplasia).

Fetal breathing movements (FBM) are a feature of normal fetal life and are used to assess fetal wellbeing (as part of a biophysical profile assessment) or the risk of hypoxic injury. FBM have an important role in the growth and development of the lung, and respiratory

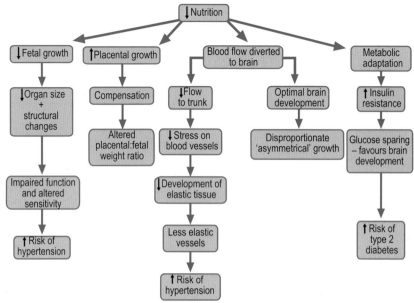

Fig. 9.15 The fetus adapts to suboptimal nutrition with strategies for survival. The slower growth rate reduces use of nutrients but affects final organ size and function. The redistribution of blood to the brain affects development of the blood vessels and predisposes to later hypertension. Altered metabolism and peripheral insulin resistance favours glucose availability for the developing brain but the 'thriftiness' predisposes to insulin resistance, obesity and type II diabetes if the individual experiences good or overnutrition in later life.

muscles (Koos and Rajaee, 2014). They oppose lung recoil and maintain the level of lung stretching and expansion and development of neural regulatory pathways that are essential for normal growth and structural maturation of the fetal lungs. Normal development of the fetal lungs is very important as there is limited capacity for later recovery. FBM are inhibited by fetal hypoxaemia, hypoglycaemia, maternal alcohol consumption, maternal smoking, intra-amniotic infection and maternal consumption of sedatives or narcotic drugs. The absence of FBM is associated with lung hypoplasia (Triebwasser and Treadwell, 2017), premature rupture of fetal membranes and oligohydramnios (decreased amniotic fluid volume). Oligohydramnios causes decreased lung growth and expansion, whereas tracheal occlusion, which prevents expulsion of lung fluid, can cause overgrowth of lung tissue (Wu et al., 2017). At term, the infant has about 50 million alveoli, half the adult number; these continue to increase in the first 8–10 years of life.

The Urinary System

The urinary and genital systems both develop from the intermediate mesoderm and are closely associated (see Chapter 5). During embryonic folding, urogenital ridges appear each side of the primitive aorta (Fig. 9.17). The nephrogenic ridge develops into the renal system of kidneys, ureters, bladder and urethra. Abnormalities of the kidneys and ureters affect 3–4% of newborn infants. Most of the abnormalities are harmless, such as variation in blood supply, abnormal position or shapes, and urinary tract duplications such as supernumerary kidneys. However, unilateral renal agenesis (one kidney failing to develop) affects 1 in 1000 live-born babies and is often discovered at autopsy. This condition is often associated with other abnormalities on the same side (ipsilateral) such as undescended testes in boys. Bilateral renal agenesis or Potter syndrome (inadequate development of both kidneys) affects 1 in 3000 fetuses and is incompatible with life. It is usually associated with oligohydramnios. Three pairs of kidneys develop during fetal development: the pronephroi, the mesonephroi and the metanephroi (singular: pronephros, mesonephros and metanephros). The pronephroi are transient nonfunctional structures that exist for only a few weeks. When they degenerate, their ducts are utilized in the next stage. The mesonephroi appear in the 4th week and function as intermediate kidneys until the end of the embryonic period, disgorging waste products into the remnants of the yolk sac. They degenerate and disappear in the 8th week, although parts of their structure persist as Wolffian ducts in males (see Chapter 5).

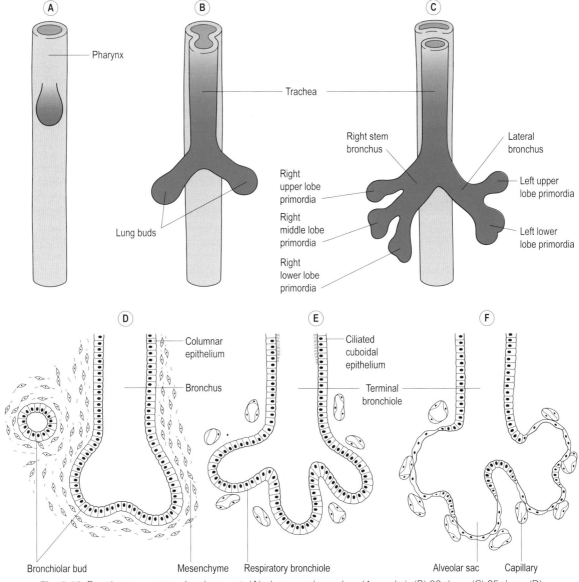

Fig. 9.16 Respiratory system development: (A) pharyngeal pouches (4 weeks); (B) 32 days; (C) 35 days; (D) pseudocanalicular phase (17 weeks); (E) canalicular phase (17–26 weeks); (F) terminal sac phase (26 weeks).

The permanent kidneys, or metanephroi, develop from the 5th week and begin to function about 4 weeks later. The kidneys start development in the pelvis and appear to migrate upwards. In fact, this observation is due to continued downward growth of the embryo. As the kidneys 'ascend' out of the pelvic area, new arteries at successively higher levels supply them. During fetal life, the kidney is subdivided into lobes, which disappear in infancy as the nephrons grow. The main increase in size is due to elongation of the proximal convoluted tubules and loops of Henlé. Disruption of normal differentiation of the nephrons during development leads to renal dysplasia, the major cause of renal failure in infants and children (Phua and Ho, 2016). Functional maturation of the kidneys occurs after birth. Renal hypoplasia is the term to describe an abnormally small kidney with relatively normal function; the reduced nephron number is often associated with essential hypertension.

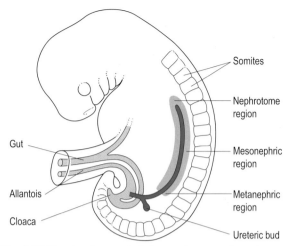

Fig. 9.17 The development of the renal system from the urogenital ridges.

Until 20 weeks' gestation, the skin is not keratinized so fluid can move through this semipermeable membrane. Essentially the outer barrier is the amnion. As the skin matures and lays down keratin, the rate of transudation decreases and the outer barrier of the fetus becomes the skin. The urine then becomes an important source of amniotic fluid. The fetus produces up to 600 mL of urine per day. Amniotic fluid is also produced by the amniotic membrane and the fetal lungs. The fetus swallows most of the amniotic fluid; the rest diffuses through the amniotic membranes to the maternal circulation. The epidermis of the skin develops from the ectoderm, which is colonized from melanocytes from the neural crest and Langerhans cells from the bone marrow. The dermis is derived from the embryonic mesoderm.

Fetal Growth

At 4 weeks, the crown–rump length (CRL) is about 4 mm and increases by 1 mm per day up to 30 mm; measures of fetal skeletal growth are similar in healthy populations in early pregnancy worldwide, provided the mother's nutritional, health, educational and other needs are met (Papageorghiou et al., 2018). Thereafter, between weeks 8 and 28, the growth increases markedly to ~1.5 mm per day, so this period is recognized as the fetal growth period. The organs and tissues continue to grow and mature. Although growth is most rapid during this period (compared with any other time in life), factors affecting growth may have their origins earlier. Environmental insults regulating growth appear to last for several generations. Fetal growth is due to interaction between the genetic drive for growth and the nutritional supplies in pregnancy to support it, which

involves a dynamic interaction between fetus, placenta and mother. There is an important difference between growth reference data and prescriptive standards. Growth references describe how individuals in a population *have grown* whereas growth standards are developed to describe how individuals *should grow* if they are healthy and receive the best nutrition and health care (Papageorghiou et al., 2018).

There are characteristic differences between the different phases of growth during development. Growth in the first 16 weeks is principally through increased cell number (hyperplasia). Then between 16 and 32 weeks, cell division or hyperplasia continues albeit at a slower rate and the cells also increase in size (hypertrophy). In the third trimester from about week 32, cell division slows further and cellular hyperplasia is dominant; there is a rapid increase in cell size. There is little variation in fetal growth up to about 16 weeks' gestation (Papageorghiou et al., 2018), after which genetic and environmental influences particularly have a more marked effect on outcome. Fat deposition, determined by nutrient availability and insulin levels, plays an important contribution to the final birthweight. There are 42 successive cell divisions between fertilization and birth, but only about five more, depending on the tissue, from birth to adult size (excluding mitotic cell division to replace dead cells).

All low birthweight (LBW) infants are potentially at some health risk. LBW is traditionally defined as being <2500 g at birth. Very low (VLBW) and extremely low birthweight (ELBW) are defined as being <1500 g and 1000 g at birth, respectively. LBW remains one of the great challenges to modern healthcare services; small size at birth can affect susceptibility to infection, rate of postnatal growth and neurocognitive development. LBW is associated with increased neonatal mortality as well as higher neonatal and infant morbidity and mortality with the most adverse outcomes arising in the most immature infants. Many chronic adult diseases are programmed in early life; they originate *in utero* as a result of fetal stress or adaptation to suboptimal quality or quantity of nutrients in order to optimize survival (Kwon and Kim, 2017). Conditions identified to be strongly related to the fetal environment include glucose intolerance, insulin resistance and type 2 diabetes mellitus, cardiovascular disease, hypertension, stroke, obstructive lung disease, hyperlipidaemia, hypercholesterolaemia, hypercortisolaemia, renal disease, osteoporosis, schizophrenia, autism and reproductive disorders.

The use of LBW as the outcome measure of the success of a pregnancy is very widespread and it can be measured with precision and validity. Infant mortality increases exponentially with lower birthweight. However, birthweight is a function of two factors (gestational length and rate of fetal growth), which have different aetiologies and different prognoses. The simple definition of an LBW infant as one who weighs <2500 g at birth does not differentiate between infants who are growth-restricted (small at term) and infants who are born prematurely. Prematurity is often complicated by IUGR (Kiserud et al., 2018). Small for gestational age (SGA) is defined as an infant with a birthweight less than the 10th centile of the mean for the age-matched population. Some SGA infants are constitutionally small rather than growth-restricted or growth-retarded. Growth in the first trimester of pregnancy affects birthweight; fetal growth restriction in the first trimester is associated with complications and increased risk of adverse outcomes such as neurodevelopmental issues and chronic health problems (McCowan et al., 2018).

LBW is associated with poor perinatal outcomes and lifelong health consequences. However, birthweight is a proxy measure of intrauterine growth and development. It is possible for suboptimal maternal body composition and nutrient intake to result in an abnormal intrauterine growth trajectory and have a programming effect on the offspring without necessarily affecting size at birth (Larose et al., 2017). Birthweight does not identify effects of nutrition on body composition and development of specific tissues and organs; a similar birthweight can be attained with different growth trajectories. Birthweight may not identify growth restriction. For instance, if an infant does not reach its potential birthweight but is born >2500 g, it may not be classified as growth-restricted. Conversely, an infant with 'normal' birthweight, such as 3.4 kg, may be growth-retarded and have long-term health risks if it was destined to be bigger under optimal intrauterine conditions. Most infants born of LBW in developed countries are born prematurely rather than growth-restricted; in most cases, the cause(s) of preterm delivery is not known. Rates of LBW babies are higher in areas with a higher level of socioeconomic deprivation and higher rates of smoking; birthweight is also related to income level and accessibility to healthcare, education and housing.

A variety of factors alter the fetal growth trajectory (Box 9.11). Fetal growth restriction affects 5–10% of all pregnancies; the fetus does not meet its growth potential. Growth restriction is a major cause of perinatal mortality and one of the most common complications of pregnancy. Growth restriction is classified as three types depending when it is identified (Nardozza et al., 2017). Type I IUGR is more serious and is often a consequence of poor placentation and marked hypoxia. Growth falters in early gestation during the cellular hyperplasia stage and the infant at birth is symmetrically small with a proportionately smaller head and abdominal circumference. Type II or late IUGR presents less of a risk for postnatal morbidity and mortality and is usually due to inadequate placental delivery

> ### BOX 9.11 Factors Affecting Fetal Size
>
> - Fetal factors
> - Maternal size (lean body mass): maternal genetic effects
> - Maternal weight gain and nutrition in pregnancy
> - Maternal age extremes
> - Maternal behavioural factors such as smoking, recreational drug use
> - Multiple pregnancy
> - Fetal oxygenation: affected by maternal anaemia, etc.
> - Maternal medical conditions such as hypertension, heart disease, infections and diabetes
> - Placental sufficiency affected by preeclampsia, uterine blood flow, etc.
> - GHs such as insulin and IGFs

of nutrients and oxygen during the cellular hypertrophy stage of growth (32 weeks onwards). The infant at birth is described as asymmetrically grown. Head circumference and femur length are usually as expected for gestational age but abdominal circumference is markedly affected and final weight is low for length. Type III growth restriction is a combination of type I and type II; growth falters in the second trimester when the hyperplasia and hypertrophy phases are both occurring. It is often associated with infections and damaging toxic agents (from pharmaceutical and illegal drugs or toxins).

Early diagnosis of IUGR means that the possible cause can be identified and monitoring and management are optimal. It is often useful to consider factors affecting fetal growth as fetal factors (such as gender, chromosomal abnormalities, inborn errors of metabolism and genetic syndromes, intrauterine infections and multiple gestation) and maternal factors (such as clinical diseases, nutritional issues, drug use, ethnicity, stress and depression). However, these factors may overlap and growth can be affected by a combination of factors. Chromosome and genetic disorders are associated with fetal or IUGR; excluding these, the dominant cause of growth retardation is due to an inadequate supply of nutrients and oxygen related either to maternal supply or to placental transfer capacity.

Fetal Factors

Gender affects growth. Male infants are on average heavier than female infants at birth. The ovaries have limited capability to synthesize steroid hormones, whereas the testes produce testosterone, which has anabolic effects. In males, the presence of a Y chromosome and higher prenatal levels of testosterone positively promotes growth of both the fetal body and the placenta (Sundrani et al., 2017).

Multiple pregnancies are more likely to be affected by growth restriction and result in smaller babies (Townsend et al., 2019). This may be due to limited haemodynamic support in late gestation or overcrowding. In monochorionic (identical) twins, selective growth restriction may be associated with twin-to-twin transfusion syndrome (TTTS); the disproportionate blood supply compromises the prognosis for both the 'donor' and the 'recipient' twin, particularly if the difference in growth rate is marked (Monaghan et al., 2019). Aneuploidy is also a risk factor for IUGR. Parity affects birthweight; first-born infants tend to be slightly lighter than second and subsequent siblings.

Fetal malformations, especially those due to chromosomal abnormality, are strongly correlated with impaired growth rates. Trisomies (13, 18 and 21) and Turner syndrome have a marked effect on birthweight (Nardozza et al., 2017). Chorionic villus sampling (CVS) indicates that in 1–2% of conceptuses tested there is a degree of confined placental mosaicism (where one or more types of placental cells have nuclei with an abnormal number of chromosomes). Confined placental mosaicism (chromosomal abnormalities affecting the placenta but not the embryo) is associated with an increased frequency of IUGR (Toutain et al., 2018).

Maternal Size

The classic experiments on horses showing that the size of offspring of hybrid crosses between small Shetland ponies and large Shire horses was most closely related to maternal size demonstrated that maternal size is a critical determinant of birthweight (Walton and Hammond, 1938). However, final adult size is also affected by paternal genetics to different degrees in different species; in humans about 5% of the variability in size is attributed to paternal influences. Historically, pregnant women were asked for their shoe size, which was thought to correlate with their pelvic size, and their husband's hat size, which was thought to be related to the size of the baby; the relationship of the two sizes was used to predict the likelihood of difficulties in delivery. A small maternal size appears to impose a constraint on fetal growth, although factors such as immaturity, social circumstances, maternal behaviour (such as smoking, recreational drug use and alcohol consumption), diseases and psychological stress all affect the outcome of the pregnancy. Shorter maternal stature is also positively correlated with lower socioeconomic status, malnutrition, chronic disease, increased levels of stress and large family size. The cycle of deprivation tends to repeat, as there is a correlation between maternal height and birthweight and between birthweight and adult size, which is not solely due to genetic influences.

The uterine environment affects fetal growth. Half-siblings who share the same mother have similar birthweights and the birthweights of babies born after ovum donation are more strongly related to gestational age and the weight of the recipient mother than to that of the donor woman (Pereira et al., 2016). These findings suggest that birth size is more strongly influenced by uterine environment than by genetics. Birthweight is also affected by assisted reproductive techniques (ART; see Chapter 6). More than one embryo may be transferred to the uterus in ART but it appears that the association is more than a result of multiple gestation; singleton ART pregnancies are also at increased risk of preterm birth and LBW. Recent analysis of the outcome of ART pregnancies suggests that the growth profile of the embryo is established early in development and related to the site of implantation (Pereira et al., 2016).

The relationship between fetal growth and maternal size led to the suggestion that there is a conflict between the maternal and paternal genes governing fetal size and that fetal growth was constrained by uteroplacental factors governed by maternal phenotype (Haig, 2015). Fetal genes of paternal origin ('patrigenes') favour fetal growth and the transfer of nutrients to the parasitic fetus; if this happens at the expense of maternal health or life, the male can choose a different mate. Fetal genes of maternal origin ('matrigenes') limit transfer to the fetus to optimize survival of the mother and her children. Matrigenes limit the depth of placental invasion of the maternal tissue in implantation (Haig, 2015). Some of the support for this hypothesis comes from examination of the extremely rare pregnancies affected by hydatidiform moles (gestational trophoblastic disease). Complete hydatidiform moles derive from fertilization of the ovum by a single sperm followed by duplication of its chromosomes (androgenetic complete mole) in 80% of cases or by two sperm (dispermy) (heterozygous complete mole) in 20% of cases. The androgenetic complete moles are always 46, XX (46,YY has never been reported) whereas the heterozygous complete mole results from dispermy and can be 46, XX or 46, XY but all chromosomes are of paternal origin. Complete moles can also (but rarely) be biparental, with both maternal and paternal genes but, due to failure of maternal imprinting, only the paternal genome is expressed. A partial hydatidiform mole usually has an associated embryo and is triploid, 69,XXX or 69,XXY. This results from fertilization of a haploid ovum and duplication of the paternal haploid chromosomes or from dispermy. Tetraploidy may also be encountered. As in a complete mole, hyperplastic trophoblastic tissue and swelling of the chorionic villi occur. If the two sperm fertilizing the ovum carried Y-chromosomes, the diandric triploid (1m:2p) conceptus exhibits placental hyperplasia (excessive placental development), whereas a digynic triploid (2m;1p) has placental hypoplasia (poor placental development). This demonstrates that proliferation of the placenta depends on the ratio of matrigenes to patrigenes and that the paternal genome promotes trophoblastic or placental overgrowth.

The father's birthweight influences placental size. Birthweights of mothers correlate with their children's birthweights and even with their grandchildren's birthweights, suggesting that the maternal constraint on fetal growth is set very early; indeed environment of the periconceptual period may be one of the most important considerations (Fleming et al., 2018). The paternal effect on the fetal growth trajectory is permitted by the lifting of the maternal constraint on growth. Therefore, fetal growth rate responds to, and is appropriate for, the prevailing nutrient availability.

Maternal constraint is a mechanism for matching fetal growth to maternal pelvis size. The evolution of a large human brain together with changes in pelvic size and shape due to bipedalism ('the obstetric dilemma') means that the fit of the fetal head in the birth canal is much tighter than in other primates (Rosenberg and Trevathan, 2018). Constraint of growth by maternal factors is important in preventing fetal overgrowth, obstructed delivery and dystocia (obstructive and difficult passage through the birth canal), which is risky for both mother and infant (and survival of the species). Interestingly, it is suggested that all human fetal growth is restrained below genetic potential to some extent to ensure maternal survival. Impaired fetal growth and excessive fetal growth present an increased risk for perinatal morbidity and mortality; the most favourable outcome for both short-term survival (of gestation and early life) and long-term health (lowest risk of adult disease) is achieved with a birthweight between the 80th between 90th centiles (Vasak et al., 2015).

There are other paternal factors that influence birthweight; infants whose fathers are older or who were born with a LBW themselves are more likely to have LBW children. Poor paternal nutrition can affect the development of sperm including epigenetic modification (see Chapter 7) of the genes, which affect protein expression and risk of disease in the offspring (Lucas and Watkins, 2017).

Growth Hormones

It has been suggested that growth in children from fetus through infancy and childhood to puberty follows a mathematical model on which three growth curves are imposed, forming a sigmoidal curve (Fig. 9.18; Karlberg et al., 1994). Phase 1, the infancy growth rate, begins in fetal life with a rapid deceleration until about 3 years of age. This is the phase of growth that seems to be regulated by insulin-like growth factors (IGFs; see Chapter 4); the effect of poor nutrition on growth may be mediated by IGFs. The childhood phase begins in the first year of life and is due to the effect of growth hormone (GH; see Chapter 3), provided thyroid hormone secretion is normal. During this period most of the growth is localized in the lower body (particularly leg length), as the long bones are very sensitive to GH. Children who have deficiency of GH or who are anencephalic have normal birthweight and early infant growth; the deficiency usually becomes apparent only after 6 months of age. The final component of growth is the pubertal growth spurt, which is stimulated by the interaction of sex hormones with GH. Although levels of GH in the fetus are high, GH receptors are expressed at low levels in fetal tissues so GH has little effect. This is supported by observations that GH-deficient fetuses or young infants have almost normal linear growth. Fetal growth is controlled by IGFs and their receptors (Reynolds et al., 2017).

IGFs are mitogens (i.e. they stimulate cell division and differentiation); they interact with two types of receptor and are modulated by a family of six binding proteins. The IGF axis controls growth before and after birth (see Chapter 15). The mechanisms involved can explain both the interaction of genetic drive and nutrient supply and the effects of maternal and paternal size. IGF-2 is the primary growth factor influencing embryonic growth and the development of fetal organs such as the brain, kidneys and liver, whereas IGF-1, produced by the fetal liver and amniotic membranes, is more important in regulating growth in late gestation. IGF-1 increases the efficiency of the placenta so fetal weight increases without a corresponding increase in placental weight. Fetal insulin, driven by fetal glucose availability, is the main regulator of IGF-1; IGF-1 is very sensitive to maternal nutrition. IGF-2 is also involved in fetal gut maturation and the development of the fetal skeleton and skeletal muscles. Both IGF-1 and IGF-2 have anabolic effects and exert their biological growth promoting actions via the type 1 receptor (IGF1R). The IGF-2 receptor (IGF2R) acts mainly as a clearance receptor to reduce circulating levels of IGF-2 by internalization and lysosomal breakdown. IGF-2 is paternally imprinted and expressed and promotes growth via the IGF-1 receptor, whereas the type 2 receptor, which is hypothesized to be maternally imprinted, causes its internalization and destruction thus limiting growth by clearing or 'mopping up' the free IGF-2 (Sferruzzi-Perri, 2018). Overexpression of IGF-2 leads to overgrowth such as in Beckwith–Wiedemann syndrome. IGF-2 deficiency is often associated with growth restriction both during gestation and postnatally. In diabetic pregnancies, fetal hyperinsulinaemia appears to cause increased proteolysis of the IGF-binding proteins, so there is more bioavailable IGF-1, which contributes to excess fetal growth

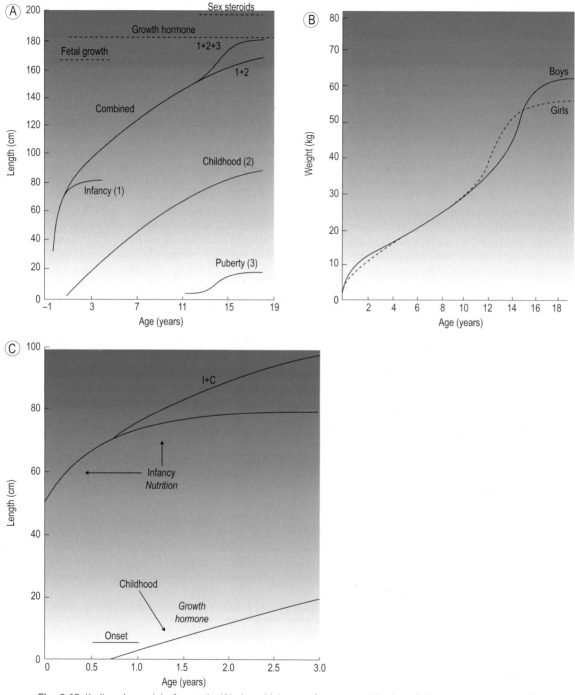

Fig. 9.18 Karlberg's model of growth: (A) sigmoidal curve from a combination of three growth curves; (B) the curve of weight increase; (C) the curve of increase in length. (Reproduced with permission from Karlberg et al., 1994.)

and macrosomia (Al-Far et al., 2016). Nutrient availability promotes IGF-1 levels and fetal growth. Thus, a balance is achieved between paternal genes promoting growth and maternal genes restricting and regulating growth.

Insulin itself has a growth-promoting effect in the fetus; it is a growth-promoting hormone, which signals nutrient availability. Its somatogenic (growth-promoting) actions are mediated via IGF-1 but it has a direct effect on fat deposition. Maternal hyperglycaemia causes increased placental transfer of glucose to the fetus. The higher concentration of glucose stimulates the fetal pancreas to produce insulin, which facilitates cellular uptake of glucose, stimulating anabolic metabolism and fetal growth. Babies of diabetic mothers are often macrosomic owing to particularly large fat stores. The macrosomia tends to be somatic so the bodies of macrosomic infants are big so their heads can appear relatively small. Fetal insulin deficiency, which is rare, can occur with nutrient deprivation or pancreatic agenesis, and results in fetal growth retardation (symmetrical IUGR) and decreased levels of body fat and muscle development (Sferruzzi-Perri, 2018).

Glucocorticoids (see Chapter 15) affect fetal growth and maturation by altering production and secretion of hormones, regulating receptor density and altering the activity of enzymes involved in activating and deactivating hormones. The fetus is usually protected from overexposure to maternal glucocorticoids because they are inactivated by the placental enzyme 11β-hydroxysteroid dehydrogenase 2 (11β-HSD2), which thus limits their transfer to the fetus (Chivers and Wyrwoll, 2017). However, maternal malnutrition (inadequate intake of nutrients, protein restriction or obesity) downregulates this enzyme so the fetus is exposed to increased glucocorticoids. This situation disrupts the growth of the placenta and fetus. However, the higher levels of cortisol enhance maturation of the lungs and other organs, promoting survival of the IUGR infant; premature delivery frequently accompanies IUGR. Thyroid hormones promote fetal development and signal energy availability.

Maternal Nutrition

Fetal growth is related to maternal size (reflecting nutrient level during her own fetal development), maternal body composition (which indicates nutrient supply), nutrient availability in pregnancy and placental efficiency. If periconceptual maternal nutrition sets the growth trajectory early in gestation, the fetal growth rate is more likely to be accommodated by nutrient availability when its demands are high in later gestation. The fetus is able to adapt metabolically to undernutrition in pregnancy by altering its growth rate and sparing nutrients for certain tissues, like the brain. This plasticity can lead to the disproportionate

organ development and fetal growth patterns, which are the basis of the Developmental Origins of Health and Disease hypothesis (Hoffman et al., 2017). At one time, it was thought that these fetal adaptations to undernutrition and the resulting increased risk of disease were permanent, but recent research in this area suggests that programming could be reversed by interventions during early critical periods of development (Reynolds et al., 2017).

Maternal nutrition stores correlate with birthweight. Pregnant women exposed to conditions of starvation during the famines during World War II were particularly susceptible to nutrient deficiency if they were subject to nutritional deficiency in the preconceptual period or in early pregnancy. Not only was the size of their own babies significantly smaller, but the prenatal growth of their grandchildren and their subsequent health were also affected (Roseboom, 2017). Nutrient deprivation later in pregnancy affected birthweights and fat deposition, but the lengths of the neonates were not affected so much and the babies appeared to regain normal weights after birth. However, the metabolic adaptation in those fetuses exposed to nutrient deprivation late in gestation is associated with persistent insulin resistance and a predisposition to develop glucose intolerance and type 2 diabetes mellitus (T2DM) later in life (Vaiserman, 2017). These effects are not always related to maternal nutrition; placental dysfunction or changes in placental resource allocation can also limit transfer of nutrients from the mother to the fetus (Sferruzzi-Perri et al., 2017).

In humans, dietary intervention studies have had disappointing results, producing improvement in fetal growth only in severely undernourished women. Part of the problem may be the methodology and ensuring that supplements intended for pregnant women are not used as alternative sources of nutrition or to feed other members of the family (maternal nutrient sacrifice). The timing of the nutritional supplements may also be important, as fetal growth trajectories may be set before the nutritional status of the mother is improved by the intervention. Women experiencing marginal diets and seasonal famine for generations appear to have evolved strategies to conserve energy by suppressing metabolic rate and acquiring little fat during the pregnancy (Durnin, 1987). The energy cost of pregnancy in affluent countries where food is plentiful may be met with little or no increase in energy intake, although economies in energy expenditure may offset the increased requirements (see Chapter 12).

Prepregnant size (body fat levels) and accumulation of adipose tissue in early pregnancy may affect the fetal growth trajectory (Perez-Perez et al., 2018); the placenta is also a source of leptin. Appropriate conditions and nutrient intakes during pregnancy may then fulfil the requirements for this trajectory to be achieved. In experimental animals, the effect of moderate maternal malnutrition over a number of generations is decreased birthweight, which is maintained for a few further generations even when food supply is restored to a good level (Stewart et al., 1980). A plentiful food supply imposed after generations of malnutrition in these animals is associated with obstructed labour, potentially caused by fetal–maternal pelvis disproportion, and poor fetal outcome.

Acute undernutrition in late gestation can cause premature delivery by stimulating signals, which promote cervical ripening and uterine contractility and cause early labour (see Chapter 13). Macronutrient balance at different stages of pregnancy may affect fetal growth (see Chapter 12). Micronutrient availability can affect the somatotrophic and insulin regulation of growth; zinc deficiency is associated with IUGR. Vitamin E and vitamin A affect insulin sensitivity and GH secretion, respectively. Folate status affects gene imprinting and methylation.

Maternal nutrition could also exert an effect on fetal growth even before fertilization. The nutritional support of follicular development prior to ovulation and fertilization may affect the growth trajectory of the embryo (see above). Nutrition of the embryo prior to implantation may be important. The composition of the culture media used in human ART is suggested to have an effect on birthweight, which is still evident in the offspring at least 2 years later (Fleming et al., 2018). In addition, the cardiovascular phenotype is different in those children conceived by ART and those conceived naturally. Studies of offspring born after ART for reasons unrelated to infertility, and in animal studies, suggest that these outcomes are not a result of parental infertility but are related to the techniques used and the embryonic environment.

Maternal Behaviour

Differences in birthweight across different socioeconomic groups may be largely attributable to differences in cigarette smoking. The birthweight appears to fall by about 14 g multiplied by the average number of cigarettes smoked per day, on average reducing fetal birthweight by about 250 g (Abraham et al., 2017). Smoking is associated with a poorer diet and other behavioural factors including the level of health care. Although effects on oxygen transfer are probably compensated for by 2,3-bisphosphoglycerate (2,3-BPG), which improves the efficiency of oxygen–haemoglobin dissociation, it is evident that the fetus is not protected from the adverse effects of environmental exposure to smoking. Smoking causes nicotine-induced vasoconstriction of the uterine vessels, carbon monoxide inhibits oxygen diffusion and cyanide affects enzyme systems. Fetal brain development is also affected by adverse environmental exposure during gestation including toxins (including alcohol), hypoxia and inflammation (Lei

et al., 2018). Although hypoxia is normal and essential in early embryonic development and plays a crucial role in placental development, angiogenesis and haematopoiesis during this time, and chronic and marked fetal hypoxia later in gestation, prevents the fetus from achieving its full growth potential (Fajersztajn and Veras, 2017). The adverse effects on growth may be accompanied by changes in gene expression affecting subsequent health status. Hypoxia is not a rare event and could result from unavoidable exposure to air pollution, high altitude and maternal anaemia (Ritchie et al., 2017).

Iron deficiency in pregnancy may affect fetal growth (see Chapter 12). Alcohol consumption is associated with effects on growth; one of the common effects of fetal alcohol syndrome is growth retardation (Del Campo and Jones, 2017). The use of illegal recreational drugs, such as heroin and cocaine, in pregnancy is associated with LBW babies but again it is difficult to dissociate the use of the drugs from the other health-related variables. Caffeine, whether from coffee or other sources such as soft drinks, also has an effect on fetal growth (see Chapter 12).

Other Factors Affecting Fetal Growth

Medical complications of pregnancy or pre-existing maternal diseases can affect fetal growth. Mild maternal hypertension does not restrict growth but severe hypertension is associated with LBW particularly if it is complicated with renal disease. Preeclampsia is a major cause of LBW; it has been suggested that IUGR of unknown cause may be due to undiagnosed or subclinical preeclampsia (see Chapter 8). Severe maternal respiratory and cardiovascular problems and chronic renal disease are also associated with fetal growth restriction. Fetal growth restriction has also been observed in women with congenital uterine abnormalities possibly due to implantation in the lower half of the uterus, which has a reduced blood supply compared with the upper fundal region.

Maternal and fetal infections, such as rubella, cytomegalovirus and Zika virus, also detrimentally affect growth. It is not clear whether HIV affects fetal growth as coexisting problems cannot be dissociated. In developing countries, malaria infection causes placental disease and affects fetal growth. The fetus is also at risk from certain types of anti-malaria drugs such as quinine, which can be teratogenic, taken by the mother. Placental supply of amino acids is close to the minimum required to support fetal protein synthesis. It is possible that the adverse circumstances limiting fetal growth do so by increasing levels of catabolic hormones, such as catecholamines, cortisol and β-endorphin, which affect epigenetic programming (Vaiserman et al., 2018).

Complications Associated with SGA

Babies who are SGA have an increased risk of perinatal complications (Box 9.12). Although some catch-up growth

BOX 9.12 Complications Associated with SGA

- Increased mortality
- Short- and long-term pulmonary morbidity
- Intrapartum hypoxia
- Hypothermia
- Hypoglycaemia
- Necrotizing enterocolitis
- Ophthalmic morbidity
- Neurological morbidity
- Delayed psychomotor development
- Polycythaemia
- Infection
- Pulmonary haemorrhage
- Sudden infant death syndrome
- Adult-onset cardiovascular and metabolic disease

CASE STUDY 9.2

Razia gives birth to a healthy female infant at term. The baby appears healthy and chubby, although she weighs 2.1 kg.
- Is the midwife right to assume that Asian babies are normally smaller than Western babies?
- What reasons would you give to argue for or against this assumption?
- What antenatal observations and measurements could be used to assess whether or not Razia's baby is at increased risk?

may occur postnatally, some of the effects of IUGR on the structure and function of physiological systems may be irreversible (Hoffman et al., 2017).

Case study 9.2 details the example of a baby with LBW.

KEY POINTS

- During the 2nd week of development, the inner cell mass differentiates into the bilaminar disc, consisting of two germ layers: the epiblast and the hypoblast. The definitive yolk sac is created and the amniotic and chorionic cavities are evident. The differentiated cells migrate and adhere and the genes are switched on and off.
- The embryonic period consists of cell growth (increased cell number and size), differentiation, organogenesis (organization of tissues into organs) and morphogenesis (development of shape). This is the period that is most susceptible to teratogens, which can cause major morphological abnormalities.
- Gastrulation is the major event of the 3rd week. It begins with the appearance of the primitive streak, results in the conversion of the bilaminar disc into a trilaminar disc, consisting of ectoderm, mesoderm and endoderm and establishes the axis for further embryonic development. The neural tube, precursor of the nervous system, and the somites also appear in the 3rd week.
- The trilaminar disc is converted into the characteristic vertebral structure by differential growth of the cell layers causing folding and fusion.

- Weeks 4–8 are the period of organogenesis, differentiation of the major organ systems.
- Fetal growth is influenced by genes and the environment, but limited by nutrient and oxygen supply. Paternal gene expression tends to favour fetal growth, whereas maternal gene expression tends to constrain fetal growth to a growth trajectory that may be set by environmental influences prior to fertilization.
- The fetus can adapt to undernutrition by altering metabolism and blood flow to protect the brain, albeit at the expense of other organs.
- Stem cell collection and storage from cord blood samples obtained immediately after delivery is becoming increasingly popular. Careful consideration is required by all health professionals, if this is requested, to ensure all legal and ethical issues are considered. Currently, it is still unclear what the benefits of fetal stem cell storage are and they are very seldom used; however, ongoing research is progressing into exploring the possible advantages of this. It is possible that some genetic conditions may be treatable with donated stem cells extracted from cord blood such as metabolic, immune and haematological disorders.

APPLICATION TO PRACTICE

- An understanding of embryonic and fetal development is required in the explanation of congenital conditions.
- Many factors, some of which are modifiable and can be affected by advice and guidance of the midwife, for example maternal smoking, drug abuse, stress and nutrition, affect fetal development and growth.
- As pregnancy progresses, most women are keen to know how their baby is developing, so the midwife should be able to describe fetal development and growth in an appropriate way.

- A basic understanding of fetal development is important in recognizing abnormal conditions in the physical examination of the newborn.
- Antenatal assessment using customized growth charts facilitates identification and earlier intervention in IUGR babies and can potentially reduce fetal and neonatal morbidity and mortality.

ANNOTATED FURTHER READING

Bianco-Miotto T, Craig JM, Gasser YP, et al.: Epigenetics and DOHaD: from basics to birth and beyond, *J Dev Orig Health Dis* 8:513–519, 2017.
A recent review of Developmental Origins of Health and Disease (DOHaD), which investigates how the environment of early life can affect risk of chronic diseases throughout life and the mechanisms involved including epigenetic mechanisms.

Burton GJ, Jauniaux E: Pathophysiology of placental-derived fetal growth restriction, *Am J Obstet Gynecol* 218:S745–S761, 2018.
A thorough consideration of the interrelationship of placental development and fetal growth by two of the best-known experts in the world.

Carlson BM: *Human embryology and developmental biology*, ed 6, Oxford, 2018, Elsevier.
A recently updated and well-illustrated textbook, which covers the molecular basis of development, cellular aspects, developmental anatomy and the progression of development. Includes recent research findings, case studies, timeline information, review questions, clinical vignettes and useful end-of-chapter summaries. The textbook is packaged with an eBook, which provides access to figures, text and animations.

Copp AJ, Adzick NS, Chitty LS, et al.: Spina bifida, *Nat Rev Dis Primers* 1:15007, 2015.
One of the excellent reviews from Nature Reviews Disease Primers, which covers all aspects of spina bifida from its aetiology, clinical implications, healthcare costs, diagnosis and prevention. An illustrated summary of the review is available from http://go.nature.com/fK9XNa.

Moore KL, Persaud TVN, Torchia MG: *Before we are born: essentials of embryology and birth defects*, ed 9, Philadelphia, 2015, Saunders.
This updated book covers normal and abnormal human development week by week from fertilization through the development of the major organs and physiological systems to birth.

Moore KL, Persaud TVN, Torchia MG: *The developing human: clinically orientated embryology*, ed 10, Philadelphia, 2015, Saunders.
This richly-illustrated book provides a comprehensive description of embryological development, targeted at medical students and clinicians, which covers new research findings and their clinical applications. It includes aspects of molecular biology, clinical cases, effects of teratogens and detection of fetal defects.

NIH National Institutes of Health: *Stem cell basics*, 2016. U.S. Department of Health and Human Services. Available at: https://stemcells.nih.gov/info/basics/1.htm.
A useful primer about stem cells, which describes the biological properties of stem cells, current research areas and the potential use of stem cells in research treating disease; includes a comprehensive glossary and good links to further information.

Sadler TW: *Langman's medical embryology*, ed 13, Philadelphia, 2016, Lippincott Williams & Wilkins.
An up-to-date text (supported by online resources), illustrated with excellent line drawings and photographs, which covers stages of human development in detail with timelines and sections on the interaction between genetics and human development; links molecular aspects including cellular signalling and experimental principles to clinical correlates.

Webster S, de Wreede R: *Embryology at a glance*, ed 2, Oxford, 2016, Wiley-Blackwell.
A large format, slim and well-illustrated textbook, which provides clear and succinct explanations of the key concepts of human development taking a physiological systems approach.

REFERENCES

Abraham M, Alramadhan S, Iniguez C, et al.: A systematic review of maternal smoking during pregnancy and fetal measurements with meta-analysis, *PLOS ONE* 12:e0170946, 2017.

Agnello M, Bosco L, Chiarelli R, et al.: The role of autophagy and apoptosis during embryo development. In Ntuli TM, editor: *Cell death – autophagy, apoptosis and necrosis*, London, 2015, InTech Open, pp 83–112.

Al-Far HFM, Tjessem IH, Lausus FF: Macrosomia and the IGF system, *Focus on Sciences* 3:1–8, 2016.

Carlson BM: *Human embryology and developmental biology*, ed 6, Oxford, 2018, Elsevier.

Chivers EK, Wyrwoll CS: Maternal malnutrition, glucocorticoids, and fetal programming: a role for placental 11β-hydroxysteroid dehydrogenase type 2. In Rajendram R, Preedy VR, Patel V, editors: *Diet, nutrition, and fetal programming*, Switzerland, 2017, Springer, pp 543–555.

Collado MC, Rautava S, Aakko J, et al.: Human gut colonisation may be initiated in utero by distinct microbial communities in the placenta and amniotic fluid, *Sci Rep* 6:23129, 2016.

Cusick SE, Georgieff MK: The role of nutrition in brain development: the golden opportunity of the 'first 1000 days', *J Pediatr* 175:16–21, 2016.

Del Campo M, Jones KL: A review of the physical features of the fetal alcohol spectrum disorders, *Eur J Med Genet* 60:55–64, 2017.

Durnin JVGA: Energy requirements of pregnancy: an integration of the longitudinal data from the five-country study, *Lancet* ii1131–ii1133, 1987.

Fajersztajn L, Veras MM: Hypoxia: from placental development to fetal programming, *Birth Defects Res* 109:1377–1385, 2017.

Ferrer-Vaquer A, Hadjantonakis AK: Birth defects associated with perturbations in preimplantation, gastrulation, and axis extension: from conjoined twinning to caudal dysgenesis, *Wiley Interdisc Rev Dev Biol* 2:427–442, 2013.

Fitzgerald MJT, Fitzgerald M: *Human embryology*, London, 1994, Baillière Tindall, pp 23, 24, 37, 42.

Flavahan NA: In development – A new paradigm for understanding vascular disease, *J Cardiovasc Pharmacol* 69:248–263, 2017.

Fleming TP, Watkins AJ, Velazquez MA, et al.: Origins of lifetime health around the time of conception: causes and consequences, *Lancet* 391:1842–1852, 2018.

Giussani DA: The vulnerable developing brain, *Proc Natl Acad Sci USA* 108:2641–2642, 2011.

Giussani DA: The fetal brain sparing response to hypoxia: physiological mechanisms, *J Physiol* 594:1215–1230, 2016.

Goodwin B: *Health and development: conception to birth*, Milton Keynes, 1997, Open University, pp 203–205. 209.

Haig D: Maternal-fetal conflict, genomic imprinting and mammalian vulnerabilities to cancer, *Philos Trans R Soc Lond B Biol Sci* 370, 2015.

Hoffman DJ, Reynolds RM, Hardy DB: Developmental origins of health and disease: current knowledge and potential mechanisms, *Nutr Rev* 75:951–970, 2017.

James DK, Stephenson T: Fetal nutrition and growth. In Chamberlain G, Dewhurst J, Harvey D, editors: *Clinical physiology in obstetrics*, ed 3, London, 1998, Gower Medical, pp 467–497.

Jauniaux E, Gulbis B, Burton GJ: The human first trimester gestational sac limits rather than facilitates oxygen transfer to the foetus: a review, *Placenta* 24(Suppl A):S86–S93, 2003.

Karlberg J, Jalil F, Lam B, et al.: Linear growth retardation in relation to the three phases of growth, *Eur J Clin Nutr* 48(Suppl 1):S25–S44, 1994.

Kiserud T, Benachi A, Hecher K, et al.: The World Health Organization fetal growth charts: concept, findings, interpretation, and application, *Am J Obstet Gynecol* 218:S619–S629, 2018.

Koos BJ, Rajaee A: Fetal breathing movements and changes at birth, *Adv Exp Med Biol* 814:89–101, 2014.

Kwon EJ, Kim YJ: What is fetal programming?: a lifetime health is under the control of in utero health, *Obstet Gynecol Sci* 60:506–519, 2017.

Larose TL, Turner SW, Hutcheon JA, et al.: Longitudinal ultrasound measures of fetal growth and offspring outcomes, *Current Epidemiol Rep* 4:98–105, 2017.

Lei J, Calvo P, Vigh R, Burd I: Journey to the center of the fetal brain: environmental exposures and autophagy, *Front Cell Neurosci* 12:118, 2018.

Lindsay KL, Buss C, Wadhwa PD, Entringer S: The interplay between nutrition and stress in pregnancy: implications for fetal programming of brain development, *Biol Psychiatry* 85:135–149, 2019.

Lucas ES, Watkins AJ: The long-term effects of the periconceptional period on embryo epigenetic profile and phenotype; the paternal role and his contribution, and how males can affect offspring's phenotype/epigenetic profile, *Adv Exp Med Biol* 1014:137–154, 2017.

McCowan LM, Figueras F, Anderson NH: Evidence-based national guidelines for the management of suspected fetal growth restriction: comparison, consensus, and controversy, *Am J Obstet Gynecol* 218:S855–S868, 2018.

Menendez-Castro C, Rascher W, Hartner A: Intrauterine growth restriction – impact on cardiovascular diseases later in life, *Mol Cell Pediatr* 5:4, 2018.

Merfeld E, Ben-Avi L, Kennon M, Cerveny KL: Potential mechanisms of Zika-linked microcephaly, *Wiley Interdiscip Rev Dev Biol* 6, 2017.

Midgett M, Thornburg K, Rugonyi S: Blood flow patterns underlie developmental heart defects, *Am J Physiol Heart Circ Physiol* 312:H632–H642, 2017.

Miranda JO, Ramalho C, Henriques-Coelho T, Areias JC: Fetal programming as a predictor of adult health or disease: the need to reevaluate fetal heart function, *Heart Fail Rev* 22:861–877, 2017.

Moffat JJ, Ka M, Jung EM, Kim WY: Genes and brain malformations associated with abnormal neuron positioning, *Mol Brain* 8:72, 2015.

Monaghan C, Kalafat E, Binder J, et al.: Prediction of adverse pregnancy outcome in monochorionic- diamniotic twin pregnancies complicated by selective fetal growth restriction, *Ultrasound Obstet Gynecol* 53:200–207, 2019.

Moore KL, Persaud TVN, Torchia MG: *The developing human: clinically oriented embryology*, ed 10, Philadelphia, 2015, Saunders.

Nardozza LM, Caetano AC, Zamarian AC, et al.: Fetal growth restriction: current knowledge, *Arch Gynecol Obstet* 295:1061–1077, 2017.

Paluch EK, Aspalter IM, Sixt M: Focal adhesion-independent cell migration, *Annu Rev Cell Dev Biol* 32:469–490, 2016.

Papageorghiou AT, Kennedy SH, Salomon LJ, et al.: The INTERGROWTH-21(st) fetal growth standards: toward the global integration of pregnancy and pediatric care, *Am J Obstet Gynecol* 218:S630–S640, 2018.

Pereira N, Cozzubbo T, Cheung S, et al.: Identifying maternal constraints on fetal growth and subsequent perinatal outcomes using a multiple embryo implantation model, *PLOS ONE* 11:e0166222, 2016.

Perez-Perez A, Toro A, Vilarino-Garcia T, et al.: Leptin action in normal and pathological pregnancies, *J Cell Mol Med* 22:716–727, 2018.

Phua YL, Ho J: Renal dysplasia in the neonate, *Curr Opin Pediatr* 28:209–215, 2016.

Reynolds CM, Perry JK, Vickers MH: Manipulation of the growth hormone-insulin-like growth factor (GH-IGF) axis: a treatment strategy to reverse the effects of early life developmental programming, *Int J Mol Sci* 18, 2017.

Ritchie HE, Oakes DJ, Kennedy D, Polson JW: Early gestational hypoxia and adverse developmental outcomes, *Birth Defects Res* 109:1358–1376, 2017.

Rosales-Reynoso MA, Juarez-Vazquez CI, Barros-Nunez P: Evolution and genomics of the human brain, *Neurologia* 33:254–265, 2018.

Roseboom TJ: The effects of prenatal exposure to the Dutch famine 1944–1945 on health across the lifecourse. In Preedy V, Patel VB, editors: *Handbook of famine, starvation, and nutrient deprivation: from biology to policy*, Cham, 2017, Springer International Publishing, pp 1–15.

Rosenberg KR, Trevathan WR: Evolutionary perspectives on cesarean section, *Evol, Med, Public Health* 2018:67–81, 2018.

Sadler TW: Establishing the embryonic axes: prime time for teratogenic insults, *J Cardiovasc Dev Dis* 4, 2017.

Scarpa E, Mayor R: Collective cell migration in development, *J Cell Biol* 212:143–155, 2016.

Semeraro R, Cardinale V, Carpino G, et al.: The fetal liver as cell source for the regenerative medicine of liver and pancreas, *Ann Transl Med* 1:13, 2013.

Sferruzzi-Perri AN: Regulating needs: exploring the role of insulin-like growth factor-2 signalling in materno-fetal resource allocation, *Placenta* 64(Suppl 1):S16–S22, 2018.

Sferruzzi-Perri AN, Sandovici I, Constancia M, Fowden AL: Placental phenotype and the insulin-like growth factors: resource allocation to fetal growth, *J Physiol* 595:5057–5093, 2017.

Sousa AMM, Meyer KA, Santpere G, et al.: Evolution of the human nervous system function, structure, and development, *Cell* 170:226–247, 2017.

Stedman HH, Kozyak BW, Nelson A, et al.: Myosin gene mutation correlates with anatomical changes in the human lineage, *Nature* 428:415–418, 2004.

Stewart RJC, Sheppard H, Preece R, et al.: The effect of rehabilitation at different stages of development of rats marginally malnourished for ten to twelve generations, *Br J Nutr* 43:403–411, 1980.

Stinson LF, Payne MS, Keelan JA: Planting the seed: origins, composition, and postnatal health significance of the fetal gastrointestinal microbiota, *Crit Rev Microbiol* 43:352–369, 2017.

Sundrani DP, Roy SS, Jadhav AT, Joshi SR: Sex-specific differences and developmental programming for diseases in later life, *Reprod Fertil Dev* 29:2085–2099, 2017.

Toutain J, Goutte-Gattat D, Horovitz J, Saura R: Confined placental mosaicism revisited: impact on pregnancy characteristics and outcome, *PLOS ONE* 13:e0195905, 2018.

Townsend R, D'Antonio F, Sileo FG, et al.: Perinatal outcome of monochorionic twin pregnancies complicated by selective fetal growth restriction according to management: a systematic review and meta-analysis, *Ultrasound Obstet Gynecol* 53:36–46, 2019.

Triebwasser JE, Treadwell MC: Prenatal prediction of pulmonary hypoplasia, *Semin Fetal Neonatal Med* 22:245–249, 2017.

Vaiserman AM: Early-life nutritional programming of type 2 diabetes: experimental and quasi-experimental evidence, *Nutrients* 9, 2017.

Vaiserman AM, Koliada AK, Lushchak OV: Epigenetic programming of human disease and aging. In Tollefsbol TO, editor: *Epigenetics in human disease*, London, 2018, Elsevier Academic Press, pp 975–992.

Vargesson N: Thalidomide-induced teratogenesis: history and mechanisms, *Birth Defects Res C Embryo Today* 105:140–156, 2015.

Vasak B, Koenen SV, Koster MP, et al.: Human fetal growth is constrained below optimal for perinatal survival, *Ultrasound Obstet Gynecol* 45:162–167, 2015.

Vaughan OR, Rosario FJ, Powell TL, Jansson T: Regulation of placental amino acid transport and fetal growth, *Prog Mol Biol Transl Sci* 145:217–251, 2017.

Walton A, Hammond J: The maternal effects on growth and conformation in Shirehorse–Shetland pony crosses, *Proc R Soc Lond B* 125:311–335, 1938.

Wigle JT, Eisenstat DD: Common signaling pathways used during development. In Moore KL, Persaud TVN, Torchia MG, editors: *The developing human: clinically oriented embryology*, Edinburgh, 2015, Elsevier, pp 487–501.

Woodley MA, Rindermann H, Bell E, et al.: The relationship between microcephalin, ASPM and intelligence: a reconsideration, *Intelligence* 44:51–63, 2014.

Wroe S, Ferrara TL, McHenry CR, et al.: The craniomandibular mechanics of being human, *Proc Biol Sci* 277:3579–3586, 2010.

Wu CS, Chen CM, Chou HC: Pulmonary hypoplasia induced by oligohydramnios: findings from animal models and a population-based study, *Pediatr Neonatol* 58:3–7, 2017.

10

Overview of Immunology

LEARNING OBJECTIVES

- To review the immune system, identifying the roles of innate, and acquired immunity.
- To recognize how pregnancy affects the maternal immune system.
- To discuss the reasons why the fetus is not rejected.
- To appreciate the importance of placental transfer of maternal immunoglobulins.
- To demonstrate an understanding of Rhesus

incompatibility and how it can be screened for and treated.
- To describe the immunological immaturity of the neonate and why this is relevant to midwifery practice.
- To describe the principles of neonatal immunization.
- To outline the effects of human immunodeficiency virus (HIV) infection on the functioning of the immune system.

INTRODUCTION

Knowledge of the immune system is important in midwifery for several reasons. First, implantation and the nurture of an immunologically foreign fetus presents some interesting questions as to the functioning of the immune system in pregnancy. Second, some causes of infertility may be related to the immune rejection of the sperm or fetus. During pregnancy, the maternal immune system is modified so the fetus is not rejected but maternal defences against infection continue to function. Pregnant women have enhanced immune responses to bacterial infections. However, they seem to develop increased susceptibility to viral infections such as seasonal influenza, and human immunodeficiency virus (HIV) so viral-related problems may increase during pregnancy.

Pregnancy affects immune-related conditions in a variety of ways: some may temporarily improve during pregnancy, such as Graves disease, whereas others may worsen and cause serious complications such as systemic lupus erythematosus (SLE), which can significantly increase the risk of maternal death (Piccinni et al., 2016). Maternal immune adaptations in pregnancy also seem to prepare for possible pathogenic contamination of the placental wound site, during the vulnerable period of the puerperium. Blood group incompatibility and the resulting immune response can compromise the wellbeing of the developing fetus. The neonate is born immunologically immature but receives some passive immunity from the mother, both during pregnancy and neonatally in breast milk.

CHAPTER CASE STUDY

Zara and James try to live a healthy lifestyle; they have never smoked and have not drunk any alcohol for many years. They follow a vegetarian diet and prefer to have organic, fresh products that are unprocessed and rely on milk products, nuts and pulses as the main source of protein in their diet. What precautions do Zara and James need to take and what particular types of food do they need to avoid and what are the reasons for this?

As part of their preparation to work in Africa, both Zara and James underwent in-depth medical screening to ensure that they were fit enough to undertake this work. Zara has the blood group AO Rhesus-negative and James has the blood group BB-negative.

- As they are both Rhesus-negative, Rhesus incompatibility is not going to occur, but what possible complications could arise in the pregnancy as a result of these different blood groups, how could they be recognized and what are the possible treatments that may be required?
- What advice would women need before, during and after pregnancy in regard to travelling to or from tropical countries?
- If Zara wanted to know what tropical disease vaccinations are safe in pregnancy, how would the midwife advise her and what appropriate referrals should be made.

The immune system is a complex network of specialized cells and chemical signals, which interact to provide a defence against infectious organisms. A number of microorganisms are associated with the body. Some, described as commensal organisms, exist within or on their host without causing any harm. These are beneficial, or symbiotic, like those inhabiting the skin and the gut.

However, some organisms, including microbes (bacteria, viruses, fungi, etc.), and larger organisms, such as tapeworms, are potentially damaging and are described as pathogens because they cause disease. The human immune system has evolved to detect and eradicate these pathogenic organisms. Pathogens are diverse and numerous and have a rapid rate of replication and gene mutation and are constantly evolving their own mechanisms to combat the host's defence mechanisms. Therefore, eradication of infectious diseases can only be achieved by ongoing human interventions, such as improved hygiene and sanitation, quality of living conditions, nutrition and vaccination. For example smallpox, a disease caused by the variola virus, was responsible for >300 million deaths in the 20th century alone and, as a result of successful vaccination programmes, was declared as eradicated by the World Health Organization in 1980, 3 years after the last reported case in the world. Refusal to have offspring vaccinated on the grounds of spurious and unsubstantiated claims of vaccine-triggered diseases like autism results in substantial risks to the population. Unlike variola, where all infected people show symptoms, avoidance of infection and quarantine to prevent the spread of diseases like polio is far more difficult, since for every person who becomes paralysed, 500 people are infected but show no symptoms.

The role of the immune system becomes evident when it is compromised, such as in acquired immune deficiency syndrome (AIDS), when HIV causes dysfunction of the immune system (Fig. 10.1). However, under less extreme conditions, both infections and poor nutrition can overwhelm the immune system. In acute infections, life-threatening sepsis (formerly known as blood poisoning or septicaemia) can occur, in which the infection triggers an inflammatory immune response, which causes damage to the body's own tissues and, in extreme cases, leads to multiple organ failure and death (overwhelming sepsis). Sepsis is still a major contributor to maternal deaths.

To some extent, both the pregnant woman and the neonate are immunocompromised, but the concept that pregnancy is a state of immunosuppression, which increases susceptibility to infectious diseases, is controversial. It does not make evolutionary sense for pregnancy to be dangerous from an immunological perspective. Reproduction is

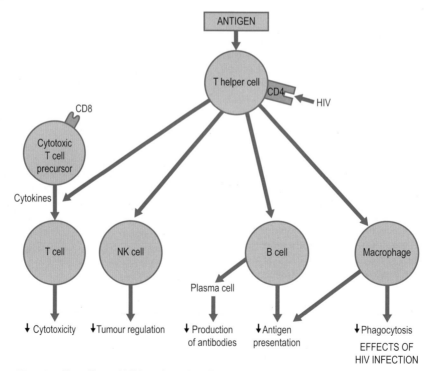

Fig. 10.1 The effect of HIV on the helper T cell and other cells of the immune system.

crucial for survival of the species; a paramount aspect of this is that the immune system, and therefore the survival of the mother and fetus, is strengthened by enhanced recognition, cell communication, mobilization of immune cells and repair mechanisms (Mor and Cardenas, 2010). It is preferable to describe pregnancy as a state of immunomodulation. An alternative explanation to the apparent increased risk of infection in pregnancy is that the mother is more readily sensitized by the changes that occur in her immune system.

THE EVOLUTION OF THE IMMUNE SYSTEM

The detection of the presence of pathogens initiates the immune response in the host, stimulating a cascade of interactions, which culminates in a counter-attack on the pathogen. There are two types of immunity: innate immunity and adaptive (acquired) immunity. As discussed below, passive immunity takes advantage of maternal adaptive immunity, using placental and lactational transfer of maternal immunoglobulins to 'bestow' immunity on the fetus and neonate.

Innate (natural) immunity pre-exists in an organism before any contact with pathogens; it is a collection of genetically encoded responses to foreign pathogens, which does not change throughout the lifespan. Innate immunity occurs throughout the plant and animal kingdom, occurring in mammals, birds, sponges and worms. It evolved in early life forms and is particularly effective against bacteria, probably the earliest form of life on earth. It mounts an immediate nonspecific response to an invading microorganism. The second type of immunity, adaptive or acquired immunity, is facilitated by mechanisms that adapt to the presence of pathogens and becomes more effective with each exposure (sensitization).

As organisms evolved and became more complex, colonizing new habitats, they were vulnerable to a broader range of more recently evolved pathogens such as viruses. Adaptive immunity occurs exclusively in higher multicellular organisms that have evolved relatively recently, such as mammals, birds and some fish (jawed vertebrates). It has evolved in response to increased pressure on survival and augments innate immunity; it is specific and effective at eliminating infections. The adaptive immune system ensures that, if an animal survives an initial infection by a pathogen, it is usually immune to further illness caused by the same or sometimes a similar pathogen, for example *vaccinia* (an orthopoxvirus causing cowpox and closely related to variola virus) will bestow immunity against smallpox; this response is exploited in medical vaccination programmes. Although the innate and adaptive systems operate differently, there are many common mechanisms and components. It has been hypothesized that the innate system, though more 'primitive', plays a critical role in viviparity (internal reproduction and embryo dependency on the mother) and toleration of the fetal allograft.

OVERVIEW OF THE IMMUNE SYSTEM

Innate Immunity

Innate immunity is inherent and does not require prior contact with a pathogen for responses to occur. The defence is nonspecific, immediate, but not long lasting. The responses are mobilized quickly and activated by receptors that generically respond to a broad range of pathogens. The first line of defence can be considered to be the physical and chemical barriers of the respiratory, reproductive and gastrointestinal systems and skin (Brostoff et al., 1991; Fig. 10.2). The skin is an almost impermeable barrier, which is shed continuously (desquamation) from the surface of the body. Commensal organisms on the skin or in the respiratory and gastrointestinal epithelium, create a naturally acidic environment, which is hostile to pathogens which they outnumber and usually outcompete to reduce the possibility of infection. The gastrointestinal and respiratory tracts utilize peristalsis and cilia, respectively, to keep potentially infectious agents moving (such as producing coughing in respiratory infections and the expulsion of frequent liquid stools in diarrhoea). In addition, secretions such as sweat, tears, saliva and secretions in the respiratory and gastrointestinal tract contain antimicrobial substances. The chemical protective mechanisms of the innate immune system include that provided by the acidity of the skin (pH 3–5) and the stomach lumen (pH 2–3), lysozyme in tears and saliva, the complement system and interferons, which block viral replication (Table 10.1). The responses of the innate immune system, such as inflammation, generate cytokines (chemical signals), which recruit immune cells to the site of infection, resulting in identification and removal of dead cells and foreign substances and also communicate with the adaptive immune system via presentation of antigens.

Cells of the innate immune system express pattern recognition receptors (PRRs), which recognize pathogen-associated molecular patterns (PAMPs), unique molecular sequences expressed on the surface of pathogenic microorganisms (Koga et al., 2009). When PRRs of the immune cells bind to PAMPs on the pathogen, an inflammatory response is generated against the pathogen. One of the main

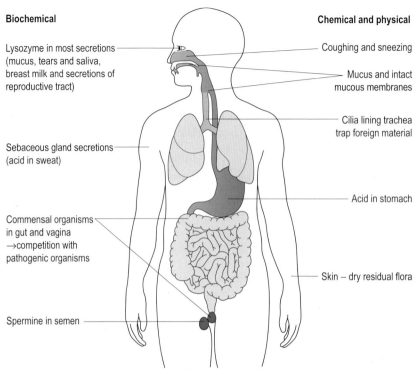

Biochemical

Lysozyme in most secretions
(mucus, tears and saliva,
breast milk and secretions of
reproductive tract)

Sebaceous gland secretions
(acid in sweat)

Commensal organisms
in gut and vagina
→competition with
pathogenic organisms

Spermine in semen

Chemical and physical

Coughing and sneezing

Mucus and intact
mucous membranes

Cilia lining trachea
trap foreign material

Acid in stomach

Skin – dry residual flora

Fig. 10.2 The main physical and chemical barriers to infection (the 'first lines of defence'). (Reproduced with permission from Brostoff et al., 1991.)

TABLE 10.1 Defensive Activity of the Innate Immune System

Phagocytosis	Neutrophils and macrophages adhere to the surface of the target organism. Adherence is enhanced by opsonins, which form a bridge between the pathogen and the phagocyte. The phagocytic cells produce pseudopodia facilitating the engulfing and phagocytosis of the pathogen into a cellular vesicle (phagosome). Lysosomes fuse with the phagosome and their digestive enzymes degrade the pathogen
Cytotoxicity	Eosinophils and NK cells adhere to target pathogens (opsonins increase efficiency). Eosinophils secrete chemicals, which damage the target cell membrane, causing cell death, and an inflammatory response, which is particularly effective against parasites. NK cells attack body cells expressing viral proteins in their membranes and some tumour cells. The NK cells adhere and release perforin, which penetrates the cell membrane causing cell death
Inflammation	The sequence of events is that the trigger (such as a bacterial signal) stimulates vasodilation and increased blood flow and delivery of blood cells (redness, heat and pain). Vascular permeability (swelling) occurs, which increases exudation and extracellular fluid (oedema), phagocyte invasion, promotion of fibrin wall enclosing infection and tissue repair

families of PRRs is the Toll-like receptors (TLRs). Eleven types of TLRs have been identified in humans. TLRs are very specific to particular PAMPs that are molecules which are evolutionarily conserved and critical to the pathogen's function (Koga and Mor, 2010). For instance, TLR4 recognizes Gram-negative bacterial lipopolysaccharide and TLR2 recognizes bacterial lipoproteins, Gram-positive bacterial peptidoglycans and fungal zymosan. TLRs also act with host cells, which display 'danger signals', for instance, express different molecules on their surface when they are apoptotic (undergoing programmed cell death), stressed or damaged, e.g. by reactive oxygen species.

Lysozyme

Lysozyme, which is sometimes described as 'the body's own antibiotic', is an enzyme that breaks down peptidoglycans, a major component of Gram-positive bacterial cell walls. It is an abundant component of body secretions such as sweat, tears, breast milk and the mucus secretions of the reproductive and respiratory tracts.

The Complement System

The complement system is comprised of a group of >30 interacting proteins, mostly synthesized by the liver, and receptors, which form an amplification cascade of defence, leading to cytolysis of bacteria (osmotic pressure-related destruction of bacteria after the cell walls have been damaged), chemotaxis (the movement of immune cells towards the chemical signals produced by the pathogen), opsonization (the tagging of the pathogen to enhance the response by the immune cells) and inflammation (a generic response that increases movement of immune cells from the blood to the injured tissue; results in heat, redness, pain and swelling).

As in the blood coagulation cascade, the components of the complement cascade exist in an inactive precursor form that can be triggered and activated. There are three pathways of activation: the classic pathway, which requires recognition of bacteria by antibodies (immunoglobulins); the alternative pathway, where the complement cascade is activated by the unique composition of an organism's cell wall (activator surface); and the mannan-binding lectin pathway in which lectins bind with very high specificity to carbohydrates on the surface of bacterial cells.

The outcome of complement activation is the formation of a membrane attack complex, cylindrical assembly of proteins that form pores in the membrane of bacterial cells. This pore or membrane attack complex (MAC) allows ions to enter cells so that fluid follows by osmosis causing the bacterial cells swell and burst. The complement cascade stimulates the release of histamine and kinins from mast cells, attracts macrophages and neutrophils to the site and enhances phagocytosis by opsonization. The complement system may be a factor in a number of diseases such as multiple sclerosis, asthma, Alzheimer's disease, type 1 diabetes (T1D) (Hewagama and Richardson, 2009) and autoimmune diseases such as SLE (Chen et al., 2010).

Interferons

Interferons are cytokines secreted by virally infected host cells that carry out a nonspecific defence, which prevents viral replication. Viruses have no ability to synthesize either DNA, RNA or proteins and, in order to replicate, they must 'hijack' the DNA/RNA/protein synthetic pathways in the host cells they have infected. Therefore, the cell is diverted to make both the viral genome (DNA or RNA) and viral proteins, which are assembled into numerous viral particles, which infect additional cells or new hosts. Interferons 'interfere' with this production of new viral genomes and proteins; they are secreted by the virally infected cell inducing the synthesis of protective proteins in neighbouring uninfected cells creating a barrier around the viral infection, which prevents the viral replication. Interferons also stimulate macrophages and natural killer (NK) cells; they can also upregulate major histocompatibility complex (MHC) expression. Interferons produced by genetic engineering are used therapeutically, for example in multiple sclerosis, various cancers and in treatment of viral infections such as chronic hepatitis.

Leukocytes and Lymphocytes

The cells of the immune system are leukocytes and lymphocytes. Although they are described as white blood cells, some of the cells spend very little time in the circulation, whereas others never enter the vascular system at all and remain in the lymphatic system, spleen or other tissues. Blood cells are derived from a single population of haemopoietic stem cells (HSCs) in the bone marrow. These precursor cells have the potential to divide into progenitor cells, which can differentiate into all cell types present in blood. After radiation for cancer treatment, the destroyed stem cells have to be replaced by stem cells from a bone marrow transplant; very few cells need to be transplanted for regeneration of a mature population of cells. This type of treatment is risky as it destroys the immune system completely and so the risk of overwhelming infection is high until the bone marrow transplant is established and functioning. Classic studies performed in mice first demonstrated that a single bone marrow-derived stem cell could repopulate the entire population of blood cells, which had been destroyed by prior radiation treatment (Krause et al., 2001).

Phagocytes

Neutrophils and macrophages are phagocytic white blood cells that can engulf and digest foreign cells and unwanted matter, such as the body's own dead and dying cells, through the processes of phagocytosis, cytotoxicity and the generation of an inflammatory response. The cells that mediate innate immunity are the granulocytes: neutrophils, monocytes, eosinophils and basophils. Neutrophils, also known as polymorphonuclear leukocytes, are the most numerous, forming about 40–70% of the circulating white blood cells.

On entering the circulation, neutrophils, which have a lifespan of a few days, cease cell division. Neutrophils are motile and exhibit chemotactic behaviour, moving through a concentration gradient towards chemical messengers, such as those released from dividing bacteria, activated platelets or other phagocytic cells, towards the site of infection. Neutrophils have multilobed nuclei (hence their original name, polymorphonuclear leukocytes), which aid diapedesis (the amoeboid movement of neutrophils through the intercellular spaces between the capillary endothelial cells). Neutrophil phagocytosis is fast. Neutrophils usually reach the site of infection and begin phagocytosis within about 90 min of the initial stimulation; they surround the unwanted material and engulf it into an intracellular vesicle or phagosome, which merges with a lysosome to form a phagolysosome containing powerful digestive and oxidative enzymes that kill the engulfed bacterium. The neutrophil can generate a vigorous oxidative burst releasing lethal reactive oxygen species or produce nitric oxide, which kills both the phagocyte itself and the engulfed pathogen. Alternately, the bacterium is killed by myeloperoxidase from neutrophil granules, which can generate hypochlorite (bleach), which is very toxic to bacteria; the green haem pigment of myeloperoxidase gives the greenish colour of bacterially infected mucous and 'pus'. Neutrophils also generate extracellular traps (or NETs), which capture and kill invading microbes.

Adherence of the phagocyte to the target cell or pathogen can be increased by opsonization. Opsonins include antibodies that bind specifically to an antigen on the pathogen surface and are then recognized by Fc receptors on phagocytes, which bind specifically to the Fc regions of the antibodies so that the pathogen is more efficiently recognized and phagocytosed. The complement component, C3, also binds to pathogens and is recognized by the complement receptor on phagocytes, thus increasing the efficiency of recognition and adherence of the phagocyte. Effectively, the opsonin acts as a bridge between the pathogen and the phagocyte, so promoting phagocytosis. Monocytes circulate for a short time in the bloodstream and then migrate to tissues and organs where they differentiate into macrophages and exhibit characteristics specific to their host tissue. Less than 7% of circulating white blood cells are monocytes, but 'resident macrophages' are abundantly distributed in the body tissues and are particularly dense around blood vessels, the gut walls, the genital tract and lungs. In some tissues, these resident macrophages are specifically named and have additional functions such as Kupffer cells in the liver and glial cells in the brain. Macrophages are oestrogen-sensitive. Monocytes are the largest white blood cell and have a characteristic horseshoe-shaped nucleus. They are also phagocytes and have a longer lifespan than neutrophils. Circulating monocytes respond more slowly than neutrophils, reaching the site of infection within about 48 h, but they have a greater capacity for phagocytosis, engulfing more material than neutrophils.

A major component of tissue homeostasis in the body is cell death and replacement by young cells, which derive from tissue stem cells. Different cell types can have very different lifespans at the end of which they undergo apoptosis and flag their imminent cell death by flipping the phospholipid, phosphatidylserine, from the inner to the outer leaflet of their cell membrane phospholipid bilayer. This apoptotic 'Eat Me' signal marks these cells for phagocytosis. Many billions of cells reach the end of their lives each day in humans and release of their contents into extracellular fluids would provoke a life-threatening inflammatory response, which is avoided by their wholesale phagocytosis and breakdown to harmless products, which can then be released.

Many pathogens have evolved mechanisms to evade phagocyte activity; these include inhabiting niches like the skin where phagocytes cannot reach, suppressing inflammatory responses, interfering with the phagocyte recognition of pathogens or interfering with chemotaxis. In addition, some bacteria can block phagocytosis or survive within phagocytes or in the phagolysosomes.

Natural Killer Cells

NK cells are cytotoxic lymphocytes, which attack compromised host cells such as virally infected and cancerous cells. Although NK cells are lymphocytes, they are part of the innate immune system. NK cells target cells expressing low levels of MHC proteins (see below), a common characteristic of both virally infected and some cancer cells. NK cells can respond rapidly compared with B and T cells, which depend on antigen specificity but have recently been shown to also have antigen-specific responses and to undergo the clonal proliferation that is generally associated with B and T cells. Not surprisingly, given their lymphocyte phenotype, they have also been shown to have a long-lived memory like B and T memory cells (Sun and Lanier 2018; Pahl et al. 2018).

NK cells (and also cytotoxic T cells, see below) release granules containing perforin and granzymes on contact with their target cell. Perforin creates pores in the target cell membrane so that the cytotoxic granzymes can enter the cell and trigger apoptosis. NK cells also secrete proinflammatory cytokines including IFN-γ and TNF-α to trigger additional immune responses.

The Acquired (Adaptive) Immune Response

The acquired immune response is highly specific to particular molecular determinants of antigens, which are recognized as 'non-self', rather than common molecular patterns that are recognized by the innate immune system.

Lymphocytes

There are three types of lymphocytes: those that mature in the bone marrow, called B lymphocytes (or B cells); those that mature in the thymus, called T lymphocytes (or T cells); and NK cells, which are innate lymphocytes (see above). Lymphocytes, which constitute ~20–40% of the circulating white blood cells, coordinate the adaptive immune responses. These small cells have relatively little cytoplasm, few organelles and no granules. T lymphocytes have secretory vesicles containing perforins and granzymes. B lymphocytes are responsible for antibody secretion, the humoral response and these immunoglobulins (antibodies) attack bacteria and viruses. Antibodies are large protein complexes of >150 kDa molecular weight, which cannot cross cell membranes to access intracellular pathogens. This is the role of T lymphocytes and cell-mediated immunity and, like NK cells, these T cells can trigger cell death of infected or tumour cells. Small lymphocytes also circulate in the lymphoid system and spend much of the time resident in lymphatic organs. The lymphoid system is the main site of the adaptive immune responses. Fluid leaks out of blood capillaries into the intercellular spaces and whereas some of the fluid re-enters the blood capillary (see Chapter 1), the remainder enters the lymphatic capillaries. This lymph fluid, therefore, has a similar composition to plasma, except that the protein component of plasma is retained within the blood vessels so lymph has a low protein content. Ultimately, the lymph is transported through lymph vessels to the thoracic duct and back into the bloodstream. The small lymphocytes 'burrow out' of the small veins as they pass through the lymph nodes and so enter the lymphoid tissue. Each lymphocyte spends minutes in the bloodstream compared with hours residing in the lymphatic system. Lymphocytes have different levels of maturity; naive lymphocytes, which are mature but have not yet encountered the antigen they will recognize; effector cells, which have been activated by an antigen; and memory cells, which have survived from past exposure to the antigen and could rapidly divide in response to subsequent exposure to the same antigenic determinant.

Antigen Recognition

Cells of the acquired immune system differentiate between 'self' and 'non-self' (foreign), and 'changed self' in host cells, which have become infected or cancerous, targeting the cells and pathogens, which are not 'self' and have evaded the innate immune response. The surface of a pathogen displays a unique combination of antigenic determinants that can be recognized by the immune cells as 'foreign' or 'non-self'. An immune response to a pathogen will normally result in multiple B or T lymphocytes recognizing multiple antigenic determinants (also termed

'epitopes') as 'non-self'. Such antigens can be displayed by the pathogen itself or can be secreted by a pathogen as in the case of bacterial toxins, or can be substances from non-pathogenic sources, such as plant pollens, resulting in allergic responses or chemicals such as synthetic vaccines. Only certain parts of the entire antigen are immunogenic; these parts bind antibodies and activated lymphocytes. Large chemically simple molecules (such as plastics) have little or no immunogenicity. Antigenicity depends on the ability of the host to identify the substance as an antigen; there are variations in individual responses.

B and T lymphocytes have high-affinity surface receptors that recognize antigens with a very high specificity. Each lymphocyte has a single type of specific antigen receptor, unlike the cells of the innate (nonspecific) immune system, which have many different types of receptor on each cell. These receptors differ between T lymphocytes (T-cell receptors) and B lymphocytes, the latter displaying on its cell surface copies of the specific antibody that each cell can secrete. Infecting pathogens will normally display multiple antigenic determinants, which are recognized as foreign by many different lymphocytes in the infected host. Antibody–antigen interaction and T-cell receptor–antigen interaction are so specific that they can distinguish between proteins, for example, which differ in a single amino acid. It is estimated that the human immune system can recognize and respond to >1 billion different epitopes via structurally different antibodies and T-cell receptors, and yet our best estimates of the number of genes in the human genome is <25,000.

The explanation for this conundrum is 'somatic recombination'; the enormous diversity of antibody and T-cell receptor specificity results from genetic recombination of a few hundred small gene segments, so that the antigen specificity of each lymphocyte is originally unique. The gene segments recombine to form unique genes. This process is known as combinatorial diversification or V(D)J (variable, diverse and joining gene segment) recombination. Exposure of the immune system to 'non-self' antigens and their presentation to lymphocytes by antigen-presenting cells (APCs) switches on the naive lymphocyte, which recognizes each antigenic determinant to enter clonal selection and divide into millions of B or T lymphocytes, each displaying identical receptors and thus mounting a massive immune response to a specific antigenic determinant. Since pathogens will always display many different epitopes, many clones of lymphocytes will be generated each of them specific for a different antigenic determinant on the pathogen. A minority of cells formed by clonal selection will become memory cells. These will remain in the body usually for years and, on reinfection by a pathogen with an identical antigenic determinant, will mount a faster and stronger immune response (Fig. 10.3).

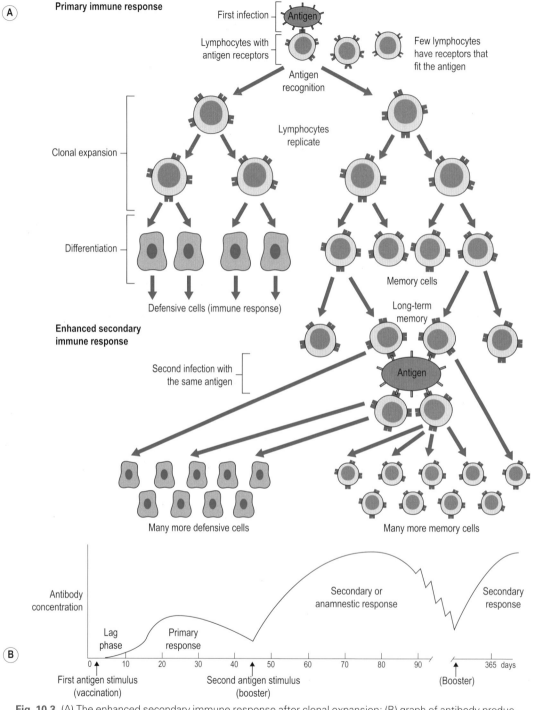

Fig. 10.3 (A) The enhanced secondary immune response after clonal expansion; (B) graph of antibody production following exposure to antigen. ((A) Reproduced with permission from Stewart, 1997.)

TABLE 10.2 Types of Acquired Immunity

Active Natural	Artificial	Passive Natural	Artificial
Clinical or subclinical disease	Vaccines: dead or extract attenuated toxoids	Congenital (across placenta) colostrum	Antiserum antitoxin gamma globulin

In the random production of antigen receptors, some lymphocytes will possess receptors, which recognize the body's own antigens and become self-reactive. 'Quality control' mechanisms ensure that before lymphocytes are released from the bone marrow or thymus they can recognize self-MHC proteins and are killed by apoptosis if they react too strongly to 'self'. Only those B and T cells that are able to recognize self MHC proteins (with or without a peptide) are allowed to mature and it is estimated that only ~2% of the lymphocytes produced are allowed to survive. This process is called 'central tolerance' and failure of these central tolerance mechanisms plays an important causative role in autoimmune disease (Goodnow et al., 2005). It seems that some of the self-reactive T cells escape central tolerance in all individuals. These may be prevented from causing autoimmune disease by a range of peripheral tolerance mechanisms. The immune system protects us from morbidity and mortality on a daily basis but it is also essential that these central and peripheral tolerance mechanisms prevent our powerful immune system from erroneously recognizing our own tissues as non-self and targeting them for destruction, as happens in autoimmune diseases.

Clonal Selection and Immunological Memory

The initial response on the first exposure to an antigen is slow to develop, perhaps taking 5–14 days, and then builds slowly to a peak ~2 weeks later. Symptoms of infection become apparent until the immune response has become effective. The secondary adaptive response, when the host subsequently encounters the same antigen, develops more quickly over 3–5 days, lasts longer and is more effective with higher antibody levels, for example, in a humoral response. This more efficient response might result in the absence of any symptoms of the infection. In the humoral response, clonal expansion produces mostly antibody-secreting plasma cells but a minority of the cells produced become memory cells, which have a long life and continue to circulate as a permanently enlarged clone of lymphocytes capable of recognizing specific antigens and mounting this more immediate response. Effectively, the initial immune response is boosted by repeated exposure, providing that the antigenic determinant that is recognized remains identical in subsequent infections. Many viruses, particularly RNA viruses (such as HIV), which require the infected host cells to produce DNA via reverse transcriptase for viral replication, have a very high rate of mutation so that the immune system may fail to recognize modified antigens in repeated or maintained infection.

Individuals have immunity to an antigen if their immune system can mount a fast and effective specific response to that antigen. The role of a vaccine is to deliberately stimulate the immune response and trigger clonal expansion of lymphocytes, which recognize the antigen that has been provided in a noninfective form. Effective vaccines can be in the form of killed whole organisms, harmless organisms, organisms that have been modified or attenuated (as in most viral vaccines), fragments of organisms (as in many bacterial vaccines), substances with similar epitopes, synthetic epitopes or inactivated toxins (Table 10.2). Some antigens are more effective at triggering clonal expansion, such as rubella (German measles) virus, which is highly antigenic; thus, after primary exposure, the host rarely acquires the infection again. Other pathogens, such as *Neisseria gonococcus* (which causes gonorrhoea) and *Treponema pallidum* (which causes syphilis), are only weakly antigenic; therefore, there are currently no effective vaccines available.

B Lymphocytes

B lymphocytes secrete antibodies that are responsible for the humoral immune response. On binding to an antigen, B lymphocytes undergo clonal expansion producing two types of daughter cells: memory B cells and plasma cells. The plasma cells are short-lived cells, which synthesize and secrete large amounts of antibodies (immunoglobulins), which are specialized glycoproteins that bind specifically to the antigen that was recognized by the B lymphocyte. These antibodies bind to their target antigens and enable other components of the immune system, such as phagocytes and complement proteins, to attack the precise organism bearing the antigen rapidly and effectively. There are five classes of antibody (Table 10.3); these differ in the structure of the 'Y'-shape of the tail, which affects whether the antibodies bind in groups or singly (Fig. 10.4). The antigen receptor on B lymphocytes is a surface immunoglobulin closely resembling the structure of the binding site on the antibodies produced that will bind to the same antigen. The binding of the B cell to the epitope is relatively straightforward in that the antigen is intact or native, whereas T lymphocytes bind only to processed antigens. However,

TABLE 10.3	Classes of Antibodies
Antibody	**Role and Characteristics**
IgG	Most abundant antibody (85% circulating antibody), found in blood and all fluid compartments including cerebrospinal fluid. Produced in large amounts at secondary adaptive response, therefore represent 'history' of past exposure to pathogens. Long lasting. Can diffuse out of bloodstream to site of acute infection and can cross placenta. Act as powerful opsonins bridging phagocyte and target cell. Important in defence against bacteria and activation of the complement system via the classic pathway
IgM	IgM molecules are groups of five immunoglobulin molecules (IgM pentamers), therefore tend to aggregate antigens into a clump that is a target for phagocytes and NK cells. Large molecules so cannot diffuse out of bloodstream. Very powerful activators of complement, important in immune responses to bacteria. First antibody produced when the body is confronted by a new antigen
IgA	Mostly in secretions such as saliva, tears, sweat and breast milk, especially colostrum (termed secretory IgA or sIgA). Link in groups of two to three. Protects body by adhering to pathogen and preventing its adherence to body cavity. Cannot activate complement or cross placenta
IgE	Tail binds to receptor on mast cells so involved in acute inflammation, allergic responses and hypersensitivity. Binding sites for antigens on larger parasites such as worms and flukes. Some people have IgE for common apparently harmless environmental proteins such as pollen, fur, house-dust mite and penicillin
IgD	Rarely synthesized; little is known about its functions. Large, found only in blood. May be involved in antigen stimulation of B cells

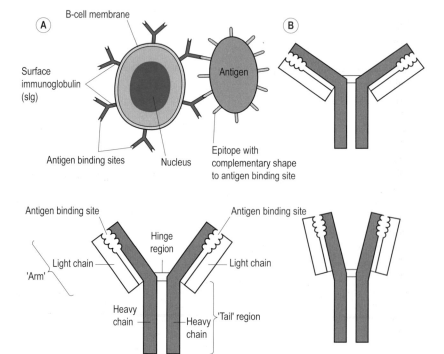

Fig. 10.4 (A) B-cell surface immunoglobulins are receptors for antigens; (B) the antibody molecule is a hinge-like structure that allows binding to two antigens. (Reproduced with permission from Stewart, 1997.)

antigen binding by a B lymphocyte usually requires helper T-cell activity before clonal expansion can take place.

Case study 10.1 looks at an example of a pregnant woman who has been exposed to German measles.

CASE STUDY 10.1

Melanie is expecting her first baby. She attends the midwives' clinic at 11 weeks' gestation concerned over the welfare of her unborn baby. Her 3-year-old nephew, Michael, whom she sees regularly, has a Rubella infection (German measles).

- What factors would the midwife need to consider in advising Melanie over her concerns?
- Would there be any specific investigations to carry out?
- If Melanie was susceptible to Rubella infection, how would this be recognized and what subsequent management and care should be planned?

MHC Proteins

Neither antibodies nor immune cells are able to access pathogens that are located within host cells so a vital component of the recognition of intracellular antigens by T cells is their translocation to the cell surface to be displayed. This is one of the roles of the MHC proteins. MHC proteins were first identified as the antigens that were recognized in transplanted tissue, which were associated with its rejection by the recipient's immune system. The underlying mechanism of this rejection was shown subsequently to be a T-cell-mediated reaction against histocompatibility proteins located on the cell membranes of transplanted tissues. This complex of proteins was subsequently termed 'human leukocyte antigens' (HLA), which are encoded by the cluster of MHC genes. MHC (HLA) proteins are recognized by T cells and, if non-self, those cells are targeted by the immune system for attack. The genes, which code for MHC proteins, are highly polymorphic with numerous forms of the same gene so that different individuals display very different complements of MHC proteins unless they are closely related, a complication in the identification of suitable donors for organ transplantation.

A major function of MHC proteins is to bind to small peptides produced from protein breakdown within a cell and then move to the plasma membrane where these peptides are displayed to T cells. MHC proteins contain a deep groove between two α-helices which are capable of binding tightly to essentially any short peptide. Two classes of these proteins, MHC I and MHC II, are associated with different cell types. MHC I proteins are expressed by essentially all nucleated cell types, whereas MHC II proteins are present in APCs, dendritic cells, B cells and macrophages. The role of these APCs is to phagocytose extracellular pathogens and degrade antigenic proteins to smaller peptides, which are then attached to MHC II proteins in the endoplasmic reticulum, then translocated to the plasma membrane where they are displayed. The MHC II–peptide complex is recognized by T helper cells, which play a vital role in regulating the immune response from all immune cell types. The MHC I–peptide and MHC II–peptide complexes must be reliably distinguished by their target cells so that, for example, virally-infected cells are killed by cytotoxic T cells, which recognize MHC I-peptide but that this must not happen with MHC II-peptide expressing cells, otherwise these essential APCs would also be lost. This discrimination is reinforced by the presence of co-receptors on T cells, which recognize an additional binding site on the appropriate MHC protein. In addition, other proteins on cytotoxic T cells including CD8 bind to regions of MHC I on infected cells and further stimulate T-cell activation. CD4 protein on T helper cells also binds to MHC II on APCs. These and many other 'quality control' mechanisms ensure that the actions of these powerful immune cells are not misdirected.

Cytokines

Cytokines are a group of small, soluble polypeptide signalling molecules that are particularly important in communication between different immune cell types. Their actions are often local (autocrine or paracrine) but can also be endocrine (see Chapter 3). Cytokines are a diverse group of molecules that include interleukins, interferons, tumour necrosis factors, some colony-stimulating factors (CSF) and lymphokines, and are secreted by a diverse range of cell types, both within and outside the immune system. Cytokines act on a variety of receptor types linked to different intracellular signalling pathways to regulate the humoral, cell-mediated and inflammatory responses and have important roles in pregnancy, parturition and disease. As such they have great potential as therapeutic tools and targets in the treatment of disease.

T Lymphocytes

There are several subsets of T lymphocytes including cytotoxic T cells (T_c), helper T cells (T_h) and regulatory T cells (T_{reg}) (formerly called suppressor T cells). A key requirement for research into the functions of these cells was to be able to unequivocally identify these different cell types so that their behaviour could be studied *in vitro* and *in vivo*. To this end, unique glycoproteins present on the cell surface, which are involved in mediating cell function as mentioned above, were used to raise highly specific monoclonal antibodies to distinguish the different subpopulations of lymphocytes. The system of nomenclature is based on the cluster of differentiation (CD) system. Cytotoxic T cells express CD8 protein markers in the plasma membrane and are sometimes referred to as CD8+ cells. They recognize and destroy cells that have become infected or malignant. Some regulatory T cells also express CD8 but express other markers as well, including CD4 and CD25, which distinguish them from other T-cell types.

T helper cells express CD4 proteins, and are sometimes called CD4+ cells. T helper cells 'conduct the orchestra' of the immune response and play important roles in its regulation. For example, they play essential roles in the control of B-cell antibody production and the activation of cytotoxic T cells and also interact with other cell types such as macrophages via the cytokines they secrete, which activate and regulate other components of the immune system. Additional T-cell types have also been recently identified including Th17 cells discussed below.

An example of the vital importance of T helper cells to immune defences comes from studies on HIV, the causative pathogen of AIDS. The receptor for HIV is the CD4 protein expressed not only by T cells but also by macrophages and possibly other cell types. HIV reduces the number of helper T cells by inducing apoptosis, so none of the immune mechanisms work effectively. Infection of macrophages shifts the profile of cytokines produced, which contributes to wasting and acute respiratory distress syndrome. Macrophages can also act as a reservoir for the HIV virus during a period of 'clinical latency', which can range from weeks to >10 years, when HIV replication and symptoms resurge before death ensues. The catastrophic impact of HIV infection reflects the enormous importance of a functional immune system, and T helper cell function in particular, to our very survival. The major cause of death in HIV/AIDS sufferers is opportunistic infections by pathogens, which would normally be destroyed by a functional immune system and would not be fatal.

T lymphocytes have antigen receptors on their surface, formed of two peptide chains that contain the binding site for a specific epitope. However, the T lymphocyte cannot bind to an epitope unless it has been processed and presented to the T lymphocyte by one of the host's own cells. Most nucleated cell types in the body routinely turnover and degrade their intracellular proteins. Peptides from this process enter the endoplasmic reticulum where they are bound to Class I MHC (MHC I) proteins. As mentioned above, these MHC I–peptide complexes are 'displayed'

BOX 10.1   The Major Histocompatibility Complex

Each person has a unique configuration of MHC antigens, which are molecules on the surface of virtually all nucleated cells (except monozygotic twins who have identical MHC). MHC molecules are a marker of 'self' and also termed 'human leukocyte antigens' (HLA). MHC molecules present antigens to T cells. There are different classes of MHC molecules, with MHC I present on all nucleated cell types and MHC II only on APCs. MHC II molecules interact with helper T cells to trigger an immune response, which is appropriate for the detected antigen. MHC proteins are also involved in rejection of transplanted tissue, which has non-self MHC molecules. Tissue grafts have increased survival if there is some similarity in MHC structure between the donor and the recipient (hence the need for tissue typing) and if drugs are used to suppress the immune response.

---

on the cell surface and, if the displayed peptide is recognized as non-self because it has originated from an intracellular pathogen, or from a mutated gene, it will activate cytotoxic T cells. These infected or mutated (cancerous) cells will be killed by apoptosis, which is triggered by the cytotoxic T cell. This process, which occurs in essentially all nucleated cell types, differs from that seen in 'professional' APCs. APCs such as dendritic cells, B lymphocytes and macrophages, bind to antigens present in extracellular fluid and phagocytose them, degrading the proteins present in phagolysosomes. APCs express Class II MHC (MHC II instead of MHC I) proteins, which bind to peptide products from the degraded pathogen. APCs migrate to the lymph nodes where these peptides are displayed in the cleft of the MHC II molecule (Box 10.1), on the surface of the APC (Fig. 10.5). Helper T and Treg lymphocytes bind only to epitopes processed in this manner and displayed on MHC II proteins on APCs, in order to switch on or suppress the immune response to peptides seen as non-self. This activation of naive T cells by 'professional APCs' requires verification by costimulatory proteins on the surface of the APCs to avoid the accidental triggering of an immune response. If verified, T helper cells will be stimulated to secrete cytokines, which trigger a humoral and/or a cell-mediated immune response, depending upon the type of pathogen present. For example, a cell-mediated response will be required to target virus-infected cells or cells expressing mutated tumorigenic proteins where non-self peptides will be displayed on the membrane on MHC

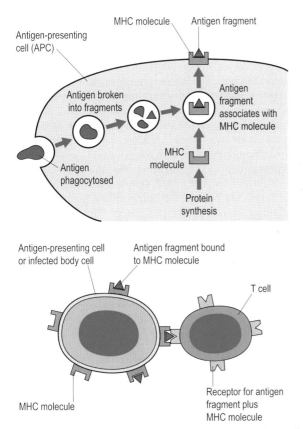

Fig. 10.5 Antigen processing by the antigen-presenting cell (APC). (Reproduced with permission from Stewart, 1997.)

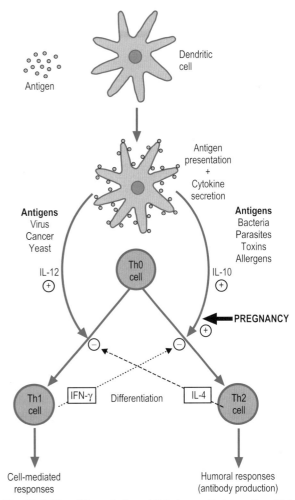

Fig. 10.6 The differentiation of T helper cells into either Th1 or Th2 cells depends on the type of antigen presented by the dendritic cells and the pattern of cytokine secretion. Th1 cells are generated in response to IL-12 secreted by dendritic cells. Once produced, Th1 cells secrete IFN-γ, which prevents the formation of Th2 cells, leading to a predominantly cell-mediated response. Th2 cells are generated in response to IL-10 secreted by dendritic cells. If Th2 cells are generated, they produce IL-4 (and IL-13) which suppresses Th1 cells leading to a predominantly humoral immune response, relying upon antibody production. Th1 and Th2 responses are mutually suppressive and define the appropriate immune response for the type of antigen detected. In pregnancy, the Th2 response is enhanced, which is important in preventing a cell-mediated fetal rejection.

I proteins and recognized by cytotoxic T cells, which will trigger apoptosis to destroy the cell. Since antibodies cannot enter cells, the humoral response would be ineffective in targeting such cells.

There are several forms of T helper cells that arise from naive T cells (Th0) that originated in the bone marrow before moving to the thymus where positive and negative selection 'quality control' mechanisms are applied. These naive T cells are activated by distinct cytokines and become polarized into different Th subsets, Th1, Th2, Th17 or Treg cells, which each secrete different cytokines. The dendritic cells present the antigen to T helper cells and direct them to differentiate into these different T-cell subsets, which essentially defines the appropriate immune response for the type of antigen detected. The pathway of differentiation is controlled by the cytokine secretions of the dendritic cell. Secretion of IL-12 by the dendritic cell drives the differentiation towards Th1, whereas IL-4 triggers differentiation into Th2 cells (Fig. 10.6).

The Th1 cells coordinate the response towards intracellular pathogens, viruses, malignant cells and intracellular bacteria (e.g. *Mycoplasma pneumoniae* or *Chlamydia*) or tumours. The outcome of the Th1 response is activation of cell-mediated immunity by the secretion of IL-2, tumour necrosis factor (TNF) β and interferon gamma (INF-γ) to activate macrophages and the clonal expansion of cytotoxic T cells, to target cells carrying intracellular pathogens or mutated genes and proteins (tumours), for which circulating antibodies would be useless. Following clonal expansion of the T lymphocytes that recognize the non-self peptide, cytotoxic T cells seek out the virally infected or mutated cells and, on contact release granules containing perforin and granzymes onto the target cell. As mentioned above for NK cells, perforin creates pores in the target cell membrane so that the cytotoxic granzymes can enter the cell and trigger apoptosis. This process will be turned off when the antigen-expressing cells have been eliminated. When the infection has resolved, most of the cytotoxic T cells die and are removed by phagocytosis; a small percentage of the T cells remain as memory cells.

Extracellular pathogens, including other bacteria, parasites (such as helminths), toxins and allergens (e.g. such as those which cause asthma), predominantly trigger a Th2 response and secretion of IL-4, IL-5 and IL-13, which activate eosinophils, leukocytes, B lymphocytes (which produce antibodies) and mast cells. The Th1 and Th2 systems suppress each other and the Th1/Th2 balance is important. For instance, some viruses produce proteins that mimic IL-10 and drive the differentiation of Th0 cells into Th2 cells, which are less effective at attacking viruses so viral survival is enhanced. In pregnancy, the Th1/Th2 balance shifts in favour of Th2; this downregulation of Th1-induced cell-mediated immunity and enhancement of the Th2-induced humoral responsiveness in the maternal immune system in pregnancy is mediated by progesterone and is important in preventing fetal rejection. This may explain why some viral infections are more severe and have higher morbidity and mortality during pregnancy (see below).

In addition to Th1 and Th2 subsets, Treg cells and Th17 cells also play vital roles in the immune system. IL-2 and TGF-β cytokines trigger differentiation of Th0 cells into inducible Treg cells, whereas IL-6 and TGF-β regulate Th17 cell numbers. Regulatory T cells (Tregs) have important anti-inflammatory and immune-regulatory roles and limit the activity of the immune response to self-antigens, maintaining immune system homeostasis and tolerance to self-antigens (peripheral tolerance) and thus preventing damage to the body's own cells. As such, they are essential in preventing autoimmune disorders. Treg cells can be of two types, natural or inducible. Natural Tregs in the thymus are responsible for central tolerance and the clonal deletion of T cells which inappropriately recognize self-antigens, whereas peripheral inducible Treg cells arise, as described, from naive Th0 cells as a result of self-antigen presentation and antigen-stimulated dendritic cell cytokines. Natural

Tregs suppress the effects of autoreactive T cells, whereas inducible Tregs are important in preventing an immune response to self-antigens in other body tissues.

Treg cells accumulate in the lymph nodes, draining the uterus and spleen in early pregnancy probably because they migrate towards human chorionic gonadotrophin (hCG) and chemokines produced by the trophoblast. Treg cells appear to be important in immune tolerance of the conceptus tissue (see below) and the sperm and oocytes as well as many other harmless molecules recognized as non-self, for which an inflammatory immune response would be counterproductive. Th17 cells are also important and the Treg/Th17 balance has implications for health issues including autoimmunity and cancer. Th17 cells produce the pro-inflammatory cytokine IL-17 and have important roles in the induction of inflammation. They are active in the immune response against extracellular pathogens and in the gut where most Th17 cells are found, and where they promote the 'tightness' of tight junctions and gut barrier function. Whereas Treg cells are important in the induction of tolerance and in suppressing the inappropriate immune responses of autoimmunity, Th17 cells appear to counter these beneficial effects and can induce autoimmune responses under some conditions. The roles of these two cells types is a major area of research interest in the search for causes and prevention of the >80 autoimmune disorders that affect humans, predominantly females in their childbearing and post-childbearing years.

Interaction of B and T Lymphocytes

B lymphocytes and T lymphocytes interact (Fig. 10.7). The B lymphocyte binds to the native (intact) antigen via B-cell receptors on its cell surface. The antigen is then internalized by the B lymphocyte and processed so fragments appear on its cell surface associated with the MHC II molecule. In this form, it is recognized by T helper cells, which are activated, producing a signal that triggers B lymphocyte cell division and differentiation. The immune system includes many such interactions between different cell types using numerous signalling molecules, an understanding of which is essential to many aspects of human health and disease.

Passive Immunity

Resistance to a specific pathogen resulting from previous exposure, or acquired via immunization, is active immunity. However, sometimes, the effect of infection can be disastrous before the immune system has time to mount a response. Passive immunization can overcome this by providing temporary resistance in the form of products from a donor source. Passive immunization causes destruction of the pathogenic cells without creating clonal expansion or making memory cells so its effects are not permanent.

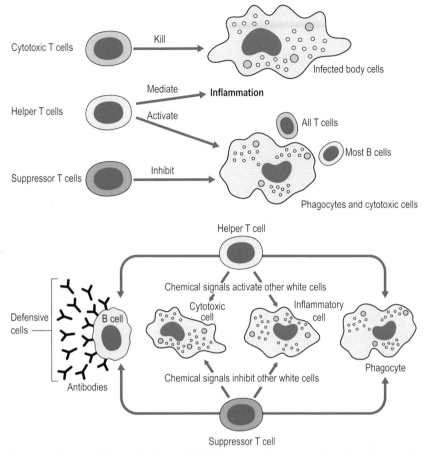

Fig. 10.7 The role of three different T cells and their interaction. Suppressor T cells and now referred to as regulatory T cells (Tregs). (Reproduced with permission from Stewart, 1997.)

An individual who has no prior immunity but is exposed to antigens of a potentially dangerous disease can be given preformed antibodies. Examples include treatment with rabies immune globulin following a bite from a rabid dog or anti-D immunization following potential exposure to Rhesus-incompatible antigens (see below). The transfer of placental antibodies (IgG) to the fetus and consumption by the neonate of maternal antibodies secreted into colostrum and breast milk (sIgA) are also examples of passive immunity, with the latter being an important source of immune protection, disease prevention and decreased mortality in breastfed infants. For this reason, the move away from breastfeeding towards formula milk products is a major concern. It was recently estimated that if breastfeeding could be increased worldwide to near-universal levels, >800,000 lives could be saved each year, mostly of children under 5 years of age, as well as >20,000 deaths prevented per annum from breast cancer in mothers (Victora et al., 2016).

Interaction of the Innate and Adaptive Immune Systems

The innate and adaptive immune systems work synergistically to protect us from disease and possible death on a daily basis. These systems utilize nonspecific protective barriers and genetically encoded receptors, versus highly specific antigen receptors respectively, in the innate and adaptive responses. Despite their many differences, these two systems are tightly interrelated so that the adaptive component relies entirely upon the innate immune system to tell it if, how, when and where to respond.

THE IMMUNE SYSTEM IN PREGNANCY

Recent evidence has demonstrated the vital importance of the maternal immune system in all aspects of pregnancy from fertilization, implantation, acceptance of the fetus, successful fetal development and the timing and triggering of parturition. In addition, the health of the neonate and even the adult offspring can be significantly impacted by the ability of the maternal immune system to control and protect fetal development and help trigger, at term, the successful completion of gestation.

ACCEPTANCE OF THE FETUS

Humans are 'outbred'. The genetic diversity resulting from sexual reproduction means that the fetus is phenotypically unique and immunologically distinct from both of its parents. The fetus has a unique combination of histocompatibility antigens and is therefore actually an allograft – foreign tissue from the same species but with different genotype and antigenic make-up. Half of the fetal antigens are derived from the father and therefore are foreign (non-self) to the maternal immune system. There is a marked antigenic difference between the maternal tissues and the maternal–paternal inherited antigens that are expressed by the fetus. If tissue from the offspring is grafted on to its mother, a strong maternal immune response is mounted and the tissue is rejected. It seems surprising therefore that the mother does not reject the fetus because of these foreign paternal antigens. Peter Medawar, a pioneer in the field of tissue and organ transplantation and Nobel laureate, proposed several possible mechanisms to explain why the fetus is not rejected: (1) since fetal tissue is antigenically immature, it may not express normal antigens; (2) the uterus may be a privileged site (or not in contact with fetal tissue) or (3) pregnancy may affect the maternal immune system and normal immune responses (Medawar, 1953). However, it is the placenta and not the fetus that is the 'transplant', and the placenta has very different characteristics from those of a transplanted tissue or organ, and the interaction of the trophoblast with the maternal immune system orchestrates cooperative modulation of the components of the immune system.

Fetal Antigen Expression

Contrary to Medawar's first suggestion, fetal tissue is antigenically mature and does express antigens and immunocompetence from an early stage (Koga and Mor, 2010). MHC class I and II antigens (see above), albeit in smaller amounts, are present on embryonic cells from the time of implantation and throughout pregnancy. The MHC proteins identify 'self' and are the molecules that are normally recognized by a transplant-recipient's immune system, which triggers the rejection of allografts (foreign tissue transplants). Nonimmune cells generally express the MHC I proteins, HLA-A and HLA-B, whereas the primary villous trophoblast cells are HLA null and the invasive extravillous trophoblast cells express a unique combination of classical HLA-C and nonclassical HLA-G and HLA-E proteins but neither HLA-A nor HLA-B (Apps et al., 2009).

Women are exposed to paternal antigens during intercourse and seminal fluid elicits an immune response. T-cell activation, cytokine secretion and immune cell recruitment are all triggered by soluble MHC proteins in seminal fluid in unprotected intercourse, to prime the maternal immune response, even before conception occurs. Interestingly, recent reports suggest a significantly improved outcome when women undergoing IVF are exposed to seminal plasma at the time of ovum collection or embryo transfer (Crawford et al., 2015). The importance of this priming of maternal immune tolerance of paternal antigens in the fetus can also be seen by the consequences of its absence in preeclampsia. Preeclampsia is a condition that can develop usually late in pregnancy, with symptoms of high blood pressure, high urinary levels of protein and swelling of the legs, feet and hands and can lead to life-threatening eclampsia. Preeclampsia is more common in first pregnancies, particularly when these occur after minimal sexual contact between the partners, or after predominant use of barrier contraceptives. Also, although previous pregnancy with the same partner protects, the likelihood of preeclampsia increases with a change in partner, or with the use of donor sperm in IVF, where no previous exposure to paternal antigens has occurred (Robertson et al., 2018). However, a change of partner is often associated with a longer interpregnancy interval, which is more strongly correlated with preeclampsia, as is a short interval between first coitus (exposure to the partner's sperm) and pregnancy. After conception, paternal antigens are already apparent in the 8-cell stage embryo and major histocompatibility antigens begin to be expressed at later stages of cell division. Dendritic cells from fetal skin are in contact with maternal blood and enter the maternal circulation; these cells express MHC antigens (Zenclussen et al., 2007). The zona pellucida and early trophoblast have glycoprotein coatings, which may limit the cell-mediated immune responses. Also, immunological problems are usually not an issue prior to implantation because the endometrium secretes immunosuppressive factors.

The Uterus as a Privileged Site

The mother, like other individuals, would reject grafts of tissue from her own fetus because fetal tissue expresses non-self MHC proteins, reflecting the contribution of the paternal genome. Maternal responses to transplanted tissue remain competent in pregnancy; a pregnant mammal will reject transplanted tissue from the father of the fetus and tissue from the fetus, when grafted to areas other than the uterus. Some tissues, such as the testis and parts of the eye and brain, lack components required in immune responses or are not accessible to them. These sites are described as 'immune privileged' and can accept transplanted tissue with fewer problems. HLA-G, which was first identified on human trophoblasts and shown to have immunosuppressive properties, is found on immune cells such as NK cells, T cells and APCs at immune privileged sites and also in certain tumours, where it exerts important tolerogenic functions. The development of ectopic pregnancies also shows that immune tolerance of the fetus is not simply a result of the uterus being a uniquely immune privileged site, as was previously suggested. The increased vascularization of the pregnant uterus allows efficient delivery of lymphocytes and other maternal immune cells so nonfetal allogenic tissue transplanted in the uterus is rejected (Beer and Billingham, 1974). Maternal and placental tissue are in close proximity and there are a number of interfaces between maternal immune cells and placental cells that change as pregnancy progresses.

The Chorion and Trophoblast as a Barrier

The fetus is separated from the mother by the placenta and fetal membranes. It is suggested that the chorionic membranes are resistant to maternal rejection and can protect the fetus from maternal antibodies and immune cells. The placenta and chorion originate from cells derived from the fertilized egg (zygote), which are therefore genetically and antigenically different to the maternal cells. Maternal blood bathes the chorionic villi (see Chapter 8) and is therefore in contact with trophoblast cells, which are derived from the zygote and thus have nonmaternal antigens. This means that maternal blood containing immune cells is in apposition with the syncytiotrophoblast (outer layer of nonmitotic cells; see Chapter 8).

Some cytotrophoblast cells (the dividing cells underlying the syncytiotrophoblast) penetrate the syncytiotrophoblast layer to form the cytotrophoblast columns, which anchor the villi to the maternal tissue (see Chapter 8). During implantation and placental development, other invasive trophoblast cells and fragments break away from the mass of placental tissue and enter the uterine veins and maternal venous system. It is this extravillous (nonvillous) trophoblast that remodels the uterine spiral arteries to allow increased maternal blood flow to the intervillous space (see Chapter 8). This extravillous trophoblast layer of cells therefore makes extensive contact with the maternal tissue. The innate immune cells, particularly macrophages, uterine NK cells and dendritic cells (DCs) are abundant in the decidua in the luteal phase of the menstrual cycle, the time when implantation starts. These cells provide growth factors, which support trophoblast invasion. Some of the cells breach the trophoblast and invade the maternal circulation, forming minute emboli,

which lodge in the pulmonary circulation where they are destroyed. However, even within the maternal circulation, the extravillous trophoblast cells do not appear to provoke a normal inflammatory or immune response. The expression of nonclassical HLA-G antigen on the trophoblast cells protects the tissue from cytotoxic T lymphocyte activity and inhibits NK cells, which recognize and lyse cells that are deficient in class I HLA expression. In addition, the trophoblast cells may actively contribute to maternal tolerance by secreting soluble factors, which modulate the maternal immune response (Zenclussen et al., 2007).

The Mother's Immune Response

The mother is tolerant to fetal antigens, not via a single mechanism as suggested by Medawar, but due to many local and systemic changes that facilitate immune tolerance. Different mechanisms operate at different stages of the pregnancy to mediate this tolerance; some of the mechanisms operate locally at the placenta to prevent the fetal antigens being recognized and other mechanisms act on T cells to suppress fetal rejection. The mother does respond immunologically to fetal antigens on the trophoblast or on the fetal HSCs that enter the maternal circulation. Both lymphocytes and antibodies that recognize fetal antigens are present in maternal blood in pregnancy. During pregnancy, maternal T cells become transiently and reversibly tolerant to paternal alloantigens both systemically and at the uteroplacental surface (Weetman, 2010).

It is suggested that a lack of maternal immune response to the fetus could be harmful. The incidence of pregnancy where the parents are closely related (consanguineous), as in incest, is far less frequent; thus, heterozygosity is promoted within the population. A close relationship between the parents means that the fetal antigens will be more similar to the maternal antigens so the maternal immunological response will be less. It has been suggested that some of the cases of unexplained recurrent pregnancy loss (RPL), also known as recurrent spontaneous abortion (RSA) or habitual miscarriage/abortion, involving more than three consecutive early pregnancy miscarriages, may be due to a failure of maternal immune responses and immunological adaptation. Other known causes of RPL include chromosome and endocrine abnormalities, anatomical and haematological problems, and uteroplacental infections. It was controversially hypothesized that increased similarities of antigens between parents (described as HLA parental sharing) would result in the fetus having a high degree of antigen similarities with its mother. The mother would then not produce such a strong immune response to fetal cells, with perhaps fewer blocking antibodies, which would prejudice the outcome of the pregnancy. However, immunotherapy treatment for RPL where women are immunized with paternal leukocytes or antibodies has not been successful.

Fetal lymphocytes inhibit replication of stimulated lymphocytes in both the mother and unrelated individuals. This may account for the increased number and increased severity of maternal viral infections, especially in the later part of gestation. Trophoblastic cells express high levels of three membrane-bound complement-regulatory proteins that thwart potential complement-mediated damage to the trophoblast by either the classic or alternative pathways.

The placenta is in contact with fluids containing high concentrations of progesterone, corticosteroids and hCG, which may act as local immunosuppressants and inhibit the effectiveness of immune cells. The uterine endometrium has a large population of white blood cells (leukocytes), constituting up to one-third of the endometrial cell number. Approximately 90% of the leukocytes present are the innate immune cells, NK cells and macrophages (Faas and de Vos, 2017). From early pregnancy, numbers and activity of monocytes and granulocytes progressively increase. The macrophages are highly activated and secrete substantial amounts of interleukin and IgE, which may play vital roles in immunosuppression and rapid nonspecific anti-inflammatory activity. T lymphocytes are present but in early pregnancy comprise <10% of leukocytes present with very few granulocytes, dendritic cells or B cells. Cytotoxic activity and interferon production by circulating or peripheral NK cells decreases; it seems that these cells migrate to the uterine tissue where they become known as uterine NK cells (uNK cells). Approximately 90% of circulating NK cells in the blood are cytotoxic cells with the remaining 10% having a regulatory function producing cytokines and are not cytotoxic. uNK cells in the endometrium and placental bed are also the regulatory cell type but unlike the circulating NK cells they are highly granulated (Faas and de Vos, 2017). Also, there seems to be two distinct populations of uNK cells, those associated with the endometrium and the more active uNK cells, which are associated with the decidua, underlying placental development. The uNK cells seem to be hormonally regulated as they occur in decidualized tissue in extrauterine ectopic pregnancies, and their association with the uterine tissue actually occurs before implantation during the secretory phase of the menstrual cycle (Manaster and Mandelboim, 2010). In early pregnancy, uNK numbers increase to reach ~70% of all leukocytes present in the uterus during the first trimester. uNK cells have low cytotoxic activity and are probably not involved in removal of damaged embryonic cells or regulation of trophoblastic invasion. The cytokines that they produce are important in immunosuppression and growth regulation. The uNK cells may also be important in the protection against viral pathogens. When uNK cells migrate to the endometrium, they proliferate and cluster around the spiral arteries where they are involved with both trophoblastic invasion and the first wave of remodelling of the uterine spiral arteries into the low-resistance vessels supplying the placenta (see Chapter 8). Activated T cells expressing progesterone receptors are present in the peripheral blood of healthy pregnant women. Progesterone stimulates these cells to secrete the protein progesterone-induced blocking factor (PIBF). PIBF is important in immunomodulation as it alters the profile of cytokine secretion by activated lymphocytes to help generate a dominant Th2-type, which is a characteristic and keeps NK-cell activity low to prevent them from targeting fetal-maternal cells. IgA, secreted from the cells lining the uterine tubes, may also be important in protecting the uterine environment. A remission of some autoimmune diseases (such as rheumatoid arthritis and multiple sclerosis) is often observed when women with these diseases become pregnant and may correspond to the modified Th1/Th2 balance. However, as mentioned above, suppression of T-cell activity increases susceptibility to viral infections and to specific intracellular pathogens such as *Listeria*.

EFFECTS OF PREGNANCY ON THE IMMUNE SYSTEM

The maternal immune response is affected by pregnancy. Many of the cells of the immune system are affected by the hormonal changes that occur. For example, macrophages and T lymphocytes have oestrogen receptors. In pregnancy, the number of white blood cells, particularly neutrophils, increases and the cells respond more readily to challenges. hCG stimulates neutrophil production and response. The high levels of oestrogen and progesterone decrease the number of helper T cells and increase the number of Treg cells. Yeast infections increase in pregnancy, possibly because of the effect of oestrogen on the commensal microbiota of the reproductive tract. Women have a much higher incidence than men of autoimmune diseases, occurring most frequently during, or after, their child-bearing years. It is notable, however, that women who are not pregnant or who have never been pregnant still have a higher incidence of autoimmune diseases than men due to the loss of self-tolerance (see above). The exposure to female sex steroids is thought to drive this increased susceptibility (Hewagama and Richardson, 2009) so women experience a higher Th1-mediated response pattern. However, an alternative explanation is that the second X chromosome may create this genetic predisposition to autoimmune diseases.

Local concentrations of corticosteroids around the fetus and placenta suppress phagocytic activity, especially in response to Gram-negative bacteria. This means that pregnant women have a decreased ability to respond to Gram-negative infections of the reproductive tract such as gonorrhoea and *Chlamydia* (Hosenfeld et al., 2009) and *Escherichia coli*. Components of the complement cascade increase from the end of the first trimester so chemotaxis and opsonization are enhanced. Changes like this, which do not occur at the beginning of pregnancy, may be delayed to protect the fetus during implantation and very early embryonic development.

The maternal immune response is important at all stages of pregnancy and may sense the reproductive fitness and compatibility of the male partner and the developmental competence of the conceptus to ensure biological benefits for the woman and her offspring (Robertson, 2010). This 'immune-mediated quality control' hypothesis proposes that the immune system expedites pregnancy loss if the pregnancy is not in the best interest of the female, for instance, because the conceptus is not developing appropriately or when external conditions do not favour the risk of investing maternal resources into pregnancy. The corollary is that pregnancy loss may not be pathological but may be a normal and beneficial part of optimal and healthy reproductive function.

Natural Killer Cells and Cytokines

Both oestrogen and progesterone play important roles in uNK cell recruitment as part of the immune responses to pregnancy. NK-cell activity around the uterus is suppressed by local increased concentrations of prostaglandin E_2 and other cellular signals. This suppression of NK cells may be important in preventing rejection of the fetus. However, maternal resistance to intracellular pathogens such as *Toxoplasma* and *Listeria* may also be reduced. The relative proportions of cytokines change in pregnancy and the association between intra-amniotic infection (chorioamnionitis) and premature rupture of membranes may be related to cytokine-mediated stimulation of proteolytic enzyme release from neutrophils.

Toll-like Receptors

TLRs are expressed by immune cells at the maternal–fetal interface and also by nonimmune cells of the trophoblast and decidua. Their expression in the human placenta is not constant and varies in a temporal and spatial manner during pregnancy (Koga and Mor, 2010). Seminal fluid contains TLR4 ligands, which stimulate an inflammatory response and recruitment of antigen-presenting dendritic cells and macrophages, which phagocytose male antigens for presentation to naive T cells in the lymph nodes. This triggers T-cell activation and expansion of circulating Treg numbers, which accumulate in the uterus. These Tregs are essential in mediating the tolerance of paternal antigens during implantation so that an imbalance between Treg and cytotoxic T cells may undermine the implantation. The expression of the TLRs increases throughout gestation, suggesting that the placenta in early pregnancy is less responsive to microbial challenges. It is suggested that pregnancy has three distinct immunological phases characterized by different immune responses and cytokine profiles (Mor and Cardenas, 2010). The first phase of implantation and placentation is an inflammatory phase (mediated by a Th1-dominant response) to ensure repair of the uterine endometrium and removal of cellular debris after the embryo breaks through and invades the maternal tissue. At this stage of pregnancy, the placental site has been likened to an 'open wound', with the cellular responses affecting the mother's wellbeing. The second phase is the period of rapid fetal development and growth and is an anti-inflammatory state (mediated by a Th2-dominant response) when the mother feels well. Then, the third phase is another inflammatory (Th1-dominant) state leading to uterine contraction, expulsion of the fetus and delivery or rejection of the placenta.

The other notable aspect is the relative lack of TLRs on the syncytial tissue compared with the villous cytotrophoblast and extravillous trophoblast, which suggests that the placental tissue only responds to bacterial and viral products that penetrate the outer layer of the placenta. It is suggested that the differential expression of TLRs is regulated by changing levels of sex steroids and that TLRs may be involved in tissue remodelling of the endometrium and preparation for implantation (Koga and Mor, 2010). Clinical observations and studies on animal models have demonstrated that TLRs are involved in a variety of pregnancy disorders, including spontaneous abortion, preeclampsia and premature labour. Activation of TLRs can inhibit trophoblastic migration, which might be linked to the incomplete remodelling of the spiral arteries by trophoblastic cells in preeclampsia. TLRs are also important in identifying and responding to pathogens in amniotic fluid (Koga and Mor, 2010).

Antibodies and B Lymphocytes

The levels of most antibodies do not change during pregnancy. However, IgG concentrations may fall. This fall may be due to haemodilution, increased loss in urine, increased placental transfer to the fetus in the third trimester and so it can increase the risk of streptococcal infection. Fetal secretion of cytokines may suppress cell-mediated immunity and enhance humoral responsiveness. SLE, an autoimmune condition causing tissue damage in the joints and kidneys, is 10-fold more common in women, has an increased 'flare-up' frequency in pregnancy and increased maternal and fetal morbidity and mortality, which may be related to enhanced activity of B lymphocytes. This enhanced responsiveness by B lymphocytes may compensate for decreased T lymphocyte activity. B lymphocytes may also produce blocking antibodies that protect the fetus from attack by maternal T lymphocytes.

T Lymphocytes

T lymphocytes are involved in graft rejection and could therefore pose a serious threat to the fetus. However, T-cell function is suppressed in pregnancy, especially in the first trimester (Koga and Mor, 2010). Circulating numbers of T lymphocytes are lower and they have decreased ability to proliferate, to produce IL-2 and to kill foreign cells. Ratios of helper and Treg cells change and the Th1/Th2 balance is shifted in favour of Th2, generating noninflammatory responses, mediated by interleukins such as IL-4 and IL-10, which are compatible with trophoblast growth, survival of the fetus, fetal and infant growth and maintenance of pregnancy. IL-10 inhibits the activity of Th1 cells (Thaxton and Sharma, 2010). A Th1 reaction in the placenta generates inflammatory responses and is associated with miscarriage; the cytokines secreted from Th1 cells are harmful in pregnancy as they inhibit embryonic and fetal development. A Th1 dominant pattern (upregulation of IL-2, IL-6, INF-γ and TNF-α) occurs in miscarriage; the inflammatory responses seem to mediate fetal rejection. An imbalance in the Th1/Th2 shift is also associated with preeclampsia and an inflammatory host response mediated by Th1 cytokines (Zenclussen et al., 2007). Trophoblastic production of cytokines promotes the change in Th1/Th2 balance as does progesterone and the decidual production of leukaemia inhibitory factor. Although the shift in the Th1/Th2 balance explains some of the changes in the immune system during pregnancy, the observations that Th2 knockout mice had normal pregnancies (Svensson et al., 2001) led to further scrutiny of the hypothesis. Furthermore, uNK cells were shown to be necessary for successful pregnancy and INF-γ was shown to be critical in remodelling of the spiral arteries (Chaouat et al., 2010). So the originally proposed model, the Th1/Th2 paradigm, has now been revised to include the new lineages of T cells, Th17 cells, which produce IL-17, a pro-inflammatory cytokine, which induces inflammation, and acknowledges the role of Treg cells in inhibiting proliferation and cytokine production from Th1, Th2 and Th17 cells. This new model has been termed the 'Th1/Th2/Th17 and regulatory T (Treg) cells' paradigm (Saito et al., 2010). The number of Treg cells in the circulation and in the decidual tissue and the lymph nodes draining the uterus increases markedly during pregnancy. Insufficient Treg numbers or impaired Treg function are implicated in infertility, miscarriage and placental insufficiency, including intrauterine growth retardation (IUGR) (see Chapter 9) and preeclampsia.

Rheumatoid arthritis, a cell-mediated autoimmune disease, frequently goes into remission during pregnancy, because of the suppression of T lymphocytes. The amelioration of symptoms in pregnancy led to the identification of glucocorticoids as anti-inflammatory agents. Hormonal changes in pregnancy may augment the suppression of T lymphocytes. However, as T lymphocytes are involved in the immune response to viral infection, pregnant women are at increased risk of viral infections and may experience more severe viraemia.

The Treg cells are also involved in acceptance of paternal antigens expressed by the semi-allogenic fetus. As mentioned above, exposure to paternal antigens during unprotected intercourse primes the maternal immune response, even before conception occurs. The Treg cells undergo expansion and migrate to the lymph nodes and then to the fetal–maternal interface after implantation. This Treg cell population, which is specific for paternal antigens, generates a tolerant microenvironment at the maternal–fetal interface throughout the pregnancy. Maternal and fetal cells are reciprocally recognized by each other's immune systems, which means that the mother can tolerate the fetal allograft and the fetus acquires a tolerogenic environment that helps to protect it against autoimmune diseases.

Treg cells are essential regulators of immune tolerance of the allogeneic fetus and placenta. The absence of Tregs in mice was shown to trigger fetal rejection and also to increase markedly the numbers of cytotoxic T cells and helper T cells, dramatically shifting the immune response towards Th1 and fetal rejection. Also, administration of antibodies against the Treg protein, CD25, shortly after mating in mice, resulted in the failure of implantation showing that the presence of tolerogenic Tregs at implantation is a key requirement for the establishment of pregnancy (Robertson et al., 2018).

Tregs appear to act via several pathways to enable implantation and the establishment of pregnancy. In addition to downregulating the cell-mediated immune rejection of the fetus and placenta via T cells, Tregs also secrete cytokines, which target macrophages and dendritic cells to shift the balance towards the tolerogenic phenotypes, decidual M2 macrophages and tolerogenic DCs (tDCs). Several cell types at the fetal–maternal interface utilize and metabolize the essential amino acid, tryptophan. Indoleamine 2,3-dioxygenase (IDO), the enzyme that catalyses the first step in tryptophan catabolism via the kynurenine pathway, is expressed by trophoblast cells, decidual stromal cells, decidual immune cells and vascular endothelial cells. Tryptophan depletion by IDO metabolism inhibits T-cell activation. Products of tryptophan catabolism, such as kynurenine, are released from cells and are thought to regulate T-cell proliferation and survival. So, IDO acts as a switch to promote the number of Treg cells and decrease the number of cytotoxic T cells. In the absence of IDO, Treg cells are reprogrammed to become pro-inflammatory Th17 cells, which also have pathogenic roles in many autoimmune diseases. The products of tryptophan metabolism prevent T-cell and B-cell activation and proliferation. IDO also suppresses complement-mediated damage.

Susceptibility to Infection

It has been suggested that as maternal immune responses are suppressed in pregnancy and the Th1/Th2 balance altered to favour acceptance of the fetus, pregnant women would have increased susceptibility to infection. Historically, pregnant women were observed to contract smallpox and poliomyelitis more readily. Today, viral hepatitis infections, particularly in developing countries, pose a major threat to pregnant women, who have 10 times the infection rate of nonpregnant women and experience higher morbidity and mortality rates. The prevention of vertical transmission to the fetus or neonate is also an important consideration. Primary infection with cytomegalovirus during pregnancy in women who lack immunity is associated with fetal congenital abnormalities and is one of the most prevalent causes of mental retardation. Pregnant women have an increased susceptibility to listeriosis, influenza (Box 10.2), varicella (chickenpox), herpes, rubella (German measles), hepatitis and human papillomavirus. In addition, a number of latent viral diseases and other infections may be of greater severity. These include malaria, tuberculosis (TB), Epstein–Barr virus and HIV-associated infections, which can be reactivated in pregnancy. Pregnancy-induced suppression of helper T-cell numbers may be permanent so pregnancy can cause a progression of HIV-related disease. Pregnant women appear to have increased immunological responses to bacterial infection. However, increased incidences of urinary tract infections are probably related to anatomical changes rather than to altered immunological responses. Similarly, the increased severity of respiratory infections is usually associated with changes in diaphragm position, which reduces the clearance of respiratory tract secretions and functional residual capacity. The immune changes in pregnancy may be responsible for the increased risk of breast cancer in the years immediately following pregnancy, particularly in women who are older at their first full-term pregnancy; however, a first full-term pregnancy at a younger age exerts a protective effect on lifetime

BOX 10.2 Seasonal Influenza

The immune changes in pregnancy mean that pregnant women who contract seasonal influenza (flu) are at increased risk of developing severe complications that can cause morbidity and mortality, especially during the third trimester. Physiological changes in the respiratory system probably contribute to the increased severity of respiratory complications. Flu viruses are classified as A, B or C types; types A and B are the main causes of mortality and type A is associated with pandemics (Toal et al., 2010). The surface antigens of flu viruses demonstrate 'antigenic drift' and change subtly due to frequent mutation so at-risk groups require annual vaccination. In the 1918 flu pandemic, one study of pregnancy showed that approximately half of the women infected with influenza developed pneumonia and about half of these women with pneumonia died – a death rate of 27%. More people died in this pandemic than in World War I, which had just ended. Surveillance of the swine flu pandemic in 2009/2010 showed that, like previous flu pandemics, pregnant women were at significant risk from the H1N1 virus (swine flu). Pregnant women who are colonized by bacteria such as methicillin-resistant *Staphylococcus aureus* (MRSA) and *Streptococcus pneumoniae* are at a higher risk of developing pneumonia if they are infected with the H1N1 influenza virus (Cheng et al., 2009). There is a higher rate of fetal abnormalities, premature delivery and stillbirths in pregnant women who contract influenza in early pregnancy, which is probably caused by high fever; however, vertical transmission of flu virus has not been demonstrated. The presenting signs of seasonal flu are usually fever, cough, vomiting, breathlessness, myalgia, sore throats and chills. The World Health Organization advises pregnant women to have seasonal flu vaccines because of the high risks associated with pregnancy. Flu vaccines are fragmented, meaning that they contain parts of the virus and are not whole or attenuated (mild form of virus). The use of antiviral drugs such as neuraminidase inhibitors (oseltamivir and zanamivir) is also advocated in pregnancy because the risks associated with their use are outweighed by the risk of novel flu virus (e.g. H1N1) infection in pregnancy. Public health measures for containing infection include hand and domestic hygiene, cough etiquette and avoiding unnecessary travel and crowds if possible.

risk of breast cancer, as does breastfeeding of the neonate (Chapter 16). Some conditions, such as multiple sclerosis, improve in pregnancy because of the expansion of the Treg cell population. The postpartum period can also be an immunologically sensitive time, as the rapid reversal of the changes that occurred in pregnancy and a rebound of inflammatory responses can cause latent or quiescent infections to become full symptomatic diseases. Thyroid autoantibody levels fall in pregnancy so conditions such as Graves disease are ameliorated, but the antibodies then peak in the postpartum period (Weetman, 2010) so postpartum thyroiditis and mild autoimmune hypothyroidism are relatively common in the first 6 months following delivery.

Microchimerism

It was assumed for decades that maternal and fetal blood never mixes, but transplacental passage of a few cells appears to be normal. Microchimerism is the presence of a small number of cells or cell fragments containing DNA within an individual, both in the circulation and in other tissues, that have come from another individual. Fetal microchimerism, the trafficking of cells from the fetus to the mother, is more common than transfer from the mother to her fetus. Low levels of fetal cells commonly persist in the maternal circulation for many years or even indefinitely and these can be blood cells or trophoblast cells, which are continually shed during pregnancy (see Chapter 8). In some cases, a maternal cellular immune response against the fetal antigens is mounted. It has been suggested that fetal microchimerism might be associated with an increased risk of miscarriage (Lissauer et al., 2009) and that the higher incidence of autoimmune diseases in women is related to microchimerism, inducing a graft-versus-host disease reaction. The transfer of cells is bidirectional and maternal cells are also transferred from the mother to the fetus, referred to as maternal microchimerism (Lissauer et al., 2009). Diseases in which fetal microchimerism has been suggested to have a possible causative role include scleroderma, Sjögren syndrome, Graves disease and SLE. Such a role would fit with autoimmune diseases being much more common in women during or after childbearing years. This hypothesis is applicable to men, children and women who have never been pregnant because, less commonly, microchimerism can result from other sources such as transplantation, blood transfusion and cells from a twin-to-twin transfer. Fetal microchimerism may also have a protective function, playing a role in tissue repair; in addition, studies have also implicated both an increased and a reduced risk of cancer associated with microchimerism (Lissauer et al., 2009). Maternal microchimerism has also been implicated in T1D in the offspring where maternal DNA levels were reported to be significantly higher in T1D patients than in unaffected siblings or healthy subjects (Nelson et al., 2007).

FETAL AND NEONATAL PASSIVE IMMUNITY

The neonate's immune system is augmented by maternal transfer of immunoglobulins across the placenta to the fetus and in breast milk. The profile of immunoglobulins transported across the placenta and secreted into breast milk depends on specific transport mechanisms for the different classes of immunoglobulin (see Table 10.3). Maternal IgG crosses the placenta into the fetal circulation via a specific active transport mechanism, which is effective from around 20 weeks' gestation but markedly increases in activity from 34 weeks. The mother will produce an immune response to antigens she encounters by producing IgG, which can then cross the placenta. Even if maternal levels of IgG are low, they will still be transported across the placenta via active transport. This means that the fetus will receive passive immunization against prevalent pathogens likely to be in the environment from birth. This passive immunity provides essential temporary protection postnatally until the neonate's own immune system matures and produces its own antibodies. Preterm babies are at risk of transient hypoglobulinaemia because they receive less IgG and they are born with immune systems that are less mature than that of a term infant. Placental dysfunction limits the transfer of IgG; therefore, SGA (small for gestational age) babies have lower levels of IgG. Neither IgA, IgM nor IgD cross the placenta but these are supplied in high concentrations in the colostrum when breastfeeding begins.

As well as beneficial IgG, potentially harmful IgG can cross the placenta. Maternal antibodies to fetal HLA will be generated as the maternal immune system encounters a few fetal cells. The maternal anti-fetal HLA antibodies will cross the placenta but do not cause any damage, as they bind to nontrophoblastic cells in the placenta, which bear fetal HLA and can sequester maternal IgG. In autoimmune diseases, however, pathogenic maternal antibodies can be transferred across the placenta. For instance, antiplatelet antibodies can cross the placenta into the fetus of a mother with autoimmune thrombocytopenic purpura. The passive transfer of autoimmune antibodies may affect fetal growth and development and can potentially cause at least transient symptoms of the disease in the neonate. The resulting increased risk of haemorrhage in babies born to mothers with thrombocytopenia means that traumatic procedures, such as fetal blood sampling and instrumental delivery, are avoided.

Some autoimmune conditions such as congenital heart block associated with SLE can cause irreversible damage to the neonate.

Preterm babies are at a higher risk of vertical infection of group B streptococci if their mothers are group B streptococcus-positive, because they do not gain passive immunity from the placental transfer of immunoglobulins until after 34 weeks' gestation. Term babies do have some degree of protection from group B streptococci and this can be extended if the infant is breastfed. The use of antibiotics in the intrapartum period does reduce the number of group B streptococcal infections in the neonate, and so any mother who is found to be group B streptococci-positive at any time, not just during the pregnancy, may be offered antibiotic therapy in labour. The antibiotics reduce the bacterial load and so the risk of infection is less, although a small number of neonatal infections may still occur. The clinical management of known group B strep in pregnant women has been the subject of much research and guidelines may vary from country to country for example universal screening, although this is not currently recommended in the UK, and intrapartum antibiotic prophylaxis (IAP) (Hughes et al., 2017).

The Rhesus Factor and Rhesus Incompatibility

In the last trimester, the placental transfer of maternal IgG will include IgG antibodies directed against the fetus's own antigens. Most of these are thought to bind to non-trophoblastic cells bearing fetal antigens within the placental villous tissue so they do not reach the fetal circulation. However, antibodies to the Rhesus antigen can cause severe complications. People who express the Rhesus antigen on their own red blood cell surface do not produce antibodies against it. These people are described as Rhesus-positive (Fig. 10.8). A mother who is Rhesus-negative does not have the Rhesus antigen on her own red blood cell surface, and her immune system has the capability of making Rhesus antibodies. About 10% of pregnancies in Caucasian populations are Rhesus-negative women with a Rhesus-positive fetus; in other ethnicities, there is a lower incidence of Rhesus-negative individuals.

The Rhesus antibody is not preformed (existing from birth) like the antibodies of the ABO blood grouping system. Rhesus antibodies are produced if the immune system is given the opportunity to recognize the Rhesus antigen as a foreign protein. In practice, this means that a Rhesus-negative mother could produce antibodies to the Rhesus antigen of fetal cells (which would recognize and attack the red blood cells of a Rhesus-positive fetus) if her immune system encountered it. The immune response can be generated from exposure to red blood cells bearing the Rhesus antigen, for instance, from transplacental leakage of Rhesus-positive fetal cells or in rare instances from a Rhesus-positive blood transfusion (see Box 10.3).

The occasion when Rhesus isoimmunization is most likely to occur is at the time of the third stage of labour. During placental separation, there is the potential for a small amount of fetal blood (perhaps half a millilitre) to cross into the maternal circulation. Fetal blood can also enter the maternal circulation earlier in pregnancy, during therapeutic or spontaneous abortion, amniocentesis, abdominal trauma and in an ectopic pregnancy. If the fetal blood entering the maternal circulation is Rhesus-positive, it could stimulate the maternal immune cells to respond by clonal expansion, developing the capacity to produce large quantities of IgG. Once a woman makes antibodies to Rhesus antigens, she is isoimmunized for life. These IgG antibodies can then be transported across the placenta to the fetal circulation late in gestation of a subsequent pregnancy. The binding of maternal Rhesus antibodies to the Rhesus antigen on the surface of the fetal blood cells stimulates lysis of the red blood cells. Mild Rhesus incompatibility can cause mild anaemia and reticulocytosis (new immature red blood cells in the circulation). Severe Rhesus incompatibility is a cause of miscarriage, intrauterine death or hydrops fetalis (abdominal ascites, generalized oedema, polyhydramnios and enlarged placenta). In the neonate, Rhesus incompatibility can result in haemolytic disease of the newborn, where profound haemolysis causes anaemia, increasing the risks of heart failure, hyperbilirubinaemia (jaundice) and kernicterus (see Chapter 15).

Treatment

Prophylactic treatment has been practised since 1967 (Box 10.3) and severe Rhesus-D alloimmunization is now rarely seen. Giving passive immunization prevents primary sensitization of the mother and the formation of cells that can produce IgG anti-Rhesus antibody. Although there is actually a complex system of Rhesus antigens, controlled by three pairs of genes (Cc, Dd and Ee), the Rhesus-D antigen predominates in incompatibility between the mother and the fetus.

In accordance with national guidelines (see Annotated Further Reading), the majority of Rhesus-negative women were offered routine anti-D administration, either two smaller doses at 28 and 34 weeks' gestation or one larger dose at around 28–30 weeks' gestation. Following delivery of the baby to a Rhesus-negative woman, the Rhesus status of the infant has to be determined. If this proves to be Rhesus-positive, then a second test is performed to estimate the amount of fetal blood in the maternal system (Box 10.4), as amounts >4 mL may require more than

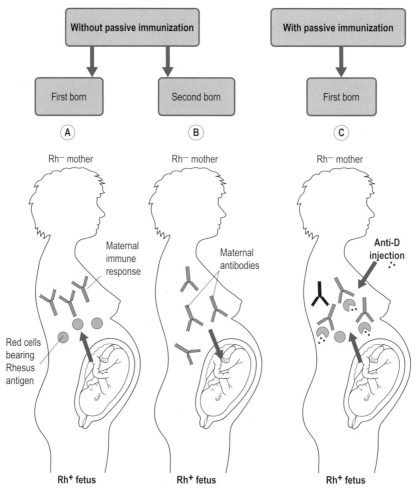

Fig. 10.8 (A) Rhesus-negative women can be sensitized when red cells from a Rhesus-positive fetus cross the placenta into her circulation. (B) Response comes after delivery of the first fetus, but in subsequent pregnancies, maternal antibodies can cross the placenta and damage the fetus. (C) Anti-D gamma globulin given to mothers immediately at delivery results in fetal Rhesus-positive cells not being recognized by maternal immune systems, so antibodies are not produced to endanger subsequent pregnancy.

BOX 10.3 Prophylactic Anti-D Immunoglobulin Treatment for Women Who are Rhesus-Negative

- Delivery of Rhesus-positive baby
- Spontaneous abortion
- Therapeutic termination of pregnancy
- Threatened abortion
- Antepartum haemorrhage
- Following external cephalic version of breech presentations
- Following CVS (chorionic villus sampling), amniocentesis or other invasive intrauterine procedure
- Following abdominal trauma

---

the standard anti-D dose of 500 international units (IU). Although if both parents were Rhesus-negative, anti-D would not be required, the guidelines do not recommend testing of the father to identify his Rhesus status, because it is recognized that the apparent father might not be the biological father, which may create a difficult situation to manage. It is difficult to justify routine anti-D administration if the father is certain that he is Rhesus-negative; however, it is prudent to observe the infant for signs of early and excessive jaundice in case the conception occurred outside of the pair bond.

If a small volume (<4 mL) of fetal blood has entered the maternal circulation at delivery, the exogenous antibodies ('anti-D') will bind to the fetal Rhesus-D antigen and cause

BOX 10.4 Maternal and Cord Blood Tests

When a mother is Rhesus-negative, a sample of the baby's blood is obtained from the umbilical cord. Two tests are performed:

1. The baby's blood group and Rhesus factor are identified; if the baby is Rhesus-negative, there is no possibility of maternal antibodies forming so the mother does not require anti-Rhesus-D antiserum (known as 'anti-D') administration.

2. If the baby is Rhesus-positive or there is another maternal/fetal antibody/antigen incompatibility, then the direct Coombs' test would also be performed. The Coombs' test enables differentiation between normal neonatal haemolysis and abnormal haemolysis caused through the action of maternal antigens. It is based on three variables and is positive when there is reduced haemoglobin in conjunction with an increased reticulocyte count and raised bilirubin levels.

Maternal blood is also taken so that the Kleihauer–Betke test can be performed. The test is based upon the resistance of fetal blood cells to be destroyed by acid (acid elution test). Not only does the test allow the presence of fetal erythrocytes to be detected but the amount of fetal blood transfused into the maternal circulation can be estimated as well. The test is not as accurate if there are maternal haemoglobinopathies present, as abnormal maternal erythrocytes (such as sickle cell disease) are also resistant to acid destruction. The test may also be falsely negative if there is an A/B incompatibility as the maternal anti-A and/or anti-B antigens quickly destroy the fetal erythrocytes, especially if the Kleihauer–Betke test is delayed, so it should be conducted within half an hour of delivery of the third stage.

It is estimated that a fetal–maternal blood transfer occurs in ~50% of pregnancies. Usually, the amount of blood is small, <0.5 mL. However, in 8% of pregnancies, it may be in the range of 0.5–40 mL and in 1%, it may well exceed 40 mL. In most cases, 500 IU of anti-Rhesus-D antiserum is enough to eradicate the misplaced fetal erythrocytes. However, if a large transfusion is suspected, then larger doses will be administered.

If an exceptionally large transfusion is suspected following the administration of anti-Rhesus-D antiserum, the Kleihauer–Betke test should be repeated, and if fetal cells are still detected, then further doses of anti-Rhesus-D antiserum would be administered.

cell lysis before the maternal lymphocytes have the opportunity to recognize the antigen and undergo subsequent clonal expansion. ABO compatibility exacerbates Rhesus isoimmunization, so ABO incompatibility offers a degree of protection against Rhesus sensitization. If the fetal blood transfused is of a different ABO grouping, the existing natural maternal IgM anti-A or anti-B antigens will rapidly eliminate the fetal blood cells before an immune response can be mounted against the Rhesus-D antigen.

Unnecessary administration of anti-D can now be prevented by identifying the Rhesus state of the fetus early in pregnancy by isolating fetal DNA markers from maternal blood (NICE, 2016). The application of noninvasive prenatal testing for fetal RhD genotype is becoming established in routine antenatal screening care programmes. Only mothers identified as carrying Rh-positive babies are offered anti-D in pregnancy. Women whose results are inconclusive are treated as carrying a Rh-positive baby until the baby's genotype is established following birth. This will further minimize the risk of exposure to blood products by limiting administration to cases where it is required (and also better utilize the donor-dependent stock of anti-D).

Other Antibodies

Most antibodies in the ABO system are IgM type so they do not cross the placenta. However, in successive ABO-incompatible pregnancies in group O mothers, a degree of neonatal haemolysis, causing mild neonatal jaundice, may occur. Haemolytic disease can potentially occur with other blood group incompatibilities such as the Kell and Duffy antigen systems. However, the density of these minor antigens on fetal red blood cells is so low that maternal IgG antibodies usually do not elicit a cytolytic effect. Women who require or have had multiple or large blood transfusions, for example, following postpartum haemorrhage, are at risk of developing antibodies to surface antigens, which could potentially put their future unborn babies at risk.

VULNERABILITY OF THE NEONATE

Neonates are born immunocompromised and are susceptible to infection. An intriguing idea is that the immaturity of the fetal immune system is an adaptive response, which helps to protect it from premature rejection by its mother (Clapp, 2006), but the cost of this is the increased risk of infections of the newborn, particularly if born prematurely. The microbiota colonize and protect the external surfaces of the body, and those membranes that appear internal but come into contact with external pathogens, such as the upper respiratory tract, gut and urinary system. The natural microbiota may protect by competing with pathogenic microorganisms for resources (colonization resistance) or by altering the local environment, making it less hospitable to pathogens. The acid mantle of the skin promotes colonization of commensal microbes and restricts growth of pathogens. The neonatal skin is particularly vulnerable to change in pH through the use of detergents, resulting in atopic dermatitis raising the risk of skin infections in the neonate (see Chapter 15).

The fetus *in utero* was generally thought to be sterile. Several recent studies have shown, however, that partial colonization occurs *in utero* with further postnatal colonization taking about 6–8 weeks from birth to be fully established. As the gut microbiota produces much of the body's vitamin K requirements, neonates have an increased risk of vitamin K deficiency until the resident population of microbiota is established. Colonization processes can be disrupted, for instance, by use of detergents, disinfectant swabs or antibiotic use. At birth, further colonization occurs with transfer of organisms from the mother's vagina, skin of her hands and breasts and the respiratory tracts of the baby's carers. Colonization of the gut can be facilitated by seeding the baby's gut, via the mouth, by using a maternal vaginal swab obtained at birth; this may be especially in babies born by caesarean section.

Neonatal skin is delicate and easily damaged and can offer a route for opportunistic infection. The umbilical cord, which becomes necrotic, presents a locus for possible infection and offers a potential pathway to the neonatal liver for pathogens. The neonatal defence mechanisms are further compromised by invasive procedures such as blood sampling or insertion of endotracheal or nasogastric tubes or intravenous cannulae.

Infants have less efficient immune systems, especially if they are born prematurely or are IUGR at birth. The cells of the immune system are immature and do not function as efficiently in early life; for instance, T lymphocytes have decreased responses and poor cytotoxic function. The phagocytes exhibit decreased phagocytosis and bactericidal activity. Their function in severe illness, such as respiratory distress syndrome or meconium-aspiration pneumonia, is further limited. The complement cascade components at birth are 50–80% of the adult levels.

Active Immunization

The immature immune system of the neonate is supported by natural passive immunization from placental transfer of IgG and the supply of IgA in breast milk, if the infant is breastfed. It is also supported by programmes of

---

> ### BOX 10.5   Principles of Immunization
>
> **Adjuvants**
>
> Examples: aluminium hydroxide or phosphate. Increases antigenic properties of a vaccine that would otherwise produce only a weak immune response, e.g. triple vaccine of diphtheria, tetanus and pertussis toxins.
>
> **Toxoid**
>
> Bacterial exotoxin treated so it does not cause a disease but still stimulates the immune cells. Examples include treatment of diphtheria and tetanus toxin with formalin.
>
> **Killed vaccine**
>
> Dead organisms such as pertussis, typhoid and paratyphoid. As with toxoid preparations, two or three doses and booster doses are required, as only a small number of antigens are introduced each time.
>
> **Attenuated vaccines**
>
> Live organisms that have been cultured to produce non-pathogenic strains. Very effective as organisms multiply within body mimicking a natural infection. Therefore, only one dose is required for full immune response (lifetime immunity), e.g. smallpox, poliomyelitis, measles, rubella, TB.

---

deliberate immunization. Active immunization requires administration of an antigen in a form that is inactivated and does not produce a disease (Box 10.5). IgG levels start to increase by 3 months so immunization is delayed after birth. However, some protection is required before the immune system is mature. Therefore, immunization programmes are often started when the baby is 2 months old. At about this age, many babies in the UK receive a combination of six vaccines for pertussis (whooping cough), diphtheria, tetanus, polio, *Haemophilus influenzae* type b (Hib) and hepatitis B antigens presented appropriately. It is also common practice to administer *pneumococcal* (PCV) vaccine, *rotavirus* vaccine and meningitis B vaccine at this time. Although theoretically only one dose is required, there are at least three strains and an effective immune response may not be produced the first time, so many of the vaccines are given as repeat doses a few weeks later. Measles vaccine is usually delayed until the infant is ~1 year old, as maternal IgG, which is present for the first 6–9 months of life, tends to destroy the attenuated organisms of the vaccine before the infant's immune system has time to recognize and respond to them. It is common for the measles vaccine to be given in combination with mumps and rubella vaccines (MMR) at 1 year of age and then repeated at between 3 years and 3.5 years of age, together with a booster combination of diphtheria, tetanus, pertussis and polio vaccines. HPV types 16 and 18 together account for 70% of cervical cancer cases. Preteen girls should be administered the HPV vaccine at around 12–13 years of age to help prevent future disease but the involvement of HPV strains in male carcinomas is a clear indicator that males should also be vaccinated. 90% of all sexually active adults are infected with at least one strain of HPV, which also causes oral, anal and penile cancers. At 14 years it is common practice to administer another booster combination vaccine for diphtheria, tetanus and polio and a multiple meningitis vaccine for types A, C, W and Y strains.

Immunization using viral vaccines may be ineffective if the individual has had a recent viral infection, such as a cold. Levels of interferon persist after a viral infection, which will inhibit viral replication in the infant so the virus provided in the vaccine preparation may not be able to reach concentrations adequate to stimulate an immune response. Therefore, immunization may not be effective until 2–3 weeks after a viral infection so administration of vaccines is delayed if an infection is suspected.

Oral doses of vaccines may be ineffective if their absorption is compromised, for instance, with diarrhoea or vomiting. High levels of steroids suppress the immune response, so steroid therapy or overactive adrenal glands can limit the effectiveness of a live vaccine and compromise the immune response. Maternal antibodies in the neonate, for instance, from placental transfer of IgG, can abrogate the young infant's immune response to vaccination but subsequent booster vaccination usually surmounts this. Infants who are themselves HIV-negative but born to HIV-positive mothers may not respond efficiently to vaccines. Allergic reactions to vaccines can occur, especially to vaccines prepared in tissue culture, or containing whole cells. Problems with allergic reactions are often associated with vaccines grown in egg-based tissue culture preparations or to which antibiotics have been added. Obviously, a severe reaction to a vaccine precludes its further use. Administration of live vaccines is not recommended in pregnancy. Immunization programmes benefit the health of the population unfortunately at the expense of the tiny minority of individuals who may have an extreme reaction to a vaccine with irreversible effects. The overwhelmingly positive statistics for vaccine use, for example the eradication of Variola virus (smallpox) infection, which caused >300 million deaths in the 20th century, has been fundamentally undermined by the unfounded scaremonger tactics of ill-informed 'anti-vaxxers'. The concept of a 'herd immunity threshold', the percentage of the population that needs to be immunized for the whole population to be protected, means that low uptake of vaccinations has a potentially devastating impact on the local population.

OTHER IMMUNOLOGICAL ASPECTS OF PREGNANCY

Antisperm antibodies can be present in both men and women. In seminal fluid, they can cause immune infertility by inhibiting spermatogenesis or fertilization. However, the Sertoli cell protects the developing sperm and seminiferous tubules from antibodies, and Treg cells secrete immunosuppressive cytokines in the epididymis. Some are coated with glycoproteins and lactoferrin, which may be why some antigen sites are evident only after sperm capacitation. Seminal fluid has potent immunosuppressive and signalling properties and can inhibit a range of immune responses. The presence of antisperm antibodies in the secretions from the genital tract, rather than in the blood, seems important particularly in male infertility. The risk of developing antisperm antibodies is increased with exposure to sperm that is excessive, as in prostitutes, or in an inappropriate site, as in homosexual men. A significant proportion of men have been shown to have antisperm antibodies associated with retention of sperm due to obstruction of the vas deferens or epididymis and so have retention of sperm, so the presence of antisperm antibodies is a useful predictor that obstruction is the primary cause of male infertility (Lee et al., 2009). Generation of antisperm antibodies may reflect a lack of immunosuppressive factors in the seminal fluid.

Endometriosis, which is deposition of endometrial tissue at nonuterine sites, can be very painful if the tissue becomes inflamed. Severe endometriosis can cause infertility, but many women have extrauterine endometrial tissue that neither causes pain nor affects fertility. The cause of endometriosis is not known, but an autoimmune aetiology has been proposed (Zondervan et al., 2018).

Concerns about the effects of HIV and AIDS in pregnancy are presented in Box 10.6 and Case study 10.2.

BOX 10.6 HIV and AIDS in Pregnancy

- HIV (human immunodeficiency virus) causes AIDS (acquired immune deficiency syndrome).
- HIV is a retrovirus, which invades cells expressing CD4, including helper T cells, monocytes and neural cells.
- A retrovirus contains a single strand of RNA, which is transcribed by reverse transcriptase in the host into a DNA copy but this enzyme lacks a 'proofreading' capability so has high mutation rates. This results in resistance to drugs and vaccines that no longer function.
- When the infected cell is activated, it will produce new viruses (viral coat proteins and RNA), which can be released and infect other cells.
- HIV infection causes decreased numbers of helper T cells, which fundamentally undermines all aspects of the immune response, so the risk of opportunistic and pathogenic infection increases.
- In Britain, women usually acquire HIV from sexual exposure and intravenous drug use. The biggest increase in HIV infection is heterosexual transmission in women.
- HIV has to evade the mechanical, chemical and biological barriers of the female reproductive tract.
- Progesterone-based contraception may accelerate HIV disease progression as progesterone inhibits cytotoxic T cells and NK cells; oestrogen may be protective.
- Coinfections in the female reproductive tract, which cause microulcerations, may increase HIV susceptibility.
- Transmission of HIV is more efficient from men to women (compared to women to men) possibly because semen transforms the local environment of the female reproductive tract, for instance, increasing pH and upregulating pro-inflammatory cytokines.
- Pregnancy can mask some of the nonspecific symptoms of HIV infection, such as fatigue, anaemia and dyspnoea.
- HIV can remain latent for years (estimated to be an average 11 years) before AIDS becomes evident.
- Progression to symptom development may be accelerated by pregnancy.
- HIV can be transmitted to the baby via the placenta, from exchange of body fluids at birth or from breast milk.
- Mothers with HIV may be advised to breastfeed their babies if the risk of fatal malnutrition is considered to be higher than the risk of HIV infection; lactoferrin is protective.

CASE STUDY 10.2

Mary is 16 weeks' pregnant. She has no fixed abode and has not previously been seen by a health professional in relation to her pregnancy. Mary attends the local hospital antenatal clinic in a state of distress. She informs the midwife that she is an intravenous drug abuser and her best friend has just died from an AIDS-related illness.

- How prepared would you be, as the midwife, to counsel and advise Mary?
- What referrals and expert advice would you seek on her behalf?
- What considerations are needed in relation to the unborn child, in relation to both HIV transmission and Mary's general situation?

KEY POINTS

- Pregnancy enhances humoral immunity and suppresses cell-mediated immunity so responses to bacterial infection are enhanced, but there may be increased susceptibility to viral infections.
- Histoincompatibility, such as the differences in fetal and maternal antigen expression, would normally lead to tissue rejection.
- The trophoblast cells lack classic HLA antigens, which prevent an antifetal response, but express HLA-G, which prevents nonspecific cytolysis.
- Fetal cells entering the maternal circulation are important in the generation of blocking antibodies, which block any immune response that does occur.

- Maternal IgG is transferred to the fetus late in gestation, which provides the neonate with passive immunization during the period of immunological immaturity. Harmful antibodies against fetal antigens are sequestered by nontrophoblastic tissue in the placenta.
- The birth of a Rhesus-positive baby to a Rhesus-negative woman can initiate an immune response. Prophylactic administration of anti-Rhesus-D immunoglobulin is therefore given after possible or actual exposure.
- The neonate is immunocompromised at birth. Immunization programmes seek to address this lack of immunity.

APPLICATION TO PRACTICE

Pregnancy results in an alteration of the immune system, so normal nonpregnant white cell count ranges cannot be applied in pregnancy. An understanding of changes within the immune system will enable the midwife to explain the consequences of such changes to the pregnant women.

An understanding of rhesus incompatibility is necessary as this is a common potential problem.

Conditions that affect the maternal immune system may complicate pregnancy, affecting not only the mother but also the fetus and the neonate. Such conditions require careful management and treatment to optimize outcomes for both the mother and the baby.

Midwives may be involved in the administration of some vaccines such as rubella and TB so an understanding of the immune system is required. The interaction of the maternal immune system and the baby is an important aspect of lactation and breastfeeding.

ANNOTATED FURTHER READING

Arora N, Sadovsky Y, Dermody TS, Coyne CB: Microbial vertical transmission during human pregnancy, *Cell Host Microbe* 21:561–567, 2017.
A recent review about how the maternal immune system responds to common congenital infectious agents and how they can breach the innate placental mechanisms that restrict their access to the fetus.

Bailey H, Zash R, Rasi V, Thorne C: HIV treatment in pregnancy, *Lancet HIV* 5:e457–e467, 2018.
A clinical review of antiretroviral treatment (ART) in pregnancy, which covers the biological mechanisms associated with adverse outcomes in pregnancy and considers barriers to the initiation and adherence to the therapeutic approaches.

Bonney EA: Immune regulation in pregnancy: a matter of perspective? *Obstet Gynecol Clin North Am* 43:679–698, 2016.
A recent review about maternal tolerance and protection of the fetus; includes succinct summaries about the roles of the components of the immune system and how they change in pregnancy.

Department of Health: *Immunisation against infectious disease – 'The Green Book'*, London, 2017, DoH.
This an updated and comprehensive reference guide about the principles, practices and procedures related to the vaccination programmes in the UK, which includes a chapter on each of the diseases, vaccinations and vaccines available; an essential reference book for all healthcare professionals.

Feder L, Hoang L: *Parents' concise guide to childhood vaccinations*, ed 2, New York, 2017, Hatherleigh Press.
This is a useful guide for parents about the pros and cons associated with immunization; includes information on vaccination schedules.

Geldenhuys J, Rossouw TM, Lombaard HA, et al.: Disruption in the regulation of immune responses in the placental subtype of preeclampsia, *Front Immunol* 9:1659, 2018.
This paper describes normal and abnormal inflammatory immune responses in pregnancy and how aberrant immune regulatory mechanisms causing hyperinflammation explain part of the aetiology of preeclampsia.

Hughes RG, Brocklehurst P, Steer PJ, et al., on behalf of the Royal College of Obstetricians and Gynaecologists: Prevention of early-onset neonatal group B streptococcal disease. Green-top Guideline No. 36, *BJOG* 124:e280–e305, 2017.
This guideline gives a full, evidence-based explanation for the treatment of group B streptococcus; for healthcare professionals.

Kagan KO, Hamprecht K: Cytomegalovirus infection in pregnancy, *Arch Gynecol Obstet* 296:15–26, 2017.
A comprehensive review of the issues about intrauterine CMG infection and the potential for fetal neurodevelopmental development to be affected.

Kinder JM, Stelzer IA, Arck PC, Way SS: Immunological implications of pregnancy-induced microchimerism, *Nat Rev Immunol* 17:483–494, 2017.
An extensive review of the implications of microchimerism and the effects of mothers being seeded with genetically foreign fetal cells in pregnancy, which suggests these cells are purposefully retained by the mothers and their offspring to promote genetic fitness because the outcomes of future pregnancies are improved.

Leeper C, Lutzkanin 3rd A: Infections during pregnancy, *Prim Care* 45:567–586, 2018.
An overview of issues to consider in relation to the common infections in pregnancy, including urinary tract infections, sexually transmitted infections, influenza, hepatitis types, HIV, foodborne infections and common viral infections including Zika.

National Institute for Clinical Excellence: *Routine antenatal anti-D prophylaxis for women who are RhD-negative*, London, 2008, NICE (Reviewed 2015).
This review forms the basis of the current use of anti-D in the United Kingdom and provides a comprehensive and referenced guide to the use of anti-D.

National Institute for Clinical Excellence: *High-throughput non-invasive prenatal testing for fetal RHD genotype (DG25)*, London, 2016, NICE. www.nice.org.uk/guidance/dg25.
This diagnostic guidance clearly presents the case for the introduction of noninvasive screening to identify RHD-neg genotype fetuses and to avoid unnecessary anti-D administration.

Playfair JH, Chain BM: *Immunology at a glance*, ed 10, Oxford, 2012, Wiley-Blackwell.
Covers a wide range of immunological topics using clear, well-labelled diagrams to summarize and simplify the mechanisms of immunological processes together with succinct written explanations on facing pages.

Sompayrac LM: *How the immune system works*, ed 5, Oxford, 2015, Wiley-Blackwell.

Clearly explained textbook, illustrated with useful diagrams, which provides a clear overview of immune concepts and the components of the immune system.

Tincani A, Dall'Ara F, Lazzaroni MG, et al.: Pregnancy in patients with autoimmune disease, *Autoimmun Rev* 15:975–977, 2016.

An interesting perspective on the issues faced by pregnant women with autoimmune rheumatic diseases now that increasingly more affected women are able to fulfil their intentions to have children.

Vanberger O, White GR, Helbert M, et al.: *Crash course: haematology and immunology*, ed 5, London, 2018, Elsevier.

This well-established textbook presents the fundamental principles of haematology and immunology in an easy-to-understand format and is a useful introductory text for healthcare professionals.

Wood P: *Understanding immunology (Cell and Molecular Biology in Action series)*, ed 3, London, 2011, Prentice Hall.

A clear, well-illustrated introductory text, which is written for students with little prior knowledge of immunology.

REFERENCES

Apps R, Murphy SP, Fernando R, et al.: Human leucocyte antigen (HLA) expression of primary trophoblast cells and placental cell lines, determined using single antigen beads to characterize allotype specificities of anti-HLA antibodies, *Immunology* 127:26–39, 2009.

Beer AE, Billingham RE: Host responses to intra-uterine tissue, cellular and fetal allografts, *J Reprod Fertil* 21:49, 1974.

Brostoff J, Scadding GK, Male D, et al.: *Clinical immunology*, London, 1991, Gower Medical.

Chaouat G, Petitbarat M, Dubanchet S, et al.: Tolerance to the foetal allograft? *Am J Reprod Immunol* 63:624–636, 2010.

Chen M, Daha MR, Kallenberg CG: The complement system in systemic autoimmune disease, *J Autoimmun* 34:J276–J286, 2010.

Cheng VC, Lau YK, Lee KL, et al.: Fatal co-infection with swine origin influenza virus A/H1N1 and community-acquired methicillin-resistant *Staphylococcus aureus*, *J Infect Dis* 59:366–370, 2009.

Clapp DW: Developmental regulation of the immune system, *Semin Perinatol* 30:69–72, 2006.

Crawford G, Ray A, Gudi A, et al.: The role of seminal plasma for improved outcomes during in vitro fertilization treatment: review of the literature and meta-analysis, *Human Reprod Update* 21:275–284, 2015.

Faas MM, de Vos P: Uterine NK cells and macrophages in pregnancy, *Placenta* 56:44–52, 2017.

Goodnow CC, Sprent J, Fazekas de St Groth B, et al.: Cellular and genetic mechanisms of self tolerance and autoimmunity, *Nature* 435:590–597, 2005.

Hewagama A, Richardson B: The genetics and epigenetics of autoimmune diseases, *J Autoimmun* 33:3–11, 2009.

Hosenfeld CB, Workowski KA, Berman S, et al.: Repeat infection with Chlamydia and gonorrhoea among females: a systematic review of the literature, *Sex Transm Dis* 36:478–489, 2009.

Hughes RG, Brocklehurst P, Steer PJ, et al., on behalf of the Royal College of Obstetricians and Gynaecologists: Prevention of early-onset neonatal group B streptococcal disease. Green-top Guideline No. 36, *BJOG* 124:e280–e305, 2017.

Koga K, Aldo PB, Mor G: Toll-like receptors and pregnancy: trophoblast as modulators of the immune response, *J Obstet Gynaecol Res* 25:191–202, 2009.

Koga K, Mor G: Toll-like receptors at the maternal-fetal interface in normal pregnancy and pregnancy disorders, *Am J Reprod Immunol* 63:587–600, 2010.

Krause DS, Theise ND, Collector MI: Multi-organ, multi-lineage engraftment by a single bone marrow-derived stem cell, *Cell* 105:369–377, 2001.

Lee R, Goldstein M, Ullery BW, et al.: Value of serum antisperm antibodies in diagnosing obstructive azoospermia, *J Urol* 181:264–269, 2009.

Lissauer DM, Piper KP, Moss PA, Kilby MD: Fetal microchimerism: the cellular and immunological legacy of pregnancy, *Expert Rev Mol Med* 11:e33, 2009.

Manaster I, Mandelboim O: The unique properties of uterine NK cells, *Am J Reprod Immunol* 63:434–444, 2010.

Medawar P: Some immunological and endocrinological problems raised by the evolution of viviparity in vertebrates, *Symp Soc Exp Biol* 11:320–338, 1953.

Mor G, Cardenas I: The immune system in pregnancy: a unique complexity, *Am J Reprod Immunol* 63:425–433, 2010.

National Institute for Clinical Excellence (NICE): *High-throughput non-invasive prenatal testing for fetal RHD genotype (DG25)*, London, 2016, NICE, www.nice.org.uk/guidance/dg25.

Nelson JL, Gillespie KM, Lambert NC, et al.: Maternal microchimerism in peripheral blood in type 1 diabetes and pancreatic islet beta cell microchimerism, *Proc Natl Acad Sci USA* 104:1637–1642, 2007.

Pahl JHW, Cerwenka A, Ni J: Memory-like NK cells: remembering a previous activation by cytokines and NK cell receptors, *Front Immunol* 9:2796, 2018.

Piccinni M-P, Lombardelli L, Logiodice F, et al.: How pregnancy can affect autoimmune diseases progression? *Clin Mol Allergy* 14:11–19, 2016.

Robertson SA: Immune regulation of conception and embryo implantation – all about quality control? *J Reprod Immunol* 85:51–57, 2010.

Robertson SA, Care AS, Moldenhauer LM: Regulatory T cells in embryo implantation and the immune response to pregnancy, *J Clin Invest* 128:4224–4235, 2018.

Saito S, Nakashima A, Shima T, et al.: Th1/Th2/Th17 and regulatory T-cell paradigm in pregnancy, *Am J Reprod Immunol* 63:601–610, 2010.

Stewart M: *Growing and responding*, Milton Keynes, 1997, Open University, pp 185, 188–191, 193, 200.

Sun JC, Lanier LL: Is there natural killer cell memory and can it be harnessed by vaccination? NK cell memory and immunization strategies against infectious diseases and cancer, *Cold Spring Harb Perspect Biol* 10(10):a029538, 2018.

Svensson L, Arvola M, Sallstrom MA, et al.: The Th2 cytokines IL-4 and IL-10 are not crucial for the completion of allogeneic pregnancy in mice, *J Reprod Immunol* 51:3–7, 2001.

Thaxton JE, Sharma S: Interleukin-10: a multi-faceted agent of pregnancy, *Am J Reprod Immunol* 63:482–491, 2010.

Toal M, Agyeman-Duah K, Schwenk A, et al.: Swine flu and pregnancy, *J Obstet Gynaecol* 30:97–100, 2010.

Victora CG, Bahl R, Barros AJD, et al.: Breastfeeding in the 21st century – epidemiology, mechanisms, and lifelong effect, *Lancet* 387:475–490, 2016.

Weetman AP: Immunity, thyroid function and pregnancy: molecular mechanisms, *Nat Rev Endocrinol* 6:311–318, 2010.

Zenclussen AC, Schumacher A, Zenclussen ML, et al.: Immunology of pregnancy: cellular mechanisms allowing fetal survival within the maternal uterus, *Expert Rev Mol Med* 9:1–14, 2007.

Zondervan KT, Becker CM, Koga K, et al.: Endometriosis, *Nat Rev Dis Primers* 4:9, 2018.

Physiological Adaptation to Pregnancy

INTRODUCTION

During the 279 days (40 weeks) of an average pregnancy (measured from the first day of the last menstrual period), maternal physiology changes remarkably to support the development of the fetus and to prepare the mother for labour, lactation and parental behaviour. The changes begin in the luteal phase of the menstrual cycle, even fertilization and implantation, as progesterone secretion from the corpus luteum is initiated. If fertilization is successful, levels of progesterone and oestrogen progressively increase. Together, they orchestrate many of the adaptations of the maternal physiological systems to facilitate pregnancy. Human pregnancy is notable in that the pregnancy, once established, requires little input from the maternal hypothalamic–pituitary–ovarian axis. The human conceptus (embryo plus placenta) is said to demonstrate 'endocrine emancipation' as it is endocrinologically independent of its mother (Johnson, 2018).

CHAPTER CASE STUDY

Zara is now in the third trimester of her pregnancy. She informs her midwife that she is not sleeping well, and James prefers to sleep in the spare room as Zara's loud snoring and frequent waking disturbs him. When Zara does sleep, she experiences vivid dreams that cause her to wake suddenly. Her sleeping is further disturbed because she often wakes up feeling hungry and thirsty

CHAPTER CASE STUDY—cont'd

and is having to make increasingly frequent visits to the toilet. Zara has now stopped working and finds that the only way she can cope is to have a rest in the afternoon. She often falls asleep sitting in front of the television for 3–4 h and says this afternoon sleep is less disturbed than the night time.

- What physiological changes could account for these changes in Zara's sleep pattern and what reasons would you give to reassure Zara that this is normal?
- Why do you think Zara is able to sleep more peacefully in the afternoon?
- Are there any advantages in these behavioural changes and might they be preparing Zara to care for her newborn baby?

ENDOCRINE CHANGES IN PREGNANCY

The physiological changes of pregnancy are largely instigated and maintained by placental hormone secretion. The trophoblastic cells produce human chorionic gonadotrophin (hCG), which stimulates secretion from the corpus luteum, increasing ovarian steroid hormone production. As the placenta develops, it takes over production of oestrogen and progesterone. However, placental endocrine function is much broader as the placenta synthesizes an extraordinary range of hormones and releasing factors, some of which are similar to those originating from the hypothalamus and other maternal endocrine organs (see Chapter 8). Placental hormones include steroid and protein hormones, hypothalamic releasing factors such as gonadotrophin-releasing hormone (GnRH) and corticotrophin-releasing hormone (CRH), pituitary hormones such as adrenocorticotrophin (ACTH), antidiuretic hormone (ADH) and oxytocin, metabolic hormones such as leptin and ghrelin, together with cytokines including inhibins, activin and insulin-like growth factors, and neurohormones. Placental products may act locally affecting placental function or they may reach the maternal and/or fetal circulation, thus regulating maternal physiology and fetal development.

Steroid Hormones

Steroidogenesis depends on interaction and biological cooperation between the mother, placenta and fetus. The mother provides precursors for placental progesterone production and the fetus is the source of some of the precursors for the production of placental oestrogens. Placental progesterone is used for fetal synthesis of testosterone, corticosteroids and mineralocorticoids. Progesterone is known as the hormone of pregnancy; it stimulates respiration, relaxes smooth muscle (of blood vessels, uterus and gut), increases body temperature, increases sodium and chloride excretion, and acts as an immunosuppressant in the placenta (see Chapter 10). It is suggested that one of the contributors to unexplained recurrent pregnancy loss (PRL or repeated miscarriages) might be associated with psychological stress or depression inhibiting the normal increase in progesterone levels (Chetty and Duncan, 2018). Stress and depression affect the hypothalamic–pituitary–adrenal (HPA) axis and increase levels of the classical stress mediators, CRH and glucocorticoids, such as cortisol. CRH can inhibit GnRH and glucocorticoids can suppress pituitary luteinizing hormone (LH) secretion and thus affect steroid hormone production.

Progesterone levels increase gradually at first (Fig. 11.1). The placenta becomes the main site of steroid hormone synthesis and is capable of producing enough progesterone to support the pregnancy by 5–6 weeks. Human and other primate pregnancies can survive ovariectomy (oophorectomy, removal of ovaries), although the corpus luteum is essential in other mammalian pregnancies (Johnson, 2018), for example marsupials. Production of 17α-hydroxyprogesterone, by the corpus luteum, normally plateaus or decreases between 6 and 9 weeks as placental production of progesterone increases. By the end of the first trimester, levels of progesterone are 50% higher than luteal levels and by term, the levels have increased threefold to about 200 mg/day. The syncytiotrophoblast uses maternal cholesterol as the substrate for progesterone synthesis. As the fetus does not contribute to progesterone synthesis,

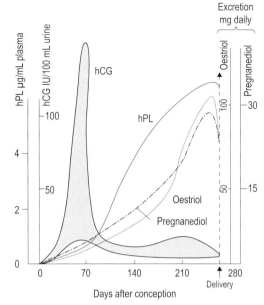

Fig. 11.1 Increasing concentrations of oestrogen and progesterone during pregnancy.

progesterone levels reflect placental but not fetal wellbeing; indeed placental production of progesterone can occur in the absence of an embryo, for instance in hydatidiform mole or choriocarcinoma.

In contrast, the production of oestrogens requires cooperation between the maternal, placental and fetal compartments. The primary oestrogen of pregnancy is oestriol, which is less potent than oestradiol 17β produced by the corpus luteum. Early in pregnancy, oestrone and oestradiol 17β levels increase but oestriol levels do not begin to rise until the 9th week when the fetal adrenal glands begin to synthesize the precursor dehydroepiandrosterone sulphate (DHEAS) from placental pregnenolone; DHEAS is the substrate for placental production of oestriol (see Chapter 3) but the placenta cannot synthesize androgens from progestagens. Maternal and placental steroids are conjugated in the fetal liver and adrenal glands into water soluble, and thus biologically inactive, forms of the hormones (so the fetus is protected from the effect of the high levels of active steroids). As the 16-hydroxyl precursor is produced only by the fetal liver, production of oestriol indicates satisfactory fetal development and wellbeing. In 'at risk' pregnancies, decreased oestriol may indicate fetal distress and the need to induce premature delivery, although as an index of placental function and fetal wellbeing, it has largely been replaced by Doppler ultrasound investigation and biophysical profiling. Oestriol measurement is part of the Bart's (triple) test for Trisomy 21 or Down syndrome (see Chapter 7).

Oestrone and oestriol levels increase about 100 times and oestradiol levels about 1000 times during the course of the pregnancy (Blackburn, 2018). Oestrogens are growth promoters; they promote the growth of the endometrium and breasts, enhance myometrial activity, increase sensitivity to carbon dioxide, increase pituitary prolactin secretion, promote myometrial vasodilation, stimulate fluid retention, alter the composition of connective tissue and increase the sensitivity of the uterus to progesterone in late pregnancy.

Human Chorionic Gonadotrophin

The main function of hCG is to maintain production of steroid hormones from the corpus luteum in early pregnancy until the placenta can take over. hCG has a very similar structure to that of LH, follicle-stimulating hormone (FSH) and thyroid-stimulating hormone (TSH); it acts on the LH receptors, prolonging the life of the corpus luteum. hCG is produced initially by the outer cells of the blastocyst, which are the cells that differentiate into trophoblast cells and subsequently into the placenta. The syncytiotrophoblast, which evolves from the trophoblast (see Chapter 8), continues to produce some hCG throughout pregnancy and the extravillous trophoblast produces a hyperglycosylated hCG, which is important in spiral artery conversion. hCG is secreted, and can be detected, before implantation in vaginal secretions and in the maternal circulation (see Fig. 11.1). As the lacunae begin to be formed by the invading syncytiotrophoblast, the hCG diffuses into the maternal blood where significant levels can be detected. Measurable hCG levels in urine are present 2 weeks after fertilization. Home pregnancy tests identifying the presence of the β-subunit of hCG are very sensitive and specific. The presence of hCG confirms successful fertilization or pregnancy as, apart from rare production by certain tumours (Groza et al., 2017), it is not produced by other tissues. hCG is produced in large amounts by hydatidiform moles (see Chapter 8); following evacuation of a molar pregnancy, urinalysis for the presence of hCG is usually continued for 2 years to exclude the subsequent development of choriocarcinoma.

Production of hCG is maximal at 8–10 weeks and then falls to a low plateau level that is maintained throughout the pregnancy. hCG levels, therefore, reflect the placental transformation from an organ of invasion to one of transfer. Persistently low levels of hCG are associated with abnormal placental development or ectopic pregnancy. If hCG is given to nonpregnant women, the corpus luteum is maintained and progesterone secretion rises. Alternatively, antibodies to hCG given to a pregnant woman would cause the corpus luteum to regress. hCG, rather than LH, can be used to induce ovulation in fertility treatment, because it has a longer half-life and is more stable therefore it requires only one injection. (There are concerns that hCG is more

likely to cause ovarian hyperstimulation syndrome than recombinant LH, which is considered to be more physiological.) By 5–6 weeks, the placenta and fetus are synthesizing significant amounts of steroid hormones and can take over the endocrine control of the pregnancy. hCG has thyroid-stimulating hormone properties, affecting appetite and fat deposition, and also affects thirst, release of ADH and other osmoregulatory changes. It also promotes myometrial growth and quiescence (inhibits myometrial contractility) and stimulates angiogenesis in the endometrium (Nwabuobi et al., 2017). The effects of hCG are summarized in Box 11.1.

BOX 11.1 Effects of Human Chorionic Gonadotrophin (hCG)

- Luteotrophic effect on corpus luteum that maintains synthesis and secretion of oestrogen and progesterone in the first trimester
- Simulates placental progesterone production
- Possesses thyrotrophic activity; stimulates maternal thyroid gland and increases appetite and fat deposition
- May be responsible for nausea and vomiting
- Increases sensitivity to glucose
- Decreases osmotic threshold for thirst and release of ADH
- Promotes immunomodulation by suppressing the maternal lymphocyte response thus preventing rejection of the placenta
- Promotes myometrial growth and endometrial and placental angiogenesis
- Inhibits myometrial contractility
- Modulates trophoblastic invasion
- Affects fetal nervous tissue development
- Affects male sexual differentiation and stimulates fetal testes to produce testosterone
- Stimulates fetal adrenal glands to increase production of corticosteroids
- Used as a component of biochemical screening protocols to detect trisomy 21
- Used clinically, outside pregnancy, to monitor tumour growth including possible development of choriocarcinoma
- Used illegally in combination with anabolic androgens to maintain normal testicular structure and function (anabolic steroids often cause testicular atrophy and suppress production of testosterone)
- Note that the use of hCG as a treatment promoting weight loss is considered to be fraudulent and improper as there is no evidence that it is effective

Human Placental Lactogen

As hCG levels fall, there is increased secretion of human placental lactogen (hPL), which is produced by the same cells of the syncytiotrophoblast that initially produced hCG. The levels of hPL increase in parallel with the size of the placenta and correlate well with fetal and placental weight. hPL has a similar structure and properties to growth hormone and prolactin; it is a single polypeptide chain and is lactogenic and stimulates growth of both maternal and fetal tissues. hPL appears to protect the fetus from rejection, and low levels of hPL are associated with pregnancy failure and spontaneous abortion. hPL is antagonistic to insulin, resulting in increased maternal metabolism and utilization of fat as an energy substrate. This diabetogenic effect of pregnancy reduces glucose uptake by maternal cells so maternal blood glucose is maintained at higher levels, thus sparing glucose so more is available for fetal use (see below). hPL is also called 'human chorionic somatomammotrophin'.

Relaxin

Relaxin is produced by the corpus luteum and, to a lesser extent, by the myometrium, endometrium and placenta. The chemical structure of relaxin is related to insulin. Levels of relaxin peak about 14 days after ovulation in a nonpregnant cycle. In pregnancy, levels of relaxin are highest in the first trimester; it plays an important role in maternal adaptation of the cardiovascular system and remodelling of blood vessels. Relaxin also has a role in the softening of elastic ligaments of pelvic bones and has been used clinically to enhance cervical ripening during induction of labour (see Chapter 13). Relaxin acts with progesterone to maintain uterine quiescence; it may also suppress oxytocin release and affect gap junction expression and permeability. The softening and relaxation of the pelvic ligaments allow mobilization and growth of the uterus into the abdomen. Sometimes women experience low-back pain in pregnancy, which is associated with the stretching of these ligaments. For some women, this results in the pelvic joints becoming unstable and in severe cases results in symphysis pubis dysfunction (SPD), which can cause severe pain on walking. Relaxin is also thought to be involved in endometrial differentiation during embryo implantation, wound healing and, possibly, tumour growth and progression. Relaxin has anti-inflammatory and anti-fibrotic properties; it is used therapeutically in patients with heart disease because it is cardioprotective and inhibits arrhythmias (Devarakonda and Salloum, 2018). Relaxin is also important in male reproduction and affects sperm motility so it has a potential role in ART (Ivell et al., 2017).

Adrenal and Pituitary Hormones

The pituitary gland increases in both size, from ~660 mg to at least 760 mg (Blackburn, 2018) and activity during pregnancy. The increase in size is predominantly due to oestrogen stimulating hyperplasia of the lactotroph cells, which produce prolactin. Occasionally, the increase in size and change in shape of the pituitary gland can cause compression of the optic chiasma (point where the two optic nerves cross over) and transient loss of vision. The proportion of lactotroph cells increases from ~20% of the cells of the anterior pituitary gland to ~60%. Prolactin levels increase by about 10-fold during pregnancy, peaking at delivery. More nonglycosylated prolactin, which is more bioactive, is produced during pregnancy; its role is to prepare the breasts for lactation (see Chapter 16). Although most prolactin is produced by the maternal anterior pituitary gland, the uterine decidua also produces some prolactin, which predominantly enters the amniotic fluid.

Oestrogen stimulates cortisol levels by inhibiting the clearance of cortisol and increasing the synthesis of cortisol-binding globulin (CBG or transcortin). Progesterone increases tissue resistance to cortisol by competing at the receptor level and binding to CBG; this also contributes to the increase in cortisol production. Cortisol levels increase 3- to 8-fold in pregnancy. CRH from the hypothalamus and the placenta affects the release of ACTH, melanocyte-stimulating hormone (MSH) and β-endorphin from the anterior pituitary gland. ACTH stimulates the adrenal gland production of cortisol. Cortisol levels increase in response to stress, including increased cardiac output and decreased fasting glucose levels in the second trimester of pregnancy. However, physiological responses to stress are blunted in pregnancy, possibly to protect the fetus (Blackburn, 2018). Both CRH and ACTH are also produced by the placenta as well as by the maternal hypothalamic–pituitary axis; the placental hormones are subject to different feedback control mechanisms and may be important in initiating labour (see Chapter 13).

The increase in circulating levels of cortisol has a positive effect on certain conditions, such as rheumatoid arthritis and eczema. This observation led to the clinical use of steroid treatments such as cortisone for these conditions. Cortisol is important in promoting the maturation of the fetal physiological systems prior to birth (Chapter 15).

Progesterone and oestrogen act synergistically to increase aldosterone production. Adrenal synthesis of androgens, oestrogen, progesterone and cholesterol is increased in pregnancy. The gonadotrophs decrease in number as the raised oestrogen concentration inhibits release of FSH and LH, which are barely detectable for most of pregnancy. MSH synthesis also increases so hyperpigmentation occurs in 85–90% of pregnant women

(Motosko et al., 2017). The melanocytes are also sensitive to the increased levels of oestrogen. Pregnant women frequently observe that they tan more deeply or that their skin develops irregular pigmented patches.

The posterior pituitary gland is also affected by pregnancy. Secretion of ADH remains in the normal range but its threshold for secretion is lowered so plasma osmolality declines during pregnancy (Blackburn, 2018). Oxytocin production from the posterior pituitary progressively increases during pregnancy; oxytocin is important in labour (Chapter 13) and lactation (Chapter 16).

Thyroid Hormones

The hypothalamic–pituitary–thyroid axis undergoes marked changes in pregnancy. Oestrogen, hCG and altered hepatic and renal function together act to change the levels of tri-iodothyronine (T_3), thyroxine (T_4) and thyroid-binding globulin (TBG); these changes are important to support the altered metabolism of pregnancy. Oestrogen stimulates hepatic synthesis of TBG by 2- to 3-fold resulting in increased total amounts of T_3 and T_4, although free concentrations remain within normal physiological limits. hCG has mild TSH activity so it stimulates both the production of T_4 and the deiodination of T_4 to T_3 in the peripheral tissues. Peripheral metabolism of thyroid hormones is also increased because the placenta produces deiodinases (Blackburn, 2018). The high concentrations of hCG in the first trimester and the consequent increased secretion of thyroid hormones results in TSH release from the pituitary gland being inhibited. This means that maternal circulating concentrations of free T_3 and free T_4 peak at the end of the first trimester requiring an increased availability of iodine (Vaidya and Chan, 2018).

If iodine is limiting, the maternal thyroid exhibits an autoregulatory response, increasing synthesis of T_3 (which requires three iodine atoms per molecule) at the expense of T_4 production. Thus, there is no change in TSH but there will be less T_4 transported across the placenta to the fetus, which could compromise neurodevelopment. Early fetal brain development requires maternal thyroid hormone input because the fetus cannot synthesize its own thyroid hormones until about 10–12 weeks old; later in gestation, both the maternal and fetal thyroid glands provide T_4. It should be noted that production of sufficient thyroid hormone requires a doubling of iodine intake compared to the prepregnancy requirement (which may mean potassium iodide supplements should be recommended; see Chapter 12).

Pregnancy mimics hyperthyroidism in a number of respects, for instance by increasing body temperature,

and stimulating appetite and feelings of fatigue. Maternal plasma iodine is decreased because urinary iodide excretion is increased due to increased renal blood flow and increased glomerular filtration rate (GFR).

The thyroid gland undergoes hyperplasia and hypertrophies as it attempts to increase uptake of iodine for hormone synthesis in pregnancy; the extent of the increase in size of the thyroid gland depends on the availability of iodine. Where diets are sufficient in iodine, hyperplasia is mild (10–15% increase in volume). In iodine-poor areas, women may experience a much more significant increase in thyroid volume and goitre may develop. Historically, the presence of pregnancy-induced goitre (thyroid gland hypertrophy) was commonly associated with pregnancy. Nowadays, maternal goitre is less common in pregnancy, partly because of improved diets and iodine supplementation of table salt, but subclinical iodine deficiency may compromise fetal brain and central nervous system development resulting in neurological anomalies, reduced cephalic size (microcephaly) and reduced intelligence quotient (IQ). Many women are at the threshold of iodine deficiency and the iodine requirements for pregnancy can compromise them further, adding support for routine iodine supplementation in pregnancy (Zimmermann, 2016). Basal metabolic rate increases by 20–25% from the 4th month of pregnancy but much of the increase is related to the increased surface area of the mother and the increased work she has to do maintaining maternal and fetal tissue requirements. Nausea and vomiting have been linked to the changes in hCG (see above) and directly to the transient rise in free T_4, which coincides with the peak of hCG in the first trimester and is due to its mild TSH activity.

Hypothyroidism is common in women of reproductive age and affects 3–5% of pregnant women. Subclinical hypothyroidism, defined as raised TSH but normal T4 levels, is more common than overt hypothyroidism (Teng et al., 2013). Women with undiagnosed or poorly managed hypothyroidism have decreased fertility. In pregnancy, overt and untreated hypothyroidism is associated with an increased risk of adverse maternal and neonatal outcomes including increased risk of pregnancy-induced hypertension, anaemia, abruptio placenta (see Chapter 8), miscarriage, stillbirth, postpartum haemorrhage (PPH), congenital malformation, fetal distress, prematurity and low birthweight (LBW) (Kroopnick and Kim, 2016). Women with pre-existing thyroid disease require prompt and close monitoring of thyroid function during pregnancy and usually require increased doses of levothyroxine due the altered metabolic demands of pregnancy. There is no consensus on whether to treat women with subclinical hypothyroidism. Hypothyroidism that develops in pregnancy is usually asymptomatic and symptoms such as weight gain, fatigue, constipation are often attributed solely to pregnancy. The presence of thyroid peroxidase antibodies is used as a marker for autoimmune disorders such as Hashimoto disease or Graves disease.

THE REPRODUCTIVE SYSTEM

The Blood Vessels

The vasculature of the uterus undergoes a number of remarkable and unique changes during pregnancy. Uterine blood flow increases from 2% of cardiac output before pregnancy to 20% by term (Blackburn, 2018); the magnitude of the increased blood flow of the uterine arteries is an extraordinary physiological adaptation (Browne et al., 2015). The vessel diameter of the 100-150 spiral arteries increases and vascular resistance falls (see Chapter 8). These essential changes accommodate the increased blood flow to the placenta, which is maintained under conditions of low blood pressure. The coursing of blood through the enlarged tortuous arteries produces a uterine 'souffle', which may be auscultated through a stethoscope, pinard horn or with a portable electronic Doppler ultrasound fetal monitor. The uterine blood flow is predominantly redistributed to the region where the placenta is implanted.

The Uterus

The uterus increases in all dimensions and also changes shape (see Chapters 2 and 13) during pregnancy. Uterine hyperplasia begins after implantation and is driven by oestrogen and growth factors; uterine growth occurs even if the embryo is implanted ectopically in an extrauterine site rather than in the endometrium (Blackburn, 2018). Early growth results in thickening of the uterine wall. The endometrium thickens into the decidua. The three layers

of the myometrium become clearly defined as the uterine muscle undergoes initial hyperplasia (development of new fibres) and subsequent hypertrophy (increase in length and thickness of existing muscle fibres). Later uterine growth is mostly due to hypertrophy and hyperplasia of the myocytes and remodelling of connective tissue, which is driven by distension as the amniotic sac containing the fetus enlarges. The muscle fibres increase in length and width as the timing and speed of the myometrial action potentials change and the muscle cells increase their content of actin and myosin, gap junctions, sarcoplasmic reticulum and mitochondria.

In early pregnancy, the uterine isthmus increases from ~7–25 mm (Fig. 11.2) in thickness and softens because of the increased blood supply. Historically, the Hegar sign (being able to compress the softened lower uterine walls) was used to detect probable early pregnancy (from ~5–12 weeks); it is no longer used having been replaced by pregnancy tests and ultrasound scanning. The Hegar sign is not a sensitive indicator of pregnancy; not being able to detect softening of the uterine consistency does not exclude pregnancy and it was not usually successful in identifying pregnancy in women who had had a previous pregnancy. From 32 to 34 weeks, the isthmus is transformed into the lower uterine segment (LUS). As effacement of the cervix commences (at ~36 weeks), the external os is incorporated into the LUS (see Chapter 13).

The blastocyst usually implants in the fundus (upper part) of the uterus. By 12 weeks, the fetus, extraembryonic tissues and amniotic fluid fill the uterine cavity and the fundus can just be palpated (felt) at the pelvic brim above the symphysis pubis. By 20 weeks, the fundus reaches the maternal umbilicus and by 8 months, it reaches the lowest part of the sternum (known as the xiphisternum). As the uterus expands during pregnancy, it loses its anteverted and anteflexed configuration and becomes erect, tilting and

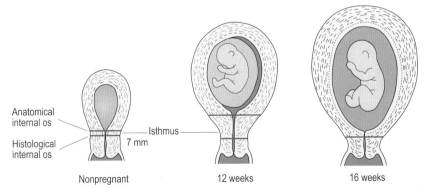

Fig. 11.2 The uterine isthmus increases from ~7–25 mm in the early part of pregnancy. (Reproduced with permission from Miller and Hanretty, 1998.)

then rotating to the right diverted by the presence of the descending colon. The uterus changes from its nonpregnant pear-shape and becomes spherical and then cylindrical. Abdominal measurement using the distance between the highest point of the fundus to the top of the symphysis pubis as a reference point is often used to assess uterine size and fetal growth as pregnancy progresses. Fundal measurements are ideally done when the woman has emptied her bladder beforehand and is in the semi-prone position.

Uterine quiescence is regulated by progesterone, relaxin, nitric oxide (NO) and prostacyclin (also known as prostaglandin PGI_2). The uterus is never completely quiescent and exhibits low-frequency activity throughout the pregnancy (as it does in the nonpregnant state). Braxton Hicks contractions are painless contractions that are measurable from the first trimester of pregnancy. These contractions do not dilate the cervix but are thought to assist in the circulation of blood to the placenta. The contractions are usually irregular and weak, unsynchronized and multifocal in origin; they exhibit a diurnal rhythm with more during the night and fewest in the early afternoon. The contractions of the circular muscles are less frequent than those of the longitudinal ones (Blackburn, 2018). The uterine ligaments soften and thicken under the influence of oestrogen, resulting in increased mobility and capacity of the pelvis.

The Cervix

The cervix increases in mass and width during the pregnancy. Oestrogen increases the blood supply to the cervix resulting in a lilac colouration and softer tissue texture; the water content of the cervix also increases as the production of hyaluronic acid increases. The collagen fibre bundles become less tightly bound (see Chapter 13). The cervical mucosa proliferates and the glands become more complex and secrete thickened mucus, which forms a plug or operculum protecting the uterine cavity from ascending infection. The plug is held laterally by projections of thickened mucus in the mouths of the mucus-secreting glands. It is this mucus plug that is released as 'the show' at the onset of labour when the cervix starts to efface and be drawn up forming the lower part of the LUS.

The Vagina

Blood flow to the vagina also increases during pregnancy, resulting in softer vaginal tissue, which is more distensible. The lilac discolouration of the vagina and cervix was traditionally recognized as being an indicator of early pregnancy (described as Jacquemier's or Chadwick's sign). The increased blood flow means that the pulsating of the uterine arteries can be felt through the lateral fornices (historically known as the Osiander sign). The increased vascularization of the vagina can result in increased sensitivity and

sexual arousal. Venous engorgement results in increased vascular transudation, which together with the increased cervical mucus production results in an increased vaginal discharge. The vaginal discharge (leucorrhoea) has a low pH (because of the effect of raised oestrogen levels on the vaginal microbiota) and is thick and white with an inoffensive odour. Oestrogen also stimulates the vaginal epithelial cell division so the cells acquire a distinctly boat-shaped appearance (which should not be mistaken for carcinoma cells). Early in pregnancy, the hypertrophied corpus luteum, which is ~3–5 cm long, distends from the ovarian surface; this may be palpated in some women or visualized during endoscopic examination in women undergoing egg retrieval for assisted reproductive technology (ART).

The Breasts

In early pregnancy, vascularization of the breasts increases. This tends to result in a marbled appearance of the skin owing to the marked dilation of the underlying superficial veins. The breasts, especially the nipple areas, may feel sensitive and tingle because of the engorgement of blood. Areolar pigmentation increases, the Montgomery tubercles enlarge and become more prominent and the nipples become more erect. (Changes to the breasts in pregnancy are described in more detail in Chapter 16.) Breast cancer is the most common cancer affecting women but diagnosis during pregnancy is not common (Durrani et al., 2018). Pregnancy following diagnosis and treatment for breast cancer is becoming more common with an increase in incidence, earlier diagnosis and delayed childbirth. Generally, the approach is to follow the guidelines for treatment of nonpregnant women with breast cancer wherever possible. Chemotherapy and radiotherapy are avoided during the first trimester when embryological development is particularly vulnerable (see Chapter 9). Although concerns have been raised about the possible promotional effects of raised oestrogen levels during pregnancy on residual metastatic disease, there is no evidence that pregnancy affects survival.

The signs of pregnancy are summarized in Box 11.2.

THE CARDIOVASCULAR SYSTEM

The most notable physiological changes occur in the cardiovascular system in preparation for the increased demands of maternal and fetal tissues (Fig. 11.3). These changes are caused both indirectly by hormones (oestrogen, progesterone, prostaglandins and other vasoactive substances) and directly by mechanical effects, as a result of changes in other systems and as a result of the increased load on the cardiovascular system. Marked haemodynamic adjustments take place in pregnancy; maternal blood volume and cardiac output increase very early in gestation

BOX 11.2 **Signs of Pregnancy**

- Amenorrhoea
- Softening of vagina and cervix
- Increased blood flow to vagina and cervix causing lilac colouration (Jacquemier's sign)
- Pulsating of uterine arteries (Osiander sign)
- Tingling and sensitive breasts with dilated superficial veins marbling surface
- Nausea and vomiting, possible changes in taste
- Increased frequency of urination as uterus compresses bladder
- Increased pigmentation of skin
- Bleeding gums
- Tiredness
- Increased appetite and thirst
- Slight rise in body temperature

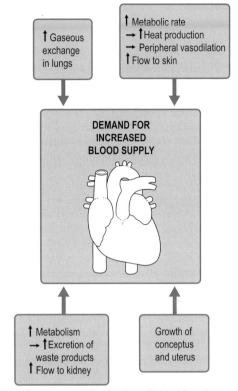

Fig. 11.3 The changed distribution of blood flow in pregnancy.

however, blood pressure falls because of the marked reduction in systemic vascular resistance (SVR; also known as peripheral resistance) and reduced blood viscosity due to haemodilution. If the cardiovascular adaptation to pregnancy is insufficient, the risk of maternal and fetal morbidity is significantly increased.

Heart disease affects 0.2–0.4% of all pregnancies and causes two deaths per 100,000 in England and Wales (and similar rates in other countries), but it is one of the main contributors to maternal death worldwide. Despite heart disease being rare, apparent symptoms (such as breathlessness, palpitations, fainting and oedema) are present in most pregnant women (Johnson and von Klemperer, 2016). Superimposed on a pre-existing cardiac disease state, pregnancy may be dangerous and even potentially fatal. Pregnancy has been called 'nature's stress test' because failure of the maternal cardiovascular system to adapt appropriately can reveal pre-existing but undiagnosed cardiac conditions (Coutinho et al., 2018). Cardiovascular issues are the most significant contributor to maternal death; older women and those who are obese or have a history of hypertension are more likely to be affected by cardiovascular pathologies in pregnancy. Diagnosis of a cardiovascular problem in pregnancy can lead to subsequent appropriate and life-saving management of the condition. Furthermore, some pregnancy-related complications, such as pre-eclampsia, gestational diabetes, gestational hypertension, arrhythmias and very preterm delivery, are risk factors for cardiometabolic disease later in life (Sanghavi and Parikh, 2017). Pregnancy offers the opportunity for early identification of women who have an underlying predisposition for cardiovascular disease.

Measurement of cardiovascular system parameters is technically difficult and notoriously variable. Measurements obviously have to be indirect and are very sensitive to changes such as emotion, exertion and posture. In the research literature, there are many inconsistencies, some of which reflect differences in standardization of conditions such as position of the pregnant woman. In the last couple of decades there has been an increased incidence of myocardial infarction (MI) in pregnancy, which partly reflects the increasing proportion of older women having babies. Pregnancy increases the risk of MI in all women but the risk of MI is 30 times higher in women >40 years compared with women <20 years of age, and is exacerbated by obesity and pre-existing diabetes (Honigberg and Scott, 2018). In addition, an increasing number of women with congenital and acquired heart disease are becoming pregnant. This reflects improvements in their medical care and the use of ART (Ashrafi and Curtis, 2017). Optimal management of pregnant women with heart disease is by a multidisciplinary care team and starts from the preconceptual stage.

Blood Volume

Total blood volume increases by 30–50% during pregnancy, and even more in multiple pregnancies and in women who are obese (Blackburn, 2018) with a concurrent fall in plasma osmolality. The rise in blood volume correlates well with birthweight and, as it begins early in pregnancy, the mechanism of these early changes in the cardiovascular system is thought to be hormonally driven. It was disputed whether the increase in volume (sodium and fluid retention) preceded the increased vascular space ('overfill' hypothesis) or whether the changes were stimulated by relative hypovolaemia (increased vascular capacity), known as the 'underfill' hypothesis. The arguments for the 'underfill' hypothesis are supported by the observation that the initial haemodynamic change is a fall in vascular resistance (Johnson and von Klemperer, 2016). By the 8th week of pregnancy, SVR has fallen by 10–30%. Often in early pregnancy women feel faint, suggesting that the physiological compensation of the underfill and restoration of adequate blood volume have yet to occur.

Oestrogen stimulates angiogenesis (formation of new blood vessels and vascular beds) and increases the blood flow to the tissues. Oestrogen affects the distribution of collagen in the tunica media of the large vessel walls, increasing venous distensibility. Oestrogen also stimulates endothelium-dependent vasodilatation, by increasing synthesis of nitric oxide (NO; a potent vasodilator) and vasodilatory prostaglandins and inhibiting the release of endothelin-I (a vasoconstrictor). Production of both prostacyclin and NO increases in pregnancy; NO is also the main vasodilator in the placenta (Zullino et al. 2018). The vasodilatory signals affect placental blood flow and remodelling of the spiral arteries (see Chapter 8). NO is also involved with implantation and early embryonic development, platelet activity in the intervillous space and placental perfusion.

Progesterone relaxes vascular smooth muscle causing systemic vasodilatation and decreased SVR, probably via vasoactive prostaglandins and enhanced NO production. The syncytiotrophoblast is an essential site of NO production, which is important in maintaining vasodilation of the uterine and feto-placental blood vessels and ensuring a high flow and low resistance blood supply to the utero-placental bed and fetus. The effect of the vasodilation is that the circulatory system increases its capacity and is relatively underfilled. One of the early effects of this is decreased glomerular arteriolar resistance, which results in increased renal blood flow (by about 50%) and increased GFR (Sanghavi and Rutherford, 2014). Relaxin production is stimulated by hCG and is also involved in renal vasodilation; it also stimulates the production

of ADH and thus water retention. The decreased vascular tone in the blood supply to the kidneys causes renal compensatory mechanisms to increase plasma volume and cardiac output. In addition, both progesterone and oestrogen increase water retention by affecting the renin–angiotensin–aldosterone system (RAAS) and oestrogen increases hepatic angiotensinogen production. This results in a rise in angiotensin II, which increases renal fluid resorption and stimulates the production of aldosterone. All components of the RAAS increase in pregnancy but there is decreased sensitivity to vasoconstrictors such as angiotensin II and noradrenaline during normal pregnancy (so blood pressure does not normally rise). Renin is produced by the uterus, placenta and fetus, as well as the kidney. Levels of renin are 2-to 3-fold higher than before pregnancy. These changes in the RAAS may mediate the oestrogen-stimulated angiogenesis and increased cell growth and division. In the first trimester, relaxin has a role in increasing vascular compliance, which contributes to the decreased SVR (Johnson and von Klemperer, 2016). The vascular actions of relaxin are largely mediated by NO (Leo et al., 2017). Relaxin increases production of ADH and oxytocin and modulates responses to angiotensin II. The increased ADH promotes water retention and thirst; the raised oxytocin promotes vasodilation and sodium excretion partly by increasing cardiac atrial natriuretic peptide (ANP) levels, which increase by about 40% in the third trimester and remain above normal postpartum (Johnson and von Klemperer, 2016).

Progesterone stimulates a 10-fold increase in the amount of circulating aldosterone. Progesterone is an aldosterone antagonist and acts on the aldosterone receptor to prevent sodium retention and protect against potassium loss (Sanghavi and Rutherford, 2014). In preeclampsia, aldosterone levels are low and the plasma volume expansion is less than optimal. Progesterone augments its effects on the circulatory volume by resetting the thirst centres in the hypothalamus and increasing thirst. Progesterone also lowers the sodium threshold for the RAAS and blocks the vasopressive activity of angiotensin II in pregnancy (Blackburn, 2018) so it promotes expansion of plasma volume without increasing blood pressure. The net result of the changes in oestrogen and progesterone is an increase in vascular resistance followed by increased sodium and water retention and expansion of the circulating volume (Fig. 11.4).

Cardiac Output

Blood volume and cardiac output increase in parallel (Fig. 11.5). Cardiac output, the volume of blood that the heart pumps into the circulatory system per minute, increases throughout pregnancy by 30–50%, an average increase

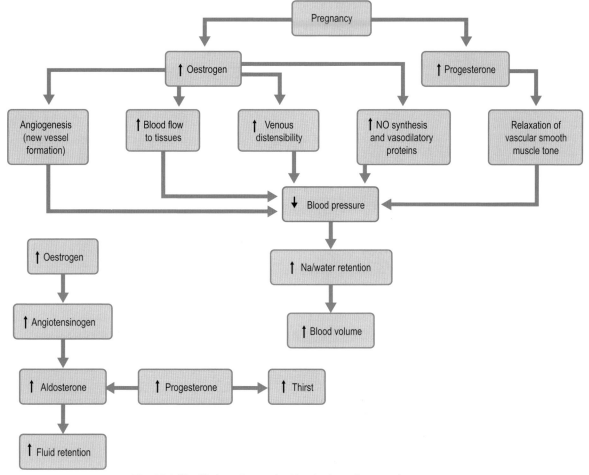

Fig. 11.4 The likely pathways for blood volume increase in pregnancy.

of 1.5 L/min from 4.5 to 6 L/min or more. Cardiac output rises quickly in the first trimester and is maintained throughout the second half of pregnancy. Increased cardiac output is evident by the 5th week of gestation and by the 8th week, it has increased by about 20% (Johnson and von Klemperer, 2016). The increase in cardiac output is greater in multiple pregnancies. Cardiac output is affected by maternal posture: when the pregnant woman lies supine, her uterus impedes venous return from the inferior vena cava resulting in significant change in cardiac output. The apparent decline in cardiac output in the third trimester, observed by a number of researchers, was most probably the result of the methods of cardiac investigation. Women with cardiac conditions that limit the increase of cardiac output usually have infants who are smaller. In labour, cardiac output increases by about 2.0 L/min, partly because uterine contractions cause a shift of some blood from the uteroplacental circulation to the systemic circulation (see Chapter 13).

Cardiac output is the result of two variables: heart rate and stroke volume (see Chapter 1). In pregnancy, both heart rate and stroke volume increase. Heart rate increases soon after implantation, by about 20% (an average of 15 beats more per min) from ~70–85 beats/min. Stroke volume typically increases gradually by ~10% from 64 to 71 mL. Steroid hormones and prolactin may affect the myocardium directly. Oestrogen stimulates an increased accumulation of components of the myocardial cells, which together with catecholamine release in response to the decreased SVR causes an increase in cardiac contractility (Johnson and von Klemperer, 2016). Heart rate is usually measured by the palpation of peripheral pulses and the

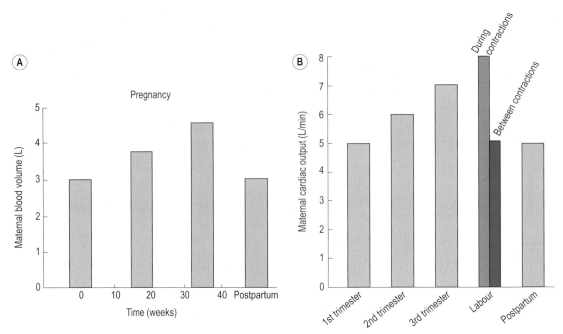

Fig. 11.5 The parallel increase in (A) blood volume and (B) cardiac output during pregnancy. Blood volume is increased up to 40%, thus increasing the load on the heart. (Reproduced with permission from Chamberlain et al., 1991. (B) After Whitfield, 1986.)

increase in stroke volume means the pulse is easier to palpate in a pregnant woman. Heart rate is affected by many things; tachycardia (fast pulse) may be caused by excitement, stress, fear, medication, illegal use of drugs, etc. and, in isolation, can be a poor indicator of physical problems such as sepsis and haemorrhage. It needs to be considered in conjunction with other abnormal observations such as raised blood pressure, temperature or respiratory rate. In pregnancy, the extra volume of blood in the circulatory system may result in women being more aware of sinus tachycardia, which is usually defined as a heart rate >100 bpm, and cardiac arrhythmias. Bradycardia is an abnormally slow heartbeat and is rare in pregnant women but can indicate heart block, raised intracranial pressure, medication and use of illegal drugs.

Heart

The changes relating to the heart occur early in the pregnancy and are caused by hormonal changes. Later, the heart is displaced upwards by elevation of the diaphragm and is rotated forward so the electrocardiogram (ECG) changes and the location of the apex beat is directed forward to the anterior chest wall. The heart increases in size by an average of 70–80 mL (~12%). This increase is due to increased filling and oestrogen-stimulated cardiac

muscle hypertrophy (an increase in the size of pre-existing cardiomyocytes). The thickness of the left ventricular wall increases by about 28% and its mass by about 50% (Sanghavi and Rutherford, 2014). The remodelling of the heart and eccentric hypertrophy that occurs in pregnancy in response to increased blood volume and workload is an adaptive response analogous to the ventricular hypertrophy of an athlete's heart in continuous training. It is an adaptation that allows increased ventricular work involved with pumping the increased blood volume, while minimizing oxygen consumption. However, heart hypertrophy can lead to cardiac disturbances such as cardiac arrhythmias (MacIntyre et al., 2018). The pregnant woman's heart is thus dilated and has increased contractility. Increased blood volume results in an increase in venous return and therefore increased atrial size. The heart sounds change because the mitral valve closes marginally before the closure of the tricuspid valve; thus, the first heart sound is louder with an exaggerated split. Many pregnant women (92–95%) develop innocent (nonsignificant) systolic murmurs in pregnancy. The increased blood flow through the mammary blood vessels may also be perceived as a possible heart murmur; this is more common in early lactation. The net result of increased contractility, increased venous return, cardiac hypertrophy, decreased

BOX 11.3 Marfan Syndrome

Marfan syndrome is a disorder of connective tissue and as a result has a high incidence of aortic aneurism due to the inherent weakness of the artery wall. Incidence of the disease is ~2 per 10,000 births and affects both men and women equally. As cardiac output is increased in pregnancy, the risk of aortic aneurism occurring is greatly increased and so the pregnant woman should have regular cardiac ultrasounds to optimize early detection of this potentially life-threatening situation. If aortic aneurism occurs, emergency surgical intervention is required, which involves the weakness of the aortic wall being strengthened by synthetic graft material.

SVR and increased heart rate is increased cardiac output. Women with known pre-existing cardiac disease must be carefully monitored during pregnancy as they may not have the physiological reserve to cope with this increased demand on the heart (Gongora and Wenger, 2015) (see Case study 11.1). Other conditions may also pose serious risks in pregnancy relating to increased cardiac output such as Marfan syndrome (Box 11.3).

Arteriovenous Oxygen Difference

The arteriovenous (AV) oxygen difference is the difference in oxygen content of arterial blood (oxygenated) supplying an organ and the venous blood (deoxygenated) draining the same organ. It is a useful way of assessing oxygen use by the uterus (and fetoplacental unit) and determining whether the maternal physiological adaptations match the increased oxygen demand. Increased cardiac output exceeds increased oxygen consumption (especially early in pregnancy when cardiac output increases considerably and oxygen consumption is relatively low) so more oxygen is returned to the heart from venous circulation compared with prepregnant values and the AV oxygen difference is smaller. The AV oxygen difference is 34 mL in mid-pregnancy rising towards term but is always less than the nonpregnant values of ~45 mL (Blackburn, 2018). The higher return of oxygen to the heart suggests that the commonly measured decrease in haemoglobin concentration is not physiologically inadequate and the relatively small increase in total haemoglobin (oxygen-carrying capacity) is more than sufficient to compensate for increased oxygen requirements. This supports the argument that the term 'physiological anaemia' is inappropriate (see p. 311). The increased AV oxygen difference, especially early in the pregnancy before oxygen consumption increases significantly, means that early fetal development and organogenesis occur in an environment, which is adequately oxygenated despite the maternal spiral arteries not connecting with the intervillous spaces in the early part of pregnancy (see Chapter 8).

Blood Pressure

Normal pregnancy has relatively little effect on arterial blood pressure. Despite increased cardiac output and increased vascular capacity, there is relatively little change in systolic pressure in pregnancy. However, diastolic blood pressure is lower in the first two trimesters and returns to prepregnant values in the third trimester. Both the development of new vascular beds and the relaxation of peripheral vascular tone by progesterone result in decreased resistance to flow. This is augmented by a change in the profile of prostaglandins produced. The levels of the prostaglandin PGE_2 and prostacyclin, which stimulate vasodilation, rise early in pregnancy. Nitric oxide (NO) plays an important role in the biology of pregnancy; it is vasodilatory and enhances blood flow (Zullino et al., 2018). Production of NO is stimulated by shear stress, platelet-derived factors and cytokines. NO deficiency is associated with pregnancy complications such as preeclampsia, hypertension and intrauterine growth restriction. Enhancing NO bioavailability, by pharmacological and nutritional approaches, may offer therapeutic strategies for pathological conditions (Cottrell et al., 2017). For much of pregnancy the pulse pressure (the difference between diastolic and systolic blood pressure) is increased. Hypotension, particularly in early pregnancy, has been associated with fatigue, headaches, dizziness and occasionally fainting, which many women experience.

CASE STUDY 11.1

Moira is a 23-year-old primigravida who, at the age of 19, underwent a heart and lung transplant as a result of cystic fibrosis. Moira and her partner had been well informed of the risks associated with a pregnancy, had planned not to have any children and so this pregnancy was unexpected.

- How should Moira's care be managed in relation to her transplant status and her pregnancy and what is the role of the midwife in this complex case?
- What are the possible complications and risks in this case and what would the midwife need to know and do to ensure early recognition, referral and intervention is optimized?
- In relation to Moira's cystic fibrosis, could her condition have any other effects upon her pregnancy?

BOX 11.4   Blood Pressure Monitoring

Hypertension in pregnancy remains one of the leading contributors for serious maternal and fetal complications. It is important that blood pressure is measured accurately using recommended techniques (NICE, 2008) such as ensuring the woman is relaxed and her arm is supported at heart level, that she has avoided recent intake of caffeine or nicotine and the cuff is of an appropriate size.

The usual definitions of hypertension are:

- Mild hypertension: diastolic blood pressure 90–99 mmHg; systolic blood pressure 140–149 mmHg
- Moderate hypertension: diastolic blood pressure 100–109 mmHg; systolic blood pressure 150–159 mmHg
- Severe hypertension: diastolic blood pressure 110 mmHg or higher; systolic blood pressure 160 mmHg or higher (NICE, 2010).

Increased surveillance is recommended if the woman has a single measurement of diastolic blood pressure of 110 mmHg or two consecutive readings of 90 mmHg at least 4 h apart and/or significant proteinuria (1+).

It is recommended that treatment should be considered if the woman's systolic blood pressure is above 160 mmHg on two consecutive readings at least 4 h apart.

Some women may not show the expected reduction in blood pressure in early pregnancy. This may be due to pre-existing renal disease or a condition causing chronic hypertension but may also be an early indicator of hypertensive disease in pregnancy. Note that preeclampsia can be superimposed on chronic hypertension. A rise in blood pressure is often associated with, but not always present in preeclampsia. Other reasons for high blood pressure may be stress and anxiety, acute renal disease such as infection, raised intercranial pressure (the significance of this is increased with a slowing pulse). The blood pressure reading needs to be considered in the context of other risk factors. A drop in blood pressure may be caused by haemorrhage (significance is increased with the presence of tachycardia), advanced sepsis (septic shock) and may be drug induced.

In pregnancy, changes in posture can cause acute haemodynamic changes (Blackburn, 2018). Blood pressure in normotensive women is higher when sitting and decreases on lying, especially in the supine position (Box 11.4). Effects on venous pressure are relatively dramatic compared with the effects on arterial pressure. As there are no valves between the return from the femoral veins to the vena cava and heart, venous pressure in the legs is similar to the pressure in the heart so, if a pregnant woman lies in a supine position, the uterus can compress the aorta and, particularly, the thin-walled vena cava and iliac veins. (The aorta is compressed as well but to a lesser degree because it has a much thicker vessel wall.) Return of blood to the heart can also be impeded by the pressure of the fetal head on the iliac veins and by hydrodynamic obstruction due to outflow of blood from the uterine vessels. Most women experience a drop in blood pressure >10% when they lie down; for some of these women this fall may be extreme, reaching up to 50%. The effect of assuming the lithotomy position in labour is to decrease cardiac output significantly; avoiding this may be particularly important in women who have pre-existing heart disease (Ashrafi and Curtis, 2017).

In advanced pregnancy, up to 80% of healthy pregnant women experience oedema of the lower extremities (see Case study 11.2) owing to the combined effects of progesterone relaxing the vascular tone, the impeding of the venous return by the gravid uterus and gravitational forces. The peripheral circulatory volume is increased by 500–600 mL per limb. Oedema is further increased in

CASE STUDY 11.2

It is the height of summer and Kathy, 38 weeks' pregnant, informs her midwife she feels fat and sluggish and cannot cope with the hot weather. Kathy's ankles are visibly swollen.

- Is the midwife right to assume that this is normal?
- What indicators would the midwife be able to use in an assessment to reassure Kathy that her symptoms are normal?
- What factors may alert the midwife to suspect that all is not well?

Three days later Kathy presents to the midwives' clinic complaining of breathlessness and chest pain.

- What should the midwife do in response to Kathy's worsening symptoms?
- What are the possible causes of these symptoms?

---

hypertensive women and tends to increase with increased maternal age (Blackburn, 2018). Fluid drunk by the pregnant woman may therefore appear as increased leg volume and the expected diuresis is likely to be delayed until she lies down, resulting in increased nocturia. The effect of increased venous pressure is to increase the incidence and severity of varicose veins of the legs, vulva and haemorrhoids (Fig. 11.6).

The tendency to develop oedema is also affected by the reduced concentration of plasma proteins (Box 11.5). The

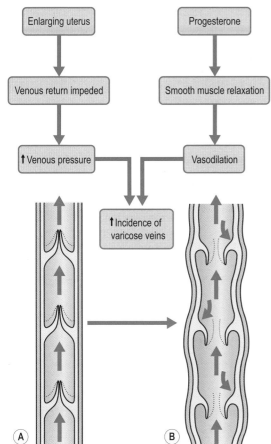

Fig. 11.6 The effect of increased venous pressure leading to increased incidence of varicose veins of the legs, vulva and haemorrhoids. (A) Normal vein with normal vascular tone; (B) varicose vein: the effects of progesterone on muscle tone cause incomplete valve closure, allowing the backflow of blood.

BOX 11.6   Exercise in Pregnancy

Exercise affects maternal physiology because there is a hormonal response, weight is redistributed and heat is generated. Many women experience very good physical health, especially early in pregnancy. However, the question is whether the adaptive response to exercise compromises fetal oxygenation and wellbeing. The ability to increase cardiac output in response to exercise progressively declines throughout pregnancy. Theoretically, redistribution of weight could affect the venous return and blood could be preferentially circulated to the skeletal muscles and to the skin for heat dissipation. Studies on animals suggest that uterine blood flow can be decreased substantially before fetal oxygen uptake or temperature regulation is compromised. It was reported that over one-third of the female medal winners in the 1956 Russian Olympic team were pregnant and their cardiovascular changes enhanced their performance. In practice, moderate exercise in normal healthy pregnancy is encouraged, as maternal and fetal health seem to benefit. However, pregnant women are advised to avoid jumping and jerky movements because of joint instability. Vigorous exercise is not recommended during hot humid weather or if the mother has a fever. It is suggested that heart rate should not exceed 140 b.p.m., strenuous exercise should be done for <15 min at a time and a pregnant woman should not allow herself to become breathless. A pregnant woman should stop physical exercise if pain, vaginal bleeding or dizziness is experienced or there are any known risk factors.

BOX 11.5   Oedema and Hypertension

The pressures in the right ventricle, pulmonary arteries and pulmonary capillaries do not change but cardiac output increases. The higher pulmonary blood flow therefore has to be absorbed by decreased pulmonary resistance and dilatation of the pulmonary vascular bed so the volume of pulmonary circulation increases to match the increased cardiac output. Conditions where pulmonary resistance is increased or fixed have a poor maternal prognosis such as Eisenmenger syndrome, which has a 30–50% mortality rate. Exercise presents an increased demand on the cardiovascular system (see Box 11.6).

---

increment in plasma volume is not matched by an increase in plasma protein synthesis so there is decreased plasma colloidal pressure. This, together with the increased venous pressure, means there is an increase in fluid loss from the capillaries. There may also be an increase in capillary permeability (Blackburn, 2018).

The effects of exercise on the cardiovascular system are summarized in Box 11.6.

Distribution of Blood Flow

Oestrogen increases blood flow to all tissues. Venous tone is affected by progesterone. The increased venous distensibility results in an increased incidence of varicose veins, venous thrombosis and thromboembolism. The uterus is the central target of the increased cardiac output and circulatory flow during pregnancy but distribution of flow to other organ systems, including kidneys, skin, lungs and breasts, increases as well. It is difficult to distinguish between blood flow to the increasing uterine tissue mass and that going specifically to supply the placenta because the uterine vessels are complex and inaccessible. AV shunts in the uterine vasculature have been identified; these allow a short circuit of the placental site after delivery of the placenta, rather than being important in increased flow during pregnancy. The increased flow to the uterus means that the proportion of cardiac output to the uterus increases from ~2% to 20%, with a flow of ~500–800 mL/min at term (Blackburn, 2018). In rare situations of maternal cardiac arrest in late pregnancy, the altered blood flow and heart position can affect the ability of external cardiac massage to provide vital organ oxygenation. In addition, the gravid uterus compresses the abdominal aorta and inferior vena cava (aortacaval compression), which can cause hypotension and loss of consciousness. In such situations, immediate delivery of the infant must be considered either by perimortem caesarean section (PMCS also known as a resuscitative hysterotomy) or an instrumental delivery if in the second stage of labour. Once delivered, the empty uterus will contract down enabling more blood to enter the central circulation improving oxygenation to the vital organs (Jeejeebhoy et al., 2015).

Blood flow to the kidneys increases by ~400 mL/min from early pregnancy, facilitating elimination of the additional fetal metabolic waste products. The increased renal blood flow promotes an increased GFR, which increases by ~40–50% above nonpregnant levels. Vasodilatory prostaglandins, NO and ANP are implicated in the peripheral vasodilation, which is particularly evident in the vessels of the breasts, hands and face. Oestrogen and progesterone depress the normal response to angiotensin II and oestrogen abrogates the vasoconstriction mediated by the sympathetic nervous system. Blood flow to the lungs increases, reflecting the increased circulating blood volume and cardiac output.

Distribution of blood to the skin is greatly increased (by ~500 mL/min) expediting heat loss and thus improving thermoregulation although it is still common for pregnant women to complain of being hot. Pregnant women usually have warm or clammy hands and feet and often complain that midwives' hands are cold. This vasodilatory effect is enhanced in smokers. Blood flow to the hands increases about sevenfold giving a very marked increase in skin temperature. The resulting peripheral vasodilation causes the capillaries to dilate and stimulates angiogenesis and may give rise to the development of vascular spiders, particularly on the face, neck and arms, and palmar erythema (redness of the palms of the hands), which is often associated with burning sensations (Alves et al., 2018). These changes

in the skin are related to high levels of oestrogen; they usually resolve after pregnancy and reappear with subsequent pregnancies. The increased blood flow to the skin means there is a decreased tendency to arterial vasospasm, and therefore conditions such as Raynaud syndrome (or Raynaud phenomenon) are often alleviated in pregnancy. (However, note that pregnant women with Raynaud syndrome may be at increased risk for other vascular complications.)

The increased blood flow to the skin stimulates the growth of nails and hair. The ratio of actively growing hair (in the anagen phase) to resting (prior to falling out; in the telogen phase) hair is altered from 85:15 to 95:5 (Motosko et al., 2017). Hair appears thicker during pregnancy because of the reduced hair loss and also because the diameter of the hair shaft increases. When this ratio returns to normal in the puerperium, vast amounts of hair can be lost; this phenomenon can be protracted lasting up to a year after pregnancy, which may cause distress. Mammary blood flow also increases (see Chapter 16). Coronary blood flow may also increase to meet the increased workload of the left ventricle, but it is thought that hepatic and cerebral blood flow are not significantly changed in pregnancy (Blackburn, 2018).

In evolutionary terms, heat dissipation from the mucous membranes had been very important in mammals (this is best illustrated by dogs panting to lose heat). The increased flow to the mucous membranes in pregnancy can result in an increased congestion of the mucosa, which is demonstrated by an increased incidence of nasal congestion, sinusitis, nosebleeds and snoring in pregnancy. It is suggested that elimination of waste products by the kidneys and heat by the skin is best fulfilled by an increased plasma volume rather than an increase in whole blood, which demonstrates the importance of the apparent physiological anaemia.

Haematological Changes

The changes in maternal blood volume and composition increase the efficiency of the transplacental circulation and exchange mechanisms, thus benefiting fetal development. The haematological changes are also part of a maternal adaptive response that protects maternal homeostasis, facilitating tolerance of a sudden blood loss and the ability to cope with placental separation. Thus, even women who have a degree of iron deficiency prior to pregnancy are protected from some decrease in haemoglobin levels at delivery. However, the adaptive responses to pregnancy potentiate the risks of iron-deficiency anaemia, thromboembolism and other clotting problems.

Plasma Volume and Blood Cell Mass/Number

Pregnancy is a state of hypervolaemia. Blood volume increases in healthy pregnant women by ~1.2–1.6 L (40–50%, with a range of individual variation). Plasma volume increases rapidly from about 6 weeks' gestation and then the rate of increase becomes slower (Blackburn, 2018). The 40–60% increase in plasma volume is not matched by increased red blood cell mass and plasma protein production, so there is a haemodilution (an apparent decrease) in haemoglobin, plasma protein concentration and other components of the blood. Red blood cell mass increases by ~15–18% in women who do not take iron supplements and by ~25–33% in women supplemented with iron (Blackburn, 2018). The differences in plasma volume and red blood cell mass are accentuated by differential timing of the increases. The expansion of plasma begins from about the 6th week. Red blood cell mass begins to expand in the second trimester and peaks in the third trimester. Plasma volume changes are related to the NO-mediated vasodilation, which stimulate the maternal RAAS so sodium and water retention are promoted to increase vascular volume. In addition, the RAAS affects red blood cell homeostasis (Kim et al., 2017); angiotensin II regulates the production of erythropoietin (see below).

The increase in blood volume is higher in multigravidae and women who are obese, have multiple pregnancies or where the pregnancy results in a large-for-gestational-age infant or gestation is prolonged. Plasma volume expansion in women having twins can be up to 70%, even more with triplets. The increment in plasma volume is positively correlated with birthweight and placental weight; preeclampsia and other complications of pregnancy resulting in recurrent abortions, stillborn and LBW babies are associated with an abnormally low increase in plasma volume and an apparent increase (or no normal decrease) in haemoglobin concentration.

There is no physiological reason that the relationship between plasma volume and blood cell mass, which are controlled by different mechanisms, should be retained throughout the pregnancy. The role of plasma is to fill the vascular space, maintaining the blood pressure, and to dissipate heat. Calculations suggest that the hypervolaemia is adequate to fill the increased vascular space of the pregnant uterus and the enlarged vascular beds of the breasts, muscles, kidneys and skin and to provide a reservoir against the pooling of blood in the lower extremities. It will also buffer the effect of the haemoglobin lost in bleeding at delivery. The decreased viscosity of the blood lessens the resistance to flow and therefore the cardiac effort required to propel the blood. Observation of a 'normal' (prepregnant) or increased haemoglobin level (rather than a lower level seen in healthy pregnancies) may therefore represent an unsatisfactory increase in plasma volume rather than a true increase in haemoglobin concentration. Levels of haemoglobin are at their lowest between 16 and 22 weeks. That haemodilution is normal and a requisite adaptation to pregnancy, rather than indicating pathological anaemia, is supported by the changes in AV oxygen difference (see above).

Most of the increase in blood cell mass is in the form of red blood cells. An initial depression of erythropoietin levels occurs, but progesterone, prolactin, hPL and angiotensin II all stimulate erythropoietin synthesis and so promote red blood cell production; however, red blood cell mass correlates best with hPL levels. The drive for erythropoiesis results in mild hyperplasia of the bone marrow and an increased reticulocyte (immature red blood cell) count. The function of red blood cells is oxygen transport; therefore, red blood cell mass will increase physiologically at high altitude and decrease with prolonged bed rest. In pregnancy, the increment in red blood cells reflects the need for more oxygen; the estimated increased requirement to supply the increased maternal tissues and conceptus is 15.0–16.5%, which is slightly lower than the measured rise of 18%.

Levels of 2,3-DPG (2,3-diphosphoglycerate) increase from early pregnancy so the oxygen–haemoglobin dissociation curve shifts to the right (see Chapter 1) thus facilitating release of oxygen from red blood cells at the peripheral tissues including the uteroplacental vasculature. Red blood cells become more spherical, with an increased diameter and thickness, because plasma colloid pressure falls and thus more water enters the erythrocyte by osmosis.

Iron Status

As plasma volume increases, haemoglobin concentration and haematocrit fall, reaching a lowest point at 16–22 weeks (Blackburn, 2018). The World Health Organization (WHO) recommends that haemoglobin concentration should not fall below 110 g/L at any point in pregnancy; others suggest it should not fall below 100 g/L. Haemoglobin concentration is regularly assessed in many pregnancies to identify women who have iron deficiency anaemia (IDA) or iron deficiency (low iron stores in the absence of low haemoglobin concentrations). IDA in pregnancy is associated with maternal cardiovascular stress, reduced physical and cognitive performance, increased risk of peripartum blood loss and, if very severe, an increased risk of maternal mortality. If maternal haemoglobin levels fall <90 g/L, there is an increased risk of intrauterine growth restriction, fetal death and premature delivery. So the WHO recommends iron supplementation programmes, which are routinely followed in many countries, usually if haemoglobin levels fall to <105–110 g/L. However, the benefits and risks of such programmes and indiscriminate iron supplementation are controversial (Friedrisch and Friedrisch, 2017). The lowest rate of perinatal mortality and highest birthweight occur when maternal haemoglobin levels are between 90 and 100 g/L (Fisher and Nemeth, 2017). Higher haemoglobin concentrations (in the normal prepregnant range) are also associated with poor outcomes such as preeclampsia, intrauterine growth retardation (IUGR), preterm birth and stillbirth. This is likely to reflect an absence of the appropriate expansion of plasma volume and haemodilution, which might be associated with poor placental perfusion and higher blood viscosity.

In pregnancy, the most accurate and appropriate method of determining iron status and anaemia is measurement of serum ferritin (SF) levels, which represent iron stores. Ferritin is the major iron-storage protein and SF becomes depleted before clinical indicators such as haemoglobin concentration reveal overt anaemia. Ferritin is secreted by macrophages, which phagocytose effete red blood cells and recycle the iron, and by hepatocytes, which are involved in storing iron; the secretion of ferritin is proportional to iron stores. SF is stable, is not affected by recent ingestion of iron and quantitatively reflects iron stores, particularly in the lower range. SF values are affected by inflammation and infection, which increase the values but low values of SF always reflect low iron stores. SF levels <50 g/L in early pregnancy are usually interpreted to indicate a need for iron supplementation and levels >80 g/L are interpreted to be likely to protect the woman from iron depletion. However, routine iron supplementation in pregnancy, of apparently healthy women with no apparent iron deficiency, results in red blood cells increasing by 30% rather than by 18% in unsupplemented women (Fisher and Nemeth, 2017). As one of the methods of assessing anaemia in nonpregnant subjects is by 'trial of iron'; observing an increase in SF or haemoglobin concentration in response to increased iron supplementation, this is often considered to be an indicator that additional iron is required.

Although the amenorrhoea of pregnancy ('menstrual savings') helps to conserve iron stores, absorption of dietary iron increases and iron is mobilized from body stores, adequate or optimal iron status in pregnancy is only likely to be achieved if the woman has sufficient iron stores prior to conception. It is calculated that ~1.2 g of additional iron is required during pregnancy (depending on maternal size; the figures are calculated for a woman of about 54 kg): 270 mg for the development of the fetus and 90 mg retained by the placenta; 450 mg for expansion of maternal red blood cell mass; 230 mg for body iron loss; and 150 mg to allow for blood loss at delivery (Fisher and Nemeth, 2017). Daily iron requirements are not uniform. Iron requirement in the first trimester is about 0.8 mg/day, which is less than the requirement before pregnancy because iron is not being lost in menstruation. Maternal blood volume expansion from the second trimester and the increasing demands of the growing fetus mean daily requirements progressively increase to 3.0–7.5 mg/day in the third trimester. Despite the demand for iron during pregnancy being fairly well understood, the recommendations for iron intake vary extraordinarily from country to country (see Chapter 12). Active transport of iron across the placenta is maximal in the last 4 weeks of pregnancy.

Iron homeostasis in pregnancy is controlled by hepcidin levels. Hepcidin is a protein released by the liver in response to adequate iron status or an infection. Hepcidin inhibits the export of iron from cells including the enterocytes that absorb dietary iron, hepatocytes that store iron and macrophages, which recycle iron from red blood cells. It does this by binding to ferroportin, the only known iron efflux transporter, to trigger its internalization and degradation. Thus, if hepcidin levels are increased, iron delivery to the bone marrow and placenta is suppressed. In healthy pregnancies, production of hepcidin by the maternal liver is low in the second and third trimesters (Fisher and Nemeth, 2017) when iron demands are high. This enhances the supply of iron to the bone marrow for maternal red blood cell production via haematopoiesis and to the placenta for the fetus to use. The secretion of hepcidin is likely to be suppressed because of the gradual development of iron deficiency as a result of haemodilution. Although inflammation usually increases hepcidin production, the mild inflammation associated with normal pregnancies is probably not high enough to increase hepcidin levels (Fisher and Nemeth, 2017). Possibly the more intense inflammation that occurs in pregnancies affected by complications may permit hepcidin secretion, which could then inhibit iron absorption and mobilization. The fetus also produces hepcidin, which remains in the fetal compartment and probably regulates the transfer of iron from the placenta to the fetus via the ferroportin transporters expressed on the syncytiotrophoblast tissue facing the fetal circulation.

Iron deficiency is the most prevalent micronutrient deficiency in the world; iron deficiency anaemia may affect 10–20% of pregnant women. It may adversely affect maternal exercise tolerance, cerebral function and wellbeing. Offspring of iron-deficient mothers may have reduced iron stores and are at risk of infantile anaemia, which may affect their mental and motor development and have long-term consequences. It is thought that iron-deficient infants tend to be disengaged and are less able to communicate their needs (e.g. for food or physical contact) to their mothers (East et al., 2017) and iron-deficient mothers are less able to interpret their infant's cries and communication and recognize what they need. Iron is required for a critical window of fetal and infant development. The first 1000 days of development, from conception until about 2 years old, encompass the time of an extraordinary level of neuronal development (see Chapters 15 and 16). Both high and low maternal iron status during this time are associated with an increased risk of adverse outcomes such as IUGR, preterm delivery, gestational diabetes and effects on the infants' long-term health including neurodegenerative conditions in ageing (Brannon and Taylor, 2017).

Haemostasis

Pregnancy is recognized to be an acquired hypercoagulable state. Clotting potential increases and there are decreased anticoagulants and decreased fibrinolysis (Blackburn, 2018). As a result of this, pregnant women are at increased risk for thrombosis and consumptive coagulopathies, such as disseminated intravascular coagulation (DIC) in which the clotting cascade is inappropriately triggered so small blood clots form, which can block small blood vessels causing pain; the outcome can be excessive and unbalanced utilization of coagulation factors so that bleeding occurs. Normal bleeding time in pregnancy decreases by about 30% because of the altered ratio of clotting and fibrinolytic (anti-clotting) factors. There is an increase in fibrinogen and other clotting factors leading to an increased generation of thrombin and a decrease in fibrinolytic or anticoagulant substances (for instance, protein S activity decreases and resistance develops to activated protein C). The number of platelets decreases slightly towards term but usually remains within the lower region of the nonpregnant range, probably due to haemodilution, for most of pregnancy. This response is variable; there may be increased platelet turnover and low-grade platelet activation (an increased number of aggregated platelets) as the pregnancy progresses, resulting in a larger proportion of younger platelets with increased volume. In preeclampsia and other conditions associated with fetal growth restriction, there is excessive activation and consumption of platelets (Gardiner and Vatish, 2017) so platelet number falls and the lifespan of platelets is reduced. This has led to clinical studies investigating the efficacy of low-dose aspirin treatment early in pregnancy to prevent preeclampsia (Roberge et al., 2018).

Low-grade chronic intravascular coagulation in the uteroplacental circulation, from about 11–15 weeks of pregnancy, is a normal part of the physiological response to pregnancy. The changed ratio of clotting activators and inhibitors facilitates the deposition of the fibrin matrix, which replaces smooth muscle and elastic tissues in the spiral arteries of the uterus (see Chapter 8). Close to term, mural thrombi (which adhere to blood vessels walls) may develop in the uteroplacental vessel walls reducing blood flow and causing the placental infarcts and small ischaemic areas, which can be seen on placental examination (Blackburn, 2018).

Synthesis of antithrombin III (the main physiological inhibitor of thrombin and factor Xa) increases in pregnancy in parallel with the increased plasma volume. Levels decrease at delivery (thus increasing the tendency to thrombosis) and increase 1 week postpartum. There is a general increase in clotting factors, particularly in late pregnancy, as demonstrated in pregnant carriers of the inherited form of von Willebrand syndrome (an autosomal dominant clotting disorder), which may improve with pregnancy. The change in amount of clotting factors seems to be compensatory in preparation for labour. The overall effect is hypercoagulability, which is augmented by venous stasis of the lower limbs, due to the pressure of the uterus on the veins in the legs and varicose veins, and endothelial injury, due to stress from the increased plasma volume. These three components (hypercoagulability, haemodynamic changes and endothelial injury or dysfunction) are recognized as Virchow's Triad of factors that predispose to thrombosis (Taylor et al., 2018). The risk of venous thromboembolism (deep vein thrombosis [DVT] and pulmonary embolism) increases fivefold in pregnancy and is the main cause of maternal death in developed countries. However, hypercoagulability is optimal in labour, meeting the demands of placental separation and protecting against excessive blood loss at delivery when normal blood loss is ~500 mL. The normal blood flow of 500–800 mL/min is staunched within seconds (aided by myometrial contraction, which decreases blood flow and rapidly closes spiral arteries). The various causes of PPH can increase this loss significantly and, in a worst-case scenario can be life-threatening. A fibrin mesh rapidly covers the placental site as 5–10% of the total circulating fibrinogen is deposited (see Chapter 11). Fibrinolytic activity decreases in pregnancy and remains low in labour. It returns to normal within an hour of delivery; the placenta produces inhibitors that block fibrinolysis. Most of the physiological changes in pregnancy are reversed quickly in the puerperium; however, the hypercoagulable state may exist for much longer (possibly over 6 weeks). This puts the woman in the early postnatal period (see Chapter 14) at a higher risk of developing DVT and pulmonary embolism from changes that occur in the antenatal period.

Table 11.1 summarizes the haematological changes in pregnancy.

TABLE 11.1	Summary of Haematological Changes in Pregnancy	
	Change in Pregnancy	**Notes**
Plasma volume	Increases by ~50% from 2600 to 3900 mL	More in second and subsequent pregnancies; correlates with birthweight
Red blood cell mass	Increases by ~18%	Increase is greater with iron supplementation (to 30%)
Neutrophil count	Both cell number and metabolic activity increase	Initial increase occurs early in pregnancy and is similar to the response to other physiological stresses
Plasma proteins	Decrease	Decreased osmotic pressure predisposes to oedema
Clotting factors	Increase	Fibrinolytic factors decrease
Platelet count	Slight fall	Coagulability increases

TABLE 11.2	Pregnancy and Physiological Reserve				
Parameter	**Normal**	**Pregnancy**	**% Increase**	**Exercise**	**% Increase**
Minute volume	7.5 L/min	10.5 L/min	40	80 L/min	1000
Oxygen consumption	220 mL/min	255 mL/min	16		
Cardiac output	4.5 L/min	6 L/min	30	12 L/min	

THE RESPIRATORY SYSTEM

Maternal respiratory effort and efficiency are increased in pregnancy to meet the increased metabolic demands of the maternal and fetal tissues. By the end of the pregnancy, 16–20% more oxygen is consumed. The respiratory system is also affected by the expanding uterine volume. In terms of physiological reserve, the stress put on the respiratory system by pregnancy is small compared with the increases that can be measured on exercise (Table 11.2). This contrasts with the much larger proportion of the cardiovascular physiological reserve required in pregnancy. The clinical implication of this is that patients with respiratory disease are much less likely to deteriorate in pregnancy than are those with cardiac disease.

Anatomy

Early in pregnancy, and therefore not secondary to pressure from the gravid uterus, the resting position of the diaphragm is displaced upwards by 4 cm (Blackburn, 2018; Fig. 11.7). The respiratory excursion of the diaphragm increases and there is an increased flaring of the lower ribs (increasing the substernal angle from 68° to 103° by late pregnancy; Blackburn, 2018). This compensatory increase in the diameter of the thorax by ~2 cm (the circumference of the chest increases by ~15 cm) means that the volume of the thoracic cavity is about the same as that before pregnancy. The diaphragm performs the major work of

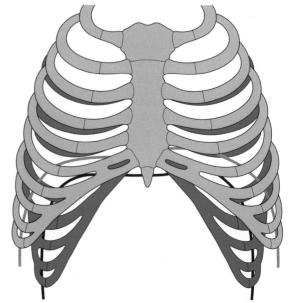

Fig. 11.7 Displacement of the diaphragm in pregnancy: the ribcage in pregnancy (light) and the nonpregnancy state (dark), showing the increased subcostal angle, the increased transverse diameter and the raised diaphragm in pregnancy.

respiration; in pregnancy, the breathing is thoracic rather than abdominal. Hormonal influences, predominantly progesterone and relaxin, cause the muscles and cartilage

TABLE 11.3   Lung Volumes and Capacities

Parameter	Definition	Normal Range	Change in Pregnancy
Tidal volume (TV)	Volume of a normal breath at rest	500 mL	Increases by 150–200 mL (25–40%) 75% increase occurs within first trimester
Respiratory rate (RR)	Number of breaths/min	12 breaths/min	Unchanged/slightly increased to 15 breaths/min
Minute volume (MV)	Total air taken in 1 min of respiration (= TV × RR)	6000 mL/min (6 L/min)	Increased by about 40% 10 L/min
Inspiratory reserve volume (IRV)	Volume of air that can be inspired above the resting tidal volume	3100 mL	Unchanged
Expiratory reserve volume (ERV)	Volume of gas that can be expired in addition to the tidal volume	1200 mL	Reduces progressively from early pregnancy to about 1100 mL
Residual volume (RV)	Volume of gas remaining in the lungs after a maximal expiration	1200 mL	Decreases progressively
Total lung capacity (TLC)	Maximum volume of the lungs (= TV + IRV + ERV + dead space)	6000 mL	Unchanged
Vital capacity (VC)	Total volume of gas that can be moved in and out of the lungs (= TLC – residual volume)	4800 mL	Increased 100–200 mL in late pregnancy? (Not apparent in obese women)
Inspiratory capacity	Total inspiratory ability of the lungs (= IRC + TV)	2200 mL	Increased ~2500 mL at term
Functional residual capacity (FRC)	Volume of gas remaining in the lungs after a resting breath (= ERV + RV)	2800 mL	Decreases progressively to 2300 mL – increases mixing efficiency
Residual volume (RV)	Volume of gas remaining after a maximal expiration (= FRC – ERV)	2400 mL	
Physiological dead space			Increases by ~60 mL
Alveolar ventilation	Difference between TV and volume of physiological dead space		Increased

in the thoracic region and the ligaments of the rib cage to relax so the chest broadens. The subsequent decrease in chest wall compliance means the thoracic wall can move further inwards so there is less trapped air and the residual volume decreases. These anatomical changes probably do not completely reverse after the pregnancy (indeed it is said that the increased flaring of the rib cage is beneficial to opera singers after pregnancy).

Progesterone is a respiratory stimulant; it lowers the threshold of sensitivity of the peripheral and central chemoreceptors for carbon dioxide (Blackburn, 2018). This effect of progesterone on the CO_2 chemoreflex means that respiratory drive is stimulated at lower carbon dioxide levels, so pregnant women breathe more deeply. As progesterone progressively increases during the pregnancy, the increased responsiveness to PCO_2 results in an increased tidal volume and therefore minute volume (Table 11.3). Hyperventilation (increased tidal volume) is normal in pregnancy. Oxygen consumption increases but arterial oxygen pressure does not change.

In pregnancy, the respiratory rate is unchanged but minute ventilation increases by 40–50% because tidal volume increases; this is apparent as early as 7 weeks. This hyperventilation exceeds the increased oxygen consumption. Alveolar gas exchange is much more efficient when tidal volume is increased rather than respiratory rate (Fig. 11.8). Alveolar ventilation is further enhanced by the decrease in residual volume. About 150 mL of an inspired breath remains in the upper airways where no gas exchange takes place (this is known as the anatomical dead

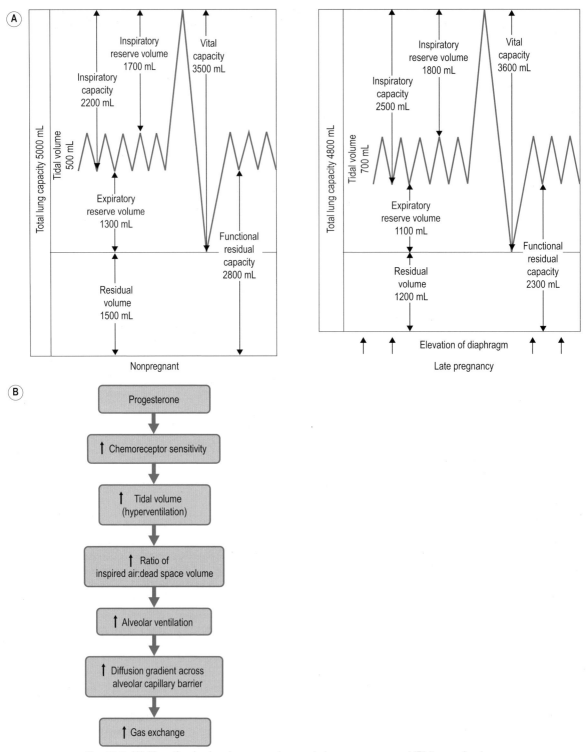

Fig. 11.8 (A) Alteration in alveolar gas exchange during pregnancy and (B) its mechanisms.

space). Although the dead space increases by ~60 mL in pregnancy because of dilation of the smaller bronchioles, the net alveolar ventilation is increased. The increased tidal volume means that the functional residual capacity is reduced, thus an increased volume of inspired fresh air mixes with a much smaller residual volume of air remaining in the lungs. Alveolar ventilation in pregnancy is thus increased by ~70% resulting in increased efficiency of mixing of gases, which facilitates gas exchange because the diffusion gradient is greater. The increased gradient of carbon dioxide concentrations between maternal and fetal blood aids transfer of carbon dioxide across the placenta and may be particularly important in adverse circumstances. Progesterone also increases carbonic anhydrase levels in red blood cells (see Chapter 1), thus further increasing the efficiency of carbon dioxide transfer.

Maternal partial pressures of oxygen increase slightly (from 95–100 to 101–106 mmHg) and levels of carbon dioxide decrease (from 35–40 to 26–34 mmHg). The small increase in PO_2 has little effect on haemoglobin saturation. Posture, however, affects alveolar oxygen levels: a supine position in late pregnancy results in a lower alveolar oxygen pressure than when in a sitting position. This change in alveolar oxygenation is probably not significant for the fetus although it may be compensatory at high altitude.

Air travel is associated with transiently increased dyspnoea and respiratory rate in response to increased altitude. The hyperventilation-associated decreased level of carbon dioxide in pregnancy results in a mild respiratory alkalosis, which facilitates transfer of CO_2 from the fetus to the mother. The change in pH also affects levels of circulatory cations such as sodium, potassium and calcium, aiding transfer across the placenta and increasing provision for fetal growth. Metabolic compensation to the relative alkalosis occurs by increasing renal excretion of bicarbonate ions. The resulting fall in serum bicarbonate, which limits the buffering capacity in pregnant women, causes maternal pH levels to increase to the upper end of the normal physiological range, from 7.40 to 7.45. Maternal ability to compensate further for metabolic acidosis is therefore limited, which may create problems in prolonged labour or where there is inadequate tissue perfusion (see Chapter 13).

Progesterone has a local relaxation effect on the smooth muscle tone of the airways and the pulmonary blood vessels and decreases airway resistance. Diffusion capacity is the ease with which gases can cross the pulmonary membranes. In early pregnancy, diffusion capacity decreases probably because of the effects of oestrogen on the composition of the mucopolysaccharides of the capillary walls, which increases diffusion distance (Blackburn, 2018). This effect may last for months after delivery. Increased water retention in the pulmonary tissues also results in a decrease in diffusion capacity. There is an increased closing volume suggesting that the calibre of the small airways is decreased; this may be due to increased lung fluid. The decreased efficiency of pulmonary gas transfer is partially compensated for by progesterone-induced relaxation of bronchiole smooth muscle, which decreases airway resistance. The decreased airway resistance means that air flow is increased. Prostaglandins also affect bronchiole smooth muscle. $PGF_{2\alpha}$, which increases throughout the pregnancy, is a smooth muscle constrictor; PGE_1 and PGE_2, which increase in the third trimester, are smooth muscle dilators. The overall work of breathing is probably unchanged as the decreased airway resistance compensates for the congestion in the bronchial wall capillaries.

Many pregnant women experience dyspnoea (awareness of breathlessness or respiratory distress), causing discomfort and anxiety, often early in pregnancy before there are changes in intra-abdominal pressure. This correlates well with PCO_2 and is likely to be due to the increased chemosensitivity to CO_2 causing hyperventilation (Lee et al., 2017). Capillaries in the upper respiratory tract become engorged, which can create difficulties in breathing via the nose and aggravate respiratory infections. Laryngeal changes and oedema of the vocal cords caused by vascular dilation can promote hoarseness and deepening of the voice, and a persistent cough. In severe cases, these changes in laryngeal thickening may cause complications should endotracheal intubation be necessary, for instance in anaesthesia. Forced expiratory volume over 1 s and peak flow rate are not usually affected in pregnancy.

In labour, pain causes an increase in tidal volume and respiratory rate (these effects are abolished by effective epidural anaesthesia). In the second stage, muscle demands result in metabolic acidosis (increased lactate and pyruvate production); this is countered to a degree by the respiratory alkalosis from hyperventilation (Blackburn, 2018). Pregnant and recently delivered women with identified respiratory risk factors or complications should have their respiratory rates monitored because increased respiratory rate can be an early indicator of physical deterioration. Oxygen saturation of arterial blood (SaO_2; the percentage to which haemoglobin in arterial blood is saturated with oxygen) monitoring should not be used in place of observing respiratory rate because a drop in SaO_2 is usually a late sign of physical deterioration. SaO_2 will often be normal in the presence of a raised respiratory rate as this initial compensatory effect maintains adequate oxygenation. If the respiratory rate is raised, SaO_2 monitoring should be used so that interventions such as oxygen therapy are observed to be effective in preventing further deterioration (Morton and Teasdale, 2018).

THE RENAL SYSTEM

Increased urinary frequency, leakage and nocturia are so common that they are considered a 'normal' part of physiological adaptation to pregnancy; urinary tract infections (UTI) are also relatively common. The marked haemodynamic and hormonal changes in pregnancy cause renal function to be altered. During pregnancy, the kidneys increase excretion of waste products in response to the increase in maternal and fetal metabolism, and retention of fluid and electrolytes is altered in response to cardiovascular changes. It is generally accepted that the increased circulating blood volume and haemodilution in pregnancy are achieved by the kidneys increasing tubular reabsorption rate of sodium, which results in increased extracellular volume. The retention of sodium is stimulated by deoxycorticosterone derived from progesterone. Fluid retention is facilitated by the action of angiotensin II. Oestrogen increases both angiotensinogen production and renin production. ADH secretion tends to be triggered at lower plasma osmolality during pregnancy, possibly affected by hCG levels (Blackburn, 2018). Likewise, the osmotic threshold for thirst decreases from early pregnancy.

The gross anatomy of the renal system is altered in pregnancy. The kidneys enlarge by ~1 cm in length and by ~30% in volume, owing to an increase in renal blood flow and vascular volume (Blackburn, 2018). Alterations in progesterone, prolactin, prostaglandin and relaxin levels all influence renal blood flow. The increased renal blood flow, due to haemodilution and these hormonal changes, causes GFR to increase by 40–60% from early pregnancy. The increased GFR means that there is more sodium, glucose and amino acids in the filtrate; however, tubular reabsorption also increases so most of the increased sodium load is reabsorbed. The sodium retention results in water accumulation. The increase in GFR also results in a fall in serum creatinine and urea levels so a 'normal' nonpregnant level of serum creatinine (of 1 mg/dL) may indicate renal impairment in pregnancy (Blackburn, 2018) or other conditions associated with a lack of plasma volume expansion such as preeclampsia. Assessment of proteinuria is also important in indicating preeclampsia and in the care of pregnant women with pre-existing kidney disease. The incidence of chronic kidney disease (CKD) is increasing in the population and, since women often choose to start a family later, it is not uncommon for kidney disease to be diagnosed for the first time in pregnancy (Gonzalez-Suarez et al., 2019). The outcome of pregnancy in women with CKD, who have mild renal impairment, little proteinuria and normal blood pressure, is good, though more severe CKD is a risk for preterm delivery and preeclampsia. Pregnancy is becoming more common in kidney transplant recipients; fertility increases markedly after transplantation though women are usually recommended to wait for at least 12 months before conceiving (Wiles et al., 2018). Routine antenatal care includes dipstick protein testing of a random urine sample to monitor proteinuria. Although this screening method has a high incidence of false-negative and false-positive results, it is much less cumbersome than a 24-h urine collection, which can be inaccurate if there is under collection.

The tendency for pregnant women to become insulin resistant in the latter part of pregnancy results in increased blood glucose. This, together with the increased GFR, results in increased glucose concentration of the filtrate, which together with an increased tubular flow rate, can mean that the maximum capacity for glucose reabsorption in the tubules is exceeded causing some glucose to be present in the urine (glucosuria). This does not necessarily indicate diabetes. Also, mild proteinuria is common and benign in pregnancy, although with coexisting hypertension it can indicate complications of preeclampsia.

There is a cumulative retention of sodium and potassium, especially in the last trimester when fetal demands for sodium are high. Urinary excretion of calcium increases but free calcium levels remain stable as dietary absorption of calcium increases. Acid–base balance is also altered in pregnancy. Hydrogen ions fall slightly primarily because of respiratory alkalosis associated with hyperventilation (see above). Although systemic blood pressure may be reduced, autoregulation (local control of glomerular blood pressure) maintains optimal renal function.

The calyces of the kidneys and the ureters become dilated and lose some of their peristaltic activity in pregnancy. The ureters elongate and become tortuous so they accommodate an increased volume of urine, which is associated with an increased risk of infection. It was generally accepted that this dilation of the ureters was primarily due to the action of progesterone on smooth muscle. However, the ovarian arteries and veins also increase in size and compress the ureters, particularly on the right side where the vessels cross over the ureter almost at right angles, whereas on the left they run approximately parallel to the ureter. This, together with the stress imposed on the ureters by the expanding uterus upon the pelvic brim, explains the extent of these morphological changes.

Bladder function is also affected in pregnancy. Urinary frequency and urgency increase early in pregnancy as the enlarging uterus in the pelvic cavity puts pressure on the bladder; fluid intake is also higher. At term, when engagement occurs, the presenting part of the fetus increases stress on the bladder. In the second trimester, the bladder is displaced upwards so urinary frequency is closer to prepregnant levels. Urinary incontinence is also relatively common during pregnancy though trauma to the pelvic floor during delivery is a significant contributor (Kissler et al., 2016). Urinary incontinence may negatively affect quality of life; it can affect hygiene, social and sexual relationships, ability to work and increases the risk of anxiety and depression. Under the effect of progesterone, bladder tone decreases during pregnancy so its capacity increases and may be up to a litre by term. The decreased bladder tone and displacement of the ureters by the enlarging uterus can affect competence of the vesicoureteral sphincters (valves created by the normal oblique angle of entry of the ureters into the bladder wall become compromised as the entry of the ureters tends to be perpendicular). The result is that urine may reflux from the bladder into the ureters, which increases the chance of ascending urinary infection, which if severe, can cause infection of the kidney (pyelonephritis). Urinary retention is not common in pregnancy but classically it occurs at the end of the first trimester; there are several predisposing factors for urinary retention including a retroverted uterus (which ~20% of women have but it usually corrects itself during pregnancy), uterine fibroids, uterine anomalies and a contracted pelvis (Cox and Reid, 2018).

The walls of the bladder become more oedematous and hyperaemic, which increases the vulnerability to infection and trauma. The relatively lax walls of the bladder may also result in incomplete emptying of urine. This urinary stasis increases the risk of a UTI as the urine, which is richer in glucose and amino acids in pregnancy, remains in the bladder allowing the usually harmless number of bacteria in the urine to reach pathological levels. UTI in pregnancy is very common and affects ~8% of women; UTI is associated with increased risk of premature rupture of membranes, fetal growth restriction and premature labour. As the pregnancy progresses the effect of posture on renal function becomes exacerbated. The structural changes of the renal system persist into the puerperium (see Chapter 14) and women who have experienced a UTI during pregnancy are at increased risk of recurrent infection in the puerperium. Women who have a positive result for Group B Streptococcal B infection (colloquially known as 'strep B') during antenatal screening may have asymptomatic bacteriuria; these women do not normally need antibiotic therapy in the antenatal period unless a symptomatic UTI develops. A UTI in these circumstances indicates an exceptionally high bacterial load, which increases the risk of transmission to the fetus during birth so should be treated (Hughes et al., 2017). It is important that a mid-stream sample of urine is used for testing (bacterial counts and strain of pathogen) because the skin of the woman's perineum may be contaminated by bowel commensal bacteria.

Case study 11.3 details an example of a urogenital tract infection.

CASE STUDY 11.3

Penny is expecting her second child and presents herself at the maternity day assessment unit at 24 weeks' gestation. Two days previously, Penny noticed her frequency of micturition had dramatically increased. Since then she has felt lower central abdominal pain radiating from her groin round to the right side of her back and has a slight fever. The midwife suspects that Penny may have a UTI. A provisional diagnosis is made on ward-based urinalysis that indicates the presence of leukocytes and nitrites.

- What is the significance of these findings and why do they indicate the presence of an infection?

The midwife instructs Penny on how to provide a mid-stream specimen of urine (MSU) and requests that the duty doctor examine Penny. Penny is prescribed a course of antibiotics with the proviso that this may be changed if the laboratory tests indicate that the antibiotic is inappropriate.

- How could the midwife explain the reasons why the UTI has occurred to Penny?
- What else besides taking the antibiotics could the midwife advise Penny to do to (1) help resolve the infection now and (2) avoid further infection in the future?
- What are the risks and possible consequences if the infection is not treated?

THE GASTROINTESTINAL SYSTEM

Maternal nutrition is very important in the outcome of pregnancy but disturbances of gastrointestinal function are the most common cause of complaints in pregnancy (Fig. 11.9). Over 50% of women experience an increased appetite (and consequent increased consumption of food) and even more an increased thirst. The changes are most marked in the first half of pregnancy; subsequently they may decline although some persist, albeit to a lesser extent. Changes in maternal appetite do not directly reflect changes in fetal growth or maternal metabolism. Appetite tends to increase in early pregnancy and may be promoted by several hormones including leptin. Comparisons with the changes in appetite during nonpregnant menstrual cycles help to identify likely culprit hormonal contributions to changed physiology in pregnancy. If nonpregnant women experience effects in the follicular phase of the cycle, the hormone causing the effect is likely to be oestrogen whereas if the effects tend to occur in the second half of the cycle (luteal phase), progesterone may be responsible. Oestrogen suppresses appetite but progesterone stimulates

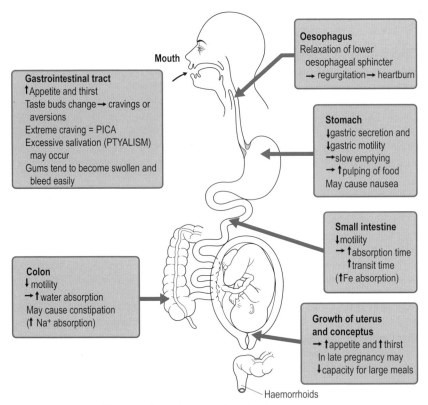

Fig. 11.9 Gastrointestinal function in pregnancy.

it, causing a shift in the central control of energy balance. Other hormones such as insulin, glucagon and leptin may also influence appetite in pregnancy (Blackburn, 2018). Leptin usually suppresses food intake but in pregnancy, leptin levels increase because hormonally induced central leptin resistance develops and leptin production from the placenta progressively increases (Perez-Perez et al., 2017). This means that despite the raised levels of leptin, food intake and thus fat deposition are increased. Adiponectin released from adipose tissue is also involved in appetite regulation; the ratio of leptin:adiponectin may be important in this respect. In advanced pregnancy, both appetite and the capacity for food intake decline owing to upward displacement of the stomach and pressure from the gravid uterus. A pregnant woman can compensate for her limited capacity by increasing the frequency of consumption of small meals and snacks. Decreased plasma glucose and amino acid levels, which are secondary to increased responsiveness to insulin, also stimulate appetite. hCG affects the hypothalamus decreasing the osmotic threshold for thirst. Thirst is increased; progesterone resets the thirst threshold by 10 mOsm so plasma osmolarity falls.

Increased angiotensin, prolactin and relaxin levels are also dipsogenic (promote thirst and fluid intake).

Food Cravings and Aversions

Changes in food habits can be deliberate, for instance avoiding fried or fatty foods that are considered less healthy. Two-thirds of pregnant women experience marked food preferences (cravings) or aversions. Sense of smell may be enhanced; pregnant women are especially sensitive to noxious smells such as nicotine and coffee. The timing of the changes in taste and smell appears to reflect secretion of hCG. The commonest cravings are for fruit and highly-flavoured foods such as pickles, kippers and cheese. The sensitivity of many of the taste buds is decreased in pregnancy so stronger tasting and highly seasoned foods may be preferred (Choo and Dando, 2017). The taste buds express receptors for many of the hormones that change in pregnancy. However, perceived intensity of bitter tastes has been found to increase in the first trimester; this enhanced 'disgust sensitivity', during the vulnerable period of embryonic development and when the maternal immune system is suppressed, is suggested to help pregnant women avoid toxins (Lieberman et al., 2018). In folklore and 'old-wives' stories from various parts of the world, the consequences of not satisfying craving resulted in the baby being born with food-shaped birthmarks; indeed in many languages, the word for birthmark means mark due to cravings. Common aversions are to tea and coffee, meat, fried foods and eggs and to caffeinated drinks, alcohol and smoking. Food cravings and aversions need to be assessed as part of a full dietary assessment; they do not necessarily have an adverse effect on dietary quality. Often dietary changes as a result of cravings cause an increase in energy and calcium intakes and those to aversions frequently result in decreased intake of alcohol, coffee and animal protein.

Pica, an extreme and persistent craving for non-nutritious substances, has been identified for coal, clay, soil and mud (geophagia), starch (amylophagia), ice (pagophobia) and other substances such as soap, charcoal, baking powder, disinfectant, toothpaste, mothballs and pencil shavings (Fawcett et al., 2016). Usually pica does not affect either maternal or fetal health. A variety of factors affect the practice of pica and what substances are craved; these include geographical region, cultural expectations and level of education or socioeconomic status. Pica in pregnancy is more common in Africa. In the southern states of America, there seems to be a social tradition of Black women eating laundry starch, chalk and clay. It was suggested that there is a relationship between iron deficiency and pica but iron-deficient or anaemic women have not been shown to be more likely to engage in pica and the foods craved are not usually iron-rich; indeed some of the substances might cause iron deficiency by reducing the bioavailability of iron (see Chapter 12).

Nausea and Vomiting in Pregnancy

Between 70% and 80% of pregnant women experience nausea and vomiting in pregnancy (NVP), making it one of the most common disorders in pregnancy. It usually occurs in the first trimester although 20% of women experience NVP throughout gestation. It may be the first physical manifestation of pregnancy; some women report nausea before or around the time of implantation. NVP is more common in Westernized urban populations and is affected by ethnicity, genetic predisposition, occupational status and maternal age (Bustos et al., 2017). The peak of NVP is usually at between 9 and 16 weeks; symptoms usually resolve by mid-pregnancy (about 22 weeks). Most women who experience NVP report that their symptoms persist throughout the day or a biphasic pattern rather than only in the mornings, so that NVP is a more appropriate term than the previously used 'morning sickness'. It is thought that women who have lower prepregnancy BMIs are less likely to experience severe symptoms of NVP compared with women with higher BMI. NVP does not necessarily mean that nutrient intake is decreased. Some women eat more as continual snacking alleviates symptoms and others alter their diet in a way that tends to usually improve dietary quality (Coad et al., 2002).

There are several theories about the causes of NVP. There is also a genetic element; that the use of medication for nausea is more similar in mothers who are monozygotic (identical) twins than dizygotic (nonidentical) twins suggest NVP is highly heritable (Bustos et al., 2017). Serum hCG peaks in the first trimester, so follows a temporal pattern with symptoms. NVP tends to be worse where secretion of hCG is higher such as in hydatidiform mole, trisomy 21, multiple gestation and where the fetus is female. However, the relationship between NVP and hCG secretion is not clearly established, possibly because particular isoforms of hCG are associated with symptoms, rather than total hCG.

The effects of progesterone on gastric smooth muscle tone, particularly where this affects either upper gastrointestinal tract motility, the patency of the lower oesophageal sphincter or delays gastric emptying, suggest the possible involvement of steroid hormones. *Helicobacter pylori* infection of the stomach is also implicated in NVP; infection is more likely in women who experience symptoms.

The unknown pathogenesis of NVP makes it challenging to treat; however, it is recommended that NVP is treated early to prevent its progression to hyperemesis gravidarum (HG) and to optimize the pregnant woman's quality of life (Erick et al., 2018). NVP is usually conservatively treated with rest and reassurance and advice to consume frequent small meals rich in easily digested carbohydrate and low in fat and to avoid foods, such as meat, and strong smells, which may aggravate NVP.

It has been suggested that NVP is an evolutionary mechanism that protects the embryo by causing pregnant women to physically expel and subsequently develop learned aversions and avoid potentially harmful foods that might contain teratogenic and abortifacient chemicals (Flaxman and Sherman, 2000). An alternative explanation is that NVP has a functional role in stimulating early placental growth by reducing maternal energy intake and suppressing maternal tissue synthesis in early pregnancy so subsequent nutrient partitioning favours the developing placenta (Coad et al., 2002). NVP is associated with an increased risk for hypertension and preeclampsia (Bustos et al., 2017). It may also negatively affect the pregnant woman's quality of life, mental health, relationships and ability to work. Although NVP may have a socioeconomic impact and create much misery, mild NVP is considered a favourable prognostic sign and is associated with a positive outcome of pregnancy, at least for the fetus, such as reduced likelihood of miscarriage, LBW and preterm delivery (Coad et al., 2002).

Intractable and persistent nausea and vomiting causing dehydration, electrolyte imbalance (hypokalaemia), metabolic disturbances (ketonuria), weight loss (of >5% or >3 kg) and nutritional deficiencies are collectively known as 'hyperemesis gravidarum'. HG affects 0.3–5% of pregnancies and is the most common reason for hospital admission in the first trimester (and second most common after threatened preterm delivery in the second trimester). HG may require hospitalization to correct the electrolyte and fluid imbalances (Abramowitz et al., 2017); pharmacological treatments or enteral feeding may be required. Risk factors for HG include first pregnancy, previous or family history of HG, hyperthyroid disorders, pre-existing psychiatric diagnosis (such as an eating disorder), molar pregnancy, gastrointestinal disorders, and multiple gestation with a female and male twin.

Mouth

Gums often become hyperaemic, oedematous and spongy in pregnancy. This is because of the effects of oestrogen on blood flow and connective tissue consistency. Gums therefore bleed more easily and are vulnerable to abrasive food and vigorous tooth brushing. Gingivitis and periodontal disease occur in a large proportion of pregnant women and are more extreme with increased maternal age and parity and where there are pre-existing dental problems. Periodontal disease is associated with an increased risk of intrauterine infection, preterm delivery and LBW. It is seeded by the oral microbiota (of the dental plaque) in the periodontal pockets, which deepen in pregnancy; then allowed to amplify by the changed immune responses in pregnancy (Tettamanti et al., 2017).

Contrary to folklore belief that a tooth is lost for every baby, there is no evidence of demineralization of dentine resulting from pregnancy as fetal calcium stores are drawn from maternal body stores (skeleton) and not from maternal teeth (Blackburn, 2018). However, there is an increase in the number of caries treated during pregnancy. This may be because changes in salivary secretion, NVP or gum changes result in an increased awareness of dental problems and, in many countries, women receive free dental care in pregnancy. Saliva becomes more acidic in pregnancy, but the volume produced does not usually change. In rare instances, excessive production of saliva, termed 'ptyalism' or 'ptyalorrhoea', may occur. It can occur in isolation or in association with HG, where swallowing of saliva induces extreme nausea and vomiting in an affected woman but ptyalism may be perceived (rather than true increases in saliva production) because of difficulty swallowing due to nausea or increased oesophageal reflux.

Oesophagus

Heartburn (medically termed 'pyrosis'), a painful retrosternal burning sensation, is common in pregnancy, affecting 30–70% women. The effects of progesterone on the tone of the lower oesophageal sphincter mean its competence is impaired and regurgitation of gastric acid into the oesophagus is more likely. Similar changes occur during the menstrual cycle and in women taking combined oral contraceptive pills. These changes are associated with increased progesterone levels and effects on smooth muscle. The risk of a hiatus hernia is increased; the sphincter is displaced and becomes intrathoracic instead of straddling the diaphragm. This usually begins in the second trimester and worsens as the pregnancy progresses. It is due to progesterone-induced relaxation of the lower oesophageal sphincter and a change in pressure gradients across the stomach. The enlarging uterus causes distortion of the stomach and changes the angle of entry of the oesophagus. Because the patency of the pyloric sphincter may also be impaired, both alkaline and acidic secretions may reflux into the oesophagus.

Heartburn is increased with multiple pregnancies, polyhydramnios, obesity and excessive bending over. Alcohol, chocolate and coffee all act directly on the lower oesophageal sphincter, reducing the muscle tone and exacerbating heartburn. Gastric reflux (gastroesophageal reflux disease; GERD) can be limited by advising more frequent intake of smaller meals, limiting fluid intake with a meal, chewing gum, and avoiding lying horizontally or bending forwards, particularly immediately after consuming a meal; women also find lying on the left side and elevating the head of the bed to be beneficial in reducing symptoms. Dietary strategies include avoiding fatty and highly seasoned (spicy) food, avoiding chocolate and mints, citrus juice, tomatoes, alcohol and caffeinated or carbonated beverages; keeping a food and symptom diary is useful to identify culprit foods. Antacid preparations are associated with a number of undesirable side-effects: aluminium salts may cause diarrhoea, magnesium salts are associated with constipation, phosphorus may affect the calcium/phosphorus balance and exacerbate cramp, sodium may affect water balance and long-term use of antacids is associated with malabsorption, particularly of drugs and dietary minerals. It may be necessary to treat gastric reflux with medication such as histamine 2 blockers (H2-receptor antagonists) or proton-pump inhibitors (PPI); although both are usually considered safe in pregnancy, concerns have been raised about whether there is a relationship between acid-suppressive drug use in pregnancy and an increased risk of childhood asthma (Lai et al., 2018) and whether vitamin B_{12} status should be monitored during treatment as these drugs affect absorption of the vitamin (Miller, 2018).

Stomach

Studies on gastric secretion in pregnancy are not conclusive but suggest acid secretion tends to decrease, which may explain why remission of symptoms of a peptic ulcer is not an uncommon event. However, the decrease in gastric acid production is small and does not reduce the effect of gastric reflux (see above). Secretion of pepsin also falls, which is secondary to the decreased acid secretion. Gastric tone and motility markedly decrease in pregnancy, under the influence of progesterone. Thus, in advanced pregnancy the stomach drapes loosely over the uterine fundus. This tends to delay gastric emptying especially following ingestion of solid foods. The delay of chyme release from the stomach may increase the likelihood of heartburn and nausea and can result in delayed absorption of glucose. The pyloric sphincter at the junction with the duodenum may also lose its tone under the influence of progesterone; this can result in a reflux of the alkaline duodenal content entering the stomach.

Intestine and Colon

Progesterone-induced relaxation of smooth muscle decreases gut tone and motility; this effect may be augmented by progesterone inhibiting the production of motilin (Astbury et al., 2015). Duodenal villus hypertrophy and an increase in villus length increases the surface area of the small intestinal mucosa and this, together with an increased transit time, increases its absorptive capacity. The activities of brush border enzymes are also increased. Absorption of several nutrients, such as iron, calcium, glucose, amino acids, water, sodium and chloride is increased (Blackburn, 2018); the increased absorption of iron in late pregnancy coincides with increased placental uptake and decreased maternal stores. However, progesterone may inhibit transport mechanisms for other nutrients such as the B group of vitamins. The effect of protracted transit time is that pregnant women may experience bloating and abdominal distension.

The relaxation of the smooth muscle in the colon leads to increased water absorption and increases the risk of constipation (Case study 11.4). The raised levels of angiotensin and aldosterone also increase sodium and water absorption from the colon in pregnancy contributing to constipation, which is experienced by 10–30% pregnant women. Other factors also predispose the pregnant woman to constipation; less physical activity, inadequate water and fibre intake, iron supplementation, metabolic disturbances and mechanical factors, which might impede movement of faecal mass in the colon such as compression from the uterus (Body and Christie, 2016). As the enlarging uterus compresses the colon, many women also experience increased

flatulence. Haemorrhoids are common in pregnancy and are worsened by constipation.

Pregnancy profoundly influences the gut microbiota, which are primarily located in the colon. Some of these changes result in the characteristics of the microbiota becoming more like those associated with obesity; decreased diversity (less variability of types of microorganisms) and an increased abundance of bacterial species capable of fermenting otherwise indigestible carbohydrates and increasing the energy yield (Astbury et al., 2015). Abnormal changes in the gut microbiota are associated with an increased risk of pregnancy complications such as intrauterine growth restriction, preeclampsia, gestational diabetes and miscarriage.

The increasing prevalence of conditions such as coeliac disease and inflammatory bowel disease (Crohn's disease and ulcerative colitis) means that more women with these conditions are facing the additional challenges of pregnancy.

CASE STUDY 11.4

Josie is 14 weeks pregnant and is suffering from constipation. She is a vegetarian and normally consumes a high-fibre diet.
- What physiological changes may account for her constipation?
- What advice could the midwife give to help alleviate this problem?

Liver and Gall Bladder

Progesterone affects the smooth muscle tone of the gall bladder resulting in flaccidity, increased bile volume storage and decreased emptying rate. Water resorption by the epithelium cells of the gall bladder is decreased so the bile is more dilute, which means that cholesterol is more likely to be sequestered because it is not solubilized. Pregnancy causes an increased production of cholesterol so the concentration of cholesterol in the bile increases. This together with the decreased gall bladder motility means there is an increased risk of cholesterol-based gall stones forming in pregnancy. Cholestasis is a liver condition sometimes observed in late pregnancy, where women complain of itchy and irritable skin (though no rash is present), typically on the palms of their hands and soles of their feet, which is often worse in the evening. The mechanism is not fully understood but the condition is related to high concentrations of steroid hormones (Wood et al., 2018), which may reduce bile acid uptake by the liver resulting in bile salts being deposited in the skin. Diagnosis is confirmed by abnormal liver function tests and raised bile acids in serum; the condition requires careful monitoring because it is associated with an increased risk of fetal distress, premature labour and fetal demise.

In many species, pregnancy-induced liver enlargement results from an increased hepatic circulation. In humans, however, morphological changes appear to result from hepatic displacement by the gravid uterus rather than an actual growth increase. Increased glycogen and triacylglyceride storage occurs in the hepatic cells. The raised level of oestrogen affects hepatic synthesis of plasma proteins, enzymes and lipids. The most marked changes are the fall in albumin (which is exaggerated by haemodilution), increase in fibrinogen (see above) and increased cholesterol synthesis. Synthesis of many binding proteins involved with transport of nutrients increases. Although epigastric pain is common in pregnancy due to reflux of gastric contents through the lower oesophageal sphincter, it may be a symptom of severe liver-related complications such as fulminating preeclampsia caused by hepatic oedema.

Changes in the liver and other physiological systems can affect drug kinetics. The changes in maternal physiology have marked effects on pharmacodynamics (the effects of the drug) and the pharmacokinetics (how the body affects the drug) of medications (Patil et al., 2017). Changes in gastric secretion and gut motility can affect absorption and bioavailability of drugs. Changes in the cardiovascular system such as plasma volume and protein binding changes can affect the apparent volume of distribution and changes in the renal system can affect drug elimination, particularly increased renal excretion of drugs without prior metabolism. Hepatic metabolism of drugs catalysed by certain isoenzymes is increased during pregnancy. Therefore, pregnant women may require different dosing regimens (changes in dose and/or timing of the dose) of various drugs. Information about the safety and effectiveness of many drugs is not available because drug trials do not include pregnant women (Blackburn, 2018).

Bariatric surgery has become one of the main methods of treating morbid obesity. Most women undergoing bariatric surgery are of reproductive age. The marked weight loss increases fertility but women are usually recommended to delay conception until at least 12 months after surgery. The effects of bariatric surgery are to improve metabolic health but also to increase the risk of protein and energy malnutrition and micronutrient deficiency (Slater et al., 2017). Optimal care for women after bariatric surgery includes preconception counselling, optimization of nutrition before and throughout pregnancy, monitoring for complications such as steatorrhoea and provision of nutritional supplements suitable for

---

BOX 11.7   Top-to-Toe Observation of a Pregnant Woman

- Hair: thicker and glossier
- Face: may have chloasma and/or oedema
- Hands: warm, may develop vascular spiders and palmar erythema
- Skin: warm, well-vascularized, hyperpigmentation (related to MSH production)
- Skin conditions, such as eczema, may improve
- Abdominal wall: pigmentation of linea nigra, lax abdominal muscles, striae gravidarum may be seen (related to cortisol production)
- Pruritus (localized itching usually of abdomen): occurs in ~20% of pregnant women in the third trimester, but earlier in pregnancy it may be a sign of pruritus gravidarum (intrahepatic cholestasis of pregnancy due to raised bile acids), which is associated with premature delivery, fetal distress and perinatal mortality
- Breasts: dilation of superficial veins, pigmentation of nipples and areola
- Legs: oedema may be evident around ankles; varicose veins may develop
- Posture and gait: lordosis, changed centre of gravity (related to effects of hormones on cartilage and connective tissue)

---

pregnancy. Some supplements may be required at levels above the normal recommendations for pregnancy such as iron and folic acid.

THE SKIN AND APPEARANCE

A number of changes can be observed in the appearance of a pregnant woman (Box 11.7); over 90% of pregnant women have notable changes in pigmentation (Blackburn, 2018). The increase in MSH means that there is a progressive increase in skin pigmentation, especially in women with dark hair and complexion. The nipple and the areola darken early in pregnancy. A dark line develops from the navel to pubis; this is the hyperpigmented linea nigra along the embryonic folding and fusion line of the abdomen (before pregnancy the line of fusion is white and called the 'linea alba'). Facial chloasma (melasma) – irregular blotchy pigmentation usually bilateral and symmetrical, often in the shape of a butterfly ('mask of pregnancy') around the eyes and forehead – is common, occurring in 45–75% of pregnant women. Freckles and recent scars may darken and many women tan more deeply in pregnancy. Pigmentation changes may remain after pregnancy in women with darker hair and skin, and chloasma may be exacerbated by exposure to the sun. Striae gravidarum (stretch marks) become more accentuated in pregnancy; these are related to changes in collagen of the connective tissue due to hormonal changes rather than being a result of actual stretching. They fade after pregnancy but do not completely disappear.

THE SKELETON AND JOINTS

Posture and gait change in pregnancy. The weight of the gravid uterus, which can increase the mass of the abdomen by up to 30% (Whitcome et al., 2007), changes the woman's centre of gravity altering the angle of inclination of the pelvic brim to the horizontal plane. The lumbar spine is naturally anteriorly convex, but the combined effects of progesterone, relaxin and the weight of the uterus on the intravertebral discs exaggerate this curve. The resulting lordosis of the lumbar spine compensates for the shift in the centre of gravity but may result in muscle and ligament strain. By the end of pregnancy, many women adopt a typical posture where they stand and walk with their backs arched and the shoulders held backwards. Lordosis is increased by poor posture generally, obesity, skeletal disorders, tuberculosis and by wearing high-heeled shoes. Oestrogen and relaxin affect the composition of the cartilage and connective tissue of pelvic joints, which soften in preparation for labour. The large diameter collagen fibres are remodelled via the action of elastin and collagenolysis to smaller diameter fibres. The symphysis pubis and sacroiliac joints become more mobile and flexible so the pelvis becomes wider resulting in a rolling unstable movement and waddling gait when walking. Pregnant women may, therefore, experience muscle and ligament strain and discomfort or pain. The incidence of backache increases particularly after the 5th month. Some women experience severe back pain, often with peak intensity at night.

Occasionally in late pregnancy the pubic bones, which are united by the symphysial joint to form the symphysis pubis, may separate. This condition, described as symphysis pubis diastasis (SPD), can cause the pregnant woman great discomfort when walking or when her legs are abducted. In severe cases, women are often observed to walk sideways as this tends to be less painful than walking with a normal forward motion or doing any weight-bearing activity. The lower back is also affected by breast changes, stretching of the round ligament and decreased tone of abdominal muscles. In the third trimester, pressure of the uterus stretching or compressing nerves and blood vessels can result in numbness and tingling of extremities. Leg cramps, especially of the calf and thigh muscles, are common in the second half of pregnancy. They may be related to mineral metabolism and increased neuromuscular irritability. Raised phosphate levels are implicated and reducing dietary intake of milk is often beneficial. About 20% of

pregnant women experience restless legs syndrome (RLS) 10–20 min after getting into bed; the cause is unknown but RLS is more common as pregnancy progresses and usually resolves after delivery (Chen et al., 2018). RLS can create sleep-wake disorders and may increase the risk of poorer fetal outcomes. Calf pain is also associated with DVT, which is not so common but there is an increased risk of DVT in pregnancy so all calf pain needs careful investigation and monitoring.

Calcium Metabolism

There is increased turnover of calcium early in pregnancy. Maternal intestinal calcium absorption increases significantly and maternal calcium metabolism changes to facilitate calcium transport to the fetus. The placenta actively transports calcium from the maternal blood during the third trimester. Placental calcium concentrations are higher than maternal levels so the fetus is protected if maternal concentrations fall. Placental efficiency is much greater than the absorptive capability of a fetus' gastrointestinal tract; thus, a baby born prematurely with immature gut function cannot absorb calcium efficiently and the skeleton is slower to mineralize. During gestation, ~30 g of calcium is incorporated into the fetal skeleton. Active transport of calcium by the placenta to the fetus increases from ~150 mg/day in mid-pregnancy to 200–300 mg/day at term (Mitchell and Juppner, 2010) so that in the last 10 weeks of gestation, the fetus obtains 18 g of calcium and 10 g of phosphorus from the maternal circulation. In addition to calcium required for mineralization of the fetal skeleton, calcium is also required for the increase in maternal blood volume.

Maternal absorption of calcium increases predominantly because there is increased production of both $1,25(OH)_2D$, the active metabolite of vitamin D, and parathyroid hormone-related peptide (PTHrP). Many other hormones also promote increased calcium absorption including oestrogen, prolactin, hPL, placental growth factor and IGF1. Gastrointestinal absorption of calcium increases before vitamin D increases and continues throughout the pregnancy even in the presence of vitamin D deficiency.

Calcitonin secretion is also increased; in the first trimester, parathyroid hormone (PTH) levels fall, then increase to normal levels by the end of pregnancy. Vitamin D levels rise early in pregnancy to double the prepregnancy level by the end of the first trimester; they then continue to increase throughout pregnancy. Calcitonin secretion is also increased; it is produced by the thyroid gland and also by breast tissue and placenta. Calcitonin inhibits mineral release from the maternal skeleton but allows the actions of PTH on the gut (to increase calcium absorption) and the kidney (to decrease urinary excretion). Maternal serum calcium levels fall progressively in pregnancy. Levels are related to haemodilution of albumin and increased urinary losses and transport across the placenta. Urinary excretion of calcium decreases after 36 weeks, which augments dietary sources of calcium.

Homeostasis, mediated by maternal hormones, means that the maternal skeleton is conserved. If dietary calcium is adequate, there is no marked change in maternal skeletal mass or bone density. There is no evidence that high parity is associated with increased fractures in later life. Calcium supplements tend to reduce blood pressure by a small amount and may be useful in the treatment of preeclampsia (see Chapter 12). A low vitamin D status in pregnancy and little exposure to sunlight are associated with osteomalacia, as demonstrated by Asian women in the UK, who have lower plasma calcium and an increased incidence of maternal osteomalacia and neonatal rickets. Low vitamin D and low calcium are both associated with an increased risk of hypertensive disorders, preeclampsia and gestational diabetes (see Chapter 12).

VISION

The changed hormonal profile of pregnancy influences the maternal nervous system. In the third trimester, mild corneal oedema is common; fluid is retained and the cornea becomes slightly thicker, which affects refraction of light. Tear composition changes; levels of lysozyme alter and tears often become greasy. This, together with altered corneal sensitivity, may cause blurring of vision or intolerance to contact lenses. Progesterone, relaxin and hCG can decrease intraocular pressure (IOP), which might slow the progression of glaucoma but, conversely, some glaucoma medications should be avoided during pregnancy or when breastfeeding. Unless they experience problems, it is wise for pregnant women to delay new prescriptions for spectacles. Women with preeclampsia and retinal oedema, and those with diabetes, are particularly prone to visual complications, which may also be associated with headaches at the back of the upper neck.

THE NOSE AND LARYNX

The nasal mucosa becomes hyperaemic and congested in pregnancy, causing nasal stuffiness and obstruction. This seems to be oestrogen-related and may interfere with sleep and sense of smell. It is associated with congestion of the Eustachian tubes (often described as blocked ears, which are unrelieved by swallowing), which may cause a transient mild hearing loss. Many women will develop snoring during pregnancy (see above). Erythema and oedema of the vocal cords can lead to hoarseness, coughing and vocal changes. Softening of the cartilage within the larynx is not usually a problem but it may make tracheal intubation harder if required. Difficult intubation in pregnant women is further complicated by obesity and so it is good practice to ensure that intubation guidelines are present in all maternity units providing both routine and emergency surgical intervention.

SLEEP

Sleep patterns change in pregnancy. As pregnancy progresses, quality and quantity of sleep decreases. An increased desire for sleep and napping in the first trimester has been reported (Blackburn, 2018). Progesterone tends to act as a sedative and to increase nonrapid eye movement (NREM) or deep sleep. Oestrogen and cortisol tend to decrease rapid eye movement (REM) sleep. Prolactin is reported to increase both REM and NREM sleep. The amount of rapid eye movement (REM) sleep increases from 25 weeks, peaking at 33–36 weeks. Stage 4 NREM sleep (deep sleep) decreases. This state appears particularly important for tissue repair and recovery from fatigue. There tends to be more night awakenings during pregnancy. In the first half of pregnancy, women tend to have more total sleep time and more napping. In the second half of pregnancy, women tend to sleep less as they are frequently disturbed by nocturia, dyspnoea, heartburn, nasal congestion, muscle aches and cramping, restless legs, stress and anxiety and fetal activity. There may be an association between sleep patterns and depression. Before the onset labour, when oxytocin levels increase, night awakenings increase and total sleep time decreases (Blackburn, 2018).

CARBOHYDRATE METABOLISM

Maternal metabolism changes in pregnancy to meet increased maternal needs, including the accumulation of maternal energy stores in readiness for labour and lactation, and to facilitate fetal growth and development (Fig. 11.10). Metabolism in pregnancy must also facilitate both the accumulation of fetal energy stores for the transition to extrauterine life (see Chapter 15) and maternal accumulation of fat stores in preparation for labour and lactation. Pregnancy is primarily anabolic: food intake and appetite increase and activity decreases. Pregnancy has been described as a 'state of accelerated starvation' (Freinkel et al., 1972) because there is an increased tendency to become ketotic. Pregnancy is a diabetogenic state; women acquire insulin resistance in later pregnancy, which appears to represent a temporary excursion into metabolic syndrome.

Early Pregnancy

Metabolism in the first trimester is predominantly anabolic with synthesis of new maternal tissues including deposition of maternal fat. It can be considered as a time of preparation for the subsequent high demands of rapid fetal growth; over 90% of fetal growth occurs in the second

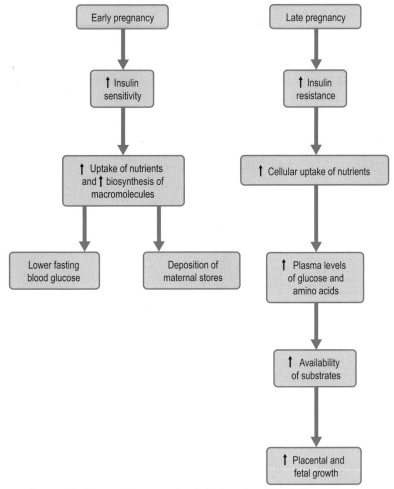

Fig. 11.10 Changes in maternal carbohydrate handling during pregnancy.

half of pregnancy. Early in the pregnancy, tissues exhibit an increased sensitivity to insulin so there is increased uptake of nutrients and synthesis of macromolecules by cells, which promotes maternal tissue growth. As pregnancy progresses, most women develop insulin resistance so levels of glucose and amino acids in the blood rise, thus increasing the availability of substrates required by the fetus and placenta.

In the first trimester, increased insulin is produced in response to glucose. Early in pregnancy, the raised levels of oestrogen and progesterone orchestrate the changes in metabolism. Oestrogen stimulates pancreatic β-cell growth (hyperplasia and hypertrophy) and therefore stimulates insulin secretion. It also enhances glucose utilization in peripheral tissues and increases plasma cortisol. So, the net effect is to decrease fasting glucose levels, improve glucose

tolerance and increase glycogen storage. Hepatic metabolism of insulin may also be altered. Lowered glucose levels between meals increases the tendency to become ketotic. Placental transfer of amino acids, increased hepatic gluconeogenesis (conversion of amino acids, particularly alanine, to glucose) and raised insulin levels, which stimulate cellular uptake, together result in lowered maternal levels of amino acids. During the first half of pregnancy, the progressive increment in insulin levels, augmented by progesterone and cortisol, stimulates hepatic lipogenesis (triacylglyceride synthesis and storage) and suppresses lipolysis (fat breakdown). An increase in the number of insulin receptors on adipocytes means there is enhanced removal of triglycerides from the circulation. Increased fat storage in early pregnancy results in hypertrophy of adipose cells. During fasting, ketogenesis is increased as the triglycerides are utilized.

Later Pregnancy

As the pregnancy progresses, the fetal-placental unit grows and levels of placental hormones, which are antagonistic to insulin, increase. Therefore, maternal tissues exhibit decreased sensitivity to insulin (insulin resistance), which means that insulin is less effective at stimulating cellular glucose uptake and utilization. Over the course of normal pregnancy, insulin sensitivity decreases by 50–60%. Pregnancy-induced insulin resistance affects adipocytes to a lesser degree. The dominant effect in the second and third trimesters is related to the high levels of hPL, but human placental growth hormone, prolactin, cortisol and progesterone are also involved. Tumour necrosis factor α (TNFα), resistin and leptin may also be involved in the increased insulin resistance that develops in late pregnancy. Levels of hPL increase markedly after 20 weeks. hPL is a very potent insulin antagonist with effects similar to those of growth hormone. Raised hPL results in decreased peripheral tissue responses to insulin and therefore increased circulating levels of glucose and amino acids, which are therefore available for transport to the fetus. hPL increases lipolysis and protein synthesis, decreases urinary potassium excretion and increases calcium excretion.

Progesterone augments insulin secretion, increasing fasting levels, but increases peripheral insulin resistance. Cortisol inhibits glucose uptake and oxidation, increases liver glucose production and possibly augments glucagon secretion. Therefore, in later pregnancy, fasting results in mobilization of maternal triacylglyceride stores leading to a marked increase in levels of fatty acids in maternal blood. This provides an alternative substrate for maternal metabolism so glucose is spared for the maternal central nervous system and for the requirements of the rapidly growing fetus. As tissue uptake of glucose is suppressed, levels of glucose are raised, which stimulate insulin release from the pancreas. Hyperinsulinaemia is a normal development in the later part of pregnancy; levels of insulin double by the third trimester. The raised level of insulin is important in stimulating protein synthesis. Raised insulin levels counteract the effect of the antagonistic hormones so maternal plasma glucose is maintained at levels similar to prepregnant levels. Insulin sensitivity rebounds after the delivery of the placenta. Women with insulin-dependent diabetes mellitus (IDDM) need to have a marked increase in insulin dose to compensate for the pregnancy-induced resistance to insulin.

In the postabsorptive states between meals, gluconeogenesis and fat mobilization provide substrates for maternal metabolism and placental transfer. Maternal cells metabolize the increased ketones and free fatty acids, thus sparing glucose and amino acids for placental uptake. As blood sugar increases in the pregnancy, it can exceed the transport maxima of the nephrons (i.e. the capacity to reabsorb the glucose from the glomerular filtrate) so some glucose is excreted in the urine. A degree of glucosuria is normal in pregnancy. As renal reabsorption of glucose is limited (so there are increased losses) and hepatic gluconeogenesis is decreased, hypoglycaemia, hypoalaninaemia and hyperinsulinaemia result.

Gestational Diabetes Mellitus

Gestational diabetes mellitus (GDM) is defined as glucose intolerance of varying severity that begins or is first recognized in pregnancy. It is the extreme end of the spectrum of normal physiological changes in pregnancy and is increasing with the increased prevalence of overweight and obesity in the population. Excessive gestational weight gain also increases the risk of GDM (Vieceli et al., 2017) although the relationship depends on factors such as the components of the weight gained (Goldstein et al., 2017). GDM is due to the inability of the maternal pancreas to increase insulin secretion sufficiently to counter the 50% decrease in insulin sensitivity, which commonly occurs in late pregnancy. Inability to produce adequate insulin at this stage of pregnancy is probably due to a limitation of the pancreatic β-cells (which may be related to the pregnant woman's own pancreatic development in utero). Inadequate secretion of insulin, and altered carbohydrate metabolism, may become evident again when there is further demand for insulin, as in a subsequent pregnancy or in later life, and is particularly associated with increased body weight. Although women who experience GDM typically return to normal glucose tolerance soon after delivery, they have a very high risk of developing type 2 diabetes later in life. GDM (or delivery of an infant weighing >4.0 kg) is also a risk factor for future pregnancies. GDM appears to reflect an unrecognized marginal ability of the mother to maintain normoglycaemia prior to pregnancy, which becomes overt during pregnancy with the demands of the fetus and the decreased insulin sensitivity. It is suggested that women who suffer GDM should be followed up, as pregnancy offers 'a window to future health' and provides an opportunity to identify women at risk of developing type 2 diabetes and cardiovascular disease in later life (Gilmore et al., 2015) who might benefit from targeted preventative interventions.

Because glucose travels across the placenta down its concentration gradient, hyperglycaemia in the mother in untreated GDM leads to fetal hyperglycaemia. This, in turn, stimulates insulin secretion by fetal pancreatic β-cells, which causes chronic fetal hyperinsulinaemia and increased fetal growth. Macrosomic babies have increased truncal fat, large shoulders and cephalo-pelvic disproportion, which can lead to a difficult delivery for both mother and offspring. Fetal birthweights and lengths in macrosomic births of >10 kg and >0.75 m have been recorded. A further consequence is that immediately after birth, the high glucose levels in the neonate disappear with placental detachment but the remaining neonatal hyperinsulinaemia can trigger life-threatening hypoglycaemia in the newborn, which should be carefully monitored. Infants of diabetic mothers and those infants with either macrosomia or born small for gestational age have an increased risk of obesity, metabolic syndrome and type 2 diabetes themselves (Goldstein et al., 2017), resulting from their intrauterine environment and possibly epigenetic changes to their genome that were triggered. In women who develop gestational diabetes, strict dietary control is important in reducing adverse effects on the fetus. A moderate energy restriction (~30% of total energy) can benefit glucose metabolism without causing ketonaemia in obese women with GDM (Metzger and Freinkel, 1987). If refractory to dietary treatment, some women with GDM may require insulin therapy as well. Diabetic women and women who require insulin therapy for GDM are at higher risk in pregnancy with problems associated with abnormal blood glucose levels such as increased risk of infection.

Case study 11.5 is an example of raised glucose levels in pregnancy.

CASE STUDY 11.5

Cathy is expecting her fourth baby. At 28 weeks' gestation, a random blood glucose test reveals a blood glucose level of 11 mol/L. Cathy looks well and, as in all her other pregnancies, says she feels exceptionally healthy. Cathy is referred to the consultant clinic for further investigation. Her previous baby was delivered at 37 weeks' gestation, weighing 4.96 kg.

- What is the provisional diagnosis and what investigations are likely to be carried out to confirm this diagnosis?
- What physiological interactions between the mother and fetus are occurring that could explain this phenomenon?
- How can the midwife best explain these to Cathy and what advice should she be given?
- What are the possible consequences for Cathy and her baby if no further investigations are carried out and no treatment advised?

KEY POINTS

- The physiological adaptation to pregnancy is mediated by the increase of steroid hormone secretion. Steroid hormones are initially produced from the corpus luteum under the influence of hCG and subsequently from the placenta.
- The maternal endocrine system is affected by the increase in steroid hormones so other hormones augment the effects of oestrogen and progesterone. For instance, secretion of MSH and cortisol increases in pregnancy, affecting skin pigmentation and improving some pathological conditions such as eczema.
- Generally early physiological changes in pregnancy are regulated by hormonal changes, whereas later changes may be due to structural effects of the enlarging uterus.
- Reproductive system: under the influence of oestrogen, the uterus increases in size and vascularization, and spontaneous uterine contractions are suppressed. The breasts undergo development in preparation for lactation.
- Cardiovascular system: physiological changes are particularly marked in this system, meeting the increased demands of the maternal and fetal tissues. The vascular system expands as progesterone stimulates vasodilation of the vascular smooth muscle and oestrogen stimulates angiogenesis and increased blood flow. The RAAS responds to the underfilled vascular system by increasing sodium and water retention; thus, blood volume increases by ~40%. Plasma expansion is greater than blood cell increase leading to overall haemodilution.
- Cardiac output increases early in pregnancy, initially as a result of increased heart rate, which is subsequently followed by increased stroke volume. Myocontractility is increased throughout pregnancy, which stimulates a degree of ventricular hypertrophy.
- Blood pressure decreases in early pregnancy, reaching a minimum in mid-pregnancy, and then returns close to prepregnant values towards term. The effects of posture on blood pressure are marked in pregnancy.
- The dilution of plasma proteins increases the formation of oedema. The ratio of clotting factors changes so bleeding time decreases.
- Respiratory system: excursion of the diaphragm alters as the rib cage flares increasing the efficiency of inspiration. Progesterone affects the sensitivity of the chemoreceptors, which increases respiratory drive. Therefore, hyperventilation is normal in pregnancy and results in lower circulating carbon dioxide levels and higher concentrations of cations, which facilitate exchange across the placenta.
- Gastrointestinal system: progesterone stimulates appetite and thirst and affects the sensitivity of the taste buds. Progesterone also affects the smooth muscle of the gut, which alters motility and transit time. This can result in increased efficiency of absorption but may also cause nausea and constipation. Decreased tone of

lower oesophageal sphincter may result in reflux and heartburn.

- Skin: the increase in MSH levels results in increased pigmentation of the nipple and areola, the linea nigra and possibly chloasma. Increased blood flow to the skin, which is important in heat regulation, affects growth of hair and nails and may cause congestion of the mucous membranes.
- Skeleton: posture is affected by changed weight distribution and altered composition of the cartilage and connective tissue resulting in an exaggerated curvature of the spine.
- Metabolism: maternal metabolism is affected by altered thyroid hormone secretion and altered responses to

insulin. In the first half of pregnancy, increased sensitivity to insulin favours deposition of maternal fat stores. In the second half of pregnancy, insulin resistance results in raised levels of substrates in the maternal plasma, which favour placental transport and fetal growth. Extremes of insulin resistance result in gestational diabetes mellitus.

- The presence of gestational diabetes, excessive gestational weight gain and conditions such as preeclampsia can be useful warnings of risk of later health issues including obesity, metabolic syndrome, type 2 diabetes and cardiovascular disease.

APPLICATION TO PRACTICE

Women experience many changes within their bodies and naturally will seek explanations and reassurance from the midwife as the changes occur. The midwife should use her knowledge of the physiological changes to aid her in assessing whether the pregnancy is progressing normally.

ANNOTATED FURTHER READING

Bates SM, Middeldorp S, Rodger M, et al.: Guidance for the treatment and prevention of obstetric-associated venous thromboembolism, *J Thromb Thrombolysis* 41:92–128, 2016.
A review about the treatment and prevention of obstetric-related pulmonary embolism and deep vein thrombosis, which are significant causes of maternal morbidity and mortality. The practical clinical guidelines are based on consensus expert opinion.
Blackburn ST: *Maternal, fetal, & neonatal physiology: a clinical perspective*, ed 5, Oxford, 2018, Elsevier.
An excellent in-depth and recently updated description of physiological adaptation to pregnancy and consequent development of the fetus and neonate that draws from physiological research studies. The chapters are clearly organized by physiological systems and link physiological concepts to clinical applications including the assessment and management of low- and high-risk pregnancies.
Goland S, Elkayam U: Pregnancy and Marfan syndrome, *Ann Cardiothorac Surg* 6:642–653, 2017.
Marfan syndrome, an autosomal dominant hereditary disorder of connective tissue, presents challenges for maternity care because the involvement of the cardiovascular, skeletal and ocular systems means there is an increased rate of pregnancy complications, which may compromise the fetus.
Guntupalli KK, Hall N, Karnad DR, et al.: Critical illness in pregnancy. Part I: an approach to a pregnant patient in the ICU and common obstetric disorders, *Chest* 148:1093–1104, 2015.
Guntupalli KK, Karnad DR, Bandi V, et al.: Critical illness in pregnancy. Part II: common medical conditions complicating pregnancy and puerperium, *Chest* 148:1333–1345, 2015.

An extensive review about the management of critically ill women in the intensive care units; considers the interpretation of laboratory and clinical parameters and possible effects of the condition and its treatment on the fetus. Part I considers obstetric disorders and part II considers medical conditions, which commonly affect women in pregnancy.
Landon MB, Gabbe SG, Niebyl JR, et al.: *Obstetrics: normal and problem pregnancies*, ed 7, Oxford, 2016, Elsevier.
Well-illustrated and clearly-written resource covering a wide range of obstetric topics from mental health to maternal nutrition and fetal programming.
Malik R, Kumar V: Hypertension in pregnancy, *Adv Exp Med Biol* 956:375–393, 2017.
Recent review about one of the most common complications of pregnancy, which is still unresolved and unpreventable. The 'deadly triad' of maternal mortality includes hypertension, sepsis and haemorrhage.
Queenan JT, Song CY, Lockwood CJ: *Protocols for high-risk pregnancies: an evidence-based approach*, ed 6, Oxford, 2015, Wiley-Blackwell.
Well-known maternal–fetal medicine textbook covering management of life-threatening challenges to the mother and fetus; offers research-based guidance to maximize outcomes and minimize risk, written in a format as though woman involved was present.
Resnik RIJ, Lockwood CJ, Moore M, et al.: *Creasy and Resnik's maternal–fetal medicine: principles and practice*, ed 8, Oxford, 2018, Elsevier.
Classic and revered textbook providing evidence-based guidelines for obstetric and fetal care including genetics, genetic testing and gene technology, fetal and placental growth and development, epidemiology, immunology, physiological adaptation to pregnancy and medical complications in pregnancy.

REFERENCES

Abramowitz A, Miller ES, Wisner KL: Treatment options for hyperemesis gravidarum, *Arch Womens Ment Health* 20:363–372, 2017.

Alves GF, Zanetti VT, Viegas RMF: Dermatology and pregnancy. In Bonamigo RR, Dornelles SIT, editors: *Dermatology in public health environments: a comprehensive textbook*, Cham, 2018, Springer International Publishing, pp 661–674.

Ashrafi R, Curtis SL: Heart disease and pregnancy, *Cardiol Ther* 6:157–173, 2017.

Astbury S, Mostyn A, Symonds ME, Bell RC: Nutrient availability, the microbiome, and intestinal transport during pregnancy, *Appl Physiol Nutr Metab* 40:1100–1106, 2015.

Blackburn ST: *Maternal, fetal, & neonatal physiology: a clinical perspective*, ed 5, Oxford, 2018, Elsevier.

Body C, Christie JA: Gastrointestinal diseases in pregnancy: nausea, vomiting, hyperemesis gravidarum, gastroesophageal reflux disease, constipation, and diarrhea, *Gastroenterol Clin North Am* 45:267–283, 2016.

Brannon PM, Taylor CL: Iron supplementation during pregnancy and infancy: uncertainties and implications for research and policy, *Nutrients* 9, 2017.

Browne VA, Julian CG, Toledo-Jaldin L, et al.: Uterine artery blood flow, fetal hypoxia and fetal growth, *Philos Trans R Soc Lond B Biol Sci* 370:20140068, 2015.

Bustos M, Venkataramanan R, Caritis S: Nausea and vomiting of pregnancy – what's new? *Auton Neurosci* 202:62–72, 2017.

Chamberlain G, Dewhurst J, Harvey D: *Illustrated textbook of obstetrics*, London, 1991, Gower Medical/Mosby, p 104.

Chen SJ, Shi L, Bao YP, et al.: Prevalence of restless legs syndrome during pregnancy: a systematic review and meta-analysis, *Sleep Med Rev* 40:43–54, 2018.

Chetty M, Duncan WC: A clinical approach to recurrent pregnancy loss, Obstet, *Gynaecol Reprod Med* 28:164–170, 2018.

Choo E, Dando R: The impact of pregnancy on taste function, *Chem Senses* 42:279–286, 2017.

Coad J, Al Rasasi B, Morgan J: Nutrient insult in early pregnancy, *Proc Nutr Soc* 61:51–59, 2002.

Cottrell E, Tropea T, Ormesher L, et al.: Dietary interventions for fetal growth restriction – therapeutic potential of dietary nitrate supplementation in pregnancy, *J Physiol* 595:5095–5102, 2017.

Coutinho T, Lamai O, Nerenberg K: Hypertensive disorders of pregnancy and cardiovascular diseases: current knowledge and future directions, *Curr Treat Options Cardiovasc Med* 20:56, 2018.

Cox S, Reid F: Urogynaecological complications in pregnancy: an overview, *Obstet Gynaecol Reprod Med* 28:78–82, 2018.

Devarakonda T, Salloum FN: Heart disease and relaxin: new actions for an old hormone, *Trends Endocrinol Metab* 29:338–348, 2018.

Durrani S, Akbar S, Heena H: Breast cancer during pregnancy, *Cureus* 10:e2941, 2018.

East P, Lozoff B, Blanco E, et al.: Infant iron deficiency, child affect, and maternal unresponsiveness: testing the long-term effects of functional isolation, *Dev Psychol* 53:2233–2244, 2017.

Erick M, Cox JT, Mogensen KM: ACOG Practice Bulletin 189: nausea and vomiting of pregnancy, *Obstet Gynecol* 131:935, 2018.

Fawcett EJ, Fawcett JM, Mazmanian D: A meta-analysis of the worldwide prevalence of pica during pregnancy and the postpartum period, *Int J Gynaecol Obstet* 133:277–283, 2016.

Fisher AL, Nemeth E: Iron homeostasis during pregnancy, *Am J Clin Nutr* 106:1567S–1574S, 2017.

Flaxman SM, Sherman PW: Morning sickness: a mechanism for protecting mother and embryo, *Q Rev Biol* 75:113–148, 2000.

Freinkel N, Metzger BE, Nitzan M, et al.: 'Accelerated starvation' and mechanisms for the conservation of maternal nitrogen during pregnancy, *Isr J Med Sci* 8:426, 1972.

Friedrisch JR, Friedrisch BK: Prophylactic iron supplementation in pregnancy: a controversial issue, *Biochem Insights* 10:1178626417737738, 2017.

Gardiner C, Vatish M: Impact of haemostatic mechanisms on pathophysiology of preeclampsia, *Thromb Res* 151(Suppl 1):S48–S52, 2017.

Gilmore LA, Klempel-Donchenko M, Redman LM: Pregnancy as a window to future health: excessive gestational weight gain and obesity, *Semin Perinatol* 39:296–303, 2015.

Goldstein RF, Abell SK, Ranasinha S, et al.: Association of gestational weight gain with maternal and infant outcomes: a systematic review and meta-analysis, *JAMA* 317:2207–2225, 2017.

Gonzalez-Suarez ML, Kattah A, Grande JP, Garovic V: Renal disorders in pregnancy: core curriculum 2019, *Am J Kidney Dis* 73(1):119–130, 2019.

Gongora MC, Wenger NK: Cardiovascular complications of pregnancy, *Int J Mol Sci* 16:23905–23928, 2015.

Groza D, Duerr D, Schmid M, Boesch B: When cancer patients suddenly have a positive pregnancy test, *BMJ Case Rep* 2017, 2017.

Honigberg MC, Scott NS: Pregnancy-associated myocardial infarction, *Curr Treat Options Cardiovasc Med* 20:58, 2018.

Hughes RG, Brocklehurst P, Steer PJ, et al.: on behalf of the Royal College of Obstetricians and Gynaecologists: Prevention of early-onset neonatal group b streptococcal disease (Green-top Guideline No. 36), *BJOG* 124:e280–e305, 2017.

Ivell R, Agoulnik AI, Anand-Ivell R: Relaxin-like peptides in male reproduction – a human perspective, *Br J Pharmacol* 174:990–1001, 2017.

Jeejeebhoy FM, Zelop CM, Lipman S, et al.: Cardiac arrest in pregnancy: a scientific statement from the American Heart Association, *Circulation* 132:1747–1773, 2015.

Johnson MH: *Essential reproduction*, ed 8, Oxford, 2018, Wiley-Blackwell.

Johnson M, von Klemperer: Cardiovascular changes in normal pregnancy. In Steer PJ, Gatzoulis MA, editors: *Heart disease and pregnancy*, Cambridge, 2016, Cambridge University Press, pp 19–28.

Kim YC, Mungunsukh O, Day RM: Erythropoietin regulation by angiotensin II. In Litwack G, editor: *Vitamins and hormones: erythropoietin*, London, 2017, Academic Press, pp 57–77.

Kissler K, Yount SM, Rendeiro M, Zeidenstein L: Primary prevention of urinary incontinence: a case study of prenatal and intrapartum interventions, *J Midwifery Womens Health* 61:507–511, 2016.

Kroopnick JM, Kim CS: Overview of hypothyroidism in pregnancy, *Semin Reprod Med* 34:323–330, 2016.

Lai T, Wu M, Liu J, et al.: Acid-suppressive drug use during pregnancy and the risk of childhood asthma: a meta-analysis, *Pediatrics* 141, 2018.

Lee SY, Chien DK, Huang CH, et al.: Dyspnea in pregnancy, Taiwan, *J Obstet Gynecol* 56:432–436, 2017.

Leo CH, Jelinic M, Ng HH, et al.: Vascular actions of relaxin: nitric oxide and beyond, *Br J Pharmacol* 174:4836, 2017.

Lieberman D, Billingsley J, Patrick C: Consumption, contact and copulation: how pathogens have shaped human psychological adaptations, *Philos Trans R Soc Lond B Biol Sci* 373, 2018.

MacIntyre C, Iwuala C, Parkash R: Cardiac arrhythmias and pregnancy, *Curr Treat Options Cardiovasc Med* 20:63, 2018.

Metzger BE, Freinkel N: Accelerated starvation in pregnancy: implications for dietary treatment of obesity and gestational diabetes mellitus, *Biol Neonate* 51:78–85, 1987.

Miller AWF, Hanretty KP: *Obstetrics illustrated*, ed 5, New York, 1998, Churchill Livingstone, p 34.

Miller JW: Proton pump inhibitors, H2-receptor antagonists, metformin, and vitamin B-12 deficiency: clinical implications, *Adv Nutr* 9:511S–518S, 2018.

Mitchell DM, Juppner H: Regulation of calcium homeostasis and bone metabolism in the fetus and neonate, *Curr Opin Endocrinol Diabetes Obes* 17:25–30, 2010.

Morton A, Teasdale S: Review article: Investigations and the pregnant woman in the emergency department – part 1: laboratory investigations, *Emerg Med Australas* 30:600–609, 2018.

Motosko CC, Bieber AK, Pomeranz MK, et al.: Physiologic changes of pregnancy: a review of the literature, *Int J Womens Dermatol* 3:219–224, 2017.

NICE: *Antenatal care for uncomplicated pregnancies (clinical guideline CG62)*, London, 2008, National Institute for Clinical Excellence, updated 2017.

NICE: *Hypertension in pregnancy: diagnosis and management (clinical guideline CG107)*, London, 2010, National Institute for Clinical Excellence.

Nwabuobi C, Arlier S, Schatz F, et al.: hCG: biological functions and clinical applications, *Int J Mol Sci* 18(ii), 2017.

Patil AS, Sheng J, Dotters-Katz SK, et al.: Fundamentals of clinical pharmacology with application for pregnant women, *J Midwifery Womens Health* 62:298–307, 2017.

Perez-Perez A, Vilarino-Garcia T, Fernandez-Riejos P, et al.: Role of leptin as a link between metabolism and the immune system, *Cytokine Growth Factor Rev* 35:71–84, 2017.

Roberge S, Bujold E, Nicolaides KH: Aspirin for the prevention of preterm and term preeclampsia: systematic review and metaanalysis, *Am J Obstet Gynecol* 218:287–293, 2018.

Sanghavi M, Parikh NI: Harnessing the power of pregnancy and pregnancy-related events to predict cardiovascular disease in women, *Circulation* 135:590–592, 2017.

Sanghavi M, Rutherford JD: Cardiovascular physiology of pregnancy, *Circulation* 130:1003–1008, 2014.

Slater C, Morris L, Ellison J, Syed AA: Nutrition in pregnancy following bariatric surgery, *Nutrients* 9(ii), 2017.

Taylor J, Hicks CW, Heller JA: The hemodynamic effects of pregnancy on the lower extremity venous system, *J Vasc Surg Venous Lymphat Disord* 6:246–255, 2018.

Teng W, Shan Z, Patil-Sisodia K, Cooper DS: Hypothyroidism in pregnancy, *Lancet Diabetes Endocrinol* 1:228–237, 2013.

Tettamanti L, Lauritano D, Nardone M, et al.: Pregnancy and periodontal disease: does exist a two-way relationship? *Oral Implantol (Rome)* 10:112–118, 2017.

Vaidya B, Chan S-Y: Thyroid physiology and thyroid diseases in pregnancy. In Vitti P, Hegedus L, editors: *Thyroid diseases*, New York, 2018, Springer, pp 673–708.

Vieceli C, Remonti LR, Hirakata VN, et al.: Weight gain adequacy and pregnancy outcomes in gestational diabetes: a meta-analysis, *Obes Rev* 18:567–580, 2017.

Whitcome KK, Shapiro LJ, Lieberman DE: Fetal load and the evolution of lumbar lordosis in bipedal hominins, *Nature* 450:1075–1078, 2007.

Whitfield CR, editor: *Dewhurst's textbook of obstetrics and gynaecology for postgraduates*, ed 4, Oxford, 1986, Blackwell Scientific.

Wiles KS, Nelson-Piercy C, Bramham K: Reproductive health and pregnancy in women with chronic kidney disease, *Nat Rev Nephrol* 14:165–184, 2018.

Wood AM, Livingston EG, Hughes BL, Kuller JA: Intrahepatic cholestasis of pregnancy: a review of diagnosis and management, *Obstet Gynecol Surv* 73:103–109, 2018.

Zimmermann MB: The importance of adequate iodine during pregnancy and infancy, *World Rev Nutr Diet* 115:118–124, 2016.

Zullino S, Buzzella F, Simoncini T: Nitric oxide and the biology of pregnancy, *Vascul Pharmacol* 110:71–74, 2018.

Maternal Nutrition and Health

LEARNING OBJECTIVES

- To review nutritional requirements and explain the basic role of nutrients in human health.
- To identify how and why nutrient requirements might change during pregnancy.
- To describe how the fetus adapts to a low nutritional plane.

- To relate undernutrition and overnutrition to the outcomes of pregnancy.
- To discuss other factors that may affect weight gain in pregnancy and birthweight.
- To discuss how maternal diet and health affect the fetus in the short and long term.

INTRODUCTION

Pregnancy often affects a woman's sense of wellbeing. Some aspects of health may be affected positively and others negatively. The role of nutrition, before, during and after pregnancy, is important for the health of both the mother and fetus. Pregnant women, and women who plan prior to pregnancy, may be receptive to advice and make changes to their diet and lifestyle, which persist after pregnancy and childbirth. Indeed, pregnancy can be viewed both as a 'window of opportunity' for making interventions on a range of health practices, which may improve the future health of the mother and/or her infant (Rodriguez-Gonzalez et al., 2018) and as a harbinger of future health issues. Maternal stressors, including perceived stress, chronic and acute stresses related to life events, work-related stress and pregnancy-related anxiety, as well as nutritional stress, are associated with adverse outcomes of pregnancy such as low birthweight (LBW), prematurity and intrauterine growth retardation (IUGR). Although stress, of all types, is a risk for preterm birth and premature labour, not all stressed women deliver prematurely suggesting that pregnant women (and/or their fetuses) have differing vulnerability to the effects of stress. Optimal fetal nutrition is implicated in a range of health outcomes affecting birthweight, growth in both infancy and childhood, and the risk of disease in adult life. The relationship between maternal and fetal nutrition is complex but the arguments that nutrient intake in pregnancy should be optimal are well founded.

Nutrient deficiencies in (or before) pregnancy impair maternal health, pregnancy outcomes and development, and long-term health of the offspring. Women may be vulnerable to nutrient deficiency because of inadequate dietary intake, lack of availability of food, lack of knowledge, lack of dietary diversity and nutrient-rich foods, and inequitable distribution of food in the household (Akseer et al., 2017). Societal norms, cultural expectations and gender discrimination may mean that pregnant women prioritize the needs of members of their family above their own needs. The most common micronutrient deficiencies in women worldwide are vitamin A, iodine. Iron, folate and zinc; they frequently co-exist (Gernand et al., 2016). Many of the targets of the 17 Sustainable Development Goals (SDGs), established by the United Nations General Assembly in 2015, are related to the importance of nutrition, especially for women of reproductive age and their children (Sabbahi et al., 2018).

CHAPTER CASE STUDY

Both Zara and James follow a vegetarian diet and try to lead a healthy lifestyle. At her first visit to the midwife, the midwife calculated that Zara had a body mass index (BMI) of 24, based on her prepregnant weight. During the pregnancy, Zara's baby appeared to be growing as expected and her midwife has measured Zara's uterine growth in centimetres using the symphysis pubis as the reference point; as expected, the fundal height has increased by 1 cm per week of pregnancy.

At 34 weeks' gestation, Zara is concerned that she only seems to have gained 4.5 kg over her prepregnant weight, unlike her sister who has put on over 10 kg and has been told by her midwife that her baby is a little bit on the small side.

- What factors could explain the differences in weight gain between Zara and her sister?
- What are the benefits of calculating the BMI of pregnant mothers and why is it preferable to calculate the BMI using the prepregnant values if they are available?
- Does Zara's smaller weight gain give any cause for concern?
- What other reasons could explain why Zara's sister appears to have gained a lot more weight than Zara has?

OVERVIEW OF NUTRITION

Growth, development and optimal health rely on good nutrition and an adequate quality and quantity of nutrients for body tissues. However, diet is influenced by many factors including wealth, religion, culture, seasonal, geographical and social factors. The insoluble macromolecules of food must be digested into soluble and small subunits in order to be absorbed by the digestive system (see Chapter 1). The major components of the diet (macronutrients), which are required in the greatest amounts, are carbohydrates, proteins and fats. They (and alcohol) can be metabolized to provide energy (ATP). Essential micronutrients are vitamins and minerals. Water is also an essential part of the diet. It is essential for life but has no nutritional value itself, however it may contain naturally occurring minerals such as calcium. As well as essential nutrients, which are required to sustain life (a deficiency of an essential nutrient will cause a deficiency disease state), food also contains nutrients, which, while not essential, may benefit health (such as the phytochemical lycopene found in tomatoes, which may have positive effects on cardiovascular health and decreases the risk of cancer).

Carbohydrates

Carbohydrates are the major energy source in the majority of contemporary human diets, but the amount and type of carbohydrate consumed varies among different population groups. With increased affluence in the Western world, there is a tendency to increase the proportion of fat in the diet at the expense of carbohydrate. The major types of carbohydrate are polysaccharides (or complex carbohydrates), simple sugars (monosaccharides and disaccharides) and oligosaccharides, which are larger polymers of monosaccharides that often have biological roles such as in cell recognition (e.g. lectins and glycolipids) and cell adhesion (e.g. selectins).

Monosaccharides, such as glucose, fructose and galactose, are not usually consumed in high quantities although fructose is found in fruit and root vegetables. The major source of carbohydrate in the diet is usually starch from plant sources, plus some glycogen from animal liver and muscle. Dietary disaccharides include sucrose (table sugar), lactose (in milk) and maltose, which occurs in malt, beer and some sprouting seeds. Most starchy foods are high in carbohydrate and low in fat. With increasing affluence, added sugars tend to contribute more to the carbohydrate content at the expense of polysaccharides; sugar-sweetened beverages (SSB) and sweet snacks may constitute a significant part of the carbohydrate intake.

Carbohydrates have differing effects on blood glucose levels and carbohydrate-rich foods can be compared using the glycaemic index (GI) ranking. GI values for different foods are calculated by comparing their effect on blood glucose with the effects of a reference food (usually glucose or white bread). Carbohydrates with high GI are digested and absorbed rapidly so that blood glucose concentration quickly rises. Carbohydrates that break down slowly and result in a slow and sustained production and absorption of glucose into the circulation have a low GI. Low GI foods prolong carbohydrate absorption, attenuate insulin secretion and increase the translocation of the insulin-responsive glucose transporter (GLUT4) to the cell membrane; they also result in more colonic fermentation of carbohydrate, which increases the beneficial production of short-chain fatty acids. High GI foods provide a rapid rise in blood glucose levels and are recommended for post-exercise energy recovery, whereas low GI foods release energy slowly and steadily and increase satiety and are appropriate for diabetics, dieters and endurance athletes. Health benefits of a low GI diet and low postprandial glycaemia (blood glucose after a meal) include reduced risk of obesity, diabetes and cardiovascular diseases and lowered incidence of certain cancers such as colorectal, endometrial and breast cancers (Augustin et al., 2015).

TABLE 12.1 Amino Acids

Essential Amino Acids	Conditionally Essential Amino Acids	Nonessential Amino Acids
Lysine	Cysteine	Alanine
Threonine	Tyrosine	Glutamic acid
Histidine	Arginine	Aspartic acid
Isoleucine	Citrulline[a]	Glycine
Leucine	Taurine[a]	Serine
Methionine	Carnitine	Proline
Phenylalanine		Glutamine
Tryptophan		Asparagine
Valine		Selenocysteine

[a]Conditionally essential or essential only at certain ages or in certain conditions.

Many carbohydrate-rich foods contain indigestible nonstarch polysaccharides (NSP or 'dietary fibre'). Dietary fibre is derived from plant sources and cannot be digested fully by digestive enzymes; it can be classified as insoluble or soluble fibre. Insoluble fibre promotes the formation of bulkier and softer faecal stools; some insoluble fibre can be fermented by colonic microbiota. Soluble fibre slows absorption of glucose and reduces blood cholesterol levels; it is associated with increased insulin sensitivity and decreased incidence of gut disease. As it delays gastric emptying, it may also increase satiety. Soluble fibre forms a viscous gel with water and so protects against constipation as this makes the stool softer. Foods rich in complex carbohydrates include cereal grains, starchy vegetables, legumes, seeds and wholegrain cereals, all of which contain reasonable proportions (3–15%) of NSP. Most other vegetables, and most fruits, contain small amounts of both starch and NSP and variable amounts of sugars. Most foods that are not highly processed, with the exception of honey and dried fruits, do not contain much sugar, whereas most processed foods contain added sugars, usually sucrose.

Proteins

Proteins are made up of 20 different amino acids linked together by peptide bonds. Indispensable or essential amino acids are those that cannot be synthesized from other amino acids in adequate amounts and, therefore, are required in the diet (Table 12.1). There are conditions, in which the requirement is high or there is a limited ability to interconvert amino acids, that result in an amino acid that can usually be synthesized (i.e. dispensable) becoming an indispensable amino acid that is required in the diet. These amino acids are described as being conditionally indispensable, for instance premature babies with immature enzyme function or under conditions of stress may require amino acids that they will be able to synthesize when they are older.

Protein quality depends on the proportion of dietary protein that is absorbed across the gut (digestibility) and the ratio of the essential amino acids in the protein. A protein that is absorbed completely and utilized completely because the indispensable amino acids are in the optimum proportions for synthesis of new proteins is described as a high-quality protein. The quality of a protein (or mixture of proteins) is scored by its Protein Digestibility Corrected Amino Acid Score (PDCAAS) or net protein utilization (NPU) value. Values of 1.0 (100%) are given to high-quality proteins. Human milk and whole egg have a PDCAAS of about 1, whereas the overall protein availability in the Western diet is typically 0.7. Diets that rely on poorer-quality proteins, such as those based on cassava (made from tapioca root), can be as low as 0.5. Proteins from animal-derived foods have higher protein quality. Consuming food with combinations of plant-derived proteins can increase the overall quality of the protein because the different composition of the two sources can compensate for each other. For instance, neither grains nor legumes are high-quality proteins in isolation but combining them can significantly increase the overall protein quality since each supplies complementary amino acids. A combination of protein sources is often the basis for some classical meals from a variety of cultures such as refried beans and corn tortillas (or baked beans on toast). Human diets rarely include a single source of protein.

In the absence of alternative sources of energy, protein can be metabolized as an energy source. Excess protein in the diet will also be used as a metabolic fuel. An adult is usually in nitrogen balance: protein intake is equal to protein breakdown so nitrogen in the diet is equal to excreted levels of nitrogen. Under conditions of growth and protein synthesis, there is a net accumulation of protein, and hence nitrogen, which is described as a state of positive nitrogen balance. States of growth, including pregnancy, result in positive nitrogen balance. Negative nitrogen balance usually indicates tissue breakdown or nutrient deficiency resulting in energy generation from protein sources. Illness and trauma cause negative nitrogen balance, which also occurs with reduced activity and decreasing muscle mass and during uterine involution (see Chapter 13).

Fat

Fat is predominantly used for energy requirements (ATP production). There is also a requirement for essential fatty acids, which cannot be synthesized by the body. These are the precursors of long-chain fatty acids and their metabolic products, prostaglandins and leukotrienes, which are important signalling molecules, for instance in parturition (see Chapter 13). Fat also provides the vehicle for absorption of fat-soluble vitamins, A, D, E and K. Within the body, there is a broad range of roles for fat including functioning as an energy store, insulating and protecting body organs, a precursor for steroid hormones and providing phospholipids, which are essential components of all cell membranes (see Chapter 1).

Most fat is present in the diet as triacylglycerides (TAG; also known as triglycerides TG); a triacylglyceride is a glycerol molecule with three fatty acids attached to the glycerol backbone by ester bonds (Fig. 12.1). There is a range of fatty acids that differ in both chain length and degree of saturation, which is related to the number of double bonds in the fatty acid molecule. Saturated fatty acids have no double bonds, monounsaturated fatty acids have one double bond and polyunsaturated fatty acids have two or more double bonds. The body handles fatty acids differently depending on their length and the degree of saturation (Fig. 12.1C). Fats in foods are predominantly triacylglycerides containing a combination of different fatty acids but are described by the predominant type. For example, olive oil is particularly rich in monounsaturated fatty acids (with single double bonds).

Saturated fats are usually solid at room temperature and are usually of animal origin, although coconut and palm oils and cocoa butter have a high level of saturated fatty acids. Saturated fats become rancid very slowly so they store well. Unsaturated fats are usually liquid at room temperature and mostly of plant origin. The C=C double bond is not very stable so it oxidizes easily and the fat becomes rancid. In food processing, unsaturated vegetable oils are hydrogenated (have hydrogen atoms added to saturate the C=C bonds), which makes the fat harder and extends the shelf-life and flavour stability. Unsaturated fatty acids from vegetable and most animal sources naturally adopt a *cis* configuration, although ruminants produce some *trans* fatty acids, which are thus found in low concentrations in milk and meat from ruminant animals. Positional isomerism is where the fatty acid has the same length and number and position of double bonds but the hydrogen atoms either lie on the same side of the double bond (*cis* configuration) or on mutually opposite sides (*trans* configuration) (Fig. 12.2). Hydrogenation and heating can convert the *cis* bonds to the *trans* isomeric forms. Many cellular processes depend on the fluidity of the plasma membranes of cells for which the types of fatty acid chains are key. Saturated fatty acids allow phospholipids to pack more tightly and are thus more ordered and rigid. The double bonds of unsaturated fatty acids produce kinks in the fatty acid, which means that the fatty acids of the membrane pack less tightly together, thus conferring a greater degree of fluidity and flexibility

to the cell membrane. *Trans* fatty acids are straighter and are more like saturated fatty acids in conformation even though they have double bonds. The ability of membrane proteins (receptors, transporters and signalling molecules) to move in the membrane and interact is dependent upon this membrane fluidity. Cholesterol also inserts into the membrane bilayer to maintain fluidity when temperature changes.

Diets high in saturated fat are associated with an increased incidence of atherosclerosis (damage to arterial blood vessels, causing hardening and plaque formation). Saturated fat stimulates hepatic production of cholesterol, which is transported from the liver to tissues in low-density lipoproteins (LDL). The cholesterol associated with these, LDL-cholesterol (LDLc), is a marker of the cholesterol being deposited in the atheromatous plaques. So the LDL-cholesterol level is a biomarker for heart disease. The cholesterol is picked up from the plaques by the high-density lipoproteins (HDL) and returned to the liver for reprocessing so HDL-cholesterol is considered 'good' as it reflects the removal of cholesterol from the plaques (Fig. 12.3). Although total blood cholesterol is considered to be a biomarker of risk for cardiovascular disease, the ratio of LDL-cholesterol to HDL-cholesterol or triacylglyceride to HDL-cholesterol is more sensitive. Diets that are higher in polyunsaturated fat are associated with increased HDL-cholesterol (HDLc) levels and an increased HDLc:LDLc ratio, which is associated with more favourable cardiovascular health. *Trans* fatty acids are implicated in increased risk of myocardial infarction and other cardiovascular problems. HDLc levels are also increased by oestrogen (so they are higher in women, which contributes to the lower risk of heart disease) and by moderate alcohol intake and exercise. The intake of dietary cholesterol has a surprisingly small effect on circulating cholesterol levels since daily production of cholesterol by the liver exceeds dietary intake and synthesis of cholesterol is reduced when intake of cholesterol is higher. Plant sources of fat do not contain any cholesterol (because a liver is required to synthesize it) but they may be rich in saturated fat and therefore increase endogenous cholesterol synthesis.

There are two polyunsaturated fatty acids that are indispensable ('essential') in the diet as they cannot be synthesized by the body. The essential aspect is the position of the double bonds. The essential fatty acids are linoleic acid (18:2, ω-6; chain length of 18 carbons and two double bonds, the first of which is at the carbon atom in the omega position 6 of the chain) and α-linolenic acid (18:3, ω-3; chain length of 18 carbons and three double bonds, the first of which is at the carbon atom in the omega position 3 of the chain). The body can further elongate (lengthen the fatty acid chain) and desaturate (add more

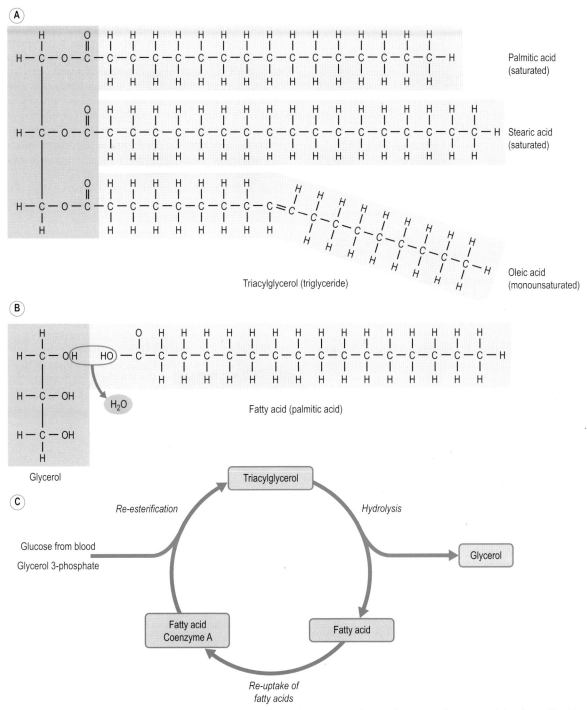

Fig. 12.1 Dietary fats: (A) structure of a typical triacylglyceride; three fatty acids each esterified to a carbon atom of the glycerol backbone of the triacylglyceride. Note that the two saturated fatty acids (palmitic and stearic acids lie straight, whereas the double bond of the monounsaturated oleic acid results in a kink). (B) Glycerol and a fatty acid can be linked by an ester bond to form a monoacylglycerol; in this case, palmitic acid will be esterified to the first carbon of glycerol to form a 1-monacylglcerol. (C) The fatty acid cycle. Triacylglycerol (as stored in adipose tissue) is hydrolysed to glycerol and free fatty acids. Glycerol can be converted to glucose in the liver (but not in the adipocytes because they do not express glycerol kinase). In the mitochondria, the fatty acids can be shortened by 2 carbon units in each cycle of β-oxidation to produce acetyl coenzyme-A, which can participate in many chemical reactions including de novo fatty acid synthesis.

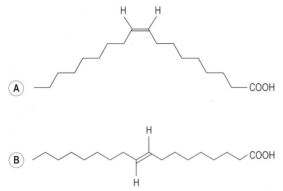

Fig. 12.2 (A) *Cis* and (B) *trans* isomerism of fatty acids. When the groups attached to the carbons of the double bond are on the same side of the double bond, a *cis* isomer forms and the fatty acid chain has a pronounced kink. When the two groups lie on opposite sides of the double bond, the *trans* isomer lies in a more linear configuration and the fatty acid behaves more like a saturated fatty acid. When the fatty acids are present in the phospholipids that comprise the plasma membranes of cells, the *cis* isomer 'kink' results in a greater special separation of adjacent phospholipids and a more fluid lipid bilayer, so that membrane proteins can move and interact more freely.

double bonds to) these essential fatty acids. However, there are two things to note. First, the fetus has limited ability to elongate and desaturate fatty acids so it is dependent on placental supply for both long-chain polyunsaturated fatty acids (LC-PUFA) and the indispensable fatty acids. Second, the enzymes involved in the pathways of elongation and desaturation of these indispensable fatty acids into their longer chain metabolites are competitive. This means that the ratio of ω-6 fatty acids to ω-3 fatty acids is important for optimal development. Oestrogen increases the expression and activation of the enzymes involved in elongation and desaturation so women are more efficient than men in synthesizing the LC-PUFA, particularly during pregnancy when the fetus requires them for development of its brain and nervous system.

Vitamins

Vitamins are organic substances required in small amounts for metabolism, growth and maintenance; they are either not synthesized at all by the body or not synthesized in adequate amounts and so are essential nutrients. Vitamins cannot be oxidized to provide energy; they predominantly act as regulators of metabolic processes. They can

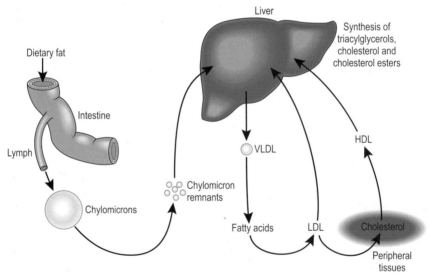

Fig. 12.3 Cholesterol metabolism. Dietary fat is absorbed in the small intestine as monoacylglycerols and free fatty acids. The enterocytes resynthesize triacylglycerol, which is packaged into chylomicrons (with other fat soluble compounds absorbed from the gut) and transported into the lacteal of the small intestinal villus. The chylomicrons are transported into the circulatory system via the lymphatic system. They circulate in the blood; the chylomicron triacylglycerol is hydrolysed by lipoprotein lipase and the fatty acids are taken up by the tissues. The chylomicron remnants reach the liver where their components contribute to hepatic synthesis of fat and cholesterol. These are packaged into very-low-density lipoproteins (VLDL), which circulate in the blood; when these are hydrolysed by lipoprotein lipase of the endothelial cells of blood vessels, glycerol and fatty acids are released and the lipoprotein loses density and becomes a low-density lipoproteins (LDL). The liver also produces high-density lipoproteins (HDL) that pick up cholesterol from the blood vessels and transport it back to the liver. Cholesterol associated with LDL is indicative of cholesterol being deposited in the blood vessels, whereas cholesterol associated with HDL indicates its removal so the ratio between LDLc and HDLc represents the net direction of cholesterol depositor.

TABLE 12.2 Water-soluble Vitamins

Vitamin	Role	Source
Thiamin (B$_1$)	Carbohydrate metabolism	Pork, wheat germ, yeast
Riboflavin (B$_2$)	Protein metabolism	Offal, milk, grains, legumes, eggs, vegetables
Niacin (B$_3$)	Production of energy from glucose; synthesis of fatty acids	Meat, nuts, legumes
Pyridoxine (B$_6$)	Synthesis and catabolism of amino acids; synthesis of antibodies and neurotransmitters	Pork, offal, grains, legumes, potatoes, bananas
Cyanocobalamine (B$_{12}$)	Reactions preceding use of folic acid in DNA synthesis	Animal and dairy products, eggs, yeast
Folate	Formation of DNA, gene expression (via epigenetics)	Liver, green leafy vegetables, kidney beans, oranges, melon
Pantothenic acid	Metabolism; synthesis of acetylcholine	Liver, egg yolk, milk, dried and spouting beans
Biotin	Synthesis of fatty acids, amino acids and purines (required for DNA and RNA)	Offal, egg yolk, tomatoes
C	Collagen formation, tissue formation and integrity, antioxidant, iron absorption	Citrus fruit, tomatoes, other fruit and vegetables

TABLE 12.3 Fat-soluble Vitamins

Vitamin	Role	Source
A	Visual perception (rhodopsin synthesis); growth of epithelial tissue and bones, antioxidant	Liver, kidney, egg yolk
D	Hormone involved in bone mineralization and calcium homeostasis	Synthesized in skin; fish oils
E	Tissue growth + integrity of cell membranes; antioxidant	Vegetable oils, grains, milk, eggs, fish, meat
K	Synthesis of blood-clotting factors; bone metabolism	Gut flora, liver, green leafy vegetables

be divided into water-soluble (Table 12.2) and fat-soluble vitamins (Table 12.3). The fat-soluble vitamins are more stable than water-soluble vitamins and are stored in body fat, so when taken in excess they are more likely to cause toxicity than water-soluble vitamins. As most B vitamins function as coenzymes in energy metabolism, requirement for B vitamins increases in parallel with increased energy consumption. Vitamins A, C and E function as antioxidants protecting cells from free-radical damage.

Minerals

Minerals regulate body function and are essential to good health. They are inorganic and become part of the body structure (Table 12.4). Excessive intake of minerals can be toxic or lead to illness indirectly, because of the competitive nature of mineral absorption in the body. For example, excess iron can lead to zinc deficiency and excess zinc can lead to copper deficiency.

PRECONCEPTUAL NUTRITIONAL STATUS

The sensitivity of the hypothalamus to environmental influences, such as nutrient availability, was probably of significant importance in promoting pregnancy in seasons when the fetus and infant had optimal chances of survival. Weight loss affects cyclical ovarian function in women. Anorexia nervosa disrupts the hypothalamic–pituitary–ovarian axis (see Chapter 4) and may cause amenorrhoea. Amenorrhoea related to inadequate nutrient intake is often reported in ballet dancers, competitive runners and other athletes. Low body fat not only affects the ovulatory cycle but also can result in low levels of oestrogens, which reduce bone density and predispose to osteoporosis. In the 1970s, Rose Frisch and colleagues observed that although the age

TABLE 12.4 Minerals

Mineral	Function	Dietary Source
Sodium (Na)	Extracellular ion essential for the generation of action potentials; required in the active transport of small molecules into the cell	Table salt (NaCl)
Potassium (K)	Intracellular ion essential for the generation of action potentials; utilized by the cell to maintain ion concentration gradients	Meat, milk, fruits, vegetables
Calcium (Ca)	Bone and teeth structural component; essential for blood clotting, muscle contraction and nerve impulse conduction	Dairy products, fortified flour, cereals, green vegetables
Chlorine (Cl)	Cation in body fluids; gastric acid excretions	Salt (NaCl)
Phosphorus (P)	Structural component of bones and teeth; essential for formation of ATP for energy storage	Meat, dairy products cereals, bread
Magnesium (Mg)	Required by some enzyme activities; present in cells, body fluids and bone	Vegetables, milk, cereals, bread
Iron (Fe)	Transfer of oxygen in haemoglobin molecule; oxidation processes; electron transfer chain	Meat, vegetables, flour
Zinc	Enzyme activity; growth and development of the immune system; spermatogenesis; tissue growth	Oysters, steak, crab meat, red meat, milk products
Iodide	Thyroid hormones	Seafood, iodized table salt
Copper	Constituent of enzymes; energy production and release	Legumes, grains, nuts and seeds, offal
Manganese	Synthesis of urea; conversion of pyruvate in TCA cycle	Plant products
Fluoride	Essential to reduce decay in bone and tooth tissues	Fluoridated drinking water
Selenium	Component of antioxidant selenoproteins; catalyst for the production of thyroid hormone	Liver, shellfish, fish meat, Brazil nuts

of menarche varied markedly in different populations, there was a much stronger relationship between body weight or body fat and the timing of menarche (Villamor and Jansen, 2016). This observation led to the hypothesis that total body fat needed to reach about 17% to trigger the onset of puberty; this hypothesis was controversial. One of the alternative explanations is that earlier progression of sexual development stimulates earlier adipose tissue deposition. However, low body weight is not always associated with amenorrhoea. Conversely, dieting, high energy expenditure, nutrient restriction or erratic eating patterns (such as crash dieting and binging) can suppress normal reproductive cycles in women even if their weight stays within a normal range (Coad, 2003).

A minimal level of nutrient intake and fuel metabolism seem to be required to maintain reproductive functions, particularly the pulse generating secretion of gonadotrophin-releasing hormone (GnRH; see Chapter 4). Fluctuations in body fat can also disturb the transport and metabolism of the steroid hormones, which are fat soluble. Nutrient deficiency may itself suppress appetite. Studies in sheep identified that the strategies to improve nutrition prior to mating (known as 'flushing') improved the ovulation rates (fertility) and number of lambs born (Robertson et al., 2015) but did not consistently improve the lamb survival or growth rate or the lamb's later reproductive potential. Similarly, it is suggested that optimal pregnancy outcome in humans may depend on long-term nutritional status rather than a short-term good-quality diet immediately prior to conception.

Although restricted nutrient intake can suppress reproductive function, excess energy intake may also be disruptive. Obesity also affects fertility and conception rate, both in men, primarily because androgens are aromatized to oestrogen in adipocytes (Hayden et al., 2018), and in women, because there is also increased aromatization of androgens to oestrogen plus insulin resistance, which leads to hyperandrogenaemia (Silvestris et al., 2018). Polycystic ovary syndrome (PCOS), which often causes anovulation (see Chapter 6), is frequently associated with insulin resistance, hyperinsulinaemia and dyslipidaemia even in the absence of obesity (Meier, 2018). However, the symptoms and effects of PCOS on reproduction are more severe with increased body weight and the presence of symptoms of metabolic syndrome (Lim et al., 2019). In PCOS, insulin resistance drives compensatory hyperinsulinaemia, which stimulates the ovaries and adrenal glands to increase androgen production (Silvestris et al., 2018). In the theca cells of the ovarian follicles, the high insulin levels amplify the response to luteinizing hormone and result in follicular arrest and anovulation. Hyperinsulinaemia also suppresses production of sex hormone binding globulin so free levels of testosterone are increased.

A woman's weight, particularly related to her height, indicates her nutritional status to some degree. Weight loss and nutrient fluctuation caused by self-imposed dieting, affecting reproductive function, may be the cause of infertility in a significant proportion of the women seeking fertility treatment. Maternal nutritional status can be assessed by calculation of body mass index (BMI; Box 12.1). BMI is used as a proxy of adiposity or fat mass (and health prognosis) but there are limitations to its use; BMI tends to overestimate fat mass in individuals who are active and have a high muscle mass relative to their body weight and to underestimate fat in individuals who are sedentary and have a high fat mass relative to their body weight. There are also racial differences in the correlation between BMI and fat mass; individuals from African and Polynesian races have less fat per BMI class compared with individuals from Caucasian races, whereas individuals from Asian races tend to have more fat for a given BMI. Whilst it is clear that the time to pregnancy is longer for underweight and overweight women, there is no consensus about the optimal BMI. A BMI of <18.5 kg/m^2 is not associated with good fertility or pregnancy outcome and is associated with ovulatory disorder infertility (Panth et al., 2018). A BMI of ≥30 kg/m^2 before pregnancy (defined as obese) increases the risk of infertility threefold compared with women whose BMI is in the normal range (18.5–25 kg/m^2).

Obese women are less likely to conceive spontaneously and take longer to conceive. Problems with fertility occur even if the obese woman has regular menstrual cycles and no clinical sign of ovulatory dysfunction. Overweight and obese women have poorer outcomes in assisted reproductive technology (ART) pregnancies; oocyte quality is often poor and there is a lower implantation rate because

---

BOX 12.1 Body Mass Index

Body mass index (BMI) is a proxy for fat mass. It is used to indicate nutritional status and risk factors associated with obesity but should be applied to populations not to individuals because there is a range of fat distribution and particular components of body composition such as muscle mass and bone mass can distort the association between fat and BMI. It is not an accurate indicator of fat in pregnancy but the prepregnant BMI is commonly used to identify risk.

BMI is the ratio of weight (measured in kg) divided by height (measured in metres, squared).

Calculation:

$$BMI = weight/height^2 \ kg/m^2$$

Interpretation:

Grade/Class	BMI	Definition
–	<18.5	Underweight
–	18.5–24.9	Desirable/normal weight
I	25–29.9	Overweight
II	30–34.9	Mild obesity
II	35–39.9	Moderate obesity
III	>40	Morbid (severe/extreme) obesity
–	>50	Super obese

A healthy shape is considered to be that usually associated with a BMI of 18.5–25 kg/m^2. Waist circumference and waist to height ratios are also used as indicators of healthy shape. A waist circumference of <80 cm is considered healthy in women and <94 cm in adult men, with waist circumferences above 88 and 102 cm, respectively, indicating risk. A waist:height ratio of <0.5 is also considered healthy with a ratio >0.6 indicating risk to health.

Note that there are ethnic specific cut-offs, which are not shown above.

---

of issues with uterine receptivity. In egg donor fertility treatment, high BMI of the donor woman has a greater effect on the outcome of pregnancy than the adiposity of the recipient woman (Fleming et al., 2018). Mouse studies indicate that obesity causes oxidative stress, hyperlipidaemia and hyperinsulinaemia, which affects the oocyte mitochondria and spindle and decreases the developmental competence and potential of the oocyte. Obese women have higher risks of miscarriage and poor outcome of pregnancy (Silvestris et al., 2018).

The higher prevalence of obesity in the general population is reflected in the increasing number of pregnant obese women who have more pregnancy-related complications such as hypertension, preeclampsia and gestational diabetes. Surgery for severe obesity is consequently becoming more commonplace. Bariatric (weight loss) surgery (such as gastric banding or gastric bypass) is an effective treatment for obesity, which can restore hormonal status and fertility but as there may be initial nutritional compromise, it is recommended that women wait 12–24 months after the surgery or 2 months after weight has stabilized before conceiving (Harreiter et al., 2018).

Maternal malnutrition (undernutrition or overnutrition) causes an imbalance of nutrients (deficiency or excess), raised levels of cortisol (a physiological stress response) and oxidative stress. Nutrient deficiency also affects male fertility by altering DNA synthesis and rates of cell division. Both embryonic development, especially early in gestation, and follicular development involve a rapid rate of protein synthesis and cell division, which are associated with a high energy and nutrient requirement. Preconceptual nutrient deficiency may retard development of the follicle and corpus luteum, affecting subsequent embryonic growth, even if the level of deficiency is not adequate to cause infertility. Excess intakes of some nutrients may increase mutation rate.

It is known that maternal protein intake affects many aspects of reproduction including gonadotrophin secretion, follicular development, and ovulatory maturation, embryonic survival, growth and development (Herring et al., 2018). Both diets with abnormally high protein content and those with very low protein content affect the menstrual cycle, fertility and pregnancy outcome.

Selenium (Se) availability is an important factor in male fertility. Selenoproteins are important for sperm function including selenoprotein P (SePP), which transports selenium to body tissues, including the testes. Male SePP-knockout mice are infertile. The antioxidant selenoprotein glutathione peroxidase-4 (GPX4) is also a structural component of the sperm mid-piece and levels have been shown to correlate with semen quality.

Whether the mother enters pregnancy with high nutritional stores can affect the outcome of the pregnancy. Placental size in humans appears to be governed by genetic growth potential, hypoxia and nutrient availability. In sheep, 'nutritional flushing' (see above), a period of poor nutrition early in gestation, may have a positive effect on the outcome of pregnancy because it increases placental size, presumably as an adaptive mechanism to increase nutrient extraction (note it may also enhance follicular development and ovulation rate) (Scaramuzzi et al., 2006). When the nutrient restriction is transient and the sheep are then returned to richer pasture transiently after conception, the increase in placental size is associated with an increase in lamb birthweight. In humans, an increased placental:fetal weight ratio is usually associated with both poorer outcome and long-term health prognosis (see Chapter 8). However, larger babies have larger placentas but in proportion to their birthweight. Morning sickness may produce a period of poor nutrition in early pregnancy, which could stimulate placental growth (Coad et al., 2002). Provided the woman entered pregnancy with good nutrient stores and the effects on nutrient consumption were limited, nausea in pregnancy could promote placental enlargement and positively affect the fetal growth trajectory. An adequate interpregnancy interval (IPI) may be important to allow replenishment of maternal stores, especially of vitamins such as folate. A short IPI is often considered to be associated with an increased risk of adverse outcome of pregnancy; an IPI of <12 months (6 after miscarriage) or >60 months is correlated with the highest risk (Palmsten et al., 2018). However, the relationship may not be causal and due to a clear-cut modifiable risk factor; it is possible that the observed relationship between short IPI and outcomes such as lower birthweight may be due to confounding factors such as unintended pregnancy or other socioeconomic factors (Liauw et al., 2019).

Case study 12.1 is an example of a midwife considering factors that might affect a pregnant woman's nutritional status.

CASE STUDY 12.1

Fiona informs the midwife at her first (booking) appointment that she has a healthy balanced diet.
- How can the midwife assess that this is an accurate statement?
- What observations can help the midwife assess Fiona's nutritional status?
- Are there any other factors that might affect Fiona's description of her diet?
- Are there any perceptions of what is a 'healthy balanced diet' that may actually be potentially harmful and if so what are they and why should they be avoided?

NON-NUTRITIONAL FACTORS AFFECTING REPRODUCTIVE FUNCTION

Food can provide nutrition but it is also the source of a number of maternal infections (Box 12.2). Pregnant women are advised to be particularly careful about food

---

BOX 12.2 Food Safety

Listeriosis

- Caused by: bacterium *Listeria monocytogenes*
- Possible effects: miscarriage, stillbirth and neonatal death, brain damage, premature delivery, maternal mortality, meconium before 37 weeks' gestation
- Sources: soil, soft cheeses, pate, raw seafood, cold meats, poultry, cook-chill food

Note: bacteria can multiply at low temperatures so women are recommended to thoroughly reheat refrigerated leftovers

Salmonellosis

- Caused by: *Salmonella enterica*
- Possible effects: maternal high fever, vomiting, diarrhoea and dehydration associated with food poisoning may increase the risk of preterm labour or miscarriage
- Source: raw meat, poultry and eggs, foods made from raw eggs such as mousses and sauces

Note: survives in soft-boiled eggs and mayonnaise, cross-contamination by uncooked foods or utensils is common

Toxoplasmosis

- Caused by: *Toxoplasma gondii*
- Possible effects: congenital mental retardation or blindness, neonatal convulsions, visual and hearing loss, haematological abnormalities, enlarged spleen and liver
- Sources: soil, raw or undercooked meat, cats' faeces and litter trays, goats' milk

Campylobacters

- Caused by: *Campylobacter jejuni* and *C. coli*.
- Possible effects: preterm delivery, intrauterine death
- Sources: undercooked poultry, unpasteurized milk

BOX 12.3 Factors Affecting Weight Gain in Pregnancy or Birthweight

- Maternal diet before and during pregnancy
- Maternal size, particularly lean body mass
- Age (younger women tend to gain more weight but pregnancy in adolescents is associated with an increased likelihood of an LBW baby)
- Birth order (first babies tend to be slightly smaller)
- Parity (multigravidae tend to gain less weight)
- Fetal sex (male babies tend to be an average of 150 g heavier)
- Nicotine (both smoking and tobacco chewing are associated with decreased birthweight)
- Alcohol (regular alcohol consumption is associated with lower birthweight)
- Hypoxia (high altitude and chronic maternal anaemia depress birthweight)

---

hygiene and food safety. Although nutrient intake and weight gain are associated with clear effects on birthweight, a number of other factors have been shown to affect fetal size and growth potential (Box 12.3).

The periconceptual period is a critical time when maternal and paternal physiology and nutrition, lifestyle, body composition and metabolism can have huge effects on both the short-term outcome of pregnancy and the risk of chronic disease in the offspring (Fleming et al., 2018). Ageing affects cell proliferation and gamete formation. Smoking, drugs, alcohol and radiation all affect cell division, probably by altering DNA methylation patterns (Witt

et al., 2018) (see Chapter 7). Indeed, smoking (including secondary smoking) remains one of the main modifiable risk factors associated with complications of pregnancy and the prevalence of LBW babies (Chamberlain et al., 2017). Maternal smoking is decreasing in high-income countries but is associated with poverty and is increasing in low- and middle-income countries.

Sexually transmitted diseases (STDs), caused by sexually transmitted infections (STIs), can cause pelvic inflammatory disease (which may affect fertility and pregnancy outcome), ectopic pregnancy and miscarriage. Each year, there are an estimated 357 million new infections with one of four STIs, chlamydia, gonorrhoea, syphilis and trichomoniasis (WHO, 2016). Chlamydia, gonorrhoea and syphilis are all caused by bacteria and are generally curable by antibiotic therapy but are frequently undiagnosed. Strains of multidrug-resistant gonorrhoea have been reported that do not respond to any available antibiotics. Untreated syphilis in a pregnant woman can be transmitted to the fetus, often causing fetal or neonatal mortality. In 2012, mother-to-child transmission of syphilis resulted in an estimated 143,000 early fetal deaths or stillbirths, 62,000 neonatal deaths and 44,000 babies being born preterm/LBW (WHO. 2016). Viral infections including human papillomavirus (HPV), HIV and herpes simplex (HSV) can also affect pregnancy outcome. More than 500 million people are estimated to have genital infection with HSV and >290 million women have a human papillomavirus (HPV) infection. Data from 2012 reported that of the 900,000 pregnant women worldwide infected with syphilis, ~350,000 suffered adverse birth outcomes including stillbirth (WHO, 2016).

NUTRITIONAL REQUIREMENTS IN PREGNANCY

Energy Requirements

There are concerns about recommendations related to increasing energy intake in pregnancy. In many developed countries, a significant proportion of women of child-bearing age are obese or overweight. Both high prepregnancy weight and excessive gestational weight gain (GWG) are risk factors for adverse outcomes of pregnancy such as gestational diabetes, preeclampsia and pregnancy-induced hypertension. Maternal obesity is a risk factor for macrosomia (and therefore caesarean section), congenital malformations, stillbirth and preterm delivery. Offspring of obese women are more likely to be obese children and adults. Excessive GWG may contribute further to obesity as some women do not return to their prepregnancy weight and progressively gain significant weight with each pregnancy.

There are two key questions: how much weight is appropriate to gain? And how much additional energy is required to support pregnancy (and achieve the desirable weight gain)? The optimal outcome of pregnancy is associated with GWG within recommended ranges of desirable weight gain, such as those published by the Institute of Medicine (IOM), but many women gain more weight than the guidelines recommend. The IOM guidelines were originally published in 1990 and were drawn from data about weight gain in women who had healthy outcomes of pregnancy. In 2009, the guidelines were revised (Rasmussen et al., 2009) to take various factors into account such as BMI cut-offs, women being heavier, having different ethnic backgrounds, being older, having multiple gestation or having chronic medical conditions. This remains a controversial area. Many women report not being given any advice about weight gain or being advised to gain outside of the guidelines. A significant proportion of women try to maintain their prepregnancy weight or to deliberately lose weight during pregnancy.

There are two approaches to determining energy requirements for pregnancy: to theoretically calculate the additional intake of energy (and other nutrients) or to observe what intakes are associated with the best outcome of pregnancy. The nutritional costs of pregnancy were theoretically calculated by using mathematical models based on estimating the cost of the new maternal tissues (particularly maternal fat deposition and also the expansion of maternal blood volume) and the tissues of the conceptus (fetus, placenta, membranes and other tissues) – the 'capital gains' – and the cumulative metabolic costs of maintaining these growing tissues – the 'running costs' (Campbell-Brown and Hytten, 1998). Tissue accrued (based on the average deposition of an extra 3.8 kg of body fat in pregnancy), converted to energy using the standard heat of combustion values accounts for about 185 MJ (50,000 kcal), and increased metabolism accounts for about 150 MJ (36,000 kcal), bringing the total absolute specific cost of pregnancy to about 335 MJ (80,000 kcal) (Fig. 12.4). Initially, the costs of pregnancy are the changes in maternal physiological systems and the deposition of maternal fat. Subsequently, fetal growth is rapid and the fetus has a higher energy requirement; this occurs when the assimilation of maternal fat is decreased and often maternal food intake is limited (see Chapter 11). This means it can be assumed that the increased nutritional requirements of the pregnancy are spread fairly evenly and the total energy cost of pregnancy can be divided by the number of days to estimate the approximate additional daily energy intake to support maternal and fetal needs. So the daily increase in energy requirement was calculated to be about 1.2 MJ (300 kcal) by dividing the total cost of 335 MJ (80,000 kcal) by 270 days of pregnancy. This approach is based on the theoretical requirements for a well-nourished woman with a normal BMI (prepregnant weight of 60–65 kg), an average GWG of ~12.5 kg and an average infant birthweight of 3.4 kg. Subsequently, the recommendations were revised and modified to take into account the stage of gestation: 375 kJ/day, 1200 kJ/day and 1950 kJ/day additional energy was estimated to be required for the first, second and third trimester, respectively (Butte and King, 2005).

As more studies about nutritional requirements during pregnancy are performed, the recommended daily allowances of energy have progressively decreased. The assumption that additional food is required to achieve the optimal weight gain has been repeatedly questioned. Meta-analyses of data from observational studies suggest that modern well-nourished women need to consume very little additional energy to sustain a healthy pregnancy to term, achieve the optimal physiological GWG and deliver a healthy infant (Blumfield et al., 2012; Jebeile et al., 2016). The average increase of reported food intake equates to 140–650 kJ/day, which is significantly lower than the recommendations in most dietary guidelines. Indeed, following the recommendations to increase energy intake by 1000 kJ/day (and often more in the third trimester) may drive excessive weight gain and an increased risk of adverse pregnancy outcomes. There are several reasons for the marked differences between the theoretical energy cost of pregnancy and the observed intakes; women may be more sedentary and reduce physical activity in pregnancy, so saving on costs of energy expenditure (Berggren et al., 2017) and there may be metabolic and behavioural adaptations, which spare energy (Jebeile et al., 2016). Insulin and leptin concentrations increase throughout pregnancy and affect

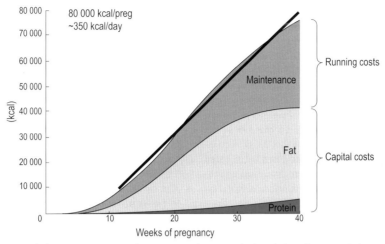

Fig. 12.4 The cumulative energy costs of pregnancy. It was calculated that the cumulative energy cost of pregnancy was about 80,000 kcal/day. The laying down new maternal and fetal tissue can be considered as a capital cost but the metabolic costs of the new tissue also need to be considered (the 'running costs'). Overall the costs are fairly linear so the additional energy required can be divided by the total number of days of the pregnancy resulting in a calculated consistent extra energy required per day. (Reproduced with permission from Hytten, 1991.)

appetite and therefore energy intake and energy balance. One of the important practical implications of a lower energy intake being able to sustain a healthy pregnancy is that there needs to be dietary changes, which result in an increased nutrient density. Micronutrient requirements for iron, calcium, folic acid and iodine are significantly increased in pregnancy and may not be met by merely increasing the intake of the prepregnancy diet even if it was nutritionally adequate for a nonpregnant woman.

Dieting or deliberate energy restriction is not appropriate for most pregnant women; it is unlikely to be beneficial and may harm the fetus. The current recommendations (Rasmussen et al., 2010) are that obese women should lose weight before but not during pregnancy because of concerns about the neurological development of the fetus and a lack of evidence to support recommendations for very low weight gain or weight loss. Low GWG is associated with increased risk of preterm delivery and small for gestational age (SGA) in all women whatever their prepregnancy weight. Though SGA at term is not associated with neurological dysfunction, preterm delivery of an SGA infant is a risk for irreversible cognitive and neurodevelopmental impairment. Insufficient energy intake may cause maternal metabolic and hormonal responses that affect fetal development. Pregnant women, even those with normal blood glucose tolerance, are predisposed to ketonaemia (raised blood levels of ketone bodies), which is usually accompanied by increased free fatty acids (FFA) and decreased glucose, insulin and certain amino acids. Although some

degree of metabolic change is commonplace, if changes are extreme or protracted, fetal development might be adversely affected.

GWG is defined as the difference between the measured weight at the first antenatal appointment, ideally when pregnancy is confirmed, and the last antenatal appointment, ideally just before delivery. In practice, the timing of these appointments can vary significantly and self-reported prepregnancy weight is often used, though this may be aspirational (usually underestimated) rather than accurate. This presents some challenges in antenatal care and making dietary recommendations particularly when antenatal care starts well into the pregnancy. In most countries including the USA, maternal weight is routinely measured throughout pregnancy and there are explicit guidelines for recommended GWG (Kominiarek and Peaceman, 2017). In other countries, such as the UK (NICE, 2010) and New Zealand, routine repeated weighing of pregnant women is not advised unless there is a nutritional concern or it is deemed to be clinically important (for instance, for obese women or those with pre-existing diabetes) and there are no evidence-based guidelines about optimal GWG. There may, however, be guidelines about the recommendations for increased energy intake, particularly that women should not 'eat for two', which is a common belief.

Routine weighing of pregnant women in the UK started in the 1940s when there were concerns about wartime food rationing providing adequate nutrients to support pregnancy (Allen-Walker et al., 2016). In the 1970s, the observation that preeclampsia was associated with excessive weight gain led to women being recommended to limit their food and energy intake and weight gain. However, energy restriction has no effect on the development of preeclampsia; excessive GWG is usually the result, not the cause, of the underlying clinical pathology (excessive water retention). It is therefore appropriate to recognize a sudden and marked increase in maternal weight as one of the signs of possible early preeclampsia. In the 1990s, the practice of routine antenatal weighing in the UK was questioned mostly on the grounds that it could not be justified because assessing weight gain was not being manipulated to a clinical advantage and it might cause unnecessary stress to pregnant women (Walker et al., 2018). This remains a controversial topic in antenatal care.

Low GWG, particularly in the first trimester, is associated with an increased incidence of LBW infants, congenital abnormalities and perinatal mortality (Kominiarek and Peaceman, 2017). Inadequate GWG is also associated with difficulties in establishing lactation. There is a strong argument that the advantages of monitoring GWG outweigh the disadvantages. Pregnant women are reported to desire appropriate information about diet and to want clear and consistent advice regarding GWG and weight management (Walker et al., 2018). They are often highly motivated to make lifestyle changes, particularly if supported by health professionals. Excessive GWG is a serious public health issue because it contributes to the obesity epidemic. It is estimated that 40–70% of women have GWG in excess of the IOM recommendations and those most at risk are those women who are overweight or obese at the time of conception (Walker et al., 2018). Those women who have excessive GWG are more likely to retain weight postpartum, which may affect the outcome of future pregnancies. Excessive GWG has other adverse maternal outcomes such as increased risk of gestational diabetes, hypertension, preeclampsia and caesarean section. There may be long-term consequences such as metabolic syndrome, type 2 diabetes and cardiovascular disease. Excessive GWG is associated with poor neonatal outcomes such as macrosomia and being large-for-gestational age (increasing risk for birth trauma), hypoglycaemia, low 5-min Apgar score, polycythaemia, meconium aspiration and seizures (see Chapter 15). Furthermore, maternal nutrition and lifestyle including GWG can influence fetal gene expression and the predisposition of the child to chronic disease in later life (Langley-Evans, 2015).

The risks for excessive GWG are similar to prepregnancy obesity and the conditions may occur together. Optimizing and/or restricting GWG is a possible intervention, which could reduce adverse pregnancy outcomes. The motivational interviewing style of counselling has had notable success in eliciting behavioural change in pregnant women who have issues with weight management or use of tobacco or alcohol (Kominiarek and Peaceman, 2017). Interventions found to be successful in preventing excessive GWG include dietary restriction advice to consume low GI foods, restrict energy intake or simple healthy eating advice and increasing physical activity. Routine weighing of *all* pregnant women by health professionals is a low cost and acceptable intervention that is easy to incorporate into antenatal care.

Protein Requirements

The optimum birthweight in humans can be considered to be within the range of birthweights associated with the lowest incidence of perinatal mortality and morbidity, that is a term weight of 3500–4500 g. Mothers of babies in the optimal birthweight range tend to eat more protein than women who give birth to babies with lower birthweight. The main regulator of fetal growth seems to be availability of nutrients, which can affect growth directly by changing the availability of substrates required for growth, or indirectly by altering hormonal control of growth.

Protein requirements increase in pregnancy, to support maternal tissue synthesis and fetal growth. Metabolic adaptations enhancing the efficiency of protein synthesis are evident from early pregnancy onwards; fewer amino acids are oxidized and used as an energy substrate, which promotes nitrogen conservation and protein deposition (Moran and Robinson, 2017). The rate of branched chain amino acid transamination falls and less urea is produced and excreted. The progressively increasing insulin resistance increases glucose availability for the fetus, sparing amino acids.

During the pregnancy, there is a fall in blood protein levels from ~70 to 60 g/L. Much of this fall is due to decreased plasma albumin concentration resulting from haemodilution. Albumin functions as a nonspecific carrier of lipophilic substances such as some drugs, hormones, free fatty acids, unconjugated bilirubin and some ions. It has an important role in maintaining the plasma osmotic pressure. The fall in plasma colloid osmotic pressure increases movement of water out of the blood vessels (see Chapter 1), thus increasing lower limb oedema and affecting glomerular filtration rate (GFR). Plasma globulins increase in pregnancy.

Protein requirements for the growth of maternal tissues and the growth of the conceptus were calculated by the factorial method to be about 925 g (Campbell-Brown and Hytten, 1998) but have since been reassessed to be closer to 500–700 g (Moran and Robinson, 2017). The increased protein synthesis, and therefore increased dietary requirement, in late pregnancy is about 6 g/day. In Britain and other developed countries, where the average NPU value is 0.7, this is equivalent to about 8–9 g of additional dietary protein being required to maintain nitrogen balance.

The normal protein intake of women in most developed countries, who regularly consume foods such as lean meat and poultry, fish, reduced-fat milk products, wholegrains and legumes as part of a balanced and varied diet, appears to be sufficient (on average 60–100 g/day) to provide the additional requirements of pregnancy. However, in the poorest developing countries, protein intake may be inadequate particularly in pregnancy. Protein-rich foods are often the most expensive component of the diet so women in the poorer sectors of affluent countries may also have difficulties meeting protein recommendations. Vegetarian and vegan women must ensure a range of wholegrains and legumes, providing complementary proteins, are consumed daily to provide adequate protein. The U.S. Dietary Guidelines (USDA, 2015) recommends an additional 25 g of protein per day for pregnancy in addition to the recommended daily intake (RDI) of 46 g of protein per day (0.80 g/kg per day), a total RDI of 71 g of protein per day for pregnant women (or 1.1 g/kg per day). Women with twin pregnancies are recommended that it is prudent to consume an additional 50 g of protein per day together with an appropriate energy increment to optimize efficient utilization of the protein.

Low maternal protein intake affects fetal programming and body composition; abdominal adiposity influences the risk of future disease in the offspring (Blumfield et al., 2012). Insufficient maternal protein intake is also associated with increased risk of IUGR, which increases neonatal mortality. IUGR infants who survive have an increased risk of cardiometabolic disease (particularly cardiovascular disease and diabetes), hormonal imbalance and abnormal development. Animal studies have identified that the early gestational period is much more vulnerable to the effects of deficiency in protein and amino acids (Herring et al., 2018).

Although low-protein diets are associated with an adverse outcome of pregnancy, it has usually been assumed that low protein intakes are unlikely in affluent developed countries. Using the indicator amino acid oxidation (IAAO) method, it was determined that protein synthesis increases by ~15% in the second trimester and 25% in the third trimester (Elango and Ball, 2016). Protein requirements therefore increase to 1.2 g/kg of body weight/day (14% of energy intake) in early gestation and to 1.52 g/kg body weight/day (17.5% of energy intake) in late gestation. These values are considerably higher than the previously determined estimated average requirement of 0.88 g/kg body weight/day (using the classic nitrogen balance method) on which most dietary recommendations are based (Stephens et al., 2015).

Plasma levels of most amino acids fall in pregnancy. The most marked falls are observed in glucogenic amino acids, which can be used to form glucose, then those involved in the urea cycle and then the ketogenic branched-chain amino acids. Amino acids are actively transported across the placenta. The transfer of amino acids across the placenta is only just adequate for fetal protein synthesis so any factor adversely affecting amino acid transport mechanisms has the potential to limit growth. Imbalances in maternal amino acid concentration will be reflected by placental uptake. For example, women with phenylketonuria (PKU) are advised to resume a low-phenylalanine diet (and take tyrosine supplements) prior to conception, as high levels of phenylalanine can harm the fetus, even if the fetus does not have PKU. High phenylalanine levels in pregnancy are associated with fetal IUGR, congenital heart disease, microcephaly and mental retardation. The amino acid methionine is involved in one-carbon metabolism; women who have higher dietary intakes of methionine are at lower risk of delivering a baby with a neural tube defect (NTD). However, the pathway, which generates one-carbon units for methylation, involves several other nutrients including folate, vitamins B_6 and B_{12}, choline and other amino acids, serine and glycine (Ducker and Rabinowitz, 2017). Good sources of methionine tend to be foods such as animal proteins that are rich in other amino acids and total protein, iron, zinc and calcium.

The intake of other specific amino acids may also be important. L-Arginine is considered to be a conditionally essential amino acid in pregnancy because of its role in embryonic growth and survival (Wu et al., 2016). L-Arginine is a precursor of nitric oxide, which is involved in the cytotrophic invasion in placental development and remodelling of the maternal spiral arteries (see Chapter 8) and vasodilation of all blood vessels (Khalil et al., 2015), which is important in the increased maternal blood volume (see Chapter 11). Nitric oxide deficiency is also implicated in the development of preeclampsia. Results from intervention studies suggest L-arginine supplementation in pregnancy may improve symptoms of preeclampsia and decrease blood pressure, improve fetal development and extend gestation (Dorniak-Wall et al., 2014). L-Arginine also has a number of other roles including regulation of protein synthesis, enhancing placental angiogenesis and for formation of urea and removal of ammonia. Lysine may also be particularly important in pregnancy; requirements are higher in late gestation (Payne et al., 2018). The implications of this may be particularly important for populations, which have a diet high in cereal-derived protein with little or no animal protein intake; animal proteins are rich in lysine, which is the first limiting amino acid of cereal proteins. Arginine, leucine and glutamine may have other functional roles in addition to protein synthesis (Manta-Vogli et al., 2018) such as in regulating gene expression, cellular signalling pathways and immune responses.

Some popular weight-restriction diets have promoted high protein intake. High protein intake (or imbalance due to an excessive intake of one or more particular amino acids) is also associated with IUGR. In experimental animals, high protein intakes have been associated with increased rates of congenital abnormalities. Increased protein breakdown can result in ammonia toxicity, which can affect placental transport of amino acids and blood flow; the vulnerable periods of organogenesis in the first trimester may be particularly vulnerable to the effects of excess ammonia. There may be competition for amino acid transporters affecting umbilical uptake of amino acids. A higher contribution of protein to the energy intake affects offspring body composition and concentrations of growth factors such as IGF-2 and insulin. IGF-2 affects nutrient availability and thus regulates placental and embryonic growth. It is therefore important that protein supplements designed for pregnant women have balanced amino acids. Women with very low energy intakes may be at risk of inadequate protein intake. The use of high-protein formulated supplements, powders or beverages is discouraged because clinical studies suggest they may be potentially harmful to the fetus. However, balanced protein and energy supplements where <25% of the energy intake comes from protein improve fetal growth and outcome of pregnancy when given to malnourished women (Ota et al., 2015).

Fat Requirements

In pregnancy, lipid metabolism alters markedly, resulting in hyperlipidaemia and accumulation of maternal fat stores. Maternal fat storage is highest early in pregnancy when maternal maintenance costs of pregnancy and fetal growth are relatively low. Levels of free fatty acids (also known as nonesterified fatty acids or NEFA), triacylglycerides (TAG), cholesterol, lipoproteins and phospholipids transiently fall in pregnancy as maternal lipid synthesis and fat storage are increased, and then rise. The changes in lipid metabolism are orchestrated by hormonal changes and are associated with changes in insulin resistance during the pregnancy (Herrera and Ortega-Senovilla, 2014). In the first two semesters, pregnant women are more insulin sensitive (see Chapter 11) and hyperphagic (have increased appetite and eat more); this is the time when maternal adipose tissue mass increases. Lipoprotein lipase (LPL), located on the endothelial cells of capillaries in adipose tissue, catalyses the hydrolysis of TAG in chylomicrons (carrying fat from the gut) and very low-density lipoproteins (VLDL, carrying fat from the liver). The products of this hydrolysis, FFA and glycerol or 2-monoacylglycerol, are taken up by

the adipocytes, which use them to resynthesize TAG to be stored. Insulin activates LPL in adipocyte capillaries and increases the expression of enzymes involved in lipid synthesis so the increased insulin response during this period of pregnancy enhances lipogenesis and fat storage. Insulin also stimulates the uptake of glucose and the activity of the enzymes involved in converting lipogenic substrates (such as glucose and fructose) into acetyl-CoA, which can be converted into TAG.

In the third trimester of pregnancy, when fetal requirements are maximal and maternal nutrient intake could be restricted by lack of availability of food or by limited capacity for eating and gastrointestinal disturbances (see Chapter 11), the maternal fat stores (on average 3.5 kg of fat equivalent to 132 MJ or 30,000 kcal of energy), can be mobilized to subsidize the energy costs of the pregnancy. This is the period of pregnancy when the woman is insulin resistant (see Chapter 11). Insulin resistance increases blood glucose levels so transfer to the fetus is enhanced. Maternal fat deposition stops for three reasons: (1) adipose tissue fatty acid synthesis decreases; (2) LPL activity decreases so the breakdown of TAG in lipoproteins is decreased, which causes maternal hypertriacylglycerolaemia (high TAG in blood); and (3) increased lipolysis in adipose tissue (Herrera and Desoye, 2016). The effects occur because although maternal insulin levels are increased, adipose tissue becomes insulin resistant and does not increase fat synthesis and breakdown of lipoproteins in response to insulin. High hPL augments the effects and promotes lipolysis.

As maternal fat is mobilized, blood levels of FFA and glycerol increase. The FFA are transported to the liver and converted into metabolic intermediates, which can be used for the synthesis of ketone bodies. Most maternal tissues can use ketone bodies as an energy substrate, sparing glucose for the maternal tissues, which have an absolute requirement for glucose (nervous tissue and red blood cells) and for placental transport to the fetus. Glycerol can be used by the liver for gluconeogenesis and contribute to maternal glucose levels.

The fetus depends on placental transfer of maternal fatty acids required for its growth and development. The fetus has a requirement for LC-PUFA, such as docosahexaenoic acid (DHA), eicosapentaenoic acid (EPA) and arachidonic acid, for neurodevelopment. Some of the fatty acid derivatives (such as eicosanoids) have signalling roles for instance in parturition (see Chapter 13). Most fatty acids in the maternal circulation are esterified in TAG and carried in lipoproteins (Fig. 12.5) with a small proportion (~3%) present as FFA. Lipoproteins do not cross the placenta intact but bind to LDL receptors on the surface of trophoblasts so that FFAs can be dissociated from

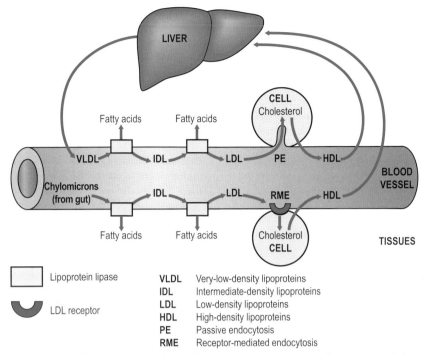

Fig. 12.5 Classification of lipoprotein complexes. Lipoproteins are composed of an outer shell of phospholipid and cholesterol surrounding a core of lipid components such as triacylglycerol, cholesterol and cholesterol esters. They transport fat soluble substances in aqueous solutions such as blood. The more fat that the lipoprotein contains, the larger and less dense it is. (Reproduced with permission from Saffrey and Stewart, 1997.)

lipoproteins by lipases present on the surface and internalized via different fatty acid transport proteins. The placenta has receptors for all the lipoproteins present in maternal plasma and expresses a broad range of lipases and fatty acid transport proteins (Lewis et al., 2018). Cholesterol, which is a precursor for placentally secreted steroid hormones, is delivered via the LDL receptor, as well as being synthesized by the placenta. Although the placenta transports the fatty acids, which fatty acids are available depends on the maternal diet (current and when the maternal fat stores were deposited) and maternal metabolism. Placental lipid metabolism releases more FFA into the maternal circulation than into the fetal circulation. In later gestation, maternal fatty acids are predominantly used for maternal metabolism and ketone body synthesis. The more mature fetus can synthesize nonessential fatty acids via de novo lipogenesis from substrates like glucose and also from ketone bodies.

Maternal plasma levels of TAG and FFA correlate with fetal lipid levels and fetal growth. Gestational diabetes causes dyslipidaemia that results in an increased transfer of maternal lipids to the fetus (Herrera and Desoye, 2016), which affects fetal body composition and metabolism, even when maternal serum glucose levels are within the normal range. Conversely, IUGR is associated with impaired placental transfer of fatty acids as well as fat soluble vitamins. LC-PUFA requirements of pregnant women are particularly high, especially in the third trimester when fetal brain and nervous tissue growth is maximal; accretion of DHA into the developing nervous system and fetal brain is high. Arachidonic acid (20:4, ω-6) is essential for neonatal growth and is the precursor for eicosanoids, prostaglandins and leukotrienes, and docosahexaenoic acid (DHA; 22:6, ω-3) has a key role in fetal brain development and visual function. Therefore, fetal demand for indispensable fatty acids (linoleic acid, 18:2, ω-6; and α-linolenic acid, 18:3, ω-3) must be met from either maternal dietary intake or be released from maternal adipose tissue. Under the influence of the high oestrogen levels of pregnancy, the synthesis of LC-PUFA from essential fatty acid precursors is facilitated so maternal phospholipids have significantly increased LC-PUFA, which can be released by placental endothelial lipase for placental LC-PUFA transfer. There is selective transfer of LC-PUFA across the placenta by specific fatty acid transport proteins (Lewis et al., 2018). Low maternal intake of these indispensable fatty acids is correlated with reduced fetal and neonatal growth. Impaired placental transport of DHA in growth-restricted or premature infants may lead to compromised neurodevelopment and long-term consequences for cognition and behaviour.

Consumption of fish, and therefore ω-3 LC-PUFA such as DHA and EPA in pregnancy, is associated with a reduced incidence of preeclampsia, LBW and preterm delivery (Makrides and Best, 2016), probably because signalling molecules derived from ω-3 fatty acids inhibit the effects of ω-6-derived eicosanoids, which are involved in cervical ripening and the initiation of parturition. Women who eat more ω-3 LC-PUFA-rich marine foods may be protected to some degree from the more serious complications of pregnancy associated with gestational diabetes, preeclampsia and IUGR (Wadhwani et al., 2018). These positive effects of fish consumption on the duration of gestation and fetal development have generated much interest with respect to the maternal dietary requirements for LC-PUFA associated with the optimal outcome of pregnancy. The balance between ω-3 and ω-6 LC-PUFA is likely to be important, as proinflammatory cytokines (derived predominantly from ω-6 PUFA) are important in early pregnancy for implantation and in late pregnancy for initiating labour. Anti-inflammatory cytokines (derived predominantly from ω-3 PUFA) are important in the middle stages of pregnancy for uterine quiescence, pregnancy maintenance and fetal brain growth (Akerele and Cheema, 2016). Supplementation with ω-3 LC-PUFA in the DOMInO (DHA to Optimize Mother Infant Outcome) trial was shown to increase the length of gestation and reduce the risk of early preterm birth and LBW, but have little effect on postpartum depression and early child neurodevelopment. It also reduced the risk of atopic eczema in the first year of life (Makrides, 2016).

Modern Western diets are relatively rich in ω-6 fatty acids but poor in ω-3 fatty acids and intake of preformed DHA is low, so the supply of DHA to the fetus may be compromised. The ratio of ω-6 fatty acids to ω-3 fatty acids is estimated to be significantly higher currently than it was in the Neolithic era when the big brain of modern man evolved. Obese women with insulin resistance and thin women with little body fat are likely to be more dependent on dietary DHA. Eating fish in pregnancy will increase DHA intake but much of the advice about fish liver oils containing vitamin A, and not consuming an excess of fish in case of heavy metal contamination, generates a complicated health message, which has led many pregnant women to avoid fish totally in pregnancy rather than increase their intake because they are pregnant.

A high fat intake is not recommended in pregnancy as there is an association between increased fat intake and increased risk of gestational diabetes (Schoenaker et al., 2016) whereas a Mediterranean diet, low in fatty foods,

seems to be protective (Donazar-Ezcurra et al., 2017). There may be also be adverse effects for the infant on the establishment of gut microbiota (Chu et al., 2016). High-fat, low-carbohydrate diets are not optimal for pregnancy and it is suggested that a diet containing <30% energy from fat and >50% energy from complex carbohydrate is associated with the best outcome of pregnancy (USDA, 2015).

Carbohydrate Requirements

Adequate carbohydrate intake is important in pregnancy to ensure sufficient glucose for maternal brain metabolism and transfer to the fetus, but normal healthy and varied diets are usually rich in carbohydrates and no change is necessary for pregnancy. Metabolism of carbohydrates and lipids changes, under hormonal influence, throughout pregnancy to ensure that the fetus receives a continuous supply of nutrients despite maternal intake being intermittent. Maternal plasma glucose concentration is maintained at a significantly higher level in later pregnancy by insulin resistance and increased hepatic glucose production in order to meet the increasing requirements of the placenta and fetus. The developing fetus utilizes glucose as its primary energy source but it can also metabolize maternally derived ketoacids.

Maternal pre-existing diabetes (type 1 or type 2, but not gestational diabetes, which develops later in pregnancy), high sucrose intake and prepregnancy obesity are all associated with an increased risk of congenital abnormalities including NTD. This is probably because the embryo does not have mature pancreatic function when the neural tube is developing and closing, so it is unable to produce insulin to regulate excess plasma glucose at this time, which may lead to oxidative stress affecting closure of the neural tube. It has been demonstrated in animal models of 'folic acid non-responsive' NTD that although fetal growth retardation is seen in the absence of several vitamins, NTD occurs only in the absence of inositol and supplemental inositol can prevent NDT (Greene et al., 2017). Inositol may ameliorate, at least to some degree, NTD induced by diabetes and folate deficiency. The developing embryo may also be vulnerable to the effects of maternal hypoglycaemia following hyperglycaemia. Thus, good control of plasma glucose levels and glucose metabolism is required in early pregnancy, which is more is likely to be achieved by a diet higher in foods with low GI, which lowers the risk of congenital abnormalities. Gestational diabetes, which becomes evident in the second half of pregnancy after embryonic development is completed, is not associated with an increased risk of congenital abnormalities. Low GI diets (rich in unrefined cereals, wholegrain breads and nuts) may be beneficial in protecting against the development of gestational diabetes in those women at risk (Zhang et al., 2018).

The modern Western diet tends to be high GI and low in fibre. Low GI diets in pregnancy tend to result in lower fasting blood glucose, which could affect fetal growth and birthweight. Studies that have investigated this find there may also be a beneficial effect on neonatal adiposity (determined by waist:length ratio), which persists into childhood.

The main sources of fructose, which is the sweetest of the naturally occurring dietary sugars, are sucrose and high fructose corn syrup (HFCS). The increasing intake of SSB appears to parallel the prevalence of obesity, type 2 diabetes and cardiovascular disease in many populations. Excess fructose consumption in adults is associated with insulin resistance, increased lipogenesis and fat deposition, and high LDL-c and TAG. Emerging research indicates that fructose consumption by pregnant women can lead to metabolic dysfunction and increased risk of metabolic disease in their offspring (Zheng et al., 2016). Consumption of foods, such as fruit, which are naturally high in fructose does not appear to have the same effect. High intakes of both SSB and artificially sweetened beverages is associated with increased risk of preterm delivery (Englund-Ogge et al., 2012).

Adequate dietary fibre is particularly important in pregnancy because the high progesterone levels affect smooth muscle tone and result in a slower rate of gastrointestinal motility and transit. This has advantages for nutrient absorption because the contents of the gut are in contact with sites of absorption for longer times however water is also absorbed to a greater extent, which often results in constipation (see Chapter 11). Recommending that pregnant women increase their intake of complex carbohydrates, such as wholemeal or wholegrain breads, cereals, legumes, fruit and vegetables, would provide low GI carbohydrate with good sources of fibre. Promoting foods high in fibre helps to address problems of constipation as well as generally increasing carbohydrate intake. Increasing intake of fibre and complex carbohydrate also has the positive outcome of displacing intakes of fat and added sugars. A high fibre, low to moderate fat diet recommended by many authorities also has the advantage of promoting greater maternal gut microbial diversity, which is associated with lower levels of inflammatory markers and a healthier lipid profile (Roytio et al., 2017).

Vitamins and Minerals

Micronutrient deficiencies are common in pregnancy because of insufficient intake and increased requirement due to pregnancy; deficiency can compromise fetal growth and contribute to placental dysfunction, which is associated with increased risk of adverse outcomes of pregnancy (Baker et al., 2018). However, supplementation needs to be evaluated carefully as nutrient–nutrient interactions can be detrimental and some micronutrients are toxic in excess. Both micronutrient deficiency and excess are associated with adverse pregnancy outcome. Maternal plasma levels of fat-soluble vitamins tend to increase during pregnancy and maternal plasma levels of water-soluble vitamins tend to fall. However, levels of vitamin A fall but levels of carotenoids rise. Fat-soluble vitamins cross the placenta more readily than water-soluble vitamins and their transport increases with gestational length; decreased levels of maternal plasma micronutrients may be due to haemodilution rather than to increased uptake by maternal and fetal tissue. Thus, lower circulating levels of nutrients in the blood of pregnant women cannot be simply interpreted as indicating a deficiency. The hormonal resetting of homeostatic mechanisms favours transfer of nutrients to the fetus (Campbell-Brown and Hytten, 1998). Low levels of nutrients in maternal plasma may limit uptake by maternal cells while optimizing placental uptake. The placenta is able to extract nutrients from maternal plasma and transfer them to the fetus, maintaining transport against a concentration gradient. Thus, fetal concentration of vitamins may be 5–10 times their levels in maternal blood. The 'pump' mechanisms of the placenta appear to be specific for vitamins; most minerals are not transported by similar mechanisms.

A good-quality maternal diet may be able to provide the increased vitamin and mineral requirements of the pregnancy, particularly if energy intake is slightly increased and the normal diet is rich in high-nutrient-density foods. However, a poor-quality diet can adversely affect both fetal growth and the establishment of adequate stores for neonatal growth. Micronutrient requirements increase slightly in pregnancy but, unless the woman is at the threshold of a deficiency, it is generally assumed that most women consuming a varied and balanced diet should have adequate reserves. The possible exceptions to this generalization are iron, calcium and iodine nutritional intakes, which should be assessed early in antenatal care. Periconceptual folate requirements are higher than can usually be provided by the diet. Vitamin A potentially presents some challenges in pregnancy, as both deficiency and excess can be teratogenic. Certain groups of pregnant women are at increased risk of vitamin D deficiency, such as Asian women.

Folate and Folic Acid

Folate (also known as vitamin B_9) is a generic term applied to dietary sources of related compounds that have the same biological activity in the body. Dietary folates are water-soluble vitamins that occur naturally in foods such as citrus fruit, legumes and green leafy vegetables; they are vulnerable to being broken down and lost during food preparation. Folic acid is the synthetic oxidized form of the vitamin used in fortified food and supplements, which is more stable. Folic acid is the monoglutamate form, which is almost all bioavailable, especially when consumed on an empty stomach so there are no other foods present to interact with it. Folate exists in plants as the polyglutamate form; it has to be digested to the monoglutamate form in order to be absorbed, so its bioavailability is about 50%.

Folate deficiency in early pregnancy is a cause of NTDs, failure of the embryonic neural tube to close in early pregnancy, which results in congenital malformations of the cranium and/or spine (Juriloff and Harris, 2018). There is a well-established protective effect of folic acid supplements that significantly reduce the incidence of NTDs and possibly other congenital malformations such as cleft lip (Li et al., 2016). Folate deficiency is also associated with other negative pregnancy outcomes including LBW, abruptio placentae, increased risk of miscarriage, megaloblastic anaemia of pregnancy, cervical dysplasia and atherosclerosis. Use of folic acid supplements also reduces the risk of developing preeclampsia and gestational hypertension (De Ocampo et al., 2018).

Folate is involved in one-carbon (1-C) metabolism reactions used in the synthesis of nucleic and amino acids, and hence the synthesis of DNA, RNA and proteins. Requirements for folate increase in pregnancy because the number of one-carbon metabolism reactions increases, for instance for nucleotide synthesis, cell division and gene expression (see Chapter 7). Blood folate levels fall in pregnancy, reflecting the high rate of DNA synthesis and cell division. Any factor that reduces DNA, RNA and protein synthesis may increase the risk of congenital malformations, which are usually associated with a reduced cell number rather than a reduced cell size.

There is considerable interaction between folate and other vitamins, such as choline and vitamins B_6 and B_{12}, which also have a role in one-carbon methyl group donation and, thus, recycling homocysteine to methionine. (Homocysteine in a nonprotein amino acid derived from a methionine molecule, which has lost its terminal methyl group.) Deficiency of any of these vitamins can contribute to hyperhomocysteinaemia (high homocysteine levels in blood), which causes endothelial damage, stimulates the production of reactive oxygen species (free radicals), increases oxidative stress and promotes coagulation pathways. Raised levels of homocysteine in pregnancy are associated with complications and adverse outcomes of pregnancy such as increased risk of preeclampsia, early pregnancy loss, placental abruption, NTDs and other congenital abnormalities, IUGR, LBW, preterm delivery and venous thrombosis (Gaiday et al., 2018). Mothers who have offspring with NTD may have higher plasma homocysteine levels (Yang et al., 2017). It is also suggested that DNA methylation patterns that are crucial to normal neurodevelopment can be perturbed by folate deficiency. The resulting defects in neuron proliferation, migration and differentiation and reduced neurite growth (of dendritic processes of the neurons) and synapse development are linked to clinical conditions such as intellectual disability, learning disorders, autism spectrum disorder and attention deficit hyperactivity disorder (Lintas, 2019).

NTDs are the most common congenital abnormality and result from failure of the neural tube to close effectively between 22 and 27 days postconception, which is often before many women realize they are pregnant. Increased intake of folic acid periconceptually overcomes apparent abnormalities in folate utilization, which are associated with folate-related gene polymorphisms of genes for enzymes in the folate metabolism pathways. The incidence of NTD is 1.6 per 10,000 live births in England and 3.1 per 10,000 in Wales; NTDs are a clinical reason for offering termination of pregnancy, so the actual incidence of pregnancies affected by NTDs is higher than the live birth rate suggests.

Folic acid supplements, of 400 µg/day in most countries, are recommended for all pregnant women and, importantly, women who are planning to become pregnant. The levels of folic acid that are associated with reduced incidence of NTD are significantly higher than those that could be easily achieved from the diet. It is difficult to increase levels of folate-rich food to the level recommended. Increased consumption of folate to reduce the risk of NTD is recommended 4 weeks before and 12 weeks after conception, which presents difficulties in many developed countries because about half of all pregnancies are unplanned. Although there are vigorous public heath campaigns about the recommendations to take preconceptual folic acid supplements, they do not always affect behaviour. Many pregnant women are aware of the recommendations but seem reluctant to follow them, at least at the critical time of planning a pregnancy and in its early stages. By the time many women start taking folic acid supplements, the neural tube of the fetus will have passed the stage of closure. Possibly, advice to supplement the diet with folic acid may appear to conflict with the usual health advice to avoid unnecessary drugs in pregnancy. Renaming folic acid as 'vitamin B_9', as is done in some parts of Europe, might alter the perception of folic acid as a drug.

Over 80 countries in the world have mandatory fortification of flour with folic acid, which has resulted in significant reductions in the incidence of NTDs (Wald et al., 2018). Folic acid supplementation and consumption of folic acid fortified food are complementary interventions to reduce NTD; consumption of fortified food alone does not provide adequate protection. The amount of folic acid added to flour is set by the tolerable upper limit (UL), which is determined as the maximum daily intake of a nutrient unlikely to cause adverse health effects in almost all individuals in the general population. One of the issues about fortifying flour is that bread consumption within a population can be extremely variable; the folic acid fortification level is set by the consumption patterns of the highest consumers in the population and the probability that their consumption could reach the UL. The UL for folic acid is hotly contested; it was determined by the Institute of Medicine in the USA based on data from patients with vitamin B_{12}-deficiency macrocytic (pernicious) anaemia. Folic acid supplementation can mask the symptoms of anaemia due to low vitamin B_{12} intake, which can delay the diagnosis of vitamin B_{12} deficiency increasing the risk of permanent neurological damage. But this should not be interpreted as an adverse effect of folic acid; it means that it is important to consider vitamin B_{12} status as well. It is vitamin B_{12} deficiency that causes neurological damage; folic acid does not have neurotoxic effects. Wald argues that the use of the UL to set fortification levels should be abandoned as withholding a benefit is a harm (Wald et al., 2018); he compared the 5 million preventable NTD pregnancies in the world since 1991 that resulted in stillbirth, infant death, disability and termination of pregnancy with the 10,000 cases due to thalidomide-induced phocomelia. Note that some women may not consume bread, for instance because they have coeliac disease, noncoeliac gluten sensitivity or other reasons to avoid bread.

Food fortification policies are sometimes criticized as an infringement of personal choice, as mass medication and unethical (Lawrence, 2013) with emotive terms such as 'nanny state' being used. However, there are other examples of actions by governments to protect the health of the population such as banning smoking in public places and legislating for compulsory use of seatbelts. The argument for supplementing a staple food, such as bread or flour, with folic acid has been strengthened by the other advantages of increasing folate consumption for individuals not planning pregnancy. Folate is important in maintaining optimal levels of homocysteine; hyperhomocysteinaemia (accumulation of circulating homocysteine) or low folate levels are associated with increased risk of cardiovascular disease, stroke, depression, Alzheimer's disease and some types of cancer.

Some drugs are folate antagonists and so increase the risk of NTDs. These include anti-epileptic drugs (such as carbamazepine and valproate), retinoids (used to treat acne) and some anti-tumour agents. Women who are pregnant with more than one fetus, breastfeeding women nursing more than one infant and those women with malabsorptive conditions (such as inflammatory bowel disease or coeliac disease), or are on chronic anticonvulsant or methotrexate therapy have increased requirement for folate. Alcohol affects folate intake and absorption. Exposure to high levels of ultraviolet light (e.g. from phototherapy or use of tanning beds) can lead to deficiency as folate is degraded by UV light (Zhang et al., 2017). It is usually recommended that women who are at higher risk for pregnancy affected by NTD (because they have previously had an NTD-affected pregnancy, have a family history of NTD, have insulin-dependent diabetes, are taking anticonvulsants known to affect folate metabolism or other risk factors) take a high-dose folic acid supplement. Those women who have already had one conception affected by a NTD are advised to consume 4 mg folic acid per day to reduce the risk of recurrence.

Obese women have a higher risk of pregnancy being affected by congenital abnormalities and NTD. It is possible that obesity affects folate metabolism; however, obesity may be a marker for socioeconomic status and a poorer quality diet. In many countries, it is recommended that obese women take a daily folic acid supplement of 4 mg. This is a controversial recommendation, as no studies have identified further risk reduction with daily doses above 1 mg. It is over 10 times the recommended intake for nonpregnant women and, at doses above 1 mg folic acid, unmetabolized folic acid can be detected in maternal and fetal blood, which raises concerns about possible adverse health effects (Dolin et al., 2018). In pregnancy, there are concerns that high folate status and low vitamin B_{12} status may act synergistically to predispose the pregnant woman to diabetes and her offspring to LBW, insulin resistance and adiposity (Paul and Selhub, 2017). Ideally, the folate status of women of reproductive age should be assessed (e.g. by measuring plasma and red blood cell folate levels) and personalized, and appropriate strategies for supplementation should be made prior to conception. However, biochemical measurements are expensive and it is easier to recommend a daily standard folic acid supplement than to assess whether plasma folate levels are >15.9 nmol/L or red blood cell folate is >906 nmol/L (Maffoni et al., 2017).

Case study 12.2 considers some of the issues related to folic acid supplementation.

Vitamin A

Vitamin A (retinal) status in pregnancy is positively correlated with outcome of pregnancy in terms of infant size and gestational length. Requirements for vitamin A are highest in the third trimester of pregnancy when fetal growth is highest. Vitamin A is involved in vision, reproduction, gene expression, embryological development, growth, immune function, integrity of the epithelium and bone remodelling. Both deficiency and excess of vitamin A

CASE STUDY 12.2

Jane seeks preconceptual nutritional counselling. She has had a previous miscarriage and is keen to improve the quality of her diet. Jane expresses concern about taking drugs in pregnancy, including folic acid, and is adamant that the human species could not have evolved requiring nutrients that could not be provided by a normal healthy diet.

- How might a midwife summarize the characteristics of a balanced diet?
- What rich sources of folate could be identified and how might consumption be increased?
- Is the connection between a previous miscarriage and diet valid?
- How could Jane's fears about folic acid supplementation be addressed?

in pregnancy can cause fetal abnormalities. Vitamin A is a nutrient that directly regulates gene expression. Vitamin A in food mostly exists in two forms: retinol (preformed vitamin A from animal-derived foods) and carotenes (provitamin A from plant-derived foods). Not all the carotenoids can be converted into retinol; the absorption and conversion of carotenoids into retinol is variable. In the body, vitamin A exists as three forms: retinal, retinol and retinoic acid. Retinol can be converted into retinal, the visual chromophore used in vision. The retinoic acid form of vitamin A is important in gene transcription. Retinoic acid binds to nuclear retinoic acid receptors (RARs), which form heterodimers with retinoid 'X' receptors. The heterodimer RAR-RXR (retinoic acid bound to RAR coupled with vitamin A in any form bound to RXR) is recognized by retinoic acid response elements (RARE) on DNA that control which genes are expressed. Heterodimers can also be formed with other ligand–receptor complexes, such as vitamin D and vitamin D receptor (VDR), to control other response elements and thus the expression of other genes. If there is vitamin A deficiency, gene expression will be altered because there is not enough vitamin A to form the heterodimers. If there is vitamin A in excess, then excess RXR homodimers may be formed (RXR-RXR), which bind to retinoid 'X' response elements (RXREs) on DNA resulting in a different pattern of gene expression. This is why both insufficient and excess vitamin A can result in perturbed embryonic development when expression of specific genes is not optimal for normal development.

Requirements for vitamin A are higher in pregnancy for fetal growth and metabolism and for maternal metabolic needs. Low vitamin A status in pregnancy is associated with increased maternal and infant morbidity and mortality,

decreased birthweight and increased risk of congenital abnormalities, compromised infant growth and development. In the third trimester, vitamin A deficiency is associated with increased risks of maternal anaemia and preterm delivery (Wiseman et al., 2017). High vitamin A intake is also associated with teratogenicity; in the first trimester, when embryological development is occurring, excess vitamin A can cause birth defects deriving from cranial neural crest cells such as craniofacial deformations (cleft lip and palate) and abnormalities of the central nervous system (not NTDs), heart and thymus.

Liver is a naturally rich source of vitamin A because vitamin A is stored in the hepatic stellate cells. However, changes in animal husbandry, and increased use of growth-promoting agents and vitamin supplements may make the livers of farmed animals excessively rich in vitamin A so pregnant women are usually advised to avoid liver and liver-based products such as pate. Isotretinoin (13-cis-retinoic acid) is a vitamin A analogue used to treat severe acne and other dermatological problems. It is a teratogen and can cause birth defects because it is structurally similar to retinoic acid and can affect gene expression. Women prescribed drugs like isotretinoin are advised to exclude possible pregnancy before they start treatment and not to conceive during treatment or for at least 1 month after ceasing treatment. They are advised to have effective contraception (not solely barrier methods) or practice sexual abstinence and may be advised to have an abortion should they accidentally become pregnant while using the drug. People taking isotretinoin are not permitted to donate blood during and immediately after treatment. Preformed vitamin A (retinal) is only available from animal-derived foods. As provitamin A from carotenoids in coloured fruit and vegetables is not efficiently converted into retinal, pregnant women who are vegetarian or vegan or avoid dairy products and meat need to consume five or more servings of fruit and vegetables per day and to select rich sources of carotenoids (from a range of yellow, orange and red fruit and vegetables). Carotenoids and vitamin A may also increase intestinal absorption of iron (Costa-Rodrigues et al., 2018). Vitamin A supplements including cod liver oil are not advised in pregnancy. No adverse effects of carotenoids from normal dietary levels of intake have been reported.

Vitamin D

Vitamin D maintains serum calcium and phosphorus concentrations within the range that optimizes bone health, by affecting the absorption of these minerals from the small intestine, their mobilization from bone and calcium resorption from the glomerular filtrate by the kidney. There are two forms of vitamin D: vitamin D_2 (ergocalciferol) made by plants and vitamin D_3 (cholecalciferol) made by animals including humans. Vitamin D_3 is synthesized in the skin on exposure to ultraviolet radiation (UVR); dietary vitamin D can be either vitamin D_2 or D_3 (where the subscript is not shown, vitamin D can be either). Interestingly, the vitamin D-folate hypothesis suggests skin colour evolved as an adaptation to UVR (Jones et al., 2018). Vitamin D is synthesized on exposure to UVR and folate is degraded by UVR. So skin pigmentation evolved to balance the levels of these two unrelated vitamins, which are both important to reproductive success. Vitamin D is also degraded in the presence of prolonged exposure to UVR, which prevents vitamin D reaching toxic levels. Possibly the lighter skin of women in all populations reflects the higher requirement for vitamin D in pregnancy.

Once formed in the skin, vitamin D_3 diffuses into the circulation and binds to the vitamin D binding protein (VDBP). Vitamin D from the diet binds to VDBP and is also packaged into chylomicrons (see Chapter 1). Vitamin D is hydroxylated in the liver to 25(OH)D (calcidiol), the biologically inactive major circulating form of the vitamin (which is the biomarker of vitamin D status that is usually measured). Many other tissues also express the 25-hydroxylase and produce 25(OH)D, which may have an autocrine effect. 25(OH)D is further hydroxylated by the kidneys to biologically active $1,25(OH)_2D$ (calcitriol), which has a very short half-life. The 1α-hydroxylase enzyme is also produced by many other tissues, which can convert the precursor into the biologically active form that has an autocrine or paracrine function. The classical role of $1,25(OH)_2D$ is to maintain calcium homeostasis but it has many other roles as well including modulating cell growth, immune and neuromuscular functions and suppressing inflammation. Vitamin D affects expression of genes (see section on vitamin A p. 353) encoding many proteins that regulate cell proliferation, differentiation and apoptosis. In addition, maternal vitamin D status may have epigenetic effects, which influence neurological development and later health of the child.

In pregnancy, vitamin D requirements increase substantially and its metabolism is markedly changed. The conversion of vitamin D to 25(OH)D seems unchanged but the conversion from 25(OH)D to $1,25(OH)_2D$ is remarkably increased. By 12 weeks' gestation, $1,25(OH)_2D$ is more than double the prepregnancy level and continues to increase up to threefold (>700 pmol/L) (Hollis et al., 2011). The concentrations reached in pregnancy would cause hypercalcaemia and be toxic outside pregnancy. The relationship between 25(OH)D and $1,25(OH)_2D$ exists both in the mother and fetus and indicates a much higher level of conversion and dependency on substrate availability than occurs in the nonpregnant state. The increase in circulating $1,25(OH)_2D$ is not related to calcium homeostasis; by week 12 of gestation, there is no increase in calcium requirement by the mother or fetus. When calcium requirements are high in lactation, this increase in $1,25(OH)_2D$ is not sustained. Instead, it seems that the role of vitamin D in pregnancy is primarily in immune tolerance to ensure the immunologically foreign fetus is not rejected (see Chapter 10). Vitamin D is known to modulate inflammation outside of pregnancy; vitamin D deficiency is associated with many inflammatory diseases such as cardiovascular disease, multiple sclerosis, sepsis, arthritis and cancer. Vitamin D deficiency is implicated in preeclampsia; animal models of preeclampsia have identified endothelial instability as the mechanistic pathway leading to placental ischaemia and administration of vitamin D causes it to insert in the membrane and stabilize the endothelium (Ganguly et al., 2018). Vitamin D also affects placental gene expression and implantation. Vitamin D deficiency affects fertility (in both men and women) and in pregnancy, is a risk factor for abnormal fetal growth, adverse birth outcomes such as preterm birth, preeclampsia, gestational diabetes, reproductive failure and childhood asthma (Wagner and Hollis, 2018).

Dietary requirements depend on exposure to ultraviolet rays so more dietary vitamin D is required for those individuals whose skin is not adequately exposed to sunlight. Women who are regularly exposed to sunlight are much less dependent on dietary sources of vitamin D. Risk factors for low vitamin D are low socioeconomic status, being covered or otherwise restricting access to ultraviolet light, and having a low educational level. Synthesis of vitamin D is also affected by the season of the year and the amount of UV light. Less vitamin D is synthesized in the skin of dark-skinned people as melanin absorbs ultraviolet light. Being housebound or not exposing the face, hands and body to sunlight for cultural or religious reasons will limit vitamin D synthesis. It is prudent to recommend that exposure to sunlight is in the morning or late afternoon to reduce the risk of sunburn and excessive exposure to harmful UV rays. It is not known to what extent the use of sunscreen affects vitamin D synthesis but pregnant women are encouraged to routinely use sunscreen during the middle of the day. Public health messages about sun avoidance to reduce the risk of melanoma have contributed to an increasing level of vitamin D insufficiency.

Pregnant women who do not receive regular exposure to sunlight (estimated to be ~30–40 min of exposure of face and arms each day) are recommended to have a supplement of 10.0 µg (or 400 IU) of vitamin D per day by many authorities. However, this level is under scrutiny. Recent research suggests that the best outcome of pregnancy is achieved when the serum level of 25(OH)D is at least

100 mmol/L (40 ng/mL) (Wagner and Hollis, 2018). It is difficult for women living in modern lifestyles to achieve this from sunlight exposure alone, so dietary supplements providing 4000 IU/day are recommended from before conception. No adverse effects of this dose have been reported by the randomized control trials (RCTs) using this dose and higher.

Vitamin K

Vitamin K is a coenzyme used in the synthesis of a number of proteins involved in bone metabolism and the blood coagulation cascade. Use of drugs that interfere with metabolism of vitamin K to reduce the risk of maternal thromboembolic disorders (see Chapter 11), such as warfarin, can increase the risk of coumarin embryopathy, fetal intraventricular haemorrhage, cerebral microbleeding, microencephaly and mental retardation. Anti-epileptic treatments can inhibit placental transport of vitamin K affecting fetal synthesis of clotting factors and increasing the risk of haemorrhage. For this reason, it is recommended that pregnant women with epilepsy take a vitamin K supplement in the month before delivery and during labour. In addition, microbial synthesis of vitamin K may be compromised by the use of broad-spectrum antibiotic therapy (particularly if taken for a prolonged period). Although vitamin K supplementation is not recommended in normal pregnancy, dietary changes over the last few decades have resulted in low stores of vitamin K being common.

Vitamin B_{12}

Vitamin B_{12} (cobalamin) is a coenzyme involved in homocysteine-to-methionine conversion in the cytosol (1C metabolism) and for the reaction that converts l-methylmalonyl-coenzyme A to succinyl-CoA in mitochondria. Vitamin B_{12} is involved in maternal and fetal erythropoiesis so requirements are increased particularly in the first two trimesters. Deficiency of vitamin B_{12} results in accumulation of homocysteine and methylmalonic acid and thus increases the risk of neurological abnormalities in the fetus. It is also required (like folate) for normal cell division and differentiation and for the development and myelination of the nervous system. Vitamin B_{12} deficiency in pregnancy is similar to the effects of folate (because both vitamins are involved in the same pathways) and is associated with increased risk of NTDs, impaired growth and neurodevelopment, preterm birth and maternal anaemia.

Absorption of vitamin B_{12} may increase in pregnancy; the fetus is dependent on maternal dietary intake. The placenta concentrates vitamin B_{12} and then transfers it to the fetus down a concentration gradient so fetal levels of vitamin B_{12} are about double maternal levels. The placenta preferentially transports newly absorbed vitamin B_{12} rather than that from maternal liver stores, so transfer to the fetus may be compromised even though the mother shows no overt signs of deficiency.

Vitamin B_{12} is synthesized by microorganisms and is found in foods of animal origin such as fish, meat especially organ meat, seafood, poultry, milk, cheese and eggs. Plants do not synthesize vitamin B_{12} so strict vegetarians and those people who consume low amounts of animal products are more likely to be deficient. Foods of animal origin are often expensive or not consumed for cultural or religious reasons. Plant foods exposed to vitamin B_{12}-producing bacteria, or contaminated with soil, insects or other substances containing B_{12} or foods fortified with vitamin B_{12} are the only dietary sources for strict vegetarians. Fetal levels of vitamin B_{12} may be compromised even if the mother has only recently become a vegetarian. Pregnant women who are strict vegetarians need to take vitamin B_{12} supplements (cyanocobalamin) or eat foods that have been fortified with vitamin B_{12}, ideally from before conception, and continue doing so while they are breastfeeding. For women with severe vitamin B_{12} deficiency, intramuscular hydroxocobalamin, which has a longer half-life than cyanocobalamin, is recommended. Infants are less tolerant to vitamin B_{12} deficiency than adults; breastfed infants may develop severe megaloblastic anaemia and neurological damage, even if their vitamin B_{12}-deficient mothers are not showing clinical signs of deficiency. The first symptoms of infant vitamin B_{12} deficiency are drowsiness, repetitive vomiting, swallowing problems, severe constipation and tremor (particularly involving tongue, face, pharynx and legs). Progression to unconsciousness, coma and, ultimately, death can be swift.

Vitamin C

Vitamin C (ascorbic acid) is a water-soluble antioxidant and a cofactor for enzymes involved in the synthesis of collagen, neurotransmitters and carnitine. It is involved in the recycling of vitamin E and also enhances absorption of nonhaem iron. Haemodilution in pregnancy results in plasma vitamin C concentration falling. Pregnant women have increased vitamin C requirements to ensure adequate transfer to the fetus and that maternal needs are met. The placenta transports ascorbate from the maternal circulation and transfers it to the fetus. Vitamin C deficiency is associated with a range of adverse outcomes of pregnancy including premature rupture of the placental membranes, preeclampsia, IUGR, preterm delivery, infection, maternal anaemia and more methylation changes due to smoking. Additional vitamin C from dietary sources is recommended for pregnant women exposed to increased oxidative stress; these include smokers and women who use recreational drugs or consume significant quantities of alcohol or regularly take aspirin. Routine vitamin C supplementation either alone or in combination with other micronutrients is not recommended, because, although it may offer protection against preterm PROM, there seems to be a slightly increased risk of term PROM (Rumbold et al., 2015).

Calcium

Calcium is the most abundant mineral in the body; it is required for bone formation, muscle contraction, normal functioning of many enzymes and hormones and intracellular signalling. Calcium requirements increase mostly in the third trimester when the fetal skeleton develops rapidly, incorporating a total of ~28–30 g of calcium. However, this is a tiny proportion of the total calcium in the maternal skeleton (~1000 g), which can act as a reservoir if maternal dietary calcium is low. However, if the mother's own skeleton is still growing, as in adolescent pregnancy, there may be competition between the maternal and fetal skeleton for calcium. Young girls who become pregnant within 2 years of starting to menstruate are most at risk as demineralization of maternal bone may be particularly detrimental when peak bone mass is being accrued.

Vitamin D concentrations rise in pregnancy, resulting in increased intestinal calcium absorption. There is also increased urinary excretion of calcium (hypercalciuria) and increased bone turnover resulting in increased mobilization of calcium (reversible loss of bone mineral density). Overall calcium retention is increased; this occurs in advance of mineralization of the fetal skeleton, which occurs predominantly in the third trimester. Serum calcium concentrations fall in pregnancy as a result of haemodilution. Calcium homeostasis is regulated by parathyroid hormone (PTH), calcitonin and $1,25(OH)_2D$. There is increased conversion of the inactive form of vitamin D ($25(OH)D$) to the active form ($1,25(OH)_2D$; see above). PTH levels change very little and remain in the normal range for those women who have adequate calcium intakes with a small increase in the third trimester when the maternal–fetal transfer is high. PTH drives the increased renal synthesis of $1,25(OH)_2D$, which acts with PTH to enhance calcium availability for placental transport. Parathyroid hormone-related protein (PTHrP) levels increase; it has PTH-like effects via the PTH receptors and stimulates placental calcium transport but its effects on calcium mobilization from bone are less than PTH so the maternal skeleton is protected. PTHrP is produced by the fetus and placenta and maintains a 1:1.4 maternal:fetal calcium gradient (Ditzenberger, 2018).

Calcium is one of the main nutrients which need to be considered in the antenatal nutritional assessment; women of reproductive age often have an intake that is below the recommended intake. In pregnancy, it is recommended that calcium intake increases by 400 mg/day. Pregnant adolescents are particularly at risk of inadequate intake of calcium as are women of all ages who do not consume dairy products. Pregnant women should be encouraged to consume at least three servings of calcium-rich foods a day. Although dietary sources of calcium are preferable, it may be necessary for women who avoid dairy produce and other calcium-rich foods to be prescribed a calcium supplement. Calcium supplementation, often administered with vitamin D, for pregnant women who have a low calcium intake, may protect against hypotensive disorders of pregnancy and preeclampsia but probably has no effect on bone mineral density (Khaing et al., 2017). Women who are prescribed both iron and calcium supplements should avoid taking them at the same time of day to maximize absorption of both.

Iron

The requirements for additional iron in pregnancy remain controversial (see Chapter 11). First trimester iron requirements are lower than for nonpregnant women due to menstrual savings but requirements are markedly higher by the third trimester. It is estimated that about 600 mg of iron are required for the fetus and placenta and blood lost at parturition (Campbell-Brown and Hytten, 1998). The expansion of maternal red blood cell mass accounts for ~290 mg of iron, but this expansion probably accommodates for the blood lost at parturition. Amenorrhoea of pregnancy saves ~120 mg of iron, which is not lost in menstruation, and iron absorption increases.

Iron depletion (low iron stores) or deficiency (anaemia) appears to be common in pregnant women and the consequences are significant for both mother and fetus. Maternal anaemia increases the risk of morbidity and mortality, and is associated with a risk of heart failure, haemorrhage and infection. The risks of fetal death, perinatal mortality, preterm delivery, lower birthweight, infant infection and gestational diabetes are also increased (Fisher and Nemeth, 2017). Maternal iron deficiency affects cognition, behaviour, motor development and activity of offspring and may affect the risk of neurodegenerative diseases in ageing (Brannon and Taylor, 2017). Infants of iron-deficient mothers are more likely to have low iron stores and be susceptible to iron deficiency themselves. Maternal iron deficiency affects the mother's physical work capacity and interaction with the infant. However, most of the attention has been focused on adverse effects of moderate and severe anaemia. It is hypothesized that the 'physiologic' anaemia due to healthy haemodilution may promote placental growth and perfusion by upregulating the expression of vascular growth factor receptors (Stangret et al., 2017);

mild ('normal') anaemia is not associated with adverse pregnancy outcome and appears to promote optimal fetal development.

There are two pathways of iron absorption; haem and nonhaem iron absorption (Fig. 12.6). Haem iron from meat is highly bioavailable and affected to a negligible degree by other components of the diet. However, most dietary iron is nonhaem iron (from most foods), absorption of which varies with other dietary constituents, particularly those which influence the reduction of the insoluble ferric iron to soluble ferrous iron. Vitamin C and other organic acids significantly enhance dietary absorption of nonhaem iron; meat, fish and poultry also increase nonhaem iron absorption, though the mechanism of this effect is not clear. Inhibitors of nonhaem iron absorption bind iron and render it less available; these include phytate (in legumes, grains and rice), polyphenols (in tea and coffee, grains, oregano and red wine) and vegetable proteins such as those in soybeans. Calcium inhibits absorption of both haem and nonhaem iron with a dose-related effect. Nonhaem iron is transported across the gut by the same divalent metal transporter (DMT1), which also transports other metals such as zinc and copper; this means that supplementation with one metal can affect the absorption of the others. The bioavailability of iron from meat is significantly higher than from plant-based foods, and since unidentified factors present in meat and other animal proteins also enhance nonhaem iron absorption, individuals who consume omnivorous diets absorb more iron than do vegans or vegetarians.

Risk factors for iron deficiency in pregnancy include depleted iron stores prior to pregnancy (usually related to menstrual loss), not eating meat, chronic use of nonsteroidal anti-inflammatory drugs (NSAIDs) such as aspirin (resulting in gastrointestinal damage), low intake of factors, which increase iron absorption (particularly vitamin C) and high intake of factors, which decrease absorption (such as phytate). Iron deficiency is more likely with low socioeconomic status, poorer educational attainment and multiple gestation; adolescent women and those with a short interpregnancy interval are also at increased risk of iron deficiency. Use of oral contraceptives prior to pregnancy tends to result in a favourable iron status because menstrual blood loss is reduced.

Pregnant women who are at risk of iron deficiency are usually prescribed iron supplements. Some women experience gastrointestinal effects in response to supplementary iron. Absorption of iron is best in the absence of other food (empty stomach) but may be associated with more side-effects. Low-dose supplements are associated with fewer side-effects and ferrous gluconate appears to be less irritating. However, iron is potentially toxic in excess; concerns

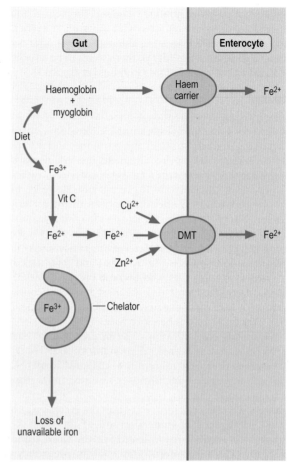

Fig. 12.6 Pathways of iron absorption. Haem iron from meat, poultry and fish is absorbed efficiently via the haem transporter, whereas absorption of nonhaem iron is affected by other dietary components. For instance, vitamin C enhances the conversion of Fe^{3+} (ferric iron) to the more soluble Fe^{2+} (ferrous iron), which is better absorbed. Some dietary components, such as phytate and polyphenols, bind to the iron and make it less available. Nonhaem iron is transported across the gut wall via the divalent metal transporter (DMT). Zinc and copper can compete for transport by DMT and therefore inhibit iron absorption.

focus on iron overload causing the generation of free radicals, which can cause cellular damage and on the possible increased susceptibility to infection of women who are not iron deficient. Thus, it is recommended that iron supplementation should always be prescribed on the basis of biological criteria rather than being administered routinely.

Haemochromatosis is the most common genetic disorder affecting Caucasian populations; it is a recessively inherited disease resulting in systemic iron overload usually caused by decreased concentration or effect of hepcidin (Brissot et al., 2018). The clinical effects of haemochromatosis, due to deposition of iron in the liver, heart and pancreas, are not usually manifest or of concern in women of childbearing age as menstrual losses (and iron losses related to pregnancy and lactation) help to maintain iron balance. However, routine assessment of blood parameters such as transferrin saturation and serum ferritin concentration in pregnant women could help to identify those women who might be at risk in later life.

To meet the additional requirements of pregnancy, women need to markedly increase their intake of iron-rich foods and the dietary factors that promote iron absorption. Nutritional assessment and dietary advice for pregnant women should take into consideration both sources of iron and the intake of factors affecting nonhaem iron absorption. Timing of consumption of foods can influence nutrient–nutrient interaction. For instance, drinking fruit juice (high vitamin C content) with a good iron source will favour absorption, and drinking tea, which has a high tannin level, should be avoided with iron sources. Vegetarian and vegan women may find it difficult to meet their iron requirements solely from food sources; they should consume grains, vegetables and legumes, and have vitamin C-rich foods or drinks (raw fruits, fruit juice or vegetables) with meals. As the absorption of iron from a vegetarian or vegan diet is lower, more iron needs to be consumed. As adolescents have a higher iron requirement, this group is particularly at risk of being unable to achieve an adequate iron intake, particularly in the latter part of pregnancy and especially if they avoid meat. Supplementation may be necessary for those with low iron stores and/or low dietary iron intakes, but supplementation must always be given in conjunction with appropriate dietary advice, and under supervision from a health professional. There are concerns about excessive intake of supplementary iron and its potential effects on free-radical generation; also, the implications of iron supplementation on zinc and copper status need to be considered.

Zinc

Zinc is an essential transition metal in humans and estimated from gene sequence analysis to be required for ~3000 zinc proteins including metalloenzymes, zinc transporters, zinc-binding factors and antioxidant enzymes. It is involved in carbohydrate and protein metabolism, cell proliferation, protein synthesis, protection from oxidative damage, apoptosis, hormone binding (by means of zinc finger proteins) and transcription and is thus likely to affect embryonic and fetal development, trophoblast differentiation and placental growth (Gernand et al., 2016). Zinc deficiency in pregnancy is teratogenic; it is associated with

increased risk of congenital abnormality (including NTDs) and fetal loss as well as other complications of pregnancy and delivery including haemorrhage, hypertension, pre- and post-term pregnancy and prolonged labour, growth retardation, retarded neurogenesis, neurobehavioural and immunological development and premature delivery (Wilson et al., 2016). Iron supplementation can decrease zinc absorption, and unbalanced zinc in excess may induce a secondary copper deficiency, as there is competition for the divalent metal transporters. Bioavailability of zinc in foods is particularly affected by high phytate content in foods such as cereal grains, legumes and nuts. Many foods rich in zinc are also rich in iron so provide both in an appropriate balance.

Selenium

Selenium is a component of selenocysteine, the 21st amino acid, which is incorporated into selenoproteins (selenocysteine has a similar structure to cysteine but has selenium in place of a sulphur atom). There are at least 25 selenoproteins, the majority of which function as antioxidant enzymes preventing cellular damage from free radicals (natural byproducts of oxidative metabolism). One of the best known selenoproteins is the enzyme glutathione peroxidase, which metabolizes hydrogen peroxide formed from polyunsaturated fatty acids. Both selenium and iodine are required for thyroid hormone synthesis.

The specific requirement for selenium is uncertain; a relatively low intake of selenium is required to prevent Keshan disease, a cardiomyopathy associated with a strain of coxsackie virus combined with a selenium deficiency, but higher intakes of selenium may be protective against cancer and cardiovascular disease, by protecting against free-radical damage. The usual recommended intake for adult women is ~60 μg/day (but varies between countries). Pregnant women have increased selenium requirements (75 μg/day) to allow for growth of the embryo and increased selenoprotein synthesis and tissue accumulation. The placenta actively transports selenium to the fetus, but it is not known whether absorption of dietary selenium increases in pregnancy. Requirements for selenium are increased with increased oxidative stress such as that caused by smoking and intense exercise. The main sources of selenium are fish and seafood, meat and poultry, eggs, dairy produce and bread. Selenium in the food supply depends on the concentration of selenium in the soil and soil–plant interactions. The soil level of selenium is greatly affected by climate–soil interactions so even minor changes in climate are predicted to increase soil loss of selenium and have negative effects on the nutritional quality of food (Jones et al., 2017). Selenium has an unusually narrow window of concentrations between deficiency and excess (selenosis), which makes it difficult to advise about the use of supplements unless existing plasma levels are known. Recommendation of dietary plant sources and amounts are also made difficult by the very marked variations in selenium content depending upon where the plants are grown.

Magnesium

Magnesium is sometimes described as being the 'forgotten' electrolyte. Magnesium forms part of the chlorophyll molecule so green leafy vegetables, grains, cereals and legumes are rich in magnesium; other sources include fruit, meat, fish and hard water. Women who consume a wide variety of foods including plenty of fruit and leafy vegetables are unlikely to be deficient in magnesium. Placental transport is significant and involves both active and passive transport mechanisms; fetal serum levels are higher than maternal levels but the fetus is not protected from maternal magnesium deficiency (Morton, 2018).

Magnesium status has been implicated in broad range of pregnancy complications including preterm labour (via uterine hyperirritability), pregnancy-induced hypertension and preeclampsia, IUGR, cerebral palsy and neurodevelopment (Zarean and Tarjan, 2017). Studies of women from poor socioeconomic backgrounds, who have a higher risk of poor pregnancy outcome, often have hypomagnesaemia. However, it is not clear whether hypomagnesaemia is a cause of adverse outcomes of pregnancy or a result of underlying disorders such as poorly controlled diabetes or a marker for other nutritional or health stresses (Morton, 2018).

Iodine

Iodine is a component of the thyroid hormones: thyroxine (T_4) and its active form triiodothyronine (T_3), which are essential in growth and development and in energy metabolism. Deficiency of iodine has multiple adverse effects throughout life; these are collectively known as iodine deficiency disorders (IDDs). Thyroid hypertrophy (goitre) is the classical sign of iodine deficiency, which represents the physiological adaptation to a low intake. Secretion of thyroid-stimulating hormone (TSH; see Chapter 3) increases when iodine intake becomes insufficient; this stimulates thyroid hypertrophy and hyperplasia. Thyroid iodine clearance increases and urinary excretion decreases.

Iodine requirements in pregnancy are increased by >50% because the pregnant woman's thyroid hormone production increases, the fetus has a high requirement and maternal urinary excretion is increased. The fetal brain is very vulnerable to maternal hypothyroidism because it is dependent on placental transport of maternal T_4 until the fetal thyroid gland starts to synthesize its own thyroid hormones at ~12 weeks' gestation (note that the thyroid gland is not fully mature until close to term). Thyroid hormones are required for neuronal migration and myelination of nerves. Maternal hypothyroidism is indicated by increased TSH and low free concentrations of T_4.

Iodine deficiency in pregnancy can cause maternal and fetal hypothyroidism; it is the most significant cause of preventable mental retardation worldwide. In pregnancy, severe iodine deficiency is associated with LBW and preterm delivery, congenital abnormalities, increased pregnancy loss, stillbirth, increased perinatal and infant mortality, and psychomotor, speech and hearing defects; the classic combination of gross mental impairment, short stature, spastic diplegia and deaf mutism is termed 'cretinism' (Zimmermann, 2012). Mild-to-moderate iodine deficiency during pregnancy is thought to adversely affects both maternal and infant thyroid function and has implications for the neurocognitive development of the infant. Marginal iodine deficiency in pregnancy may be associated with impaired development but small effects on mental development such as IQ score reduced by a few points are difficult to assess, particularly as it is difficult to measure dietary salt and therefore iodine intake and the studies are usually confounded by other factors affecting child neurodevelopment or coexisting nutrient deficiencies. Several other nutrients are required for synthesis of thyroid hormones including selenium, iron, zinc, copper and vitamin A.

The most cost-effective way of improving iodine status in regions affected by iodine deficiency is by iodized salt consumption; in some countries it is mandatory to fortify table-salt. In many countries, individuals are consuming less salt for well-founded health reasons (usually related to hypertension), consumption of commercially produced and processed foods that do not contain iodized salt has increased and there is reduced use of iodophors for cleaning equipment in the dairy industry. Pregnant women and women planning pregnancy are advised to take an iodine-containing supplement of ~150 µg/day to optimize development of the fetus; this supplement is prescribed to all pregnant women in many countries.

UNDERNUTRITION IN PREGNANCY

Undernutrition is the lack of one or more nutrients. Malnutrition includes undernutrition (nutritional deficiencies), excess or imbalance in energy or nutrient intake. In experimental animals, maternal undernutrition in pregnancy usually leads to decreased birthweight. Maternal weight gain in human pregnancy is positively associated with birthweight and developmental outcome. However, in nutritional assessment it is important to determine pre-pregnancy weight from objective data and to assess the level of oedema. Women who are underweight (or anaemic) have an increased risk of pregnancy loss or delivering small babies that have increased morbidity and mortality. It is difficult to dissociate the effects of a poor diet in pregnancy from other variables. Women who consume a poor diet in pregnancy are likely to have consumed a poor diet before pregnancy, to do so after pregnancy, and more likely to have had a poorer diet during their own growth and development. There is an intergenerational cycle of malnutrition; it is difficult to identify the best place to intervene and break this cycle. Many undernourished women are shorter than average and a poor diet is often associated with an increased prevalence of smoking. Maternal shortness is also associated with a poorer social background, young maternal age and less formal education. Paradoxically, poor maternal nutrition resulting in a LBW infant can programme metabolic changes that predispose the infant to be at increased risk of obesity and cardiometabolic disease in later life. The 'double burden of malnutrition' refers to the concurrent presence of obesity and underweight in the same populations or same communities (or even the same families). Concerns about the public health implications of these problems has led to initiatives such as '1000 Days', which promotes good nutrition between conception and the child's second birthday (270 + 365 + 365 = 1000) and encompasses the vulnerable period of critical brain development and the related UN-led 'Scaling Up Nutrition' (SUN) movement, which aims to address maternal and child undernutrition.

Diet Quality

Although many nutritional studies have focused on energy requirements and consumption in pregnancy, the quality of the diet as well as the quantity is also important. In Britain, nutrient-deficiency diseases are rare but the quality of the diet varies markedly (see below). Mothers of LBW babies have not only low energy intakes but also diets of low nutrient density. Even in affluent countries, many women have daily intakes of B vitamins below the recommended level. Lifestyle changes, such as adopting more sedentary behaviour, may result in energy requirements decreasing. However, nutrient requirements may not fall in parallel; indeed, pollution and smoking increase requirements of certain nutrients. This means that, although energy consumption may need to decrease to match reduced energy expenditure, the density of nutrients within the diet may need to increase to ensure that requirements are met.

Supplementation

Nutrient supplementation studies of the diet in pregnancy have often produced inconsistent and inconclusive results. Balanced protein:energy supplementation reduces the risk of a SGA infant (Ota et al., 2015) but high protein supplementation significantly increases the risk of SGA (da Silva Lopes et al., 2017). Lower concentrations of protein have very small effects. Oral supplementation of pregnant women indicates that low-dose calcium, vitamin A, zinc, multiple micronutrient (MMN) supplements, nutritional education and the use of preventative antimalarial drugs decreased the likelihood of LBW, whereas supplementation with high-dose calcium, zinc and omega 3 fatty acids and nutrition education decreased the risk of preterm delivery (da Silva Lopes et al., 2017). The effects are more likely to be significant if the women were markedly deficient in the nutrient being supplemented. Many of the studies are small and some may be methodologically flawed. Supplementation in the second and third trimesters of pregnancy may also be too late to have an effect on birthweight; however, it may benefit maternal health and work potential and improve breastfeeding efficiency. Earlier supplementation may have a greater effect because nutrient support of early follicular development and maternal nutrient stores prior to conception may programme the fetal growth trajectory. More research studies to investigate the effectiveness of supplementation with essential nutrients on the outcomes of pregnancy (nutrition-specific interventions) and to address the underlying causes of undernutrition (nutrition-sensitive interventions) are warranted.

Fetal Adaptation to Undernutrition

Subjected to inadequate substrate levels of either nutrients or oxygen, the fetus exhibits developmental plasticity to adapt to what is available by changing its metabolic activity in order to survive *in utero* and to optimize chances of surviving after birth in a nutritionally poor environment. Slowing of growth and reducing energy expenditure (e.g. metabolic rate) are part of this adaptation. Growth accounts for a large proportion of energy expenditure. Adapting to a lower growth trajectory means that nutrient requirement decreases and available nutrient levels may then be adequate. The placenta, which has a high nutrient and oxygen requirement itself, may also adapt. Although a number of adult-onset diseases are associated with impaired fetal nutrition (Fig. 12.7), they tend not to affect reproductive ability as they cause pathological problems late in life. Animal studies have demonstrated that marginal malnourishment for many generations requires optimal nutrition for several generations before normal size and behaviour are expressed. This intergenerational effect may be one of the reasons why dietary supplementation in pregnancy has such a small effect on outcome. It is clear that parental and environmental factors such as diet, body composition, metabolism and stress markedly influence subsequent patterns of health and disease throughout life; a concept

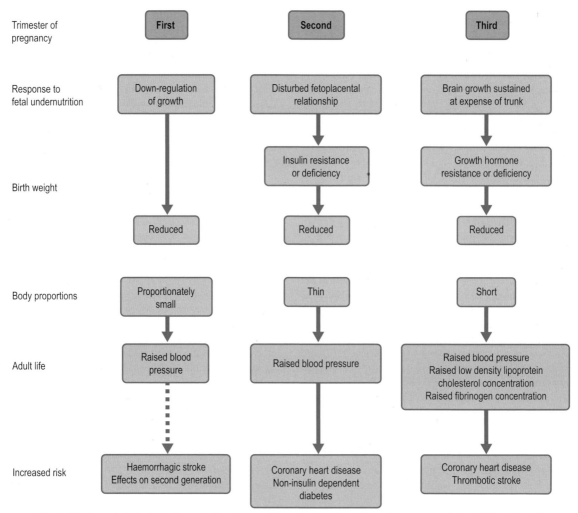

Fig. 12.7 Association of adult-onset diseases and impaired fetal nutrition. The response to nutritional insult in different trimesters of pregnancy has a differential effect on the growth of the fetus (and therefore body weight and body proportions at birth) and on the risk of adult-onset disease. In practice, fetal undernutrition is unlikely to affect fetal growth for a single trimester only.

encapsulated as the Developmental Origins of Health and Disease (DOHAD) model (Fleming et al., 2018).

Malnutrition

Interesting results come from studies looking at the effect of nutrient deprivation on previously well-nourished women (summarized by Roseboom, 2017). The Dutch Hunger Winter, from September 1944 to May 1945, was due to the Nazi blockade of food supplies, exacerbated by very severe winter weather conditions. The severe nutritional deficiency affected fertility and birthweights and the birth rate fell dramatically, by about 50%, 9 months later. This was due both to effects on ovulation and an increased

incidence of pregnancy failure. Congenital malformation rate increased among babies conceived during the famine and in the following 4 months (with adequate food supplies), which demonstrates the importance of good preconceptual nutrition. However, many women were already pregnant at the time of the food shortage. If the women were deprived of energy in the second half of their pregnancy, the birthweight of their babies was reduced by 350 g on average. These babies were thin but of normal length. They appeared to develop and grow normally. However, in adulthood the male babies who had been exposed to deficiency late in development had lower rates of obesity compared with those who had experienced restricted nutrient levels early in development. Young women who had been exposed to nutrient deficiency early in gestation, but not later, had normal birthweights themselves. However, their babies were smaller than expected. Adults of lower birthweight have increased risk of developing type 2 diabetes mellitus, heart disease, hypertension, obstructive lung disease, hypercholesterolaemia and renal disease. However, results from the longer, more severe Leningrad siege do not show any association between intrauterine malnutrition and glucose intolerance and coronary heart disease in adulthood.

Transient nutrient deficiency may alter fetal growth patterns without affecting final birthweight very much. Birthweight is a crude outcome measure of optimal gestational growth and development. Suboptimal maternal body composition and nutrient intake can have a long-term effect on the offspring without necessarily affecting size at birth; there may be time for recovery and catch-up growth. Birthweight does not differentiate between the subtler effects of nutrition on body composition and development of specific tissues and organs. It may not identify growth restriction; a similar birthweight can be attained with different growth trajectories. For instance, if an infant does not reach its potential birthweight but is born above 2500 g, it will not be classified as being of LBW even though its growth is not optimal. Nutrient deprivation before pregnancy or early in gestation affects brain growth and development in animals, which suggests that 'programming' of later brain growth is determined by nutrient availability before the demand for nutrients occurs. Lung growth is affected by later nutritional deficiency; lung weight and composition, muscle function, defence mechanisms and surfactant production are all susceptible to nutritional insult in late pregnancy.

MATERNAL OBESITY

Maternal obesity (usually defined as prepregnancy BMI >30 kg/m^2) complicates all aspects of pregnancy; it is associated with larger babies, macrosomia and increased perinatal mortality. Large-for-gestational-age babies are usually no longer in length but have increased deposition of adipose tissue. Routine antenatal care is more difficult in obese women, and labour is more likely to be prolonged and unsuccessful. Obese women are at higher risk of disorders such as hypertension, thromboembolism, preeclampsia and gestational diabetes. Obese women tend to have increased problems during delivery with more caesarean sections and associated problems; operative delivery is more complicated and there is increased risk in the puerperium (Dolin and Kominiarek, 2018. Maternal obesity is also associated with an increased incidence of congenital

malformations in the infant (Persson et al., 2017), particularly NTD (folic acid is less effective), and is a significant determinant of the infant's later risk of obesity, type 2 diabetes, cardiovascular disease and asthma (Godfrey et al., 2017). Ideally, obese women who are planning pregnancy should be encouraged to lose weight before conceiving.

LIFESTYLE ISSUES

Alcohol

Prenatal alcohol exposure (PAE) can cause fetal alcohol spectrum disorders (FASD), a group of conditions, which include fetal alcohol syndrome (FAS), partial fetal alcohol syndrome (pFAS), alcohol-related birth defects (ARBD) and alcohol-related neurodevelopmental disorder (ARND). Alcohol readily crosses the placenta so maternal alcohol levels determine alcohol levels in fetal blood. Alcohol is teratogenic and affects embryonic development, growth, fetal brain function and later behaviour. Exposure of the fetus to alcohol can cause dramatic and irreversible term behavioural and developmental problems; particular periods of embryonic development may be more vulnerable than others and patterns of drinking (such as regular or binge drinking) may determine the extent of the effect, which is affected by other dietary factors and genetics. For many years, there was an ongoing discussion about whether there was a 'safe' limit of alcohol exposure during pregnancy. Modern research methods using 3-dimensional imaging of craniofacial phenotyping, animal studies and epigenetic analysis confirm that there is no safe period or safe level of PAE (Sarman, 2018).

Fetal alcohol syndrome, the most easily recognizable outcome of fetal alcohol exposure, is characterized by intrauterine and postnatal growth retardation, characteristic unusual facial features and adverse effects on brain function leading to mental retardation and/or behavioural disturbances. Alcohol exposure during embryogenesis causes apoptosis of the cranial neural crest cells perturbing the sequence of events that establish the facial bones and neurons (Smith et al., 2014). More extreme outcomes occur if the fetus is exposed to regular heavy alcohol intake or to very high alcohol concentrations at critical periods in development. However, fetuses exposed to lower amounts of alcohol are also affected with fetal alcohol spectrum disorder, which results in a range of symptoms that can be more difficult to diagnose definitively. These symptoms include impaired growth, microcephaly and facial features: short palpebral fissures (eye width is decreased), smooth philtrum (the grove between the nose and mouth is flattened) and narrow vermillion (the upper lip is thinned) (del Campo and Jones, 2017) (Fig. 12.8) The extent of

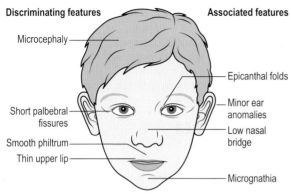

Discriminating features

Microcephaly

Short palpebral fissures

Smooth philtrum

Thin upper lip

Associated features

Epicanthal folds

Minor ear anomalies

Low nasal bridge

Micrognathia

Fig. 12.8 Facial characteristics of fetal alcohol syndrome.

brain damage is correlated to the distinctiveness of the facial characteristics. Infants exposed to alcohol *in utero* may demonstrate withdrawal symptoms after birth such as hyperactivity, excessive crying, irritability, weak sucking, disturbed sleep, tremors and seizures.

Alcohol consumption is commonly under-reported and, in recent years, 'standard' serving sizes and usual alcohol content of alcoholic beverages such as wine and lagers have increased making the recommendations based on alcohol units difficult to follow. It can be difficult to reassure women who have had a small amount of alcohol before realizing that they were pregnant and still maintain advocacy for abstinence. Treatment such as child–parent and behavioural therapies, nutrition and drug treatments may improve the outcomes for the affected child.

Smoking

Although some women stop or reduce smoking when they become pregnant, a significant proportion continue to smoke throughout pregnancy. Smoking (and environmental or secondhand tobacco smoke) is associated with increased early spontaneous abortion and placental complications such as miscarriage placental abruption, sudden infant death syndrome, growth restriction (particularly head size and femur length) and decreased birthweight, preterm delivery and long-term behavioural and psychiatric disorders. The effects are more marked when maternal smoking continues beyond the first trimester (Abraham et al., 2017). The physiological mechanisms are not clear but both nicotine and carbon monoxide are vasoconstrictors and may affect blood flow to placental and fetal tissues. Nicotine can increase maternal blood pressure and heart rate, which may compromise uterine blood flow. Carbon monoxide binds to haemoglobin forming carboxyhaemoglobin, which can cause fetal hypoxia and is implicated in sudden infant death syndrome. Cigarette smoke also contains lead, cadmium and thiocyanate, all

of which are potentially hazardous to the fetus. Cigarette smoke is a source of free radicals and oxidative stress. Smoking is also thought to affect absorption of micronutrients and to increase nutrient utilization. Thus, smoking increases maternal micronutrient requirements but may also decrease the appetite and food consumption. Smokers are more likely to consume alcohol and other substances that interact with nutrient metabolism and are less likely to take nutrient supplements. Many women who smoke in pregnancy, or who quit smoking during pregnancy and resume in the postpartum period, may be influenced by weight concerns. The most effective therapies for smoking cessation in pregnancy are behavioural interventions but many other approaches are being investigated.

Caffeine

Consumption of caffeine is topical and health and safety messages about it are often confusing. Caffeine is a pharmacologically active mild stimulant present in beverages, such as coffee, black and green tea and cola-type drinks, energy chocolate and medications such as cold remedies, allergy preparations, headache medications, diuretics and stimulants. New caffeine-containing products have been introduced such as chewing gum, doughnuts and syrups. Caffeine in pregnancy is associated with increased risk of fertility problems, implantation and placental problems, congenital abnormalities, pregnancy loss, IUGR, and behavioural problems in the children exposed to caffeine during development. In rat studies, fetal exposure to caffeine is associated with decreased bone mineralization.

Caffeine is lipid soluble and readily crosses the placenta but the enzymes involved in caffeine metabolism are not expressed by the placenta or fetal tissues, so caffeine accumulates in the fetus. There are genetic and individual differences in caffeine metabolism: some individuals metabolize caffeine more slowly (so fetal exposure would be higher). In pregnancy, oestrogen affects the clearance of caffeine so the half-time of caffeine metabolites can reach 18 h in the third trimester.

It is difficult to establish a safe dose of caffeine for human pregnancy as there are difficulties in assessing intake (in observational studies), identifying whether the woman is a fast or slow metabolizer of caffeine (genetic test) and ethical issues related to possible intervention studies. There is no international consensus about a safe intake but in many countries, it is currently recommended that pregnant women limit their caffeine consumption to about 200 mg/day. This varies between countries but the range is 100 to 300 mg/day, though some researchers suggest all caffeine consumption be avoided (Chen et al., 2016). The caffeine content of tea and coffee ranges markedly (with type of coffee bean, its processing and how it is prepared) but 200 mg caffeine is roughly equivalent to two mugs of instant coffee, one and a half mugs of filter coffee, four average mugs of tea, five cans of regular cola drinks, about two and a half cans of 'energy' drinks or 200 g of plain chocolate (caffeine in milk chocolate is about half that in plain chocolate). Most pregnant women report reduced consumption of caffeine.

Drug Use, Medication, Herbs and 'Smart' Drinks

Most medications prescribed to pregnant or breastfeeding women will have been evaluated for safety and the maternal benefit weighed against the risk of the drug being transported across the placenta and affecting the fetus. No drug is without side-effects and anxiety about birth defects is a major parental concern. Anti-anxiety drugs, antidepressants, and neuroleptic drugs may affect neurotransmitter function of the developing central nervous system. Many recreational drugs such as amphetamines, heroin, cannabis (marijuana) and hallucinogens are harmful in pregnancy. It is important that pregnant women discuss their conditions, concerns or plans to self-medicate with health practitioners including pharmacists.

Many women use herbal and complementary medicine during pregnancy, possibly because they want to control their health without using conventional medication, which may be considered riskier (Bruno et al., 2018), or because friends or health practitioners have recommended them. They are often easier to access and are perceived to be safe; use of the internet has brought more information about their use into the public domain. A number of herbs have pharmacological actions, and the safety and effectiveness of these and others are not known; there are also concerns about quality control, adulteration and contamination. Some herbs are known to be unsuitable in pregnancy; for instance, raspberry leaf tea can stimulate contractions and is used to induce labour. Other herbs that should be avoided in pregnancy include black cohosh, pennyroyal, mugwort, and Ma Huang (ephedra). Pregnant women are recommended to choose herbal teas made with ingredients that are a normal part of their diet such as mint, blackcurrant or orange extracts and avoid unfamiliar substances. Herbal teas should preferably be purchased from reputable sources.

Carbonated drinks are not harmful for pregnant and breastfeeding women per se; carbonation itself does not present problems. Carbonated drinks maybe SSB; these are usually not nutrient dense. They can significantly increase the intake of sucrose or fructose contributing to energy intake and may displace drinks that could provide more nutrients. The consumption of artificially sweetened beverages (ASB) is increasing; the implications for pregnant women are not known. Other ingredients in 'smart' drinks (also known as 'new age', 'designer' or 'energy' drinks) may be of concern. High levels of caffeine are commonly added to energy drinks. Guarana, a Brazilian berry extract, is a stimulant related to caffeine. Ginseng is also not recommended for pregnant women. Many of the smart drinks also contain higher levels of amino acids and vitamins than are considered optimal for pregnant women.

Exercise

Historically, there was a concern that exercise in pregnancy would constitute a threat to fetal wellbeing by creating a competition for energy substrates between the mother and her fetus. Extensive research over the last 50 years has demonstrated that not only is this not the case but also that exercise in pregnancy is beneficial. Physiological adaptations of the cardiovascular and glucometabolic systems ensure the fetus is protected during exercise and that placental and fetal tissue perfusion and oxygenation and nutrient delivery are maintained (Newton and May, 2017). Exercise begun in early pregnancy enhances placental development and fetal growth. Pregnant women who exercise have reduced fat gain, more rapid weight loss after pregnancy, improved mood, improved sleep patterns and a lower risk of gestational diabetes and hypertensive disorders (Gregg and Ferguson, 2017). It is suggested that there is a shorted first stage of labour and less likelihood of a need for caesarean section in women who exercise. However, women tend to decrease their activity as pregnancy progresses. It is recommended that women should be encouraged to begin or continue low-volume or moderate-intensity exercise (20–30 min/day or at least 150 min/week) throughout pregnancy.

The aim should be to maintain a good fitness level during pregnancy rather than to reach peak fitness or train for competitive events. Moderate aerobic and strength-conditioning exercises (such as swimming, yoga, stretching, biking and walking) as part of a healthy lifestyle are considered safe and beneficial for both healthy normal- and overweight pregnant women. Exercise, on its own or part of a lifestyle programme, may also be useful in the prevention and treatment of maternal and fetal complications of pregnancy such as gestational diabetes and preeclampsia. Activities that minimize the risk of loss of balance and falls that might cause fetal trauma are recommended, whereas activities that result in respiratory stress (hyperventilation) or hyperthermia should be avoided. Prolonged and excessive anaerobic exercise could create hyperthermia and dehydration and have the potential to affect uterine activity (Newton and May, 2017). Certain activities such as contact sports and walking or running on rocky or unstable ground should be avoided (as joint laxity and centre of gravity are affected by pregnancy). In late pregnancy, exercises that involve lying on the back are best avoided as the weight of the uterus can impede venous return to the heart and may cause postural hypotension (see Chapter 11). Women are advised to seek advice before starting an exercise programme in pregnancy and to seek immediate advice for any injury. Pregnant women with certain conditions such as a history of bleeding or preterm labour, placenta praevia (where the placenta is low in the uterus), anaemia, preeclampsia or hypertension, and medical conditions that limit cardiovascular reserve should be assessed before starting exercise programmes. Pregnant women taking part in physical activity should be fed and well hydrated, wear appropriate footwear, take frequent breaks and avoid exercising in extremely hot or humid weather (Gregg and Ferguson, 2017).

There are differences in physiological responses to exercise in pregnant women who are acclimatized and have physiological tolerance to high altitude (live at high altitude) and pregnant visitors to high altitude (Davenport

et al., 2018). Fetal oxygenation does not seem to be affected by air travel but unaccustomed and excessive exercise at high altitude may be associated with hyperventilation and pregnancy complications such as dehydration, bleeding and preterm labour.

Work and Physical Stress

Strenuous work and physical stress can potentially influence micronutrient status and outcome of pregnancy. Women in employment may be at risk of compromised diets because they have less time for shopping and cooking. Peak energy expenditure, length of time spent standing (which has been shown to affect patterns of meals consumed) and type of activity (for instance, lifting may result in greater intra-abdominal pressure) may be more significant. Particular occupations, long and/or irregular working hours and shift work may be associated with a poorer outcome of pregnancy.

KEY POINTS

- The diet before pregnancy, as well as that consumed during pregnancy, can affect the nutrient status of the woman.
- The increased energy requirements of pregnancy can be met by a combination of increasing intake, decreasing activity and changing metabolism.
- A good-quality, nutrient-dense diet can supply most of the additional protein, vitamin and mineral requirements of pregnancy.

- Energy restriction and obesity affect reproductive function, both male and female fertility and fetal growth.
- Pregnancy-induced hormonal changes, including insulin resistance, affect transfer of nutrients to the placenta and fetus.
- Adaptation to poor nutrition in pregnancy results in changes in growth *in utero* and birthweight and may be linked to disease in adult life.

APPLICATION TO PRACTICE

Advice on nutrition in pregnancy is important before and during pregnancy, and also for subsequent pregnancies.

Women who have a poor history of nutrition are at risk and the midwife needs to be aware of this to aid in the detection of problems associated with poor dietary intake.

Women with low body fat may have problems conceiving and so active weight gain may need to be encouraged to optimize conception.

Women with high body fat may also have problems conceiving. Obese women are at much higher risk from complications during pregnancy, delivery and the postnatal period.

ANNOTATED FURTHER READING

Kaiser LL, Campbell CG, Academy of Nutrition and Dietetics: Practice paper: nutrition and lifestyle for a healthy pregnancy outcome, *J Acad Nutr Diet* 114:1447, 2014.
A comprehensive summary of the nutritional requirements in pregnancy, designed to inform health practitioners.
Gluckman P, Hanson M, Seng CY, Bardsley A: *Nutrition and lifestyle for pregnancy and breastfeeding*, Oxford, 2015, Oxford University Press.
This builds on the work of David Barker and considers how lifestyle choices including nutrition affect fetal development and risk of later disease; includes birth outcomes and development in early childhood.

Griffin IJ: *Perinatal growth and nutrition*, Boca Raton, 2017, CRC Press.
This comprehensive book is divided into three sections: the first section concentrates on the growth and dietary recommendations for preterm infants; the second section focuses on the literature exploring the causes of IUGR and its effects in later life; the third section explores ways to reduce incidence of extrauterine growth retardation and to optimize catch-up growth.
Kapoor D, Teahon K, Wallace SVF: Inflammatory bowel disease in pregnancy, *Obstetrician, Gynaecologist* 18:205–212, 2016.
A review of the management and risk of complications during pregnancy in women with inflammatory bowel disease (Crohn's and ulcerative colitis).

Mottola MF, Davenport MH, Ruchat SM, et al.: 2019 Canadian guideline for physical activity throughout pregnancy, *Br J Sports Med* 52:1339–1346, 2018.

An extensive consideration of the best practice about exercising in pregnancy; a thorough consideration of research studies leading to the best guidance for women.

Moussa HN, Nasab SH, Haidar ZA, et al.: Folic acid supplementation: what is new? Fetal, obstetric, long-term benefits and risks, *Future Sci* 2:FSO116, 2015.

A comprehensive review of the state of knowledge about folic acid and neural tube defects, which includes a history of the research underlying the recommendations, other health benefits, concerns about drug interactions and the effects of fortification.

Saccone G, Berhella V, Sarno L, et al.: Celiac disease and obstetric complications: a systemic review and meta-analysis, *Am J Obstet Gynecol* 214(2):225–234, 2016.

An in-depth meta-analysis evaluating risks of obstetric complication associated with untreated and treated coeliac disease.

Slater C, Morris L, Ellison J, Syed AS: Nutrition in pregnancy following bariatric surgery, *Nutrients* 9:1338, 2017.

A review of the types of bariatric surgery and the nutritional challenges that they can present; particularly important given that most bariatric surgery in women is for those of reproductive age, many of whom were not able to conceive before surgery.

REFERENCES

Abraham M, Alramadhan S, Iniguez C, et al.: A systematic review of maternal smoking during pregnancy and fetal measurements with meta-analysis, *PLOS ONE* 12:e0170946, 2017.

Akerele OA, Cheema SK: A balance of omega-3 and omega-6 polyunsaturated fatty acids is important in pregnancy, *J Nutr Intermed Metab* 5:23–33, 2016.

Akseer N, Al-Gashm S, Mehta S, et al.: Global and regional trends in the nutritional status of young people: a critical and neglected age group, *Ann N Y Acad Sci* 1393:3–20, 2017.

Allen-Walker V, Woodside J, Holmes V, et al.: Routine weighing of women during pregnancy-is it time to change current practice? *BJOG* 123:871–874, 2016.

Augustin LS, Kendall CW, Jenkins DJ, et al.: Glycemic index, glycemic load and glycemic response: An International Scientific Consensus Summit from the International Carbohydrate Quality Consortium (ICQC), *Nutr Metab Cardiovasc Dis* 25:795–815, 2015.

Baker BC, Hayes DJ, Jones RL: Effects of micronutrients on placental function: evidence from clinical studies to animal models, *Reproduction* 156:R69–R82, 2018.

Berggren EK, O'Tierney-Ginn P, Lewis S, et al.: Variations in resting energy expenditure: impact on gestational weight gain, *Am J Obstet Gynecol* 217:445, 2017.

Blumfield ML, Hure AJ, MacDonald-Wicks L, et al.: Systematic review and meta-analysis of energy and macronutrient intakes during pregnancy in developed countries, *Nutr Rev* 70:322–336, 2012.

Brannon PM, Taylor CL: Iron supplementation during pregnancy and infancy: uncertainties and implications for research and policy, *Nutrients* 9, 2017.

Brissot P, Pietrangelo A, Adams PC, et al.: Haemochromatosis, *Nat Rev Dis Primers* 4:18016, 2018.

Bruno LO, Simoes RS, de Jesus SM, et al.: Pregnancy and herbal medicines: an unnecessary risk for women's health – A narrative review, *Phytother Res* 32:796–810, 2018.

Butte NF, King JC: Energy requirements during pregnancy and lactation, *Public Health Nutr* 8:1010–1027, 2005.

Campbell-Brown M, Hytten FE: Nutrition. In Chamberlain G, Broughton Pipkin F, editors: *Clinical physiology in obstetrics*, ed 3, Oxford, 1998, Blackwell, pp 165–191.

Chamberlain C, O'Mara-Eves A, Porter J, et al.: Psychosocial interventions for supporting women to stop smoking in pregnancy, *Cochrane Database Syst Rev* 2:CD001055, 2017.

Chen LW, Wu Y, Neelakantan N, et al.: Maternal caffeine intake during pregnancy and risk of pregnancy loss: a categorical and dose-response meta-analysis of prospective studies, *Public Health Nutr* 19:1233–1244, 2016.

Chu DM, Antony KM, Ma J, et al.: The early infant gut microbiome varies in association with a maternal high-fat diet, *Genome Med* 8:77, 2016.

Coad J: Pre- and periconceptual nutrition. In Morgan JB, Dickerson JWT, editors: *Nutrition in early life*, Chichester, 2003, Wiley, pp 39–71.

Coad J, Al Rasasi B, Morgan J: Nutrient insult in early pregnancy, *Proc Nutr Soc* 61:51–59, 2002.

Costa-Rodrigues J, Sa-Azevedo R, Balinha J, Ferro G: Vegetarianism during pregnancy: risks and benefits, *Trends Food Sci Technol* 79:28–34, 2018.

da Silva Lopes K, Ota E, Shakya P, et al.: Effects of nutrition interventions during pregnancy on low birthweight: an overview of systematic reviews, *BMJ Glob Health* 2:e000389, 2017.

Davenport MH, Steinback CD, Borle KJ, et al.: Extreme pregnancy: maternal physical activity at Everest Base Camp, *J Appl Physiol (1985)* 125:580–585, 2018.

Del Campo M, Jones KL: A review of the physical features of the fetal alcohol spectrum disorders, *Eur J Med Genet* 60:55–64, 2017.

De Ocampo MPG, Araneta MRG, Macera CA, et al.: Folic acid supplement use and the risk of gestational hypertension and preeclampsia, *Women Birth* 31:e77–e83, 2018.

Ditzenberger GR: Calcium and phosphorus metabolism. In Blackburn ST, editor: *Maternal, fetal & neonatal physiology: a clinical perspective*, Oxford, 2018, Elsevier, pp 571–588.

Dolin CD, Deierlein AL, Evans MI: Folic acid supplementation to prevent recurrent neural tube defects: 4 milligrams is too much, *Fetal Diagn Ther* 44:161–165, 2018.

Dolin CD, Kominiarek MA: Pregnancy in women with obesity, *Obstet Gynecol Clin North Am* 45:217–232, 2018.

Donazar-Ezcurra M, Lopez-Del BC, Bes-Rastrollo M: Primary prevention of gestational diabetes mellitus through nutritional factors: a systematic review, *BMC Pregnancy Childbirth* 17:30, 2017.

Dorniak-Wall T, Grivell RM, Dekker GA, et al.: The role of L-arginine in the prevention and treatment of pre-eclampsia: a systematic review of randomized trials, *J Hum Hypertens* 28:230–235, 2014.

Ducker GS, Rabinowitz JD: One-carbon metabolism in health and disease, *Cell Metab* 25:27–42, 2017.

Elango R, Ball RO: Protein and amino acid requirements during pregnancy, *Adv Nutr* 7:839S–844S, 2016.

Englund-Ogge L, Brantsaeter AL, Haugen M, et al.: Association between intake of artificially sweetened and sugar-sweetened beverages and preterm delivery: a large prospective cohort study, *Am J Clin Nutr* 96:552–559, 2012.

Fisher AL, Nemeth E: Iron homeostasis during pregnancy, *Am J Clin Nutr* 106:1567S–1574S, 2017.

Fleming TP, Watkins AJ, Velazquez MA, et al.: Origins of lifetime health around the time of conception: causes and consequences, *Lancet* 391:1842–1852, 2018.

Gaiday AN, Tussupkaliyev AB, Bermagambetova SK, et al.: Effect of homocysteine on pregnancy: a systematic review, *Chem Biol Interact* 293:70–76, 2018.

Ganguly A, Tamblyn JA, Finn-Sell S, et al.: Vitamin D, the placenta and early pregnancy: effects on trophoblast function, *J Endocrinol* 236:R93–R103, 2018.

Gernand AD, Schulze KJ, Stewart CP, et al.: Micronutrient deficiencies in pregnancy worldwide: health effects and prevention, *Nat Rev Endocrinol* 12:274–289, 2016.

Godfrey KM, Reynolds RM, Prescott SL, et al.: Influence of maternal obesity on the long-term health of offspring, *Lancet Diabetes Endocrinol* 5:53–64, 2017.

Greene ND, Leung KY, Copp AJ: Inositol, neural tube closure and the prevention of neural tube defects, *Birth Defects Res* 109:68–80, 2017.

Gregg VH, Ferguson JE: Exercise in pregnancy, *Clin Sports Med* 36:741–752, 2017.

Harreiter J, Schindler K, Bancher-Todesca D, et al.: Management of pregnant women after bariatric surgery, *J Obes* 2018:4587064, 2018.

Hayden RP, Flannigan R, Schlegel PN: The role of lifestyle in male infertility: diet, physical activity, and body habitus, *Curr Urol Rep* 19:56, 2018.

Herrera E, Desoye G: Maternal and fetal lipid metabolism under normal and gestational diabetic conditions, *Horm Mol Biol Clin Investig* 26:109–127, 2016.

Herrera E, Ortega-Senovilla H: Lipid metabolism during pregnancy and its implications for fetal growth, *Curr Pharm Biotechnol* 15:24–31, 2014.

Herring CM, Bazer FW, Johnson GA, Wu G: Impacts of maternal dietary protein intake on fetal survival, growth, and development, *Exp Biol Med (Maywood)* 243:525–533, 2018.

Hollis BW, Johnson D, Hulsey TC, et al.: Vitamin D supplementation during pregnancy: double-blind, randomised clinical trial of safety and effectiveness, *J Bone Miner Res* 26:2341–2357, 2011.

Hytten FE: Nutrition. In Hytten F, Chamberlain G, editors: *Clinical physiology in obstetrics*, ed 2, Oxford, 1991, Blackwell, p 153.

Jebeile H, Mijatovic J, Louie JCY, et al.: A systematic review and metaanalysis of energy intake and weight gain in pregnancy, *Am J Obstet Gynecol* 214:465–483, 2016.

Jones GD, Droz B, Greve P, et al.: Selenium deficiency risk predicted to increase under future climate change, *Proc Natl Acad Sci USA* 114:2848–2853, 2017.

Jones P, Lucock M, Veysey M, Beckett E: The vitamin D-folate hypothesis as an evolutionary model for skin pigmentation: an update and integration of current ideas, *Nutrients* 10, 2018.

Juriloff DM, Harris MJ: Insights into the etiology of mammalian neural tube closure defects from developmental, genetic and evolutionary studies, *J Dev Biol* 6, 2018.

Khaing W, Vallibhakara SA, Tantrakul V, et al.: Calcium and vitamin D supplementation for prevention of preeclampsia: a systematic review and network meta-analysis, *Nutrients* 9, 2017.

Khalil A, Hardman L, Brien O: The role of arginine, homoarginine and nitric oxide in pregnancy, *Amino Acids* 47:1715–1727, 2015.

Kominiarek MA: Peaceman AM: Gestational weight gain, *Am J Obstet Gynecol* 217:642–651, 2017.

Langley-Evans SC: Nutrition in early life and the programming of adult disease: a review, *J Hum Nutr Diet* 28(Suppl. 1):1–14, 2015.

Lawrence M: *Food fortification: the evidence, ethics, and politics of adding nutrients to food*, Oxford, 2013, OUP.

Lewis RM, Childs CE, Calder PC: New perspectives on placental fatty acid transfer, *Prostaglandins Leukot Essent Fatty Acids* 138:24–29, 2018.

Li K, Wahlqvist ML, Li D: Nutrition, one-carbon metabolism and neural tube defects: a review, *Nutrients* 8, 2016.

Liauw J, Jacobsen GW, Larose TL, Hutcheon JA: Short interpregnancy interval and poor fetal growth: evaluating the role of pregnancy intention, *Paediatr Perinat Epidemiol* 33:O73–O85, 2019.

Lim SS, Kakoly NS, Tan JWJ, et al.: Metabolic syndrome in polycystic ovary syndrome: a systematic review, meta-analysis and meta-regression, *Obes Rev* 20:339–352, 2019.

Lintas C: Linking genetics to epigenetics: The role of folate and folate-related pathways in neurodevelopmental disorders, *Clin Genet* 95:241–252, 2019.

Maffoni S, De GR, Stanford FC, Cena H: Folate status in women of childbearing age with obesity: a review, *Nutr Res Rev* 30:265–271, 2017.

Makrides M: Understanding the effects of docosahexaenoic acid (DHA) supplementation during pregnancy on multiple outcomes from the DOMInO trial, *OCL* 23, 2016.

Makrides M, Best K: Docosahexaenoic acid and preterm birth, *Ann Nutr Metab* 69(Suppl. 1):29–34, 2016.

Manta-Vogli PD, Schulpis KH, Dotsikas Y, Loukas YL: The significant role of amino acids during pregnancy: nutritional support, *J Matern Fetal Neonatal Med* 1–7, 2018.

Meier RK: Polycystic ovary syndrome, *Nurs Clin North Am* 53:407–420, 2018.

Moran VH, Robinson S: Pregnancy and lactation. In Geissler C, Powers H, editors: *Human nutrition*, Oxford, 2017, OUP, pp 337–355.

Morton A: Hypomagnesaemia and pregnancy, *Obstet Med* 11:67–72, 2018.

National Institute for Health and Clinical Excellence (NICE): *Weight management before, during and after pregnancy*, London, 2010, NHS.

Newton ER, May L: Adaptation of maternal-fetal physiology to exercise in pregnancy: the basis of guidelines for physical activity in pregnancy, *Clin Med Insights Womens Health* 10:1179562X17693224, 2017.

Ota E, Hori H, Mori R, et al.: Antenatal dietary education and supplementation to increase energy and protein intake, *Cochrane Database Syst Rev* 6:CD000032, 2015.

Palmsten K, Homer MV, Zhang Y, et al.: In vitro fertilization, interpregnancy interval, and risk of adverse perinatal outcomes, *Fertil Steril* 109:840–848, 2018.

Panth N, Gavarkovs A, Tamez M, Mattei J: The influence of diet on fertility and the implications for public health nutrition in the United States, *Front Public Health* 6:211, 2018.

Paul L: Selhub J: Interaction between excess folate and low vitamin B12 status, *Mol Aspects Med* 53:43–47, 2017.

Payne M, Stephens T, Lim K, et al.: Lysine requirements of healthy pregnant women are higher during late stages of gestation compared to early gestation, *J Nutr* 148:94–99, 2018.

Persson M, Cnattingius S, Villamor E, et al.: Risk of major congenital malformations in relation to maternal overweight and obesity severity: cohort study of 1.2 million singletons, *BMJ* 357:j2563, 2017.

Rasmussen KM, Abrams B, Bodnar LM, et al.: Recommendations for weight gain during pregnancy in the context of the obesity epidemic, *Obstet Gynecol* 116:1191–1195, 2010.

Rasmussen KM, Catalano PM, Yaktine AL: New guidelines for weight gain during pregnancy: what obstetrician/gynecologists should know, *Curr Opin Obstet Gynecol* 21:521–526, 2009.

Robertson SM, Clayton EH, Friend MA: Reproductive performance of ewes grazing lucerne during different periods around mating, *Anim Reprod Sci* 162:62–72, 2015.

Rodriguez-Gonzalez GL, Castro-Rodriguez DC, Zambrano E: Pregnancy and lactation: a window of opportunity to improve individual health. In Guest PC, editor: *Investigations of early nutrition effects on long-term health*, New York, 2018, Humana Press, pp 115–140.

Roseboom TJ: *The effects of prenatal exposure to the Dutch famine 1944–1945 on health across the lifecourse, Handbook of famine, starvation, and nutrient deprivation: from biology to policy*, Springer, 2017, pp 1–15.

Roytio H, Mokkala K, Vahlberg T, Laitinen K: Dietary intake of fat and fibre according to reference values relates to higher gut microbiota richness in overweight pregnant women, *Br J Nutr* 118:343–352, 2017.

Rumbold A, Ota E, Nagata C, et al.: Vitamin C supplementation in pregnancy, *Cochrane Database Syst Rev* 9:CD004072, 2015.

Sabbahi M, Li J, Davis C, Downs SM: *The role of the sustainable development goals to reduce the global burden of malnutrition; In advances in food security and sustainability*, Oxford, 2018, Elsevier.

Saffrey J, Stewart M, editors: *Maintaining the whole. SK 220 Human biology and health Book 3*, Milton Keynes, 1997, Open University Press.

Sarman I: Review shows that early foetal alcohol exposure may cause adverse effects even when the mother consumes low levels, *Acta Paediatr* 107:938–941, 2018.

Scaramuzzi RJ, Campbell BK, Downing JA, et al.: A review of the effects of supplementary nutrition in the ewe on the concentrations of reproductive and metabolic hormones and the mechanisms that regulate folliculogenesis and ovulation rate, *Reprod Nutr Dev* 46:339–354, 2006.

Schoenaker DA, Mishra GD, Callaway LK, Soedamah-Muthu SS: The role of energy, nutrients, foods, and dietary patterns in the development of gestational diabetes mellitus: a systematic review of observational studies, *Diabetes Care* 39:16–23, 2016.

Silvestris E, de PG, Rosania R, Loverro G: Obesity as disruptor of the female fertility, *Reprod Biol Endocrinol* 16:22, 2018.

Smith SM, Garic A, Berres ME, Flentke GR: Genomic factors that shape craniofacial outcome and neural crest vulnerability in FASD, *Front Genet* 5:224, 2014.

Stangret A, Skoda M, Wnuk A, et al.: Mild anemia during pregnancy upregulates placental vascularity development, *Med Hypotheses* 102:37–40, 2017.

Stephens TV, Payne M, Ball RO, et al.: Protein requirements of healthy pregnant women during early and late gestation are higher than current recommendations, *J Nutr* 145:73–78, 2015.

USDA: *2015–2020 Dietary Guidelines for Americans*, ed 8, U.S. Department of Health and Human Services and U.S. Department of Agriculture, 2015.

Villamor E, Jansen EC: Nutritional determinants of the timing of puberty, *Annu Rev Public Health* 37:33–46, 2016.

Wadhwani N, Patil V, Joshi S: Maternal long chain polyunsaturated fatty acid status and pregnancy complications, *Prostaglandins Leukot Essent Fatty Acids* 136:143–152, 2018.

Wagner CL, Hollis BW: The implications of vitamin D status during pregnancy on mother and her developing child, *Front Endocrinol (Lausanne)* 9:500, 2018.

Wald NJ, Morris JK, Blakemore C: Public health failure in the prevention of neural tube defects: time to abandon the tolerable upper intake level of folate, *Public Health Rev* 39:2, 2018.

Walker R, Kumar A, Blumfield M, Truby H: Maternal nutrition and weight management in pregnancy: a nudge in the right direction, *Nutr Bull* 43:69–78, 2018.

WHO: *Global health sector strategy on sexually transmitted infections 2016–2021: toward ending STIs*, Geneva, 2016, World Health Organization.

Wilson RL, Grieger JA, Bianco-Miotto T, Roberts CT: Association between maternal zinc status, dietary zinc intake and pregnancy complications: a systematic review, *Nutrients* 8, 2016.

Wiseman EM, Bar-El DS, Reifen R: The vicious cycle of vitamin a deficiency: a review, *Crit Rev Food Sci Nutr* 57:3703–3714, 2017.

Witt SH, Frank J, Gilles M, et al.: Impact on birthweight of maternal smoking throughout pregnancy mediated by DNA methylation, *BMC Genomics* 19:290, 2018.

Wu Z, Hou Y, Hu S, et al.: Catabolism and safety of supplemental l-arginine in animals, *Amino Acids* 48:1541–1552, 2016.

Yang M, Li W, Wan Z, Du Y: Elevated homocysteine levels in mothers with neural tube defects: a systematic review and meta-analysis, *J Matern Fetal Neonatal Med* 30:2051–2057, 2017.

Zarean E, Tarjan A: Effect of magnesium supplement on pregnancy outcomes: a randomized control trial, *Adv Biomed Res* 6:109, 2017.

Zhang M, Goyert G, Lim HW: Folate and phototherapy: what should we inform our patients? *J Am Acad Dermatol* 77:958–964, 2017.

Zhang R, Han S, Chen GC, et al.: Effects of low-glycemic-index diets in pregnancy on maternal and newborn outcomes in pregnant women: a meta-analysis of randomized controlled trials, *Eur J Nutr* 57:167–177, 2018.

Zheng J, Feng Q, Zhang Q, et al.: Early life fructose exposure and its implications for long-term cardiometabolic health in offspring, *Nutrients* 8, 2016.

Zimmermann MB: The effects of iodine deficiency in pregnancy and infancy, *Paediatr Perinat Epidemiol* 26(Suppl. 1):108–117, 2012.

Physiology of Parturition

LEARNING OBJECTIVES

- To describe uterine changes in pregnancy and its preparation for labour.
- To discuss theories of the initiation and timing of parturition in humans.
- To relate factors thought to be involved with initiation of labour to methods for inducing and augmenting

labour, possible causes and treatment of preterm labour.
- To describe the effects of labour on maternal and fetal physiology.
- To outline the physiology of pain in relation to childbirth and the rationale for choice of pain relief.

INTRODUCTION

The success of pregnancy and, ultimately, the survival of the species, depend on the baby being born healthy and mature enough to survive. In pregnancy and labour, the uterus has to fulfil two very different functions. It has to grow but remain quiescent during pregnancy to allow fetal development and then, at the appropriate time, commence the powerful and coordinated contractions, which result in the birth of the infant at parturition. However, successful pregnancy also requires the maturation of the fetal systems essential for extrauterine survival. The mother also needs to be physiologically prepared for lactation. Therefore, the maturation of the fetus and the onset of labour need to be synchronized. Asynchrony leads to preterm birth (≤37 weeks' gestation). Most human fetuses are capable of surviving birth and are born at term (defined as between the end of the 37th week (notation: 37^{+0} or 37 0/7 weeks of pregnancy) and ~42 weeks (notation: 41^{+6} or 41 6/7), when the probability for neonatal survival is optimal. Preterm birth (<37 completed weeks or <259 days since the first day of the women's last menstrual period) is the leading cause of death in children under 5 years of age, accounting for about one-third of the 3.1 million neonatal deaths annually and occurs globally in 8–12% of all pregnancies, with rates increasing in developed countries. In 2010, an estimated 15 million births worldwide were preterm, ~11.1% of all live births (Blencowe et al., 2012). In 2012, complications associated with preterm birth resulted in the death of ~1 million babies worldwide as well as long-term disabilities

in those children that survived (Lawn 2014). The rates of preterm births in 2010 ranged from ~5% in several European countries to 18% in some African countries, and the USA was ranked 6 in the world with 12% (Blencowe et al., 2012). Modern practices such as women giving birth at a later age and fertility treatment (often associated with subsequent multiple pregnancies) have increased the incidence of preterm birth (Lee et al., 2019). In addition, people of certain ethnicities, low socioeconomic status, or having low body mass index, as well as conditions like bacterial vaginosis or other infections (e.g. periodontal disease), inflammation, vascular disease, uterine overdistension, stress, smoking and a history of preterm delivery and abortion are all risk factors for spontaneous preterm birth (Vogel et al., 2018). The causes of preterm birth are not well understood, which limits effective obstetric and neonatal care. Therapeutic approaches currently focus on arresting or slowing the progress of established preterm labour and promoting fetal survival, however, early diagnosis, treatment and primary prevention of preterm birth are surprisingly unsuccessful, reflecting a lack of understanding of the physiological mechanisms involved in the triggering of parturition and how these go wrong.

Most early neonatal deaths that are not associated with a lethal deformity are associated with prematurity and preterm infants have an increased risk of complications not just in the neonatal period but in the long term (Luu et al., 2017). Long-term consequences include cognitive and motor neurodevelopment disabilities that include cerebral

CHAPTER CASE STUDY

While working in Africa, Zara had been able to assist several of her African friends during childbirth, all of which had occurred at home and were attended by mostly female relatives who had informed Zara that they would only call the local midwife if they felt things were going wrong. All her friends had had uncomplicated deliveries and Zara felt quite privileged to have witnessed childbirth in such a different way to how it is presented within most modern Western societies.

Zara is keen to have a waterbirth at home and wants to avoid all forms of pharmacological pain relief. She also wants her sister and some of her close friends who are also heavily pregnant to be present if possible. As Zara has had all her antenatal care from her midwife, she particularly wants her midwife to care for her in labour, especially as her midwife has extensive experience of waterbirth.

- What factors do you think will be a positive influence on enabling Zara to have a normal birth?
- Would you encourage Zara to write a birth plan and, if so, what would you suggest she should do to facilitate the birth?
- Would you be able to discuss and explain the potential benefits and risks of Zara's birth plan?
- What would you advise her and James to do in preparation for the birth?

palsy, neurocognitive impairment, deafness, blindness, learning disabilities, chronic lung disease and possibly an increased risk of disease in adult life. The shorter the gestation, the poorer the prognosis. Even though extremely low-birthweight (LBW) babies (i.e. those born below 1000 g) may now survive, it is generally associated with high rates of morbidity and much emotional stress for their parents, as well as a high financial burden on neonatal intensive care units. There are also long-term health and education costs associated with physical and learning disabilities and neurodevelopmental complications. It can be argued that one of the principal objectives of obstetrics is to reduce the incidence of preterm labour. The survival rate of premature infants born alive with borderline viability has improved over the last decade; however, improved survival rates have not been matched by a proportional decrease in the incidence of disability (Helenius et al., 2017).

In what are classified as 'extremely preterm' births (<28 weeks' gestation) a crucial stage of fetal development exists where the boundary between viability and long-term morbidity and mortality is encountered. Studies on the survival rates among 600,000+ live births in England and Wales in 2005 reported that survival to the age of 1 year rose from 5.3% to 15.6% and 41.8% in offspring born at 22, 23 and 24 weeks' gestation, respectively (Moser et al., 2008). A narrow, 2-week window of fetal viability seems to exist, therefore, between 22 and 24 weeks' gestation whereby the likelihood of survival of the offspring to 1 year is increased by approximately eightfold, for reasons which are, as yet, unclear.

There are three categories of causes of preterm birth: iatrogenic or indicated, where complications of pregnancy such as eclampsia, severe preeclampsia or intrauterine growth retardation trigger obstetric intervention and the deliberate induction of premature delivery (30–35% of cases) to improve fetal viability; preterm premature rupture of (fetal) membranes (PPROM), which may be associated with infection (25–30% of cases); and spontaneous or idiopathic preterm labour (SPTL; 40–45% of cases), presumably due to unknown maternal or fetal factors but are potential therapeutic targets (Govindaswami et al., 2018). Effective prevention of SPTL has enormous potential to lower the incidence and adverse health consequences of preterm birth but requires a much better understanding of the mechanisms which trigger parturition in order that these may be targeted therapeutically while minimizing the effects of any drugs used on non-uterine tissues. For example, the suppression of preterm uterine contractions by tocolytic drugs such as oxytocin receptor (OTR) antagonists (e.g. Atosiban) has no dangerous side-effects on other tissues, unlike the widespread effects of β-adrenergic agonists across multiple maternal and fetal tissues. Tocolytic drugs can sometimes delay delivery to allow time for corticosteroid administration and to allow patient transfer to a hospital with intensive care facilities, but their widespread use to prevent SPTL awaits an understanding of the triggering mechanisms of parturition, which has been sadly lacking for decades. Approximately one-third of preterm births are a consequence of intrauterine infection; these pregnancies are frequently terminated irrespective of gestational age because of possible serious consequences for the fetus or mother. The failure of spontaneous labour is also not well understood; prolonged pregnancy (gestation >42 weeks or 294 days) is also associated with increased fetal morbidity and mortality but is now relatively uncommon because of obstetric intervention.

The factors orchestrating the transition from ongoing pregnancy to labour are not completely understood but are very important, both in determining the possible causes of preterm labour and their prevention, and in understanding how to induce labour successfully without eliciting fetal distress. The factors that control the onset of human (and primate) parturition remain elusive. There are marked differences between human and other mammalian species in the cascade of events that lead to parturition. Humans have a very high rate of premature birth compared with

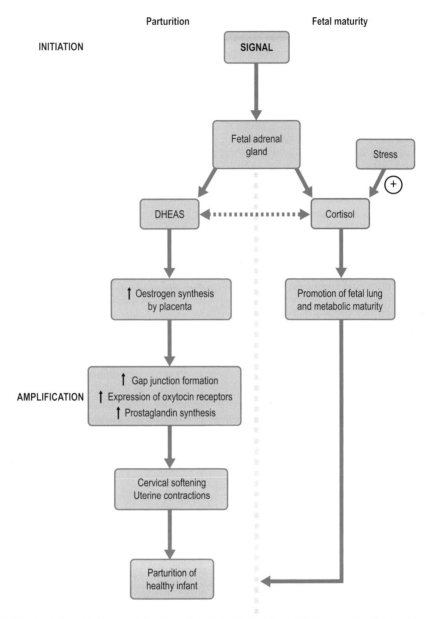

Fig. 13.1 The two distinct pathways controlling parturition and fetal development in the human. DHEAS, dehydroepiandrosterone sulphate.

other species. For most domestic and laboratory animals the duration of gestation is remarkably constant; for example, there is <1% variation in sheep (Heck et al., 2018). Theoretically, the length of gestation does not matter to the mother. The crucial aspect is that the baby can survive from birth. It has become clear, therefore, that the fetus contributes significantly to controlling the length of gestation, together with maternal and uteroplacental signals.

Certainly, in some experimental animals, e.g. sheep, there is proven fetal involvement in the timing of labour but it is difficult to obtain such evidence in humans.

In other species, it seems that the same signal that controls fetal maturation also triggers the onset of labour so fetal developmental state and parturition are synchronized. In humans, the two pathways seem to be separable (Fig. 13.1). The human fetus appears to undergo lung maturation 4–6 weeks before labour, unlike other species in which the signals initiating labour also ensure fetal organ maturity. It is not clear why the events leading to parturition should be so complex in humans; however, it seems plausible that a variable length of gestation is advantageous. The complexity of control of parturition in humans might allow a transfer of control from mother to fetus. Thus, in early pregnancy, it may be physiologically expedient for the mother to terminate the pregnancy if it is harmful for her long-term health to continue. Spontaneous termination of a pregnancy that is unlikely to be completed, for example because maternal nutrient intake is insufficient, prevents needless maternal investment. Later in gestation, once the fetus is mature enough to survive, fetal control of parturition would allow the fetus to remain in the uterus if the environment was favourable. The fetus could respond to stress by switching from cell division and growth to accelerated maturation and earlier initiation of parturition. This would suggest that intrauterine growth restriction is part of an adaptive response to fetal stress, which increases survival as long as the stressor is not too early or too severe. It is not surprising, therefore, that many of the signals involved in parturition are also involved in physiological stress responses. Midwifery and obstetric management of women in labour is often interventionist. This chapter covers the physiology of parturition; for information about clinical management, readers are referred to midwifery texts in the list of further reading.

STAGES OF LABOUR

From a clinical point of view, labour is often divided into three stages (Fig. 13.2). However, physiologically there is no abrupt transition between these stages. The events leading to the onset of labour are gradually and inconspicuously initiated earlier in the pregnancy, and the three stages overlap. Occasionally, labour can be very short (combined first and second stage <2 h) with only a few strong contractions required to expel the baby; this is clinically referred to as a precipitate delivery. It is more likely with multiparous woman who have either very strong contractions or a relaxed tone of the pelvic floor muscles; it can appear to occur if the early stages of labour were pain-free and not noticed. Precipitate delivery usually does not give the uterine tissues time to stretch so lacerations and haemorrhage are common.

The first stage is that of progressive cervical dilation (or dilatation) timed from the onset of regular coordinated contractions accompanied by progressive effacement (thinning) and dilation of the cervix. Assessment of cervical effacement is subjective, as effacement may occur before

the onset of labour especially in multiparous women where the cervix thins but does not actively dilate until the onset of regular, effective contractions. The end of this stage is marked by the full dilation of the cervix as the uterine contractions pull the entire tissue of the cervix upwards until it becomes incorporated into the lower uterine segment (LUS), continuous with the cylindrical uterine wall. This stage lasts an average of 12–14 h in primiparous women but tends to be shorter in multiparous women. The second stage is fetal expulsion, from full cervical dilation until the delivery of the baby. The contractions are usually regular and strong, aided by the respiratory muscles, primarily the diaphragm. The second stage may take over an hour in primigravidae and as little as a few minutes in multiparous women. The third stage of labour involves separation and complete expulsion of the placenta and membranes, and control of bleeding from the uteroplacental circulation. The return to the prepregnant state is described as the puerperium (see Chapter 14).

From a physiological point of view, it is useful to think of labour being related to phases of uterine myometrial activity. For most of pregnancy, the uterus is in phase 0, the quiescent phase. Under the influence of progesterone (the literal meaning of progesterone is 'pro-gestation', i.e. promoting and sustaining pregnancy), the uterus is relatively quiet (quiescent) and has a low response to stimuli. Other factors involved in promoting quiescence are prostacyclin, nitric oxide, relaxin, parathyroid hormone-related peptide, calcitonin gene-related peptide and vasoactive intestinal peptide (Amini et al., 2019). All these factors act to either increase cyclic adenosine monophosphate (cAMP) (or cGMP) concentrations in endometrial smooth muscle or to prevent increases in intracellular Ca^{2+} that would trigger myometrial contraction. In late pregnancy, the uterus changes from being quiescent (having a low level of muscle activity) to being activated; this is known as phase 1, the activation phase. This transition to activation 'marks' the initiation of labour; labour results from activation and then stimulation of the myometrium. The receptors and signalling pathways are modulated so they respond to contractile stimuli. Activation is partially stimulated by mechanical stretch of the uterus together with changes in signalling via endocrine and paracrine pathways, possibly resulting from an increased activity of the fetal hypothalamic–pituitary–adrenal (HPA) axis. Increased levels of oestrogen and corticotrophin-releasing hormone (CRH) lead to an upregulation of genes that code for contraction-associated proteins (CAPs), including genes for the gap junction protein connexin 43, prostaglandin production and oxytocin receptors. The increased production of oestrogen may be due to increased availability of fetally derived precursors. In the third phase of parturition, phase 2 – stimulation, the

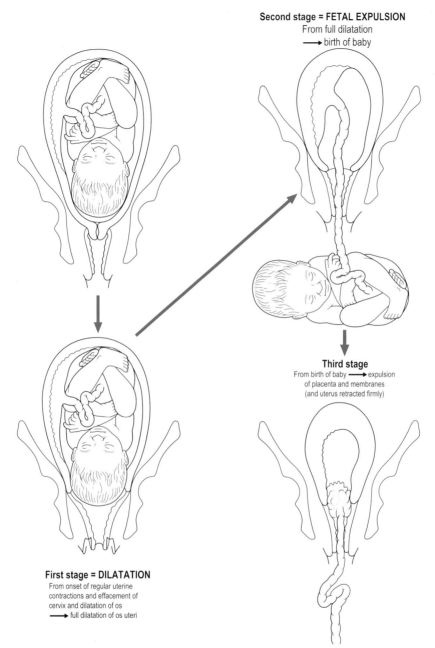

Second stage = FETAL EXPULSION
From full dilatation
⟶ birth of baby

Third stage
From birth of baby ⟶ expulsion
of placenta and membranes
(and uterus retracted firmly)

First stage = DILATATION
From onset of regular uterine
contractions and effacement of
cervix and dilatation of os
⟶ full dilatation of os uteri

Fig. 13.2 Stages of labour.

activated uterus is spontaneously excitable and responsive to uterotonins such as prostaglandins, oxytocin and CRH; so it develops coordinated, effective, regular and forceful contractions. The activation of the uterus in this stimulation phase initiates a positive feedback loop whereby the initial signals become further amplified and the uterus

becomes increasingly stimulated facilitating progression of the first and second stages of labour. This phase is accompanied by inflammatory-like biochemical changes. It is now realized that the population of immune cells that reside in the decidua, immediately adjacent to the fetal membranes, play a vital role in several aspects of both the

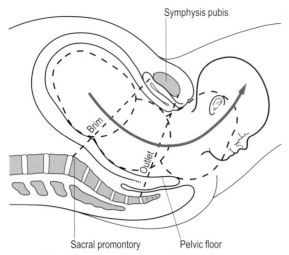

Fig. 13.3 Expulsion through the birth canal.

maintenance of pregnancy, the tolerance of the 'foreign' (allogeneic) paternal antigens expressed by the fetus (see Chapter 10), and the triggering of parturition. Leading up to parturition, this decidual population of immune cells changes with an increasing secretion of proinflammatory cytokines. This is seen in both term and preterm labour. This inflammatory signalling cascade results in an increased expression of genes that promote myometrial contractility and the production of proteases, which are involved in remodelling and ripening (softening and shortening) of the cervical tissue. The uterus is able to perform a remarkable mechanical effort to expel its contents – the baby, placenta and associated membranes and fluids – through the birth canal (Fig. 13.3). The final phase is the uterine involution phase resulting in the remodelling of the uterus and its return to a near prepregnant state and size (see Chapter 14).

THE UTERUS AT TERM

Uterine Growth in Pregnancy

The uterine muscle undergoes exceptional growth throughout pregnancy to accommodate the growing fetus and prepare for birth. The prepregnant weight of the uterus is about 50 g in a nulliparous woman and about 60–70 g in a multiparous woman with a capacity of about 10 mL. During pregnancy, uterine size increases 20-fold, to about 800–1200 g and a capacity of about 5 L.

Initially, the uterus grows by hyperplasia (increasing cell number). This is under the influence of oestrogen and, unlike later growth, occurs regardless of the site of implantation. By the 4th month, the uterine wall has thickened from 10 mm to 25 mm. Subsequent growth is due to hypertrophy (an increase in cell size) and stretch stimulated by uterine distension. The uterine wall thins and the smooth muscle cells increase markedly in length (from 50 μm to 500 μm long and from 5 μm to 15 μm wide) as they accumulate the increase in contractile proteins. The increased overall size is accompanied by a change in uterine shape from an ovoid sphere to a slightly tapered cylinder. By term, the organization of the myometrial cells is such that they develop the intrinsic capability to produce coordinated, strong and effective contractions. The uterine muscle is innervated by adrenergic, cholinergic and peptidergic fibres, which are more abundant in the cervix and uterine tubes. The uterus also has many sensory nerves.

By the third trimester, the uterine wall is thin, ~5–10 mm by term; the fetal movements are visible and the fetus can be palpated through the abdominal and uterine walls (Blackburn, 2018). The uterine fundus, at this stage, almost reaches the liver and displaces the stomach and intestine. The blood vessels in the nonpregnant uterus are extremely tortuous and coiled (see Chapter 2); this allows them to adapt to the increased requirements of the expanding uterine tissue. Uterine blood flow increases in pregnancy as the blood vessel diameter increases and resistance to flow decreases. This makes auscultation of the uterine blood flow easier and is referred to as the uterine or placental soufflé. It is usually heard in the second trimester and is synchronous with the maternal pulse.

Uterine Muscle Organization

The uterus is predominantly comprised of bundles, each containing 10–50 myometrial (smooth muscle) cells, separated by connective tissue formed of collagen and elastin. The distribution of the smooth muscle varies throughout the length of the uterus. The smooth muscle density is highest in the fundus of the uterus (an approximate ratio of smooth muscle fibres:connective tissue of 9:1) and gradually declines until the cervix where the ratio is 1:4. Associated with the myometrium are leukocytes, which produce cytokines. Procontractile proteins such as oxytocin receptors and connexin 43 are preferentially expressed in the fundal region of the uterus so that contraction moves the fetus down towards the cervix and birth canal. The isthmus, which forms the lower segment of the uterus, has a lower smooth muscle content. The lower segment forms at about weeks 28–30 of pregnancy. Caesarean sections late in gestation are usually via the lower segment of the uterus (lower-segment caesarean section, LSCS), whereas the incision in an emergency 'classic' caesarean section earlier in pregnancy usually is on the midline of the uterus and is likely to dictate the use of caesarean sections for future deliveries. Contractile

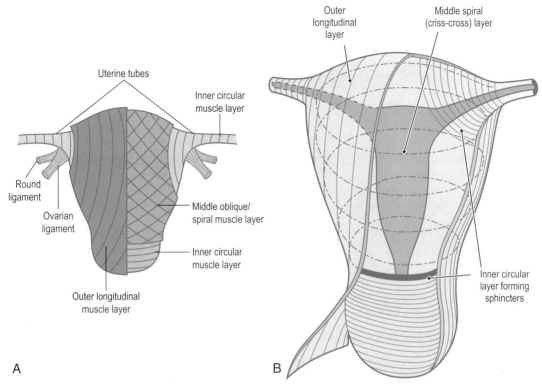

Fig. 13.4 Uterine muscle layers: (A) the inner and outer muscle layers; (B) spiral organization of central smooth muscle fibres. ((A) Reproduced from Macdonald S, Johnson G. *Mayes' Midwifery*, ed 15, Elsevier 2017, Fig. 24.13; (B) Stillerman E, *Prenatal massage: a textbook of pregnancy, labor, and postpartum bodywork*, Elsevier 2008, Fig. 5.33.)

strength is related to the proportion of smooth muscle and the degree of its stretch (Young and Barendse, 2014). Therefore, the upper part of the uterus contracts strongly and the lower segment, which has a diminishing proportion of muscle, contracts weakly and passively (see Fig. 13.10) so that, at delivery, the fetus is pushed towards the birth canal.

The uterine muscle forms three distinct anatomical layers, which are more evident with the hypertrophy of the uterus that occurs in pregnancy (Fig. 13.4). The innermost layer has muscle mostly in a longitudinal orientation. The myometrium has more muscle fibres in the inner layer than it does in the outer layers. The outermost layer has longitudinal and circular fibres. The middle layer of uterine muscle has spiralling fibres and is particularly well vascularized. It is this middle layer that ensures the blood vessels in the uterus are occluded in the third stage of labour as the crisscrossing spiralling fibres contract around the blood vessels, acting as 'living ligatures'. The LUS has a high expression of CRH receptor type I, which is involved in relaxation and of the enzymes involved in cervical ripening.

The Myometrium

The myometrium is formed of myometrial smooth muscle cells embedded in a collagen-rich connective tissue matrix, which has blood vessels interspersed within it. The cytoplasm of the myometrial cells or myocytes is packed with long random bundles of actin and myosin. Compared with skeletal muscle, the concentration of actin is higher and the myosin has longer filaments, which increases the maximum shortening of the contractile cells. Unlike the terminally differentiated skeletal and cardiac muscle cell types, smooth muscle tends to be much more 'plastic' and able to change its growth patterns and contractile responsiveness. The myosin family of proteins are ubiquitous in cells and one member of this family, myosin II, is the motor protein responsible for smooth muscle contraction. It is both a structural protein and a Mg-ATPase, an enzyme that can hydrolyse ATP and utilize the energy released by this hydrolysis for movement. When ATP is hydrolysed, actin and myosin cross-bridges form so that actin filaments slide past each other, shortening the cell so that the muscle contracts (Fig. 13.5). Myosin is made up of two long heavy chains, which

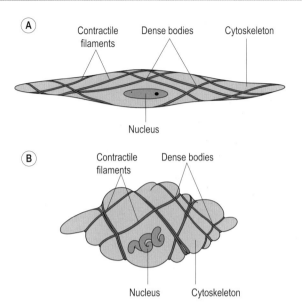

Fig. 13.5 Cell shortening and myosin contractile elements in myometrial muscle contraction: (A) relaxed; (B) contracted.

interact with other myosin molecules and each chain contains a globular head unit containing the ATPase activity. The two myosin heavy chains are associated with two copies of each of two light chains, which bind calcium and undergo phosphorylation. Phosphorylation is the incorporation of a phosphate group into the protein, catalysed by myosin light-chain kinase (MLCK), which effectively activates the protein. Factors that negatively affect myometrial contractility may be important in maintaining uterine quiescence through pregnancy; those that increase contractility may be important in facilitating the progression of labour.

The Role of Calcium

Our understanding of the signalling pathways involved in myometrial contraction comes mostly from research conducted on rats and mice, since availability of human tissue is very limited and even when small biopsies are available from caesarean section this is prior to the important physiological changes that accompany labour. Muscle contraction is triggered by a rise in the intracellular calcium ion (Ca^{2+}) concentration that results from action potentials triggered in myocytes. Electrical activity, calcium ion influx and development of myometrial tension are precisely synchronized. Calcium ions bind to the calcium-binding protein calmodulin (CAM), which regulates the activity of many of the intracellular enzymes, generating a cascade of reactions leading to binding of actin and myosin (Wray et al., 2015). Binding of calcium to CAM forms a Ca–CAM

complex that activates MLCK. MLCK is inhibited when calcium levels are low. The activated MLCK undergoes a conformational change, which exposes the catalytic site so the protein can be phosphorylated and will interact with actin, initiating contractions. Removal of calcium results in dephosphorylation of myosin by myosin light-chain phosphatase and causes muscle relaxation. Smooth muscle contraction can therefore be increased either by activating MLCK or by inhibiting myosin phosphatase. In the case of premature labour, drugs, which inhibit the transfer of calcium into the myometrial cells, are used to try to prevent contractions (see below).

Calcium enters the myometrial cell from the extracellular fluid and is released from intracellular organelles including the sarcoplasmic reticulum of the myometrial cells. Calcium released from the sarcoplasmic reticulum can prime contractions that need to be sustained by calcium influx. Recording of membrane potential using tiny glass microelectrodes inserted into contracting myometrium showed that bursts of brief action potentials could initiate brief and relatively small contractions; bursts of multiple action potentials were required for the generation of strong and sustained contractions. The underlying mechanism of these action potentials is Ca^{2+}-entry via voltage-operated calcium channels. Calcium-activated potassium channels set the threshold of activation of the cell membrane. There is a good correlation between intracellular calcium concentration and the muscular force developed, with calcium ion concentrations (denoted $[Ca^{2+}]_i$) increasing from ~0.1 μM to 0.5 μM during contraction. Uterotonins (substances that stimulate myometrial contractility), such as prostaglandins and oxytocin, increase calcium influx and mobilize intracellular calcium stores, therefore increasing intracellular calcium concentrations and MLCK phosphorylation and increasing myometrial contraction. Agents that inhibit myometrial activity, such as progesterone, β-mimetics, relaxin and prostacyclin, decrease intracellular $[Ca^{2+}]$ by promoting calcium uptake into the intracellular stores, particularly the sarcoplasmic reticulum, so that free calcium levels in the cytosol decrease and the uterine muscle relaxes. Calcium channel blockers, such as nifedipine, prevent calcium entry into the cells promoting relaxation of the uterus.

The Control of Myometrial Contractions

Myometrium is an excitable tissue with a resting membrane potential that is negative (inside relative to outside the membrane). The smooth muscle cells generate action potentials independently of neural stimulation and are therefore termed myogenic. The pacemaker for this electrical activity remains uncertain. Intracellular calcium levels (and myometrial activity) are controlled by various

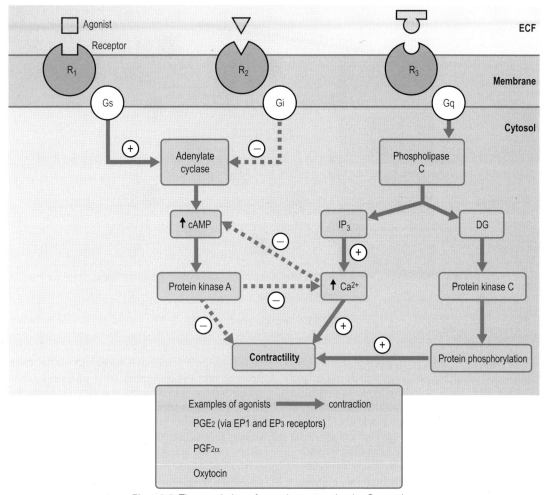

Fig. 13.6 The regulation of muscle contraction by G-proteins.

receptors on the myometrial cell membrane. Most hormones that affect myometrial contractility bind to receptor sites that are coupled to one of two G-proteins: $G_\alpha s$ or $G_\alpha q$ (see Chapter 3). The G-proteins act as transducers between the receptor and the effector regulating the cellular response by coupling the receptor to different signal-generating enzymes within the cell. These enzymes, in turn, generate an amplifying cascade of second messengers. The G-proteins allow the myometrial tissue to respond to a large number of agonists, which contribute to either relaxation or contraction (Fig. 13.6). One of the G-proteins ($G_\alpha q$) is linked to the enzyme phospholipase Cβ (PLCβ) and the inositol trisphosphate pathway (see Chapter 3). Binding of agonists (uterotonins) to receptors coupled to this G-protein activates phospholipase C (PLC), generating inositol trisphosphate and diacylglycerol. Inositol trisphosphate triggers the release of calcium ions (Ca^{2+}) from the sarcoplasmic reticulum raising cytosolic [Ca^{2+}], and diacylglycerol activates the enzymes protein kinase C and phospholipase A. The latter releases arachidonic acid from membrane phospholipids, which is the precursor of prostaglandins. The rise in cytosolic [Ca^{2+}] triggers smooth muscle contraction. The other G-protein pathway ($G_\alpha s$) activates adenylyl cyclase, the enzyme that generates cAMP. cAMP inhibits the release of calcium and therefore blocks muscle contraction. Agonists that stimulate this pathway, such as β-adrenergic receptor agonists and prostacyclin, will cause decreased release of Ca^{2+} from intracellular Ca^{2+} stores and dephosphorylation of myosin (so MLCK cannot bind Ca–CAM) and will therefore maintain uterine relaxation (Amini et al., 2019).

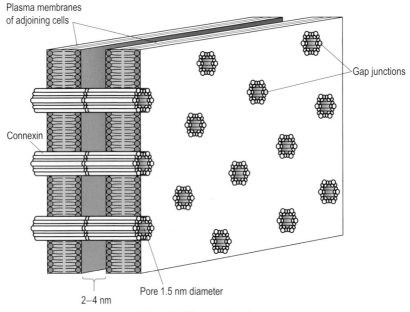

Plasma membranes
of adjoining cells

Gap junctions

Connexin

Pore 1.5 nm diameter

2–4 nm

Fig. 13.7 The gap junctions.

One of the many difficulties scientists have faced in trying to identify the signalling pathways, which trigger parturition, is that changes in hormone levels as pregnancy progresses to labour are only one part of the story. The effects of these hormones will change markedly if the type of receptor expressed by tissues changes and if these receptors are coupled to different signalling pathways. Such is the case with CRH (see below), which acts on different receptors coupled to different G-proteins at different stages of pregnancy to either maintain myometrial quiescence or, contrarily, trigger myometrial contractility and labour (Grammatopoulos, 2008).

Gap Junctions

The onset of regular uterine contractions is usually gradual, especially in primiparous women. As pregnancy progresses, the resting potential of the myometrial cells falls so that action potentials are generated with greater ease. Initially spontaneous uterine contractility is inhibited but becomes significant by mid-gestation. At about 20–24 weeks, hardening (or 'tightening') of the uterus can be felt as muscle contractions start. Initially, uterine activity is mostly of low amplitude and high frequency, with peak activity at night. This circadian rhythm stops at about 3 weeks before delivery, and may be mediated by cortisol or melatonin (Man et al., 2017). At first, small groups of myometrial cells contract together causing small fluctuations in intrauterine pressure. As pregnancy progresses, adjacent cells begin to contract synchronously so the contractions become more coordinated. This increased coordination results from cell–cell coupling and is due to the formation of gap junctions between adjacent cells.

Gap junctions are formed from bundles of proteins, called 'connexins', that align to form pore-like symmetrical channels across both plasma membranes of adjacent cells, so allowing the passage of small molecules from one cell to its neighbour and therefore communication. Gap junctions exist in other tissues where cells act together in a coordinated fashion, such as in the intercalated discs between adjacent cardiac muscle cells and between identical cell types in pancreatic islets. In the open state, gap junctions allow rapid transmission of signals such as electrical stimuli and second messengers such as Ca^{2+}, cAMP and inositol trisphosphate (Fig. 13.7). This means that depolarization and smooth muscle contraction in one cell are quickly communicated to adjacent cells so there is a synchronous contraction of multiple cells resulting in an increased contractile force.

There is an increase in the synthesis of the gap junction protein, connexin 43, and the number of gap junctions increases during gestation to ~1000 per myometrial cell. Physiological regulation of connexins and formation of gap junctions is by prostaglandins and steroid hormones; oestrogen and some prostaglandins increase and progesterone and nitric oxide suppress gap junction formation (Vannuccini et al., 2016). Gap junction density can be determined by measuring intercellular electrical resistance, which decreases just before parturition to about half of that in the nonpregnant uterus showing that the cells become very well coupled. Gap junction formation increases further prior to spontaneous labour, resulting in increased synchronization and coordination of high-amplitude high-frequency myometrial contractions, so intrauterine pressure is generated (Kidder and Winterhager, 2015). This is why palpation, especially near to term, can stimulate uterine tightening; palpation initiates the first stimulation of the uterus, which then spreads throughout the myometrium. Often fetal movements will trigger uterine tightening for the same reasons. Suppression of gap junctions may be important at the time of implantation and in early pregnancy.

Uterine Contractions and Quiescence

The uterus exhibits spontaneous, intrinsic contractility. A freshly biopsied specimen of uterine tissue, placed in a physiological solution, will contract involuntarily every 2–5 min without external stimulation. During the menstrual cycle, three distinct patterns of uterine contractility have been described. At the beginning of the cycle (menstruation), all layers of the myometrium contract exerting anterograde (from fundus to cervix) expulsive forces; these contractions may be associated with painful cramps (dysmenorrhoea). During the receptive window, in the late follicular phase, uterine contractility involves only the inner layers of the myometrium and is gentle and not perceived by women; this facilitates retrograde (cervix to fundus) transport of sperm towards the uterine tubes where fertilization usually takes place (see Chapter 7). As progesterone levels rise after ovulation, the uterus reaches a stage of quiescence. In pregnancy, progesterone continues to increase and to dampen the rhythmic activity of the uterus. Progesterone decreases the expression of genes for contraction-related proteins, stimulates the relaxant pathways and suppresses the stimulatory pathways of the myometrium and inhibits the binding of oxytocin to its receptors. Other inhibitors of uterine contractions early in pregnancy include relaxin, prostacyclin and nitric oxide, all of which increase intracellular cAMP and/or decrease intracellular calcium levels. It is also suggested that human chorionic gonadotrophin (hCG) inhibits myometrial contractility (see Chapter 3).

However, the uterus is never completely quiescent. From about 7 weeks, the contractions, or 'contractures', are irregular, not synchronized and nonfocal in origin; they have a very high frequency and a very low intensity (Wray et al., 2015). From mid-gestation, the contractions increase gradually in intensity and frequency until ~6 weeks before term when their intensity increases markedly. The early

Braxton Hicks contractions can be perceived but, although strong, they are not normally painful as the cervix remains closed. In labour, the contractions become synchronized, regular and more intense with increased duration. In primate models, in the few days before delivery, uterine contractions become synchronized during the night and disappear during the day until delivery. This pattern has not been observed in humans but women do have periods of active contractions, which then cease, suggesting there is also a degree of reversibility in the early stages of human labour.

The characteristics of the myometrium change markedly during pregnancy (Wray et al., 2015). In early pregnancy, there is a proliferative phase when the expression of IGF proteins is increased and an anti-apoptotic pathway is upregulated. This is followed by a synthetic phase of growth and remodelling involving cellular hypertrophy and increased synthesis of extracellular matrix proteins. In the third phase, the myometrial cells develop a contractile phenotype exhibiting increased excitability and sensitivity to calcium, spontaneous activity and enhanced responses to agonists. In the final phase of pregnancy, the myometrial cells are highly active and committed to labour. The cells are more excitable, there is increased connectivity between the cells and there are changes in the contractile proteins. In this phase, the myometrial cells actively participate in the inflammatory process by producing proinflammatory cytokines. There is a further stage of postpartum uterine involution where all the above changes are mostly reversed (see Chapter 14).

The Cervix

The consistency of the cervix changes in pregnancy to become softer and compliant in preparation for labour. For most of pregnancy, the cervix is a rigid cylindrical structure ~4–7 cm long, which forms a closed canal though in women who have had a previous vaginal delivery, the cervix may be slightly shorted with an internal diameter of ~1 cm. The cervix consists mostly of collagen fibrils, elastic connective tissue and blood vessels with some smooth muscle fibres. Connective tissue changes affect the whole uterus but are more evident in the cervix (due to its higher content). The uterine contractions imposed on the softened cervix result in it changing shape. During the pregnancy, the role of the cervix is to act as a closure for the uterus, containing its contents and protecting them from ascending infection. Prior to the delivery of the baby, the cervix loses its structural rigidity and is pulled by the uterine contractions so it changes from being a tubular closure to becoming a wide inverted-cone-shaped canal with very thin edges that is continuous with the rest of the uterine structure. In primigravida women, this shape change occurs in two distinct stages.

The first stage of cervical change is effacement, where the cylindrical shape is transformed into an inverted cone, but the internal sphincter, or os, is still patent and closed. The longitudinal muscle fibres of the cervix shorten. The differential localization of the fibres means that the outer margins of the cervix develop more tension so maximum uptake of the cervix occurs at the lower end and the external os and softer cervical tissue move upwards into the LUS. During vaginal examination, a midwife might feel an 'effacement ridge' of the cervical tissue undergoing effacement (Fig. 13.8) the ridge is the dissipating form of the external os. As the external os opens, usually the cervical mucus plug is lost, often associated with light bleeding from the rupture of superficial surface capillaries. This 'show' is often heralded as a sign of approaching labour but can occur quite a long time before labour is established.

The second stage begins when full dilation is reached (the edges of the internal os can no longer be felt); the uterus and vagina form one continuous 'sleeve' opening for the exit of the fetus. In multiparous women, the transition from one stage to the other is far less abrupt so effacement and dilation usually occur simultaneously. Dilation is due to the retraction or shortening of the upper part of the uterus, rather than pressure from the descending presenting fetal part. Therefore, if there is no effective presenting part, as in a transverse lie, cervical dilation still occurs. The dramatic changes in the cervix result from a combination of structural changes in the tissue and forces exerted by the uterine contractions.

The cervix is predominantly composed of fibrous connective tissue plus some smooth muscle and fibroblasts together with blood vessels, epithelium and mucus-secreting glands. The rigidity of the cervix is related to its high content of collagen, particularly type I and type III collagen. There are two elements to cervical softening: increased vascularity and water content, and structural changes in the connective tissue. At term, 90% of the weight of the cervix is water. Connective tissue is formed of collagen fibres and elastin held together by an extracellular matrix, or ground substance. The ground substance is predominantly composed of proteoglycans, which coat the collagen fibres and modify their physical properties, determining the water content of the tissue. Hormones that promote cervical softening affect the composition of the ground substance. Prior to the onset of labour, there is increased expression and activity of matrix metalloproteinases (MMP), which leads to a progressive breakdown of the collagen matrix; the composition of the proteoglycans changes so that dermatan sulphate decreases and hyaluronic acid and glycosaminoglycans increase. Dermatan sulphate binds collagen fibrils tightly, whereas hyaluronic acid has a lesser affinity for collagen and attracts water.

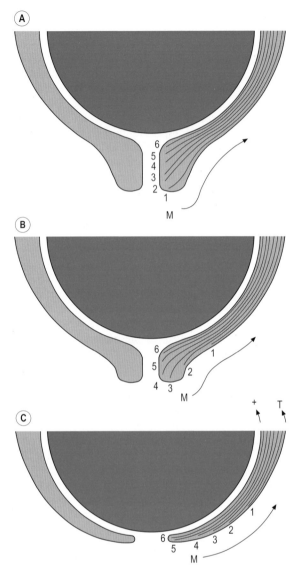

Fig. 13.8 The differential movement of tissue planes at the time of cervical effacement and early dilatation. M, direction of movement of collagen bundles; T, differential tension across the myometrium. Before labour (A), early effacement (B) and complete effacement (C). (Reproduced with permission from Sweet and Tiran, 1996.)

Although the proteoglycans are a minor constituent of the cervix, they have an amazing ability to bind water: 1 g of hyaluronic acid can bind ~1 L of water (Uldbjerg and Malstrom, 1991). The increased level of hyaluronic acid may act as a signal to activate resident macrophages and neutrophils to secrete interleukins. Interleukins increase prostaglandin activity and neutrophil migration and degranulation (releasing collagenase and elastase). Two other glycoproteins are also involved in cervical changes. Decorin binds and immobilizes the collagen fibres thus stabilizing the structure of the extracellular matrix in early pregnancy. Concentrations of decorin fall in late gestation. Fibronectin binds dermatan sulphate and collagen, protecting collagen from collagenase and stabilizing the extracellular matrix. Hyaluronic acid weakens the interaction of collagen with fibronectin. Levels of fibronectin obtained from cervical swabs can be used as a predictor for the onset of labour, which is especially useful in the management of preterm labour and prelabour rupture of membranes.

The mechanical strength of the ground substance changes as the water content increases and the number of crosslinks between elements of the connective tissue diminishes. The collagen increases in solubility and becomes disorganized and weakened (like a fraying rope) so it is more vulnerable to enzymatic digestion. Collagen is resistant to most proteases except collagenase from fibroblasts and neutrophil elastase. Amounts of neutrophil elastase in the cervix significantly increase at term. The association between intrauterine infection and premature labour may be linked to neutrophil infiltration and activation, which increase elastase levels. The effects of oestrogen on cervical ripening are mediated by insulin-like growth factor I (IGF-I). Collagenolysis is a complex balance between availability of free collagenase and the inhibitory proteins. Connective tissue in the body of the uterus also changes at term altering uterine compliance. The level of elastin increases throughout the pregnancy. It provides the elastic recoil that coordinates the contraction–retraction cycle and is important in the return of the uterus to its near-prepregnancy shape after delivery.

Although the cervix has relatively little smooth muscle tissue, it may have an important functional role as a sphincter. The cervix constricts with uterine contractions in early labour. This coordinated muscular activity may be important in the maintenance of cervical integrity during Braxton Hicks contractions before labour.

Cervical ripening is predominantly an inflammatory process. Macrophages and neutrophils infiltrate the cervical tissue towards term. They produce cytokines and elastases and collagenases, which digest the extracellular matrix proteins.

Assessment of Cervical Effacement

In practice, the cervix can be assessed by using a simple scoring system, the Bishop's score (Table 13.1). This is particularly useful prior to induction of labour and for

TABLE 13.1 Bishop's Score			
Bishop's Score	0	1	2
Station of presenting part	−3	−2	−1
Position of cervix	Posterior	Mid	Anterior
Consistency	Firm	Soft	Very soft
Length	3–4 cm	1–2 cm	<1 cm
Dilation of cervix	0	1–2 cm	>2 cm
Total =	(Bishop's score)		

monitoring the changes in the cervix as the induction/early labour progresses. If the cervix is soft, effaced and has started to dilate, induction may be implemented by artificial rupture of the membranes, which augments endogenous prostaglandin production. If the cervix is less favourable, prostaglandin E_2 (PGE_2) is administered into the posterior fornix of the vagina to facilitate effacement. However, PGE_2 should be used with caution in multiparous women because they have a greater sensitivity to it. Labour may also be stimulated by the insertion of a transcervical balloon catheter into the cervix (Gommers et al., 2017). The inflation of the balloon stretches the cervical tissue stimulating the production of natural prostaglandins.

The cause of these structural changes in the cervix is not clear. It is thought to be hormonally controlled. Relaxin has been shown to be important in cervical ripening in rodents and has been used clinically to promote cervical ripening in humans. However, the levels of endogenous relaxin in pregnant women seem to be highest at the beginning of the second trimester. Oestrogen affects the synthesis of connective tissue components *in vitro* but has limited success when used pharmacologically as an induction method. PGE_2 induces cervical softening or 'ripening' and is produced naturally by both the cervix and the fetal membranes. PGE_2 appears to act by increasing collagenolytic activity rather than by changing the composition of the ground substance, which probably precedes prostaglandin use in successful induction of labour. This may explain why early induction of labour (before term) using PGE_2 fails or takes much longer than 'beyond term' inductions. Following delivery, glycoproteins that bind strongly to collagen are reformed so the rigidity of the cervix is re-established; however, it never completely regains its original form (see Chapter 14). Damage to the cervix may have long-term consequences (Box 13.1).

Longitudinal fibres allow full dilation of the cervix to be achieved without the pressure of a presenting part, for instance in the case of a transverse lie. Artificial dilation of an unprepared cervix may damage the collagen fibres. This can result in the cervix failing to remain patent during subsequent pregnancies, resulting in habitual spontaneous abortion, usually in mid-pregnancy. Preoperative preparation to avoid this involves the administration of a prostaglandin derivative, which induces cervical softening and aids artificial dilation of the cervix. This method is used prior to procedures involving exploration of the uterine cavity such as termination of pregnancy, evacuation of retained products of conception, surgical ablation of the endometrium and investigation of infertility.

INITIATION OF PARTURITION

Animal Models of Parturition

Fetal maturation during gestation to the stage where survival after birth is optimal is a key evolutionary requirement in all mammalian species. For this reason, it seems likely that 'readiness' signals from the fetus will play an important role in the triggering of parturition. Because of the technical difficulties and ethical issues in studying the mechanisms of gestation and parturition in humans, a variety of animal models have been extensively used. One such model is the sheep in which parturition has been studied in detail. Based on the assumption that mammals are likely to share similar physiological mechanisms for the onset of labour, clinical procedures derived from understanding the mechanisms of parturition in sheep were developed, both for inducing labour and for inhibiting preterm labour in humans.

The timing of parturition in sheep is highly consistent and is controlled by the activity of the fetal HPA axis. Expression of proopiomelanocortin (POMC), the precursor of adrenocorticotrophic hormone (ACTH), progressively increases in the sheep pituitary from mid-gestation as the fetal brain matures. Regulation of secretion of pituitary ACTH in the fetal lamb is by antidiuretic hormone (ADH, also known as vasopressin) and CRH. Thus, the first indicator of impending labour in sheep is a sharp rise in fetal cortisol levels (the 'cortisol surge') due to the maturation of ACTH secretion from the pituitary gland, together with an increased sensitivity of the target tissue of ACTH, the adrenal cortex. The cortisol surge in sheep not only triggers the functional maturation of various organ systems that will be essential for survival after birth, but also decreases the production of progesterone by the placenta. Progesterone is essential for myometrial quiescence and pregnancy maintenance in sheep and the fetal lamb, therefore plays a crucial role in the triggering of uterine contractions and the timing of labour. Ablation or abnormal development of the pituitary gland in fetal lambs prevents the onset of labour so that the extended growth of the fetus eventually causes maternal gut obstruction and death. Conversely, infusion of ACTH, cortisol or dexamethasone (a cortisol analogue, frequently administered as an anti-inflammatory drug) into the sheep fetus induces labour at any stage of pregnancy. Fetal stress such as hypoxia and undernutrition can stimulate preterm birth in sheep by increasing fetal HPA maturation.

The effects of raised cortisol levels are important in both the promotion of fetal organ maturity (functional maturation of the fetal lungs and other systems) and the initiation of labour. Cortisol induces 17α-hydroxylase activity in the placenta that promotes the conversion of C21 steroids to C18 steroids. Thus 17α-hydroxylase converts progesterone to oestrogen so that the progesterone:oestrogen ratio alters in favour of oestrogen. This increases prostaglandin ($PGF_{2\alpha}$) synthesis by the placenta and myometrium. The alteration in oestrogen and progesterone levels can be measured prior to the onset of labour. Exogenous oestrogen induces labour and infusion of progesterone inhibits labour in the sheep. Increasing oestrogen or decreasing progesterone levels stimulates the synthesis of $PGF_{2\alpha}$. Prostaglandins increase myometrial sensitivity to oxytocin. $PGF_{2\alpha}$ is also important in cervical softening and increases uterine contractility. A positive feedback mechanism, known as the Ferguson reflex, amplifies these signals. The pressure of the fetal presenting part on the cervix activates a neurohumoral reflex, whereby afferent nerves from the cervix impinge on the hypothalamus and increase oxytocin release from the posterior pituitary gland. Oxytocin stimulates uterine contractions and causes further release of $PGF_{2\alpha}$ from the uterus.

Initiation of labour in the human is different in a number of respects from that in the sheep. The sheep appears to have the single mechanism described for triggering parturition whereas the situation in humans is much more complex. Note that pregnancy in some species, such as goats, rabbits and rodents, depends on progesterone secretion; the maternal corpus luteum is the source of progesterone in these species, not the placenta. Luteolysis, mediated by $PGF_{2\alpha}$, causes a fall in progesterone and initiation of parturition in these species and the fetus does not seem to play such an important role in the timing of parturition as it does in sheep. Again, as in humans, this may be explained by the nonseasonal breeding pattern of these species.

Initiation of Parturition in Humans

The mean length of human gestation is 39.6 weeks and the majority of births occur between 38 and 42 weeks. Such a wide range of gestation times in normal pregnancy suggests the timing mechanism is not precise, possibly because it is affected by a number of factors including external influences. A complex system of multiple (redundant) pathways appears to regulate human parturition making the process difficult to study. Labour invariably ensues after fetal death has occurred, although it might be delayed by a few weeks (and therefore be pre-empted by surgical removal of the products of conception). Labour occurs sooner if placental damage has occurred. The critical events permitting extrauterine survival are adequate maturation of the fetal lung and nervous system. The fetal brain may monitor this maturation and influence the timing mechanism. Mothers of fetuses with brain abnormalities still progress into labour spontaneously but with a much wider range of gestation (see below). This suggests that the fetal brain affects the precise timing of labour in humans, rather than controlling the exact length of gestation, as observed in seasonal breeding species.

Hormonal Changes Associated with Parturition in Humans

The Role of the Fetal Pituitary–Adrenal Axis

Term pregnancy in humans has a relatively wide window (37–42 weeks); pre- and post-term births are common. Human fetal malformations such as anencephaly (no cerebrum), malformed pituitary glands or hypoplasia of the adrenal glands are associated with an increased range of gestation length (both longer and shorter) but women still undergo spontaneous labour. In sheep, similar fetal malformations, either accidental or deliberate, result in significantly prolonged gestation, which adversely affects the fetus. This implies that the fetal–adrenal axis has a supportive rather than a direct role in parturition, acting to fine tune the gestational length in humans, rather than functioning as the 'timer' for the initiation of labour, as seen in sheep.

Cortisol

It is evident that the human fetal anterior pituitary gland undergoes maturational changes in the last weeks of gestation as the profile of hormonal release changes. However, there are no defined changes measurable in the maternal circulation prior to the onset of labour. The raised cortisol levels in the cord blood of infants, who have experienced a spontaneous delivery rather than an induced one, or delivery by caesarean section, are maternally derived and are secondary to maternal pain. Labour itself, whether spontaneous or induced, causes stress and therefore an increased production of cortisol, which can cross the placenta. It is possible to differentiate between cortisol of maternal origin and cortisol of fetal origin by comparing the levels in umbilical cord arterial blood with those in the cord vein. Blood in the vein flows from the placenta to the fetus so if cortisol levels are higher in the vein than in the arteries this suggests the source of cortisol is maternal.

Exogenous corticosteroids (such as dexamethasone and betamethasone) given to a pregnant woman at 24–34 weeks to promote fetal lung maturation (see Chapter 15) do not initiate parturition, although oestrogen and cortisol levels fall. Pharmacological doses of glucocorticoids introduced into the amniotic fluid increase uterine activity and induce labour; however, this effect is not observed with physiological doses. Most research studies have not been able to measure an increase in cortisol prior to the onset of labour, nor an effect on placental hormone production. Therefore, it now seems unlikely that cortisol is important in initiating labour in humans, although it has a vital role in the maturation of fetal lungs and other organs. Several factors may affect physiological responses to cortisol; these include corticosteroid-binding protein (CBP), which would influence the relative concentration of free cortisol, metabolism of cortisol to inactive cortisone by 11β-hydroxysteroid dehydrogenase and modification of corticosteroid receptor expression.

Progesterone:Oestrogen Ratio

In all animals that give birth to live young that have developed within their body (viviparous) that have been studied, parturition is characterized by changes in the myometrium from a quiescent to an excitable state. In most animal models, a fall in plasma progesterone levels is the trigger for this transition. In the sheep, fetal cortisol affects steroidogenesis so progesterone levels fall and oestrogen levels increase. This is a result of increased expression and activity of placental 17α-hydroxylase (see above). Across almost all species, the fall in plasma progesterone concentration is a common endocrine event leading to parturition. However, progesterone levels do not fall prior to labour in humans but continue to rise as they have done throughout pregnancy. In humans, the placenta does not express inducible 17α-hydroxylase activity and therefore cannot convert progesterone to oestrogen. However, increases in free oestriol levels have been observed in saliva of women before the onset of labour, both preterm and at term.

High progesterone levels inhibit myometrial activity during implantation and favour uterine quiescence throughout the remainder of pregnancy until parturition, via multiple effects on gene expression as well as nongenomic pathways. Among the former, progesterone decreases the expression of oxytocin and $PGF_{2\alpha}$ receptors and gap-junction proteins. This suppression of myometrial activity is essential to the maintenance of pregnancy, although parturition begins without a measurable decrease in maternal peripheral progesterone levels. Large doses of progesterone are relatively unsuccessful in inhibiting preterm labour in humans. However, mifepristone, the progesterone receptor antagonist previously known as RU-486, inhibits the action of progesterone and can induce labour at any stage of human pregnancy, suggesting that this progesterone-induced myometrial quiescence is also a crucial component in maintaining pregnancy in humans. Mifepristone is used clinically as an effective abortifacient drug (to cause abortion). It also has anti-glucocorticoid activity and can cause ripening of the cervix and increase sensitivity to contractile prostaglandins.

As the uterus enlarges during pregnancy, the part of the uterine wall distal to the site of implantation and therefore furthest away from the major source of progesterone production may re-establish uterine contractions and trigger the onset of labour. Measurement of absolute progesterone levels may therefore be misleading as the biological effects will be altered by receptor density, levels of binding proteins or postreceptor changes. The fetal membranes and maternal decidua can both metabolize progesterone and produce cortisol. Cortisol is antagonistic to progesterone and can increase the synthesis of CRH. Fetal membranes, therefore, offer a mechanism for local control of progesterone concentration. Prior to labour, the major products of the paracrine steroid hormone synthesis could be progesterone and oestrone (a weak oestrogen) and following the onset of labour the major products could be less active progesterone metabolites and biologically active oestradiol. It has also been suggested that in humans there is a regionalization of uterine activity and high progesterone levels are important in promoting relaxation of the LUS, while contractions in the fundal area facilitate the descent of the fetus. The altered progesterone receptor profile is postulated to modulate oestrogen effects (and hence oxytocin responses) via expression of oestrogen receptors. The human progesterone receptor exists in several isoforms produced from a single gene. PR-B is the full-length isoform, which is the major mediator of progesterone effects whereas PR-A lacks the N-terminal region of the protein that contains one of the functional domains, so it tends to have effects that oppose those of PR-B. There are also PR-C and two other truncated isoforms. For most of pregnancy, the human myometrium expresses mostly the PR-B receptor subtype, which maintains myometrial quiescence and cervical closure. In labour, predominantly the PR-A receptor is expressed and this PR-A dominance

promotes myometrial contractility (Merlino et al., 2007). Thus, although humans differ from other mammalian species by having no fall in progesterone levels prior to parturition, there is a functional removal of progesterone-induced quiescence and progesterone still appears to be an important signal. The increased synthesis of PR-A may be mediated by inflammatory factors and Toll-like receptors (Keelan, 2018); this pathway may be increased in some cases of preterm labour associated with infection.

Human placental production of oestrogen increases throughout labour and the rate seems to increase in the latter part of gestation. In sheep, increased oestrogen causes increased expression of CAPs and upregulation of prostaglandin synthase and consequent increased synthesis of PGE_2, promoting a positive feedback on myometrial contractility. However, spontaneous labour in humans can occur in the absence of measurable changes in oestrogen concentration. Exogenous oestrogen infusion in humans causes a transient increase in uterine activity and decreases the oxytocin threshold of the uterus but does not induce premature delivery or fetal membrane changes.

Synthesis of placental oestrogen depends on fetal cooperation in the provision of the precursors, and could thus potentially provide an opportunity for the human fetus to manipulate the progesterone:oestrogen ratio and uterine activity. The fetal adrenal gland in humans and higher primates is a relatively large percentage of body mass compared with the adult and has three zones: the outer adult zone produces mostly aldosterone; the unique fetal zone produces dehydroepiandrosterone sulphate (DHEAS) and the transitional zone produces mostly cortisol. This large fetal zone of the adrenal gland disappears in the neonatal period and may be regulated by hCG levels. DHEAS is the fetal adrenal C19 steroid precursor for placental oestradiol-17α and oestrone synthesis, which are implicated as having a role in labour. DHEAS is converted to oestrogens by placental sulphatase, aromatase and other enzymes (see Chapter 3). Production of DHEAS is controlled by ACTH from the anterior pituitary, which is itself regulated by hypothalamic CRH. CRH of placental origin can also stimulate production of DHEAS from the fetal zone (see below). However, women who have placental sulphatase or aromatase deficiencies and produce very little placental oestrogen can have normal pregnancy and labour. Thus, the changing ratio of oestrogen to progesterone may facilitate effective uterine contractions but is probably not critical for the induction of labour.

Corticotrophin-releasing Hormone

Hypothalamic CRH controls the function of the pituitary–adrenal axis in response to stress. CRH stimulates the anterior pituitary gland to secrete ACTH, which then stimulates the cortex of the adrenal gland to release cortisol. However, even in the presence of significant stress, levels of CRH are relatively low compared to the levels reached in pregnancy. CRH is expressed abundantly in the syncytiotrophoblast cells of the human placenta (but not in nonprimate placentas) and CRH receptors are expressed in the primate placenta and myometrium. Placental CRH seems to have an important role in the initiation of parturition in higher primates and humans. CRH is synthesized by the placenta and released predominantly into the maternal circulation although some enters the fetal circulation (Keelan, 2018). Levels of CRH steadily increase in the maternal circulation from mid-term (~90 days before the onset of labour) until about 35 weeks when levels sharply rise and are usually particularly high in pregnancies ending with premature labour and those complicated by preeclampsia. CRH activity is attenuated by CRH-binding protein (CRH-BP), which is synthesized by the liver, placenta and brain so most CRH present in blood is in the bound (inactive) form during pregnancy. However, towards term, when levels of CRH increase, levels of CRH-BP simultaneously fall and the capacity of the CRH-BP is saturated so circulating levels of physiologically active, free CRH increase markedly. The maternal adrenal CRH receptors are downregulated so the ACTH response to CRH is blunted in late pregnancy; this protects the maternal pituitary–adrenal axis from overstimulation.

The stress hormone, cortisol, has a negative feedback effect to inhibit CRH secretion and thus ACTH and cortisol secretion as part of the HPA axis. The opposite situation occurs with placental CRH where cortisol has a positive feedback effect to further increase CRH release by the placenta. This positive feedback is further augmented by increased prostaglandin production (Petraglia et al., 2010), which also increases placental synthesis of CRH. Fetal stresses such as hypoxia and hypoglycaemia result in increased plasma CRH concentrations. CRH is a vasodilator in the placental vascular bed so increased CRH should result in increased blood flow and abrogation of the fetal insult. However, if the insult persists, then CRH would increase fetal ACTH secretion and increase DHEAS production thus increasing oestrogen synthesis, which leads to myometrial activation. Thus, CRH appears to be a key component in the endocrine control of parturition and a mechanism by which a compromised fetus can precipitate labour when intrauterine life becomes unfavourable. The pathway by which CRH in the fetal circulation increases pituitary corticotrophin production, which subsequently stimulates cortisol secretion by the fetal adrenal gland, is important in the maturation of the fetal lungs and other organs particularly the central nervous system (CNS) and gut (see Chapter 15). The

maturing fetal lungs increase their production of surfactant proteins, which can then enter the amniotic fluid; these surfactant proteins together with phospholipids and inflammatory cytokines are thought to stimulate inflammation in the fetal membranes and underlying myometrium and contribute to the amplification of the signals leading to labour. It has been suggested that the ratio of placental CRH and CRH-BP acts as a placental 'clock', which controls the length of gestation and allows a distressed fetus to 'wind-on' the clock to initiate premature labour (Smith et al., 2012) when intrauterine conditions are unfavourable.

CRH acts via a family of receptors coupled to different G-proteins in different tissues and at different stages of pregnancy, to stimulate different intracellular signalling pathways. So, for most of pregnancy, myometrial CRH acts via the CRHR1 receptor to activate adenylate cyclase via G_s proteins and increase cAMP. The increase in cAMP also stimulates membrane-bound guanylyl cyclase to raise cGMP levels and activates nitric oxide synthase. These pathways culminate in the maintenance of myometrial quiescence. Near term, the expression of CRH receptors changes and CRH acts via the CRHR2 receptor via the Gq G-proteins to stimulate the PLCβ/inositol trisphosphate pathway, triggering myometrial contractility and labour (Grammatopoulos, 2008).

The involvement of a physiological stress pathway in the onset of labour could explain the relationship between maternal stress and reproductive failure and the interesting possible relationship between maternal periconceptional nutritional status and the timing of parturition. Maternal stress would stimulate the maternal pituitary–adrenal axis resulting in increased maternal cortisol production, which would stimulate placental CRH release (Smith et al., 2012). Myometrial contractility is also enhanced by upregulation of oxytocin receptor expression and crosstalk between the oxytocin and CRH receptors.

The Timing of Parturition Involves Several Different Clocks and Timers

Preterm birth is the major cause of neonatal morbidity and mortality throughout the world so an understanding of the mechanisms involved in the physiology and pathophysiology of the 'timers' and 'clocks' of pregnancy is crucial to successful intervention in preterm births. The mechanisms that underlie the maintenance of pregnancy and the signals that trigger the timing of parturition are still uncertain. Thus, despite numerous advances in obstetric practice, the incidence of preterm births has actually increased over the last 30 years and although advances in obstetric care have improved preterm neonatal survival, preterm birth is still the leading cause of infant mortality across the world.

Diagnosis of imminent preterm birth is unreliable so that >30% of all women presenting with symptoms consistent with preterm labour will proceed with pregnancy and deliver at term. Also, no currently available therapeutic intervention is able to halt the progression to labour, improve the long-term neonatal outcome or be devoid of deleterious fetal and maternal side-effects. Until recently, the only intervention shown to improve neonatal survival and outcome after preterm delivery was antenatal corticosteroid administration to drive fetal lung and tissue maturation in preparation for neonatal life. The main aim of tocolytic therapy has been to maintain pregnancy for at least 48 h so that antenatal corticosteroids can be administered and exert their effect. Significant progress in the prevention of cerebral palsy (CP), the most common neurological disorder associated with preterm delivery, has recently been made through antenatal administration of the neuroprotectant, magnesium sulphate, to females before 32 weeks' gestation. Magnesium sulphate treatment is now widely accepted and recommended by the World Health Organization (Chollat et al., 2019).

In humans, signals from both the mother and fetus, and from several different tissues in both, regulate the timing of parturition (Menon et al., 2016). These 'clocks' include:

1. *The endocrine clock:* changes in the patterns of secretion of fetal and placental hormones, and in the expression of their specific receptors on target tissues. This would include the secretion of CRH by the placenta and its effects on the secretion of cortisol from the fetal adrenal gland, as well as the changing patterns of receptor subtypes for CRH on myometrial cells, as discussed above. In addition to CRH, oxytocin is also produced by the hypothalamus to be secreted by the posterior pituitary, but also produced by placental membranes and the fetus. Its powerful effects on uterine contractions at term also reflect a dramatic rise in oxytocin receptor expression in the upper uterus in late gestation and labour. Other endocrine and paracrine effectors including prostaglandins and cytokines show modified patterns of secretion and action as pregnancy progresses and also contribute to the endocrine timing of parturition. Study of these factors is inherently difficult in human pregnancy but also complicated by their 'ectopic' secretion by the placenta and fetus, with immediate access to their sites of action, so that monitoring their concentrations in peripheral blood may not reflect their important roles.

2. *The decidual clock:* the decidua lies adjacent to the fetal membranes and develops from the endometrium of the uterus following trophoblast invasion at implantation. It has a complex cellular composition with endometrial stromal cells, fibroblasts, infiltrating immune cells and other cell types. These decidual immune cells at the fetal–maternal interface are thought to be intimately involved in implantation, the establishment and growth of the early embryo, the immune tolerance of the fetal allograft and, after suppressing inflammation for almost the entirety of pregnancy, the generation of inflammatory signals that activate parturition.

3. *The myometrial clock:* refers to the loss of myometrial quiescence to activate uterine contractions when levels of progesterone decrease or, as happens in human pregnancy, the subtypes of progesterone receptor expression are changed, as discussed above.

4. *The membrane clock:* it has recently been suggested that the senescence of fetal membranes in the final stages of pregnancy provides additional signals, which trigger parturition (Menon et al., 2016).

5. *The fetal clock:* is driven by glucocorticoid-induced fetal lung maturation, which increases secretion of surfactant, components of which (surfactant protein A (SP-A) and platelet-activating factor (PAF)) have been suggested to signal parturition (Mendelson et al., 2017). This may provide one of several signalling pathways through which the fetus can influence the initiation of labour by signalling to the mother that its lungs have achieved sufficient maturity for survival in the outside world (Mendelson et al., 2017).

Other Factors

Labour is an inflammatory process but the relationship between the immune system and parturition is still not entirely clear. It is clear that significant intrauterine infection can trigger parturition and cause preterm birth. Proinflammatory cytokines, such as interleukin 1β (IL-1β), IL-6 and tumour necrosis factor-α (TNF-α), may have an important role in parturition.

Some aspects of adaptive immunity are decreased during pregnancy, such as T-cell and B-cell numbers and the ability of naive CD4+ T cells to produce T helper cells and Th1 and Th2 cytokines (as discussed in Chapter 10). In contrast, specific innate immune responses are increased during pregnancy such as those of natural killer (NK) cells. The immune system is diffusely dispersed in the body and, as such, very difficult to study in humans, particularly during pregnancy. Recently however, Aghaeepour et al. (2017) used sophisticated mass cytometry techniques to study the changes in the maternal immune system over the duration of pregnancy with single-cell resolution. The abundance and functional responses of all major immune cell subsets were quantified in serial blood samples collected throughout pregnancy and this approach offers great promise for future studies.

Signal Amplification

Once labour has been initiated and the myometrium is activated, there is a positive feed-forward stimulation of myometrial activity. This signal amplification is mediated by prolabour factors, known as contraction-associated proteins. These include uterotonins such as prostaglandins and prostanoid receptors, oxytocin and oxytocin receptors, gap junctions and ion channels, which transform the uterus from a quiescent to a labour phenotype. It has not been easy to discriminate between those hormones and signals that initiate labour and those that amplify the triggering signals.

Prostaglandins

Prostaglandins (PGs) of the 2-series are known to be important in the feed-forward signal amplification and progression of labour; they promote myometrial contractions, cervical dilatation and membrane rupture. Prostaglandins are present in the maternal circulation in low concentrations and are cleared in the pulmonary circulation so they are difficult to measure as they have paracrine activity and a short half-life.

Prostaglandins can be formed as a consequence of tissue trauma (including labour itself and any manipulative or tactile stimuli). In late pregnancy, prostaglandin synthesis is readily stimulated by minor local stimuli, such as coitus, vaginal examination, sweeping the membranes or amniotomy, which are all associated with inducing labour. Exogenous prostaglandins can be used therapeutically to ripen the cervix and to induce uterine contractions and labour. Mid-trimester abortion can be induced by procedures, such as intra-amniotic injection of hypertonic saline, that result in the increased synthesis and release of prostaglandins. Increasing DHEAS or oestrogen concentration and decreasing progesterone concentration increase production of prostaglandins (Vannuccini et al., 2016). An increase in myometrial expression of prostaglandin receptors, particularly the receptor of $PGF_{2\alpha}$, is implicated in the causes of some preterm labour and PGE_2 and its analogues are used to induce labour (Peiris et al., 2017).

Prostaglandins are synthesized in the fetal membranes, decidua, myometrium and cervix; levels fall abruptly following placental separation. Cleavage of the fatty acid in position 2 of phospholipids is the rate-limiting step of prostaglandin production. The activity of the enzyme involved, phospholipase A_2 (PLA_2), may regulate the level of arachidonic acid, which is the precursor of prostaglandins and may be important therefore in initiating labour (see Chapter 3). Increased oestrogen (or decreased progesterone) stimulates the release of PLA_2 from decidual lysosomes and therefore increases free arachidonic acid and subsequent prostaglandin synthesis. Arachidonic acid can also be produced indirectly via PLC activity. Alternatively, the activity of cyclooxygenase (COX) may be rate-limiting (Besenboeck et al., 2016). The chorion produces prostaglandin dehydrogenase (PGDH), the enzyme that inactivates prostaglandins; this is potentially a therapeutic target to control preterm labour (Kishore et al., 2017). In late pregnancy, chorionic PGDH activity decreases so the levels of PGE_2 rises.

The two most important prostaglandins in labour appear to be $PGF_{2\alpha}$ and PGE_2. At term, concentrations of PGE_2 and $PGF_{2\alpha}$ are higher in the decidua and myometrium (but these tissues are subject to tissue trauma so some authors believe raised prostaglandin levels are caused by increased uterine activity). PGE_2 is involved in cervical ripening, by mediating the release of MMP, and is metabolized by the myometrium to produce $PGF_{2\alpha}$.

Maintenance of human pregnancy may depend on the synthesis of PGE_2 being inhibited and this inhibition of prostaglandin synthesis being attenuated at the onset of labour. Prostaglandin concentrations in the pregnant uterus are very low (~200 times lower than at any stage in the menstrual cycle) but increase sharply in the maternal circulation from 36 weeks' gestation probably in response to the increasing level of CRH (Vannuccini et al., 2016). Arachidonic acid, the precursor, is plentiful but synthesis of prostaglandins is inhibited, even if the pregnancy is extrauterine. Progesterone or the fetus may directly or indirectly moderate synthesis or metabolism of prostaglandins. Endogenous inhibitors of prostaglandin synthesis have been identified in maternal plasma; levels fall towards the end of gestation. Inhibitors of the COX enzymes, such as aspirin and indomethacin, block prostaglandin synthesis and are used therapeutically to try to arrest preterm labour. Prostaglandin synthesis is upregulated by cortisol (and dexamethasone), oestradiol, CRH and the inflammatory cytokines IL-1β and TNFα (Li et al., 2014).

Low doses of prostaglandins, particularly $PGF_{2\alpha}$, increase myometrial responsiveness to prostaglandins and oxytocin, possibly by increasing the formation of gap junctions. In vitro, PGE_2 has a biphasic effect, stimulating at nanomolar concentrations and inhibiting at micromolar concentrations. It also has a dual action: when its effects are mediated by the EP_1 and EP_3 receptors, PGE_2 increases intracellular calcium concentration, but the EP_2 receptor is coupled to adenylyl cyclase so PGE_2 acting at this receptor decreases intracellular calcium and favours relaxation. Variations in regional prostaglandin synthesis may also occur.

Prostacyclin (PGI_2) is synthesized in the myometrium and cervix. It promotes myometrial quiescence. It has an important role in maintaining uterine blood flow in labour; it causes vasodilation of smooth muscle and inhibits platelet aggregation, potentially inhibiting thromboembolic complications. Myometrial relaxation between uterine contractions in labour prevents occlusion of the uterine arteries, which could result in hypoxia and uterine or labour dystocia (abnormally slow progression of labour) (Morton et al., 2017). Placental thromboxane (TxA_2) has opposing effects to PGI_2 and is important in the closure of the fetal ductus arteriosus and haemostasis after delivery. In preeclampsia, levels of prostacyclin are low and levels of thromboxane are high. This is the rationale for aspirin treatment of preeclampsia. Aspirin-like drugs, by inhibiting the COX enzymes and thereby prostaglandin synthesis, restore thromboxane levels in preeclampsia. Trials using aspirin caused a slight prolongation of gestation and diminution of uterine contractions, but also increased the risk of premature closure of the ductus arteriosus and postnatal bleeding problems in the mother. Synthetic prostaglandins can be used clinically to trigger parturition and also to prevent closure of ductus arteriosus in newborns with certain cyanotic heart defects (see Chapter 3).

Prostaglandins are metabolized by the enzyme PGDH, which is located in the fetal membranes. Deficiency of PGDH is associated with preterm labour. Expression of PGDH is upregulated by progesterone and IL-10 and suppressed by cortisol (and dexamethasone), oestradiol, CRH, IL-1β and TNFα. Parturition is, therefore, essentially an inflammatory process. The association between inflammation and/or infection in the fetoplacental unit and preterm labour is thought to be due to the release of phospholipases from bacterial organisms (Gilman-Sachs et al., 2018), which cause an increase in arachidonic acid release and so promote prostaglandin synthesis. Decidual macrophages respond to bacterial products by releasing proinflammatory cytokines. Bacterial endotoxins, such as lipopolysaccharide, can either increase prostaglandin release directly or further stimulate release of cytokines, which then increase prostaglandin synthesis. Lipopolysaccharide also contributes to premature rupture of the membranes (PROM).

Prostaglandins also have an important role in the establishment of a neonatal circulatory pattern (see Chapter 15). Respiratory distress syndrome is associated with high levels of $PGF_{2\alpha}$ in the infant's circulation, and patent ductus arteriosus with high PGE_2 levels. PGE_2 can prevent the ductus arteriosus from closing and inhibitors of prostaglandin synthesis, such as aspirin, can promote its closure. Exogenous PGE_2 can be used therapeutically to maintain fetal circulation after birth in conditions such as ductus dependent congenital heart disease, until corrective surgery can be performed.

Oxytocin

Oxytocin is a peptide synthesized by the hypothalamus and released from the posterior pituitary gland (see Chapter 3). A synthetic form (such as Syntocinon) is used extensively for induction and/or augmentation of human labour and can limit postpartum bleeding or haemorrhage, which results from poor contraction of the uterus following childbirth or partial placenta retention. Endogenous oxytocin production can also be stimulated, for instance by nipple stimulation, with a favourable outcome. However, it is not certain whether oxytocin is important in the initiation of labour. As oxytocin receptors are generally localized to the uterus, mammary glands and pituitary, oxytocin antagonists and agonists have few systemic effects. Maternal oxytocin levels are very low and do not change very much before labour. Maternal pituitary production of oxytocin dramatically increases in the first stage of labour. However, focusing on circulating levels of oxytocin may be misleading. The concentrations of oxytocin receptors in the myometrium and decidua rise dramatically (by 100–200 times) during late pregnancy so the sensitivity of the uterus increases. This means the uterus can be stimulated by low concentrations of maternal oxytocin levels that previously had no effect (hypersensitivity). Therapeutic doses adequate to augment labour are very variable, which may reflect individual differences in receptor expression. If used to augment labour, infusions of oxytocin analogues should be commenced on low dosage, which is gradually increased until regular, strong contractions (~3 in every 10 min time period) are present to ensure hyperstimulation of the myometrium is reduced. The pattern of oxytocin release changes at the onset of labour, with an increased frequency of pulses (Fuchs et al., 1991). It may be important that maternal oxytocin levels stay low during the pregnancy so the sensitivity of the uterus to oxytocin is maintained.

Oxytocin antagonists, such as atosiban, have been used to inhibit uterine contractility in preterm labour (see Table 13.2) but are not always effective. Delaying delivery by even a few days allows antenatal corticosteroids to be administered to the mother, which will facilitate fetal lung maturation; however, atosiban should be used with caution as it affects pancreatic insulin secretion (Mohan et al., 2018). Note that all tocolytic medications have side-effects, some of which can be extreme and potentially life-threatening, so these should be administered with caution and careful monitoring (Younger et al., 2017).

Exposure of decidual cells to oxytocin increases the release of prostaglandins. Vaginal examination in late pregnancy may stimulate the Ferguson reflex so oxytocin is released from the posterior pituitary, which stimulates uterine prostaglandin production. Earlier in pregnancy,

TABLE 13.2 Intervention in Labour

Drug/Treatment	Effect	Notes
Treatment of Preterm Labour (Tocolytic Agents)		
Progesterone and related compounds	May relax uterus or block inflammatory pathways	Possibly reduce late preterm birth but not associated with reduced perinatal mortality or morbidity
β-Adrenergic agonists (betamimetics or 'β-agonists'), e.g. terbutaline, fenoterol	Inhibit uterine contractions	Effects often short-lived; unpleasant side-effects (cardiovascular, metabolic and neuromuscular)
Magnesium sulphate	Inhibits myometrial contractility by competing with calcium entry and inhibiting actomyosin interaction	Limited usefulness as a tocolytic agent but useful as cerebroprotective agent
Oxytocin receptor antagonists, e.g. atosiban, barusiban	Competitive inhibition of oxytocin	Clinical trials taking place; potentially useful as oxytocin receptors have limited distribution. Some side-effects as acts on vasopressin receptors
Prostaglandin synthase inhibitors, e.g. indomethacin	Inhibit preterm contractions. Reduce connectivity between myocytes	Serious neonatal complications in infants born <30 weeks. Adverse effects on fetal renal function, associated with oligohydramnios
Calcium-channel blockers, e.g. nifedipine	Decrease intracellular calcium, cause uterine relaxation	May affect placental and uterine blood flow; cardiovascular side-effects (hypotension and tachycardia); nonsteroidal anti-inflammatory agents
Alcohol		Risk of aspiration, intoxication, depression and incontinence
Treatment of Post-term Labour (Methods of Induction)		
Oxytocin	Used to augment labour; oxytocin has little effect on unripe cervix	Production of endogenous oxytocin can be increased by nipple stimulation
PGF2 agonists, e.g. dinoprostone, Cervidil, Prepidil	Cervical ripening, induction of labour	Effects depend on expression of receptors
Misoprostol (Cytotec)	Synthetic PGE, analogue; used to reduce acid in the stomach	Can cause the uterus to contract; nausea and diarrhoea
Mifepristone (RU-486; Mifegyne)	Antiprogestin	Primarily used to induce first trimester abortion

this response does not occur, presumably because there are inadequate oxytocin receptors. Women who go into preterm labour seem to have an increased expression of oxytocin receptors and higher myometrial sensitivity to oxytocin. Failed induction of labour is associated with a reduced number of oxytocin receptors. Therefore, the initiation of labour depends on mechanisms that induce the expression of oxytocin receptors in the myometrium rather affect the oxytocin level itself. Both oestrogen and prostaglandins increase uterine responsiveness to oxytocin.

Oxytocin is also synthesized by the decidua, corpus luteum, placenta and fetal membranes and may act locally. The fetal posterior pituitary produces both oxytocin and ADH (vasopressin). In spontaneous labour, fetal secretion of oxytocin is high and transferred across the placenta at levels comparable with those used to induce uterine activity (Arrowsmith and Wray, 2014). The increment in oxytocin levels is greater in the umbilical arteries than in the umbilical vein and is much higher than maternal levels, suggesting it is synthesized by the fetus and transferred across the placenta. Initiation and maintenance of human labour may therefore be influenced by fetal oxytocin production. ADH (vasopressin) is produced at even higher concentrations than oxytocin and may regulate prostaglandin production.

Relaxin

Relaxin is a polypeptide hormone produced by the corpus luteum, and decidua and placenta in pregnancy, which promotes tissue remodelling during reproduction. It has been found to inhibit myometrial contractility and promote vasodilation, via nitric oxide synthesis, until late pregnancy. It also appears to promote cervical ripening at parturition. Concentrations of relaxin appear to be highest in the first trimester and then fall. A very early fall is associated with preterm labour. Histologically, the number of cells staining positively for relaxin is much less after spontaneous delivery compared with caesarean section. Relaxin may inhibit PGE_2 production during pregnancy but favours its production in labour. It may act synergistically with progesterone during the pregnancy, maintaining uterine quiescence and inhibiting oxytocin release.

The Maternal Endocrine System

Functioning ovaries are not necessary for the initiation of labour. Hypophysectomized women (who have no pituitary glands) and women with diabetes insipidus (a posterior pituitary defect) go into labour at term. However, the posterior pituitary stores oxytocin, which is synthesized in the hypothalamus. In the absence of a functional pituitary gland, oxytocin may be secreted directly by the hypothalamus. Adrenalectomized women on corticosteroid maintenance therapy go into labour spontaneously but women with Addison disease, where adrenal cortex steroid production is impaired, tend to have prolonged pregnancy.

The Maternal Nervous System

There is a higher density of adrenergic and cholinergic innervation towards the cervix. The nonpregnant uterus contracts in response to both adrenaline and noradrenaline but, at term, noradrenaline increases uterine contractions and adrenaline causes relaxation. α-Receptor antagonists, such as phentolamine, decrease uterine activity and inhibit the response to noradrenaline so adrenergic drugs are used to suppress contractions in preterm labour; β-receptor antagonists, such as propranolol, increase uterine activity. Catecholamines both stimulate and inhibit uterine activity, acting via the α_2-receptors and β_2-receptors, respectively. The α_1-receptors increase intracellular calcium concentrations and promote contractile activity. However, labour occurs normally in paraplegic women (who have no nervous input to the uterus), suggesting that the onset and progression of labour is under hormonal, rather than nervous, control. Neural control appears to modulate uterine activity but is subordinate to hormonal control.

Stretch

In a normal pregnancy, growth of the uterus keeps pace with the growth of its contents and the limit of stretchability is probably not reached. In fact, mechanical stretching of the uterine wall by the growing fetus induces smooth muscle hypertrophy and increases its tensile strength. However, overstretching, for instance with multiple pregnancy and polyhydramnios, is associated with a shorter gestation period. The probable mechanism is that stretching of the muscle fibres increases their excitability and that mechanical stress can increase responsiveness to uterotonins. In most smooth-muscle containing tissues in the body, stretching leads to reflex contraction. Multiple gestation and polyhydramnios are associated with overdistension of the uterus and a higher incidence of preterm labour. Distension of the uterus causes myometrial stretching and also stretching of the fetal membranes that line the inner surface of the uterus.

THE TIMING OF PARTURITION

The human fetus possibly has the potential to survive birth as early as the 24th week of gestation. Most babies are delivered after the 37th week of gestation. However, there is a range of gestational periods producing healthy babies capable of survival. It is suggested that this variation in apparently normal gestation could allow changing environmental conditions to influence the precise timing. One suggestion is that the time of the lunar month could affect the timing after 37 weeks. Other suggestions are that gestational length may be linked to the length of the individual woman's ovarian cycle or may have a familial pattern. Women with longer menstrual cycles may have a lower level of oestrogen, which could affect the initiation of parturition (see above).

Mammals tend to labour most effectively during the period of the day in which they normally rest. This timing may be because the effect of the parasympathetic nervous system is then dominant; labour is inhibited by sympathetic stimulation. Both the start of labour and the actual time of delivery occur more frequently at night and in the early hours of the morning (Mark et al., 2017). Circadian rhythms occur in several variables including pregnancy-associated hormones and prelabour myometrial activity. Uterine activity and oxytocin levels are higher at night until about 3 weeks before delivery. The maternal circadian system or melatonin secretion may entrain fetal cooperation.

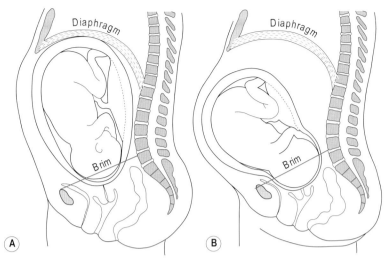

Fig. 13.9 (A) Prior to lightening: the fundus is in close proximity to the diaphragm and the lower uterine segment (LUS) is still firm so the fetal head remains high. (B) After lightening (2–3 weeks before the onset of labour): the LUS has softened and dilated so the fetal head descends and the fundus sinks below the diaphragm, easing breathing. (Reproduced with permission from Bennett and Brown, 1999.)

THE EVOLUTIONARY CONTEXT OF HUMAN LABOUR

Humans have large and complex brains and are the only living mammal that habitually walks on two legs. They have a complicated mechanism of labour and in modern societies seek assistance when they give birth. The development of bipedal locomotion has resulted in an altered pelvic morphology and physiology. Whereas the large pelvic aperture and small fetal head size in chimpanzees allows the fetus to face the mother at delivery (occipitoposterior position), the human pelvis is barely large enough to allow the passage of the fetus with its comparatively large fetal brain. The human fetus emerges from the birth canal facing away from the mother (occipitoanterior position) making unassisted birth more of a challenge. The relatively straight cylindrical pelvis of our forebears has evolved into a tilted conical birth canal. Pelvic size has decreased to enhance adaptation to the upright posture and swift movement.

It is thought that the upright stance of human ancestors led to thickening and lengthening of the pelvic bones and the forward curvature of the sacrum; this stance imposes extra pressure on the pregnant cervix and pelvic floor. Humans have a particularly high concentration of cervical collagen compared with other species and a highly muscular pelvic floor. The increased muscle resistance of the pelvic floor is important as it facilitates rotational movements of the presenting part of the fetus during labour to negotiate passage through the true pelvic cavity. Unlike most other animals, where the cervix remains firmly closed until just before delivery, there is usually some degree of cervical softening relatively early in human pregnancy (Fig. 13.9); partial dilation of the cervix occurs much earlier in gestation (Rosenberg and Trevathan, 2014). Because there is such a wide variation in the cervical changes among pregnant women, cervical assessment in isolation of other signs is an unreliable indicator of the imminence of labour. Towards the end of the first stage of labour, the changing shape of the cervix means that its tissue becomes integrated with the lower segment of the uterus (see Fig. 13.8).

The shape of the pelvis and, therefore, the birth canal varies across different mammalian species depending on locomotion and the size and shape of the neonate. The evolution of the human brain resulted in cephalization, the marked enlargement of head size in relation to overall body mass. Adaptations for bipedalism, which evolved ~5–7 million years ago, had an impact on the shape of the pelvis (Trevathan, 2015). The articulation of the skull in relation to the spine is also different in bipedal primates, which has resulted in an exaggerated range of movement of the head at the neck compared with quadrupeds. These maternal and fetal factors create the potential problem of an increased incidence of obstructed labour, which occurs at a much higher rate in humans compared with other animals. The fetus has to negotiate rather than simply pass through the pelvic cavity. Furthermore, the hypermobility of the fetal head adds to the problem a deflexed or abnormally tilted position (asynclitism) is adopted.

It seems that humans have adapted to this by the fetus completing *in utero* development at a relatively early stage and being born at a much smaller proportion of the adult weight. Cephalization has resulted in secondary altriciality, the infant being born at an immature and helpless state of development. Human infants are born with a smaller proportion of adult brain size than other primates. This has significant implications for parental behaviour and social relationships as well as placing a higher emphasis on the importance of nutrition in providing for development of the nervous system and protective parenting in the first postnatal year.

Because of mechanical differences in the birth process, the human fetus has to go through a series of rotations within the pelvic cavity and is usually born in an occipitoanterior position (facing the opposite direction from the mother) making it difficult for the mother to reach to clear a breathing passage or remove the umbilical cord from the infant's neck. Thus, human mothers actively seek assistance in childbirth and birth is a social rather than a solitary occurrence.

Whereas most primates squat during delivery, unless women are used to squatting, the semi-upright positions of kneeling and sitting are thought to be optimal. The upright position (standing, squatting or sitting) results in a shortened second stage of labour and more favourable maternal and infant outcomes. Being upright allows maternal effort to be aided by gravity. The presenting part bears the force of the neonate. The occiput has well-developed cranial plates and is best able to withstand the stress.

It is suggested that the physiological control of birth is mediated by hormones that are derived from archaic brain structures such as the hypothalamus and pituitary gland and that labour is facilitated by an environment that promotes these primitive pathways. The neocortex, on the other hand, is thought to inhibit the primitive pathways. The neocortex responds to bright light and to language. Thus, it is suggested that bright lights, feelings of being observed (use of cameras and monitoring equipment) and use of language, which stimulate neocortical activity, might interfere with the primitive physiological processes and impede the progress of labour. This may explain why relaxation techniques may progress labour. Often women appear to become detached from their surroundings indicating that neocortex activity is suppressed as they inwardly focus on their body activity and dampening down their responses to external stimuli. Birthing in a dimly lit environment may also facilitate labour for the same reason. Fear is an archaic emotional response; women often cry out and express emotional fear in advanced labour suggesting the archaic brain activity is dominant. Maternal levels of catecholamines peak towards the end of labour, which increases maternal awareness and alertness as the baby is born. This is suggested to be an evolutionary advantage, promoting maternal behaviour and protectionism, even aggressiveness. This idea is encapsulated by the fetal ejection reflex first described by Niles Newton in the 1960s, which considers the role of the environment in the progression of labour. If the early stages of labour occur in a calm environment without interruption and catecholamines are released in the late stages of labour, the fetal ejection reflex will result in a smooth delivery. If the mother is stressed and catecholamines are released in the early stages of labour, labour will be slowed to allow the maternal fight-or-flight reflex to be initiated (Odent, 2001).

THE FIRST STAGE OF LABOUR

Uterine Contractions in Labour

If softening of the cervix has taken place, the coordinated uterine contractions exert a steady pull thus thinning the cervix. This effacement of the cervix often takes place before the contractions become completely regular so it may occur a week or so before labour. In multiparous women this effacement is often 'silent' or not perceived as painful. As the cervix effaces, the presenting part of the fetus, usually the head, descends into the cavity of the pelvis. The fetal position alters, the fetal head becomes increasingly more flexed, transnavigating the pelvic cavity initially by the anterior posterior diameter aligning with the lateral diameter of the maternal pelvis, so that it fits well; this is engagement. In some women, especially multiparous women, it is common for engagement not to occur until labour is established as the strong contractions promote flexion of the head thus facilitating it to start negotiating through the pelvic cavity.

Contractions are involuntary and will therefore occur in an unconscious woman. However, they can be temporarily abolished by emotional disturbances including moving from home to hospital and by a change in staff shifts (orchestrated by the adrenalin-driven fight-or-flight reflex). The frequency and strength of the contractions can be increased by enemas, prostaglandins and oxytocin preparations, and by stretching of the cervix or pelvic floor by the presenting part of the fetus. Contractions are regular and intermittent. The intermittent nature is important as it allows recovery of both the uterus and the labouring woman and a resumed oxygen supply to the uterus and fetus, enabling recovery from transient hypoxia induced by the reduction of maternal blood flow during a contraction.

Contractions begin to feel painful as labour proceeds, usually once the internal os of the cervix starts to dilate. Backache often precedes cervical dilation. The pain is thought to be due to ischaemia in the muscle during the contraction because the uterine blood vessels are compressed (similar pain occurs for the same reason in spasmodic dysmenorrhoea). Uterine pain is analogous to myocardial pain in angina when blood flow in the coronary arteries supplying the cardiac muscle is restricted. Baseline tone in labour is ~10–12 mmHg (Blackburn, 2018). An increase in intrauterine pressure of about 10–20 mmHg can be palpated abdominally and perceived by the women at 15–20 mmHg. Pain is often perceived when the pressure rises >25 mmHg. Pressures may rise to 50 mmHg in the first stage and to 75–100 mmHg in the second stage. Weak contractions have a shorter duration with longer intervals between each contraction. The sensation of pain is related not just to the strength of contraction and the interval between each contraction but also to the well-being of the mother and position of the fetus. An anxious or tired woman experiences pain at lower uterine pressure intensity (see below). Maternal position and use of analgesics may influence the strength and timing of contractions. A woman whose baby is in an occipitoposterior position, which commonly presents with a deflexed head (often described as an 'abnormal attitude' or 'military position' – eyes forward, not looking down as in full flexion), also tends to have greater backache as there is increased pressure on the sacral bones and posterior joints of the pelvis.

Contraction Waves

The uterus is also analogous to the heart in another respect, in that it appears to exhibit intrinsic pacemaker activity, although specific pacemaker cells have not been localized. Specific areas that depolarize more rapidly have not been identified, although it was believed that they were each side of the fundus, near the uterotubal junctions or cornuae. All myometrial cells have spontaneous pacemaker activity. The contractions tend to originate from cells near the fundus and spread as a wave, as the electrical activity moves through the gap junctions of the muscle fibres (Fig. 13.10). The waves are strongest at the fundus, which has the highest density of muscle fibres, and take about 15–30 s to travel down the length of the uterus (Blackburn, 2018). There is a polarity of wave contraction with rhythmic coordination between the upper segment, which contracts for longer and retracts, and the lower segment, which contracts slightly later, to a lesser extent and then dilates. This is described as fundal dominance; it is similar to the peristaltic waves generated by smooth muscle in other viscera. If the wave pattern is abnormal, for instance if the lower part contracts first or more strongly, the waves become erratic and uncoordinated and labour does not progress efficiently. This weak and ineffective pattern of contractions is described

as 'incoordinate uterine activity'. Fundal dominance is established in the active first stage of labour, whereas incoordinate activity is often observed in nonestablished labour.

The uterine myometrium relaxes between contractions, which is important for oxygenation of the fetus and uterine tissues. The upper part of the uterus does not relax fully between contractions but retracts instead. This means that the muscle fibres do not return fully to the original length but progressively and gradually get a little bit shorter and thicker with each contraction (Fig. 13.11). This is achieved by these fibres being much longer than normal fibres and the predominant lateral arrangement of the fibres running anterior to posterior of the uterus achieving a 'downward' pressure on the fetus. This means that the less active lower segment is pulled up towards the shortening upper part of the uterus. (If the uterine muscle relaxed completely following each contraction, the uterus would remain the same size and labour would not progress.) The weakest points are the os and cervix, which are effaced and dilated, enlarging the opening of the uterus as they become incorporated into the lower segment by the exertion of the myometrial fibres.

Formation of Hindwaters and Forewaters

As the lower segment stretches and the cervix starts to efface and change its position, the chorion becomes detached from the uterine wall. The operculum (mucus plug) tends to become dislodged from the receding cervical canal. The loss of this mucus closure ('show'), which may be blood-streaked (caused by the rupture of tiny superficial blood vessels during detachment of the mucus plug), indicates the external os has started to dissipate and that active dilation of the internal os is imminent. As the lower segment stretches and the cervix starts to efface and change its position, the chorion becomes detached from the uterine wall as the interior os starts to open. The membranes are extruded through the opening cervix by the pressure of the amniotic fluid (Fig. 13.12). The head of the fetus tends to act as a ball-valve separating the amniotic fluid pushing through the cervix (forewaters) from the remainder of the fluid (hindwaters). The forewaters transmit the pressure generated from the waves of contraction, spreading the force evenly over the cervix, which aids its further effacement and dilation. The hindwaters help to cushion the fetus from the contraction pressures, as the pressure is evenly distributed by the amniotic fluid. As the fundus exerts pressure on the upper aspect of the fetus (usually breech) during contractions, the pressure is transmitted through the fetal body (via the spine) to the lower segment and cervix (this is known as the fetal axis pressure) and facilitates complete flexion of the fetal head, especially in

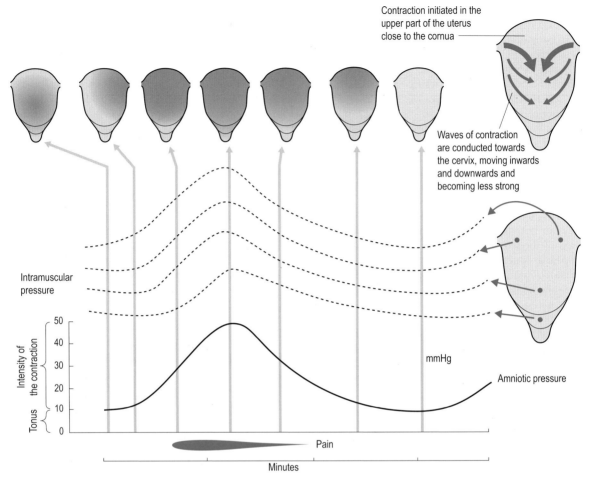

Fig. 13.10 Contraction and retraction of uterine muscle cells. (Reproduced with permission from Sweet and Tiran, 1996.)

a occipitoanterior position. As uterine contractions progress, the pressure of the fluid in the forewaters rises and the membranes tend to rupture; in spontaneous uncomplicated labour this tends to be near or at the start of the second stage of labour. When the fetus is in an abnormal position (e.g. in a breech or posterior and deflexed cephalic position), the pressure of the forewaters is not as great because the presenting part does not plug the cervix as effectively. This explains why a 'soft and floppy bag' of forewaters is associated with abnormal presentations.

Membrane Rupture

As well as an increase in the pressure of the forewaters, the fetal membranes may also rupture when the contractions cause the presenting part to distend them. There is a loss of lubricant between the chorion and amnion leading to increased shear force and cell rupture (Blackburn, 2018). In

5–10% of pregnancies, PROM occurs spontaneously before the onset of uterine contractions as the earliest sign of labour; ~60% of these are classified as term gestation. Spontaneous rupture of the membranes before 37 weeks' gestation often culminates in premature labour and delivery. Early rupture of the membranes as the first event in the course of labour is a cause for concern as it may indicate an ill-fitting presentation or high head at term in a primigravida, polyhydramnios or chorioamnionitis (a local infection, which may be due to *Chlamydia* or *Streptococcus*).

Rupture of the amniotic membrane is associated with collagen degradation in the membrane. Usually coordinated contractions and dilation of the cervix follow rupture of the membranes but if there is a delay the fetus is at risk from ascending infections so clinical intervention may be necessary if labour has not followed within 24 h. There is controversy about artificial rupture of membranes

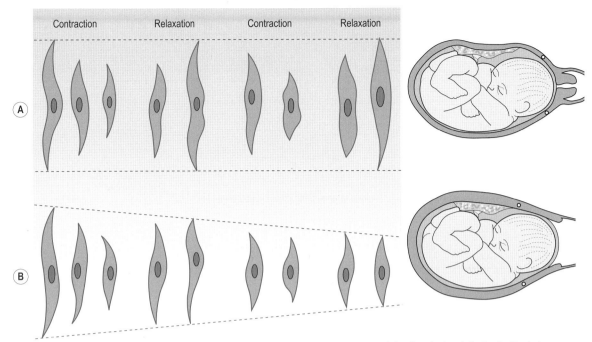

Fig. 13.11 Uterine muscle contraction. Rather than the uterine myometrial cells relaxing fully (as in A), during labour the myometrial cells in the upper segment of the uterus retract getting progressively shorter (as in B). The LUS and the cervix dilate in response to the forces of contraction generated by the shortening upper segment; thus the fetus is expelled.

(amniotomy) and the effect it has on speeding up labour; it is thought that labour may progress more abruptly and painfully and that it could lead to adverse effects and a need for further intervention in labour (Smyth et al., 2013).

Size Changes in the Uterus and Cervix

As the size of the upper segment of the uterus gradually diminishes because of the repeated cycles of contraction and retraction, the fetus is pushed further into the lower segment so its presenting part (Box 13.2) exerts pressure on the opposing maternal tissues, thus displacing these tissues. This results in increased oxytocin release from the posterior pituitary gland, which increases uterine activity by positive feedback mechanisms (see Chapter 1). Later in labour, when the baby has been born and the placenta has been expelled, retraction aids the uterine walls to come together so the cavity is obliterated as the uterine walls are brought into apposition. A physiological retraction ring forms at the junction between the thick retracted segment of the upper segment and the thin distended wall of the lower segment. Under normal conditions, this ring is not visibly evident or palpable by abdominal examination. A visible 'Bandl's ring' is the pathological consequence of advanced obstructed labour and is a sign of imminent uterine rupture.

The rate of cervical dilation is not constant; initially the cervix dilates slowly, but early changes are reinforced by

BOX 13.2 Terms Used for Fetal Presentation

- Attitude: relationship between fetal head and limbs and fetal trunk
- Lie: relationship of fetus to long axis of uterus
- Presentation: part of fetus presenting in lower aspect of uterus
- Presenting part: part of presentation immediately inside internal os
- Position: relationship of presentation, or presenting part, to maternal pelvis
- Denominator: part of presenting part marking position

positive feedback mechanisms and the rate accelerates. The latent phase of the first stage is slower and can take up to 12 h (Box 13.3; Fig. 13.13). It is during this stage, when dilation to 3–4 cm is achieved, that the cervix positively contracts in response to oxytocin. This facilitates effacement, especially around the internal os, which acts as an 'anchor' facilitating the uptake of the external os as it is drawn up to and incorporated into the LUS. After a transition stage of ~15 min when the cervix does not contract, the cervix then dilates in response to myometrial contractions during the faster active phase.

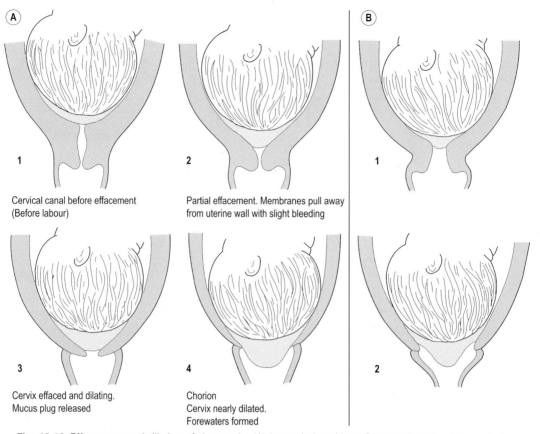

Fig. 13.12 Effacement and dilation of the cervix: (A) in a primigravidae; (B) occurring simultaneously in a multigravidae. (Reproduced with permission from Sweet and Tiran, 1996.)

1. Cervical canal before effacement (Before labour)
2. Partial effacement. Membranes pull away from uterine wall with slight bleeding
3. Cervix effaced and dilating. Mucus plug released
4. Chorion
   Cervix nearly dilated.
   Forewaters formed

BOX 13.3   Progression of Labour

The medical model of care in labour has defined an acceptable rate of progress in labour. Failure of labour to progress at this rate is described as abnormal and used as the rationale for medical intervention. Progress in labour is assessed through the use of a partogram. Cervical dilation at the rate of 0.5 cm/h is accepted as normal. Intervention (such as amniotomy or use of oxytocinon) is usually recommended if the rate of progress falls below 2 cm of the expected progress in 4 h. If in a further 4 h, following the use of oxytocinon, further progress is less than a further 2 cm, then surgical intervention should be considered (NCCWCH, 2014; updated 2017). However, this prediction or rule of progress is now being challenged.

CASE STUDY 13.1

Martha is a para 3; her previous pregnancies and labour were uneventful. She was admitted to the labour ward and confirmed to be in labour as her cervix was 6 cm dilated at 13:00 h. Four hours later on a repeat vaginal examination there was no further dilation, the membranes were intact, and cephalic presentation at the spines was judged to be in a direct occipitoanterior position. Martha was coping well and there were no concerns raised over the fetal condition.

- Should the midwife refer Martha for an obstetric opinion?
- Is the fact that Martha has made no progress enough to justify intervention?
- How could the midwife justify her decision to leave Martha alone, if she felt that this were appropriate?
- What physiological processes/influences may be contributing to this situation?
- What could Martha do to promote her labour to progress effectively and how could the midwife facilitate this?

Table 13.2 summarizes some of the possible types of intervention in labour.

Case study 13.1 is an example of a woman in the first stage of labour.

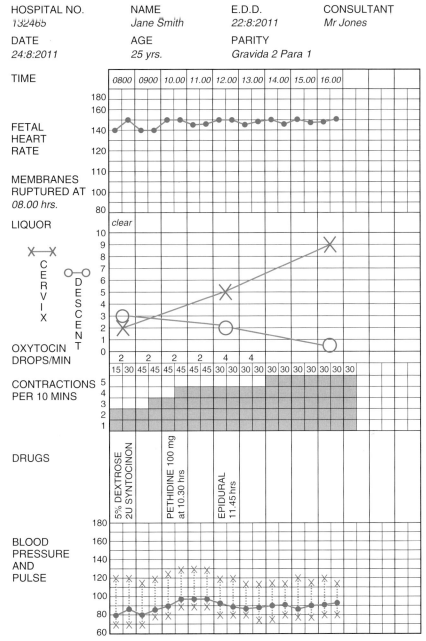

| HOSPITAL NO. | NAME | E.D.D. | CONSULTANT |
| 132465 | Jane Smith | 22:8:2011 | Mr Jones |

| DATE | AGE | PARITY |
| 24:8:2011 | 25 yrs. | Gravida 2 Para 1 |

Fig. 13.13 The partogram is a complete visual record of measurements made during labour and delivery. (Reproduced from Macdonald S, Johnson G, *Mayes' Midwifery*, 15 ed, Elsevier 2017, Fig. 36.6.)

THE SECOND STAGE OF LABOUR

By the end of the first stage of labour, the LUS, the cervix and vagina, supported by the pelvic floor, and the vulval outlet form one continuous dilated birth canal. The forces required to expel the fetus are both from the uterine muscle activity and from the secondary muscles of the maternal abdomen and diaphragm, which augment the contractions of the uterus. The forces generated by the uterus can be described as the primary power and the complementary force from the voluntary movement of the respiratory muscles as the secondary power, although this is normally an instinctive behavioural action, not necessarily under conscious control. By this stage, the uterus is markedly retracted and undergoing a pattern of strong, regular and repetitive contractions. The mother is compelled involuntarily to bear down or push. As she inspires before pushing, the diaphragm is lowered and the abdominal muscles contract, augmenting the contractile forces of the uterus. Bearing down by the mother helps to overcome the resistance of the soft tissues of the vagina and the pelvic floor. The fetal attitude (see Box 13.2) extends as it is directed through the birth canal, which aids the efficiency of the uterine contractions. The pain experienced in the second stage of labour is often less as cervical dilation is complete and the woman is aware that progress is more rapid.

As the fetal head passes through the pelvis, the pressure on the maternal sacral nerves may be associated with cramp in the legs and pain from the trauma to the tissue through stretching, compression and displacement. The fetus distends the vagina as it descends, and contacts and displaces the pelvic floor. The anterior part of the pelvic floor is drawn up causing the urethra to elongate and become compressed. The bladder is therefore repositioned within the protective environs of the abdomen. At this point, as the women pushes, involuntary leakage of urine may occur if the woman has a full bladder. Posteriorly, the pelvic floor is stretched forward in relation to the presenting part and the rectum is compressed, which may lead to defecation as the presenting part descends further down the vagina (which is often a sign the second stage has commenced). The perineum is flattened, lengthened and thinned by the presenting part of the fetus as it reaches the introitus.

During a contraction, the presenting part (usually the fetal head) advances forward and, if not in a direct anterior position, rotates forwards facilitated by the 'gutter' shape and resistance of the pelvic floor. If the fetal head is completely flexed, then the top of the head (the flexion point) meets the resistance of the pelvic floor optimizing rotation. Pressure on the pelvic floor causes it to contract exerting an opposing force to the contraction force thus rotation is facilitated by these opposing two forces. In the interval between contractions, the presenting part recedes slightly and may rotate back but, as the uterine muscle retracts with each contraction, progression in the forward direction is maintained by the pelvic floor resistance. This progression has been likened to taking two steps forward and one step back. Once the flexion point is positioned over the uretogenital hiatus (vaginal opening), the fetal head starts to distend the perineum and the vagina begins to open. At this point, rotation stops as the presenting part no longer meets the resistance of the pelvic floor and moves 'forward' as the vaginal opening offers less resistance to the contractile forces. When the widest part of the fetal head (the biparietal diameter, when head is fully flexed) distends the vulva, the stretching of the perineum and introitus is at its maximum, hence pain may be severe at this point. This is described as 'crowning' of the head.

The intensity of the pain may cause a labouring woman to gasp and inhale sharply. The momentary break in the bearing-down movement has an important role in protecting the perineum from too much trauma, which can cause tearing of the tissue. Once the head is delivered, in an unflexing movement, it realigns itself with the original internal position of the fetal body (so the baby's head moves from facing the maternal anus to face either one of the maternal buttocks); this is called 'restitution'. Following restitution, the next contraction forces the anterior shoulder to contact the perineum and therefore further external rotation of the head occurs with the fetus facing at right angles with the maternal midline. The birth of the baby is usually accomplished with the next contraction following 'crowning' with the posterior shoulder leading. A gush of amniotic fluid escapes signifying the loss of the hindwaters. The fetus undergoes a pattern of a passive corkscrew movement as it follows the shape and curvature of the true pelvis (curvature of Carus). The gutter shape of the pelvic floor facilitates the rotation of the presenting part enabling the widest diameters of the pelvis to accommodate the largest dimensions of the fetal head and shoulders (Fig. 13.14). In breach presentations, the anterior buttock of the fetus contacts with the perineum first and so rotates forward and once the anterior buttock lies over the urogenital hiatus the breech will distend the perineum and vaginal opening as it is born.

Influences of Pelvic and Pelvic Floor Morphology and Parturition

The passage of the fetus through the pelvis is described in practice as the mechanisms of labour. Engagement describes the initial descent of the presenting part into the true pelvic cavity; the term relates to the widest transverse diameter of the fetal skull having negotiated the pelvic brim or inlet. If the baby has a cephalic (head-first) presentation, this is described in terms of number of fifths palpable (Fig. 13.15). Verification of the degree of engagement can be achieved through vaginal examination. With a cephalic presentation, the level of the biparietal prominences is judged in relation to the pelvic brim and the pelvic outlet at the level of the ischial spines. Engagement may occur long before the onset of labour, or may occur during or even late in labour (more common in multiparous women). In a primigravida, engagement usually occurs at about 36 weeks' gestation in response to effacement of the cervix. Engagement does not indicate cavity and outlet measurements.

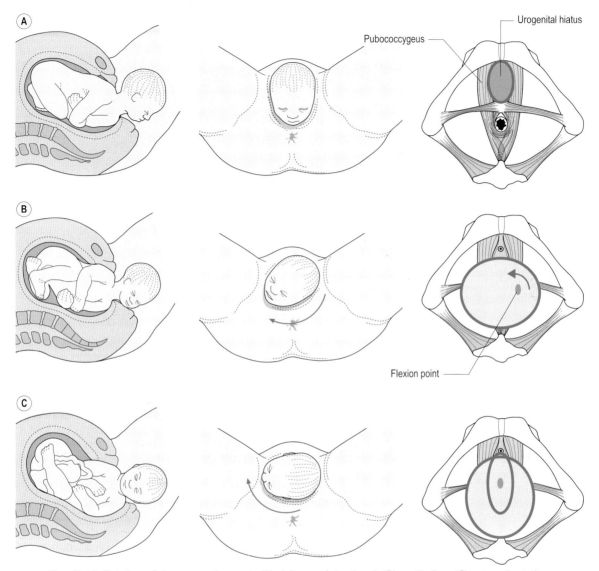

Fig. 13.14 Rotation of the presenting part: (A) delivery of the head; (B) restitution; (C) external rotation. (Adapted with permission from Bennett and Brown, 1999.)

In the abnormal pelvis, where the anterior posterior diameter is diminished, engagement of the fetal skull can still be facilitated by asynclitism (lateral tilting of the fetal head). The head enters the pelvis in a tilted position and becomes engaged as the fetus untilts its head. Posterior asynclitism is more favourable as the posterior curve of the sacrum facilitates untilting. Anterior asynclitism is less likely to untilt as the head is hindered by the pubic arch. Asynclitism can be detected by vaginal examination by determining the position from digit examination of the fetal skull landmarks and in extreme cases the anterior ear can often be felt under the pubic arch. Abnormal pelvic diameters can cause labour dystocia (arrest of progress) and/or shoulder dystocia (failure to deliver the fetal body following delivery of the head as the fetal shoulder prominences impact on the maternal pelvic brim).

THE THIRD STAGE OF LABOUR

With expulsion of the fetus, the third stage begins, in which the placenta separates from the wall of the uterus and is expelled with the fetal membranes and umbilical cord.

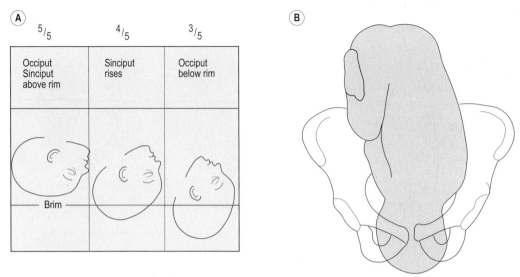

Fig. 13.15 (A) Flexion and descent of the presenting part into the pelvic cavity; (B) engagement of the head. ((A) Reproduced with permission from Bennett and Brown, 1999. (B) Reproduced with permission from Sweet and Tiran, 1996.)

Before separation, the placental extracellular matrix is degraded and remodelled by proteolytic enzymes including MMP produced by the decidua and fetal membranes (Geng et al., 2016). The uterus retracts markedly and bleeding from the placental wound site is constrained, this is facilitated by the near empty state of the uterus.

Following the safe delivery of a healthy baby, the third stage of labour still presents a number of potential, life-threatening, hazards for the mother. Should all or part of the placenta and/or membranes be retained, control of bleeding is likely to be impaired and a life-threatening postpartum haemorrhage (PPH) could ensue. Retained products of conception (RPOC) complicate 1–5% of routine vaginal deliveries and could become the focus of infection if not treated, potentially resulting in bacterial sepsis. PPH is the major cause of maternal death during pregnancy with >50,000 deaths/annum worldwide.

Immediately after delivery, the uterus markedly contracts down in size. Then the pattern of contractions is interrupted for a minute or so, until contractions resume at a slower rate. As the uterus retracts, the placental site is greatly diminished. The placenta is not elastic; thus, it tends to wrinkle and buckle and be sheared off the elastic uterine wall (like a paper label coming away from a deflating balloon). It is at this stage that some fetal blood from the placental circulation can enter the maternal circulation (feto–maternal transfusion or haemorrhage), potentially causing problems, for example, if there is Rhesus incompatibility (see Chapter 10). The marked retraction of the uterus impedes the venous drainage of the maternal

intervillous spaces. Separation usually begins in the centre of the placenta and the extravasculated blood forms a haematoma or retroplacental clot between the placenta and decidua aiding its separation as the clot adds to the placental weight peeling the membranes from the uterine wall as it 'sinks' into the lower region of the uterus and then passes into the vaginal cavity. This is often associated with a fundally located placenta where the uterine contractibility is at its greatest. As the uterus retracts, its progressively shortening muscle fibres tighten around the maternal vessels, forming 'living ligatures', which impede the blood flow. This restricts the flow of maternal blood to the uterus and placental wound site, preventing excessive blood loss.

It is the commencement of spontaneous or stimulated uterine contractions following the completion of the second stage of labour that causes the placenta to separate from the uterine wall. The weight of the placenta completes the detachment of the membranes, which peel off and are expelled (Fig. 13.16). The site of placental implantation determines the speed of separation and the method of placental expulsion. The fetal membranes are expelled with the maternal or fetal surface prominent. The Schultze method of expulsion, whereby the fetal side presents, is most common and is associated with a fundal site implantation and the Matthews-Duncan expulsion (whereby the placenta slips out sideways like a button through a buttonhole) is more likely with a lateral and/or low implantation. In some cultures, the placenta has important significance and women keep it for ritual ceremonies. In Western societies, the practice of placental encapsulation for oral

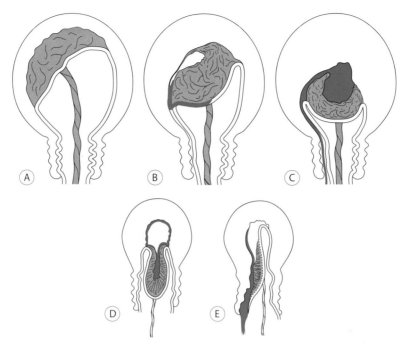

Fig. 13.16 The mechanism of placental separation and expulsion: (A) uterine wall partially retracted but not sufficiently to cause placental separation; (B) further contraction and retraction thicken uterine wall, reduce placental site and aid placental separation; (C) complete separation and formation of retroplacental clot (note: the thin lower segment has collapsed like a concertina following the birth of the baby); (D) Schultze method of expulsion; (E) Matthews-Duncan method of expulsion.

consumption (placentophagy) is a growing trend. The reasons include accelerated recovery after birth and enhanced lactation, improved mood and wellness, protection against postpartum depression and nutritional benefits. The usual method of preparing the placenta involves the tissue being dehydrated, ground up and encapsulated. The commonly used methods of preparation reduce the hormone concentration and bacterial contamination (Johnson et al., 2018).

Active Management

The third stage of labour can be physiologically managed (passive management), taking about 20–30 min to complete, but active management is widely practised by midwives and obstetricians, shortening the time of placental delivery to a few minutes. Active management involves the injection of an anti-tocolytic agent such as Syntometrine or Syntocinon (see below) at the birth of the anterior shoulder or shortly after the delivery of the baby and delivering the placenta and membranes by controlled cord traction (CCT; also known as the Brandt–Andrews manoeuvre). The sheared-off placenta is actively extracted by the midwife rather than passively expelled by the mother if active management of the third stage of labour is implemented.

The use of CCT is subject to some discussion and is not practised in all countries. The placenta should be separated and the uterus should be well contracted before CCT to ensure that it does not cause uterine inversion.

Syntometrine is a combination of oxytocinon (also called Syntocinon; synthetic oxytocin) and ergometrine, which is used to reduce the risk of PPH. Oxytocinon acts within 2–3 min following intramuscular injection, by causing intermittent contractions. These effectively continue the retraction process behind the placental site, thus encouraging separation and early expulsion. Ergometrine becomes effective about 5–7 min after administration. By this time, aided by CCT (which should be commenced as soon as the uterus contracts down, stimulated by the Syntocinon), the placenta has been extracted. The midwife applies cord traction by gripping the umbilical cord with one hand and applying a downward traction (Fig. 13.17) to compensate for the 'upward' curve of Carus. The other hand is placed on the lower abdomen, thumb and index finger stretched out to provide a line of contact, applying pressure to avoid inversion of the uterus by compressing the LUS. Ergometrine produces a sustained uterine contraction, which promotes and prolongs the haemostatic

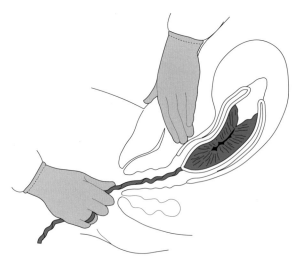

Fig. 13.17 Controlled cord traction (Brandt–Andrews method). (Reproduced with permission from Bennett and Brown, 1999.)

action of the living ligatures. It is essential, therefore, to deliver the placenta before ergometrine stimulates closure of the cervix as this could result in retained placenta and membranes. The third stage of labour can also be managed using intramuscular injections of oxytocinon only following delivery as it has fewer side-effects. Syntometrine should not be used if there is a history of hypertension because ergometrine can increase blood pressure further.

Physiological management of the third stage of labour involves no routine use of anti-tocolytic drugs, not clamping the umbilical cord until pulsations cease, no uterine manipulation or CCT. The delivery of the placenta and membranes is solely by maternal effort and should be completed within 1 h of birth. Skin-to-skin contact and early breastfeeding may facilitate the delivery of the placenta in the third stage by stimulating endogenous maternal oxytocin release. Women are encouraged to empty their bladders and adopt an upright position because gravity aids delivery of the placenta. During this time, palpation of the uterus should be avoided but careful observation is required especially of vaginal blood loss to identify and differentiate between signs of separation and haemorrhage. As placental separation occurs, there is usually an increase in blood loss but this is reduced as the uterus contracts down and the presence of the placenta in the vaginal cavity (upper part of the birth canal) stimulates the mother to bear down. This may stimulate more oxytocin release due to Ferguson's reflex. Division of the umbilical cord should not be rushed unless the baby needs attention; ideally the cord should not be cut until it has stopped pulsating. If the cord is not clamped prematurely, blood continues to flow from the placenta through

the cord. Up to a third of the fetal blood volume can be in the placenta at birth; allowing placental transfusion to continue means that a significant proportion of this can re-enter the neonatal circulation (Anton et al., 2018). This is important for neonatal transition and infant iron status (see Chapter 15) and also facilitates spontaneous delivery of the placenta, as it is easier for the placenta to pass through the birth canal.

THE EFFECTS OF LABOUR ON MATERNAL PHYSIOLOGY

Cardiovascular System

The stress of labour prepares the woman for the inevitable blood loss at delivery and limitation of bleeding after placental separation. Dehydration and muscle activity increase the haemoglobin concentration. Erythropoiesis and white blood cell number also increase as part of the normal response to stress. Concentrations of clotting factors increase; clotting times shorten and fibrinolytic activity is decreased on completion of the third stage of labour. The placenta and decidua are very rich sources of thromboplastin, which can activate coagulation (see Chapter 1). About 5–10% of the total body fibrin is deposited as a haemostatic endometrial mesh over the placental wound site (Blackburn, 2018). This hypercoagulable state is further developed in the puerperium (see Chapter 14).

The cardiovascular system is affected by pain, anxiety, apprehension, maternal position and anaesthesia, as well as by the muscular activity of the uterus itself and the dramatic increase in catecholamine production during labour. Uterine contractions progressively increase cardiac output as venous return and circulating volume are increased. Each contraction can contribute 300–500 mL of blood to the circulation (Blackburn, 2018), which significantly increases cardiac output and blood pressure. In the supine position, stroke volume and cardiac output tend to be lower and heart rate raised.

Catecholamines affect vascular tone and increase blood pressure; this effect is reduced with anaesthetics. Pain and anxiety result in tachycardia (increased heart rate) and also affects blood pressure. During a contraction, systolic blood pressure increases by at least 35 mmHg and diastolic blood pressure may increase between 25 and 65 mmHg (Blackburn, 2018). The increment in blood pressure precedes each contraction and falls to baseline between contractions. The greatest haemodynamic changes occur in women delivering their baby vaginally, which is an important consideration for women who have been diagnosed with cardiac disease.

The Respiratory System

Labour affects the respiratory system as the muscular work increases metabolic rate and oxygen consumption. Respiratory rate and depth of respiration increase. Anxiety, drugs and use of a gasmask mouthpiece can all affect respiratory rate. There is a tendency for a labouring woman to hyperventilate. Hyperventilation is a natural response to pain. Contractions occurring at high frequency can affect oxygenation causing muscular hypoxia and acidosis. Hypoxia can increase the amount of pain experienced.

The increased ventilation causes a progressive and marked decrease in partial pressure of carbon dioxide (to ~25 mmHg), particularly if the contractions are painful. In early labour, hyperventilation can cause respiratory alkalosis and increased blood pH. This can result in the woman experiencing dizziness and tingling of her fingers and toes, and possibly developing muscle spasms. At an extremely low partial pressure of carbon dioxide ($PaCO_2$), blood flow can be affected and the oxygen–haemoglobin dissociation curve (see Chapter 1) shifts to the left so release of oxygen from haemoglobin is impaired. The remedy of breath counting to slow respiratory rate, especially if the woman counts them with her partner or a midwife who deliberately slows down counting, can prevent or correct hyperventilatory effects.

By the end of the first stage, maternal acidosis due to isometric muscle contractions is likely and is compensated for, to a degree, by the respiratory alkalosis. The muscle contractions reduce blood flow to the uterine muscle, which becomes hypoxic and undergoes anaerobic metabolism. Flow to the intervillous space also decreases so fetal levels of carbon dioxide increase and the fetus tends to become acidotic. During bearing down, when the mother's accessory respiratory muscles are involved, mild respiratory acidosis is likely. In the second stage of labour lactate levels increase, thus pH falls. There is usually no physiological compensation for this metabolic acidosis.

The Renin–Angiotensin System

Labour and delivery affect the renin–angiotensin system of both fetus and mother. Levels of renin and angiotensinogen increase, which are important in maintaining blood flow, but can also affect handling and excretion of drugs. Glomerular filtration rate, renal blood flow and sodium excretion are also affected by raised catecholamine levels or general anaesthetic. Oxytocin has structural similarities with ADH and has inherent antidiuretic properties; therefore, fluid retention is increased in labour. Women in labour can be at risk of iatrogenic water intoxication due to loss of electrolytes, overuse of oxytocinon (which has ADH like properties) or excessive intravenous fluid administration (fluid overload).

Metabolic Rate

Maternal glucose utilization markedly increases in labour to provide the energy required by the uterus and skeletal muscles. Glucose and triacylglycerides are used as energy sources. Oxytocin has some insulin-like properties. An increased body temperature during labour may indicate dehydration or infection. It is common for women to experience a transient postpartum chill ~15 min after the birth of the baby or delivery of the placenta. In the following 24 h, postpartum women frequently have a slightly raised temperature secondary to dehydration.

NUTRITION IN LABOUR

Food and drink consumption in labour is sometimes controversial. There are two conflicting arguments. The first is that a woman in labour might possibly require a general anaesthetic and therefore should be treated as a preoperative patient at risk of gastric aspiration. Pulmonary aspiration of gastric acid (aspiration pneumonitis or Mendelson syndrome) or particulate food matter, although rare, was a major cause of morbidity and mortality for women in labour. The risks of gastric aspiration were thought to be greatly reduced if oral intake is limited. Pregnant women have a slower gastric emptying rate (see Chapter 11), which is further delayed by labour, and decreased tone of the lower oesophageal sphincter but it is not known whether this delayed gastric emptying predisposes to gastric aspiration.

The opposing view is that a more liberal policy may be more beneficial and that women are being needlessly deprived of food. It is argued that general anaesthesia is relatively rare with a greater use of regional anaesthesia and that obstetric anaesthesia techniques have improved, which make aspiration of gastric contents unlikely. It is argued that prolonged fasting could have detrimental psychological and physiological effects, including increased anxiety and stress, which might prolong labour.

Pregnant women are predisposed to ketosis, particularly in labour. Pregnancy is a ketotic state, and fasting in pregnancy is invariably associated with ketonuria. It is estimated that a woman in labour has an energy requirement of about 2950–4600 kJ/h (700–1100 kcal/h). When glycogen stores are exhausted, adipose tissue is mobilized. Fatty acid oxidation increases ketosis, an excess of ketone bodies in the plasma, which are excreted into the urine. Lipolysis provides fatty acid substrates for maternal energy needs and spares glucose for the fetus. The critical question is whether ketosis is detrimental to the progress of labour. Ketones can increase acidity, cause excessive renal excretion of sodium and cross the placenta to the fetus. Although the length of labour is correlated with the degree

TABLE 13.3 Fetal Behavioural States	
State 1F (1 fetal); quiet sleep	Fetal quiescence with brief gross startles; high-voltage electrocortical activity; no eye movement; FHR accelerations; minimal heart rate variability; isolated fetal heart rate
State 2F (2 fetal); active sleep	Paradoxical/irregular sleep; frequent and periodic stretches; retroflexion and movements of extremities; low-voltage electrocortical activity; continuous eye movements; increased FHR variability with frequent accelerations
State 3F (3 fetal); quiet awake	Absence of gross movements; continuous rapid eye movements; stable, but widely oscillating FHR, no accelerations
State 4F (4 fetal); active awake	Vigorous and continual movements; rapid eye movement; unstable heart rate – large, long accelerations and tachycardia

of ketosis, it is not clear whether longer labour results in increased ketosis or whether ketosis prolongs labour (Singata et al., 2013).

It is suggested that fasting in labour can increase the need for medical intervention, be unpleasant for the labouring woman or affect her subsequent interaction with her newborn baby. Allowing women to eat in labour reduces the plasma level of ketones, which may aid the progress of labour. Ketonuria can be treated by administration of intravenous dextrose but this is associated with fluid and electrolyte imbalance. A number of women experience nausea and vomiting in labour. But, in practice, most maternity units have adopted a liberal policy allowing women to eat what they want or offering a nonparticulate diet while using antacids and H_2-antagonists to reduce gastric pH and decrease volume of gastric contents, thus minimizing the risk of aspiration and lung damage.

THE EFFECTS OF LABOUR ON THE FETUS

Labour has profound effects on the fetus and is important in aiding fetal adaptation to extrauterine life (see Chapter 15). Understanding the effects of labour on the fetus is important in differentiating between normal healthy responses and diagnosing fetal distress.

Behaviour of the Fetus during Pregnancy

The use of ultrasound led to the observation that, after 36 weeks, the fetus exhibits a number of clearly definable behavioural states, which are analogous to the neonatal states (see Chapter 15). These states have characteristic patterns of fetal heart rate (FHR), fetal breathing movements (FBM), eye movements, voiding and mouthing movements (Table 13.3). The patterns of fetal behaviour change with gestational age and are assumed to reflect the activity of the fetal CNS and can potentially be used to recognize a compromised fetus (Borsani et al., 2018). The movements evidently demonstrate fetal ability to respond to external stimuli. Many factors such as time of day, meals, smoking,

etc. affect fetal behaviour. Most of the movements that are discernible in the third trimester can be traced back to the first trimester. Both the movements and the periods of quiescence between them are important.

FBM can be detected from the 10th week of pregnancy and increase with gestational age (Koos and Rajaee, 2014). FBM are more regular in state 1F than in state 2F, they occur more frequently in state 2F and are present but irregular in states 3F and 4F (see Table 13.3). FBM are more likely to be state-dependent when maternal glucose levels are lower. There is a postprandial increase in FBM and smoking diminishes them. Fetal voiding movements are inhibited in state 1F but occur at the transition to state 2F. Sucking and swallowing can be seen from the end of the first trimester. Regular or rhythmic mouthing movements are most often observed in state 1F, when they occur in bursts of 10–20 min, whereas powerful sucking movements can be seen in state 3F. Both regular mouthing and sucking can entrain FHR patterns, which can bewilder clinical interpretation.

States 1F and 2F account for about 90% of fetal life in late gestation. FHR patterns during these four behavioural states may mimic fetal distress. The fetal behavioural states and the transitions between them can be observed throughout labour. States 1F and 2F predominate as they do before labour. It is thought that diminished FHR variability and absent accelerations in a healthy term fetus probably represent fetal sleep rather than fetal distress but prolonged periods (over 25 min) are more likely to be caused by fetal compromise. In the deep sleep state, 1F, FHR pattern is usually unaffected even by strong uterine contractions. A period of low fetal heart variability (FHV) or tachycardia may indicate that fetal oxygenation is being compromised. In the second stage of labour, the length of the behavioural cycles decreases; this is related to the gamut of sensory stimuli and head compression incurred during this stage of labour.

FBM increase in frequency and in length of episode as gestation progresses. By the third trimester, FBM occur for 30% of the time and are closely associated with behavioural state, especially active sleep (2F). A few days before the onset of labour, FBM are depressed, probably because increased levels of prostaglandin, especially PGE$_2$, inhibit the fetal respiratory centre. During the latent stage of labour, FBM occur for about 10% of the time but almost cease in the active stage. In preterm labour, the decrease in FBM is less acute. FBM may be affected by changes in oxygenation and pH. FBM require energy so the fetus decreases FBM in response to hypoxia as an adaptive response to conserve oxygen. The hypoxia-induced decrease in FBM is more marked near term possibly because the responses to hypoxia have become more sensitive as the respiratory centre becomes more mature.

Although hypoxia normally decreases FBM, deeper, sustained inspiration or gasping is stimulated synergistically by raised carbon dioxide levels in the presence of hypoxia. In perinatal aspiration, this gasping can cause meconium inspiration. In practice, infants born with a history of prolonged fetal distress in the presence of meconium stained liquor require close monitoring to exclude meconium aspiration for around 48 h following birth. Paradoxically, maternal hyperventilation decreases FBM. Hypoglycaemia and CNS depressants, such as ethanol, barbiturates and diazepam, decrease FBM. Theophylline increases FBM and is used to treat postnatal apnoea and bradycardia in premature infants. Prostaglandin inhibitors, such as indomethacin, stimulate FBM but have to be used with caution because of their effects on fetal vascular function.

Changes in fetal behaviour over the course of pregnancy are summarized in Box 13.4.

BOX 13.4 Changes in Fetal Behaviour during Pregnancy

First Trimester
- Specific sequence of movements
- Continual activity
- Coordinated and graceful quality

Second Trimester
- Body movements diminish
- Breathing movements increase
- Quiescence increases
- Rest–activity cycles develop

Third Trimester
- Clear fetal behavioural states
- Specific combination of variables
- Stable with state transitions
- Breathing is state-dependent

Changes during Labour

The stress of labour causes a reflex increase in maternal catecholamine levels well above those seen in nonpregnant women or pregnant women before labour. The physiological stress and hypoxia associated with the pain and anxiety increase adrenaline secretion. The physiological work of labour, which is highest in the second stage of labour, increases noradrenaline release. Placental metabolism of maternal catecholamines reduces the transfer to the fetus. However, maternal catecholamines can affect placental blood flow and also affect the fetus in labour. Animal studies show that adrenaline is associated with vasoconstriction and a reduction in uterine blood flow. As the rise in adrenaline level is associated with maternal stress in labour, there is a clear advantage to limiting maternal psychological distress and pain.

Normal labour and delivery are associated with increased (and beneficial) physiological stress resulting in raised cord levels of catecholamines in the neonate. This increase in fetal catecholamines may be a response to fetal compression, mild acidosis and other stimuli experienced during the birth. Catecholamine levels in newborns were found to be about 20 times higher than levels in the venous blood of either resting adults, exercising adults and even adults with pheochromocytoma (a catecholamine-producing tumour) (Lagercrantz and Slotkin, 1986). This perinatal surge of catecholamines is clearly important since interference with it can result in cardiorespiratory collapse in the newborn. It is suggested that this is an adaptive response that facilitates extrauterine adaptation. The increased catecholamines stimulate breathing, increase fluid absorption from the lungs, stimulate surfactant release, enhance irritability, and play a role in metabolism by mobilizing glucose and fatty acids (Riviere et al., 2018).

Fetal tissues are metabolically active; heat dissipation is via the placenta to the mother. Cord exclusion in animal models results in an increase in fetal temperature. It seems likely that uterine contractions affecting uterine blood flow will impair heat transfer, particularly in active labour. At delivery, there is a transition from a heat-producing fetus, challenged to lose heat, to a neonate dependent on heat generation, challenged to preserve heat. *In utero*, PGE$_2$ and adenosine derived from the placenta may have a role in suppressing the activity of brown adipose tissue and therefore minimizing heat production by the fetus. Occlusion of the umbilical cord is the signal to increase heat generation. Nonshivering thermogenesis by brown adipose tissue is under the control of noradrenaline released during labour.

A healthy term fetus has good energy stores and a normal base excess (the amount of base present in the blood, which increases in metabolic alkalosis) so it can tolerate temporary reductions in uterine perfusion in labour. There is a marked increase in fetal glycogen storage in the last month of gestation. The fetus also has the enzymes required for glycogenolysis. However, under normal uterine conditions, placental transfer of maternal glucose means that the fetal glucose pool is of maternal origin. Until labour, the fetus still depends on maternal sources of glucose. The changes in catecholamine secretion boost neonatal metabolism.

The placenta also provides the route of oxygen transfer and carbon dioxide removal. Maternal hyperventilation in labour increases carbon dioxide diffusion across the placenta, therefore increasing respiratory alkalosis (increasing pH). However, respiratory depression caused by oversedation or magnesium sulphate, used to treat preterm labour, could have the opposite effect. In the presence of a reduced oxygen supply, anaerobic metabolism will cause metabolic acidosis. Lactate diffusion across the placenta is slow and the fetal kidney is not efficient at clearing organic acids. It seems likely that the respiratory alkalosis related to maternal hyperventilation compensates for at least some of the metabolic acidosis, owing to anaerobic glycolysis, thus restoring fetal pH to a normal range. Normal labour nevertheless will cause a gradual decrease in fetal blood pH, oxygen and bicarbonate ions and a corresponding rise in the partial pressure of carbon dioxide (pCO_2).

Uterine blood flow is largely determined by maternal blood pressure, cardiac output and uterine muscular tone. Labour compromises uterine blood flow. The maternal spiral arteries, which perfuse the intervillous spaces, are occluded and venous drainage of the spaces is obstructed during uterine contractions. Doppler measurements show that blood flow through the uterine arteries is gradually reduced during a contraction and gradually returns when the uterus relaxes. Most animal models demonstrate that the placenta has an anatomical redundancy; over 70% of the placental capillary bed must be occluded before impedance to gas exchange rises significantly. If placental reserve is reduced, uterine contractions may have a significant effect on fetal hypoxia and acidosis. Even with a healthy placenta and normal uterine blood flow, contractions with excessive strength or frequency can cause fetal hypoxia and bradycardia. Maternal conditions may exacerbate this by reducing uterine perfusion; supine posture can reduce venous return, therefore cardiac output and regional anaesthesia can cause vasodilation so decreasing maternal cardiac output.

Labour promotes the clearance of fluid from the fetal lungs. Transient rapid breathing (tachypnoea), caused by residual lung fluid, is more common in babies born by elective caesarean section than in those experiencing a vaginal delivery. Chest compression mechanically expels a small volume of fluid. Late in gestation, the pulmonary epithelial cells actively secrete chloride ions, and this creates a gradient, which drives water movement by osmosis and maintains adequate lung volume *in utero*. Before birth the lung epithelial cells change from being predominantly chloride-secreting to being sodium-absorbing, which draws fluid into the interstitial spaces. The sodium-pumping activity is increased in spontaneous labour; this may be related to the catecholamine surge.

A mature sucking pattern is evident from 36 weeks' gestation. Although fetal swallowing can be observed as early as 11 weeks' gestation, near-term discrete episodes of swallowing occur, probably triggered by 'thirst', gastric emptying or changed composition of amniotic fluid (Brace and Cheung, 2014). This swallowing may be important for gut development and maturation. In labour, there is some evidence that swallowing increases. Meconium passage is rare until about 38 weeks when the control of intestinal peristalsis is more mature. Early meconium passage is associated with listeriosis. Meconium-stained amniotic fluid (MSAF) occurs in about one-third of pregnancies beyond 42 weeks. Hypoxia induces vasoconstriction of the fetal gut, hyperperistalsis and anal sphincter relaxation, so passage of meconium is associated with fetal distress (Vain and Batton, 2017). However, it is possible that MSAF could reflect normal maturity of the fetal gut function rather than fetal distress. Less than 2% of babies born with MSAF go on to develop severe meconium aspiration syndrome (MAS). It has been suggested that the primary cause of MAS is pulmonary epithelial damage or airway obstruction, which results in ineffectual clearance of meconium. The residual meconium can interfere with surfactant dispersal and increase the severity of the respiratory problems.

THE FETAL SKULL AND FETAL PRESENTATION

The dimensions of the fetal head correlate well with those of the maternal pelvis. Examination of the shape of the baby's head soon after delivery shows how it passed through the pelvis (Fig. 13.18). The bones of the fetal skull are relatively mobile and mould under compression during labour. The sutures and fontanelles (Fig. 13.19) allow the skull bones to overlap partially so the dimensions of the presenting part can be reduced by ~0.5–1 cm. Diameters that are not compressed elongate to compensate for those that are reduced. If the pressure generated against the cervix impedes the circulation in the scalp then oedema may occur forming a caput or swelling. The area of the caput and the degree of moulding indicate the degree of head compression endured in labour. The caput is usually absorbed within a few days of delivery and requires no treatment. If the head is compressed to an abnormal diameter, or if the moulding

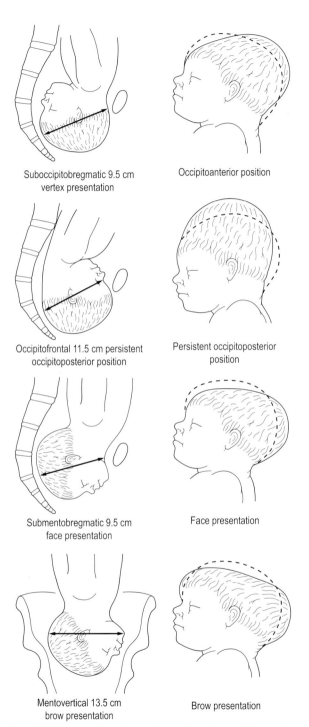

Fig. 13.18 The relationship between the shape of the baby's head and the moulding of the fetal skull.

Suboccipitobregmatic 9.5 cm vertex presentation

Occipitoanterior position

Occipitofrontal 11.5 cm persistent occipitoposterior position

Persistent occipitoposterior position

Submentobregmatic 9.5 cm face presentation

Face presentation

Mentovertical 13.5 cm brow presentation

Brow presentation

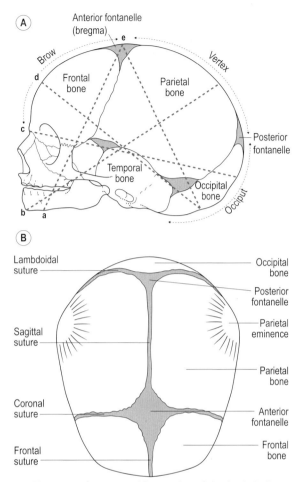

Fig. 13.19 Sutures and fontanelles of the fetal skull.

is too excessive or rapid, the dura mater forming the falx cerebri may be pulled from the tentorium cerebellum resulting in rupture of the venous sinuses and intracranial haemorrhage (tentorial tear) (Fig. 13.20).

The position of the fetus (see Box 13.2, for an explanation of terms) is determined on abdominal examination in later pregnancy and early labour (Fig. 13.21). The midwife can gently palpate the pregnant woman's abdomen to determine how the fetus is lying and how the presenting part of the fetus relates to the pelvis. The degree of engagement of the fetal head into the brim of the pelvis can also be ascertained. Auscultation of the fetal heart confirms the initial findings. The lie of the fetus describes the relative position of the long axis of the fetus to the long axis of the uterus and maternal spine. Usually the lie is longitudinal, rather than oblique or transverse, particularly in the last weeks of pregnancy. The attitude is the degree of flexion of the fetus. In the fully flexed

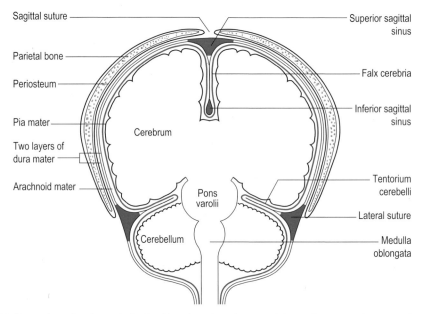

Fig. 13.20 Coronal section through the fetal head to show intracranial membranes and venous sinuses. (Reproduced with permission from Bennett and Brown, 1999.)

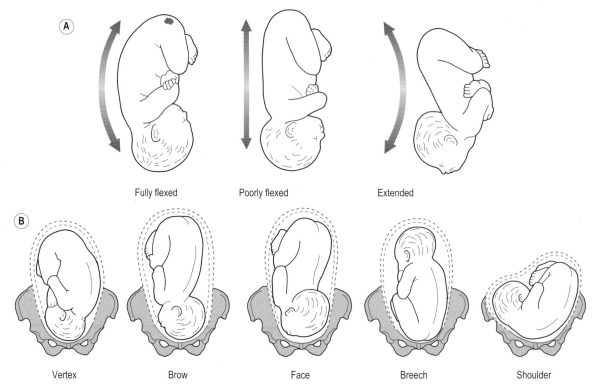

Fig. 13.21 (A) Attitude and (B) presentation of the fetus. (Reproduced with permission from Sweet and Tiran, 1996.)

attitude, the fit of the fetus in the uterus is comfortable. The presentation describes the presenting part of the fetus. Cephalic presentation occurs in most pregnancies. The fetal position is described by the relationship of the denominator (anatomical point on the presenting part) to areas of the maternal pelvic brim. The pelvic areas are left and right, anterior, lateral or posterior areas. The occiput (the bone at the back of the fetal skull) is the denominator of a well-flexed cephalic position so the fetus could, for instance, be described to be in a right occipitoanterior position. Anterior positions are more common because the fetal spine is against the mother's abdominal wall. Occipitoposterior positions tend to result in the fetus assuming a deflexed attitude, which can result in less-effective contraction, prolonged labour, uneven cervical dilatation, increased risk of trauma to the perineum and unfavourable compression of the fetal head.

PAIN IN LABOUR

Many women experience severe pain in labour. Pain is a complex and personal phenomenon. Although it is easier to understand the neurophysiological aspects of tissue damage, the experience of pain is always subjective and is related to psychological state and past experience. Pain can be defined as a sensation (sensory and emotional experience) usually evoked by tissue damage or inflammation that stimulates the activity of specific receptors transmitting information to pain centres in the brain. Although pain can often be considered to be part of a protective mechanism (a rapid warning system) against tissue damage, there are some exceptions. For instance, pain associated with radiation (as in sunburn) or tumour growth tends to occur well after the tissue damage has occurred so it does not function as a warning. Chronic pain associated with degenerative diseases, such as arthritis, also cannot be regarded as a protective reflex. In labour, some aspects of pain experienced can be protective, such as the pain due to stretching of the soft tissue as the baby's head is crowned, which causes the woman to gasp.

The perception of pain depends on a number of physiological and psychological factors. The location and intensity of the stimuli affect the quality and severity of the perceived pain; generally, the higher the intensity of the stimuli, the greater is the pain experienced. However, psychological and cultural factors are important in the perception of pain (Box 13.5). Mood and personality type are important; generally, anxious or tired people are less able to tolerate pain but emotional arousal limits pain perception.

BOX 13.5 Factors Affecting Pain Perception

- Anatomy
- Physiology
- Psychology
- Sociology
- Culture
- Cognition
- Learning
- Previous experience and perceptions of childbirth

TABLE 13.4 Fast and Slow Pain Receptors

Fast Pain	Slow Pain
Bright, sharp, localized sensation	Dull, intense, diffuse unpleasant feeling
Aδ fibres	C fibres
2–5 μm diameter	0.4–1.2 μm diameter
Myelinated	Nonmyelinated
Conduct at 12–30 m/s	Conduct at 0.5–2 m/s
Terminate on neurons in laminars I and II	Terminate on neurons in laminars I and V
Spinothalamic tract	Spinorectal tract
Somatic pain	Visceral pain

Pain Receptors

Pain or nociceptive receptors respond to stimuli that cause tissue damage. They are specific, responding to chemical mediators of tissue damage, such as plasmakinins, acetylcholine, histamine and substance P. Pain receptors are distributed unevenly with a higher density in skin, dental pulp, some internal organs, periosteum, meninges, arterial walls and joint surfaces. Pain receptors are free nerve endings that form part of small afferent myelinated Aδ fibres and larger (but unmyelinated) C fibres (Table 13.4). There is controversy over the pain being caused by overstimulation of other receptor types such as those that respond to temperature and pressure (Box 13.6).

Pain Transmission

Transmission of pain depends on the type of fibre in which the nerve ending triggers the impulse. In general, the speed of transmission is faster in larger fibres and those that are myelinated. Sharp stabbing sensations are thought to be conducted by Aδ fibres and dull aching or burning pain

BOX 13.6   Pain Receptors

Large

- Aα (Ia and Ib) (myelinated): position proprioception, touch, pressure, vibration
- Aβ (II) (myelinated): fine discriminative touch, pressure, vibration
- Aγ (myelinated): burning sensation

Small

- Aδ (III) (myelinated): well-localizable sharp pain, temperature
- C (IV) (unmyelinated): dull aching pain, temperature

by the slower unmyelinated C fibres. Myelinated fibres are more sensitive to ischaemia. Small unmyelinated fibres are more susceptible to local anaesthetics such as procaine, which is effective at blocking aching pain.

The nerve fibres enter the spinal cord and terminate in the grey matter of the dorsal horn (Fig. 13.22). Aδ fibres have a relatively direct route of transmission, synapsing with neurons in the dorsal horn to the brain stem and via the spinothalamic tract to the thalamus and cerebral cortex. Therefore, the pain is perceived as sharp and is easy to localize. The unmyelinated C fibres synapse in the grey matter of the spinal cord as well but are routed through the spinoreticular tract and reticular formation to the thalamus

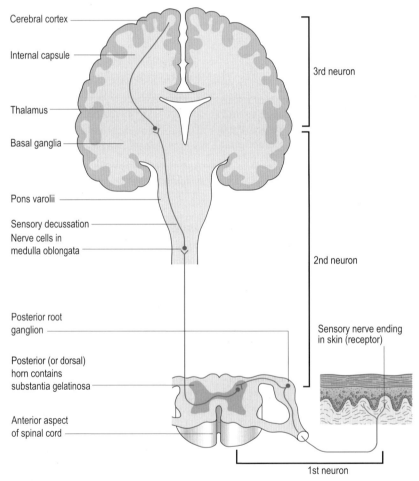

Fig. 13.22 Pathways of pain transmission. (Reproduced with permission from Bennett and Brown, 1999.)

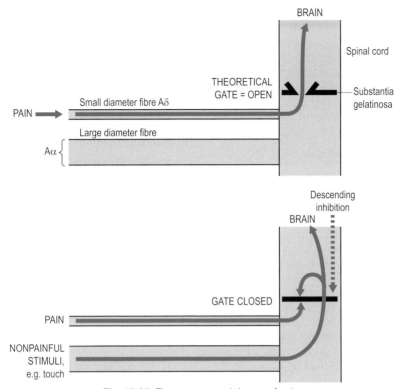

Fig. 13.23 The gate control theory of pain.

and cortex. Within the reticular formation, a number of physiological processes take place, stimulating the nervous system and affecting electrical activity in the brain, wakefulness and attention. The state of excitement that is generated means the pain is difficult to localize and produces unpleasant symptoms. The limbic system (which includes the hypothalamus and the amygdala) at the base of the brain is stimulated, which affects emotional responses such as fear, anger, pleasure and satisfaction. The thalamus integrates the sensation of pain and relays the information that tissue damage has occurred. The somatosensory cortex discriminates and identifies the precise position of the tissue damage and the parietal cortex is involved in interpreting the information and relating the learned meaningfulness to past experience. The main excitatory neurotransmitter in pain perception is glutamate.

The Gate Control Theory

There is a relationship between the pain receptors and the touch receptors at the level of the spinal cord. The pain gate control theory, proposed by Melzack and Wall (1965), suggests that interneurons in the substantia gelatinosa of the dorsal horn of the spinal cord can regulate the conduction of the ascending afferent nerve (Fig. 13.23). Input from the large-diameter myelinated fibres from the touch receptors can inhibit the impulses from the smaller-diameter fibres from the pain receptors, acting as a gate. This means that touch, like massage, can inhibit transmission from the pain receptor unless activity along the smaller fibres markedly increases. Descending fibres from the brain can also modify transmission of pain signals, thus 'opening' or 'closing' the gate. This explains the relationship between psychological factors and pain perception. If a labouring woman is feeling relaxed and confident, the descending inhibition is high so less pain is perceived. If she becomes tired or anxious, the descending inhibition is reduced. Transcutaneous electrical nerve stimulation (TENS) acts both to stimulate the large-diameter touch afferent nerves and possibly to stimulate powerful descending inhibitory pathways.

Pain from Muscle Contractions

Both visceral pain from the uterus and somatic pain from trauma to the soft tissues of the birth canal are experienced in labour. Visceral pain tends to predominate in the first stage of labour when the uterus is contracting and the cervix is stretching and dilating. Rhythmic muscle contraction in the presence of an adequate blood flow does not usually cause pain. In labour, uterine contractions compress blood vessels and reduce flow; the ischaemic pain persists until the flow is restored. It is hypothesized that a chemical mediator reaches critical levels when flow is limited and stimulates the pain receptors. When flow is restored, the chemical mediator is diluted or metabolized. This is similar to exertion causing myocardial ischaemia and angina pain, which is relieved by rest and decreased myocardial oxygen requirements. Initially, pain is transmitted by the afferent fibres entering the spinal cord at T11 and T12, spreading to T10 and L1.

Referred Pain

In referred pain, damage from one part of the body is experienced as though it had occurred in another part of the body. The pain fibres from the damaged area enter the spinal cord at the same level as the afferent nerves from the referred area. Usually the pain is referred to another tissue or structure that developed from the same embryonic structure or dermatome in which the pain originates. For instance, development of the diaphragm begins in the neck but, as the lungs develop, the diaphragm and the phrenic nerve migrate towards the abdomen. The afferent fibres in the phrenic nerve enter the spinal cord with the afferent fibres from the tip of the shoulder. Irritation of the diaphragm is therefore referred as a pain in the shoulder. However, previous experience is important in referred pain. Pain from the abdominal viscera including the uterus is usually referred to the midline. But in patients who have experienced abdominal surgery, such as a caesarean section, the pain is often referred to the scar site. Pain during this stage arising from the uterus and cervix may be referred. A labouring woman may experience pain over her abdominal wall, between the naval and pubic bone, radiating down her thighs and in the lumbar and sacral regions.

Somatic Pain

Somatic pain caused by the presenting part impinging on the birth canal, vulva and perineum tends to occur in the transition and in second stage of labour. Pain is transmitted by the pudendal nerves S2, S3 and S4. Hence, a local anaesthetic injected into these nerves is termed a pudendal block. The conscious sensation of pain is accompanied by a number of physiological responses including increased ventilation and cardiac output, inhibition of gastrointestinal function, increased oxygen demand and metabolic rate and increased catecholamine release. The increased catecholamine release may detrimentally affect placental perfusion and uterine contractions. Nonpharmacological methods of pain relief, such as imagery, relaxation techniques and provision of information about the progress of labour, probably decrease anxiety and stress and responses mediated by the sympathetic nervous system. Women with epidurals in situ may experience pain during the second stage of labour even if the epidural has been effective earlier. This is because epidurals are more effective at blocking visceral pathways than the somatic pathways. Following delivery with an epidural still in situ, if perineal repair is required, it is good practice to ensure the women remains pain free and this often requires local anaesthetic even if the epidural is topped up.

Endogenous Opiates

The endogenous opiates are of particular interest in pain perceived in labour. These include β-endorphin, enkephalins and dynorphin, which are analgesic peptides. They bind to the presynaptic receptors on the neuron membrane and block pain transmission. Enkephalins comprise two short peptide chains (consisting of five amino acids) that are very unstable and have a half-life of <1 min. Enkephalins are fragments of β-endorphin, which is more stable and also binds to opiate receptors; β-endorphin is a fragment of the pituitary hormone β-lipotrophin. β-Lipotrophin and ACTH are both derived from the same large precursor protein, POMC.

Endogenous opiates inhibit prostaglandin synthesis. Prostaglandins are chemical mediators of pain and a target of the analgesic aspirin, which inhibits their synthesis. Endogenous opiates also inhibit the actions of a number of other pain transmitters. β-Endorphin levels increase throughout pregnancy, peaking at delivery, and may be further stimulated by the stress of labour. It is suggested that it is this high level of endogenous opiates that allows women to tolerate surprisingly high levels of pain during delivery; this phenomenon is known as 'pregnancy-induced analgesia'. Acupuncture may increase enkephalin activity. Placebo responses, where pain relief occurs as a result of expectation of pain relief, rather than because of being given an analgesic, may be due to release of endogenous opiates and genuine analgesia.

Pain Relief

Pain relief in labour needs to work rapidly and effectively relieve the pain without slowing down the course of labour. It needs to be safe for the mother and fetus and not adversely affect the neonate or impede the progress of labour. There is no ideal analgesic (Table 13.5); all have some side-effects but pain also can adversely affect the fetus and maternal behaviour. Maternal analgesia can alter the balance of factors promoting effective uterine contractions and can potentially result in increased effects of oxytocin, promoting tetanic (sustained) uterine contractions, decreasing oxygen delivery and causing transient fetal bradycardia. There are three main mechanisms of pain relief, blocking either the pain receptors, the propagation of the

TABLE 13.5 Types of Analgesics

Pain Relief	Example	Mechanism	Disadvantages/Advantages
Opioids	Pethidine	Depression of CNS	Nausea, vomiting, sedation; potentiate effect of epidural
Paracervical block	Spinal	Action potentials blocked from nerves	Repeat block increase the risk of fetal injection; could provide surgical anaesthesia
Epidural	Bolus, intermittent or continuous infusion	Inhibition of neurotransmission across synapses	Maternal hypotension, motor blockade

action potential or the perception of pain within the CNS. Mild analgesics block at the pain receptor level. The sensitivity of the pain receptors is increased by prostaglandins. Drugs that inhibit prostaglandin synthesis, such as aspirin, decrease levels of prostaglandins both at the receptor and where prostaglandins are involved in pain transmission higher in the pathway.

Local Anaesthetics

Local anaesthetics prevent the propagation of action potentials by blocking the sodium channels. They are particularly effective in blocking pain carried by the C fibres, possibly because unmyelinated fibres allow easier penetration. For instance, lidocaine, a local anaesthetic, injected into the perineum is effective at blocking the pain of episiotomy. Local anaesthetics are also used in performing a pudendal nerve block, which is used for assisted deliveries such as mid-cavity forceps delivery.

Centrally Acting Opiates

Centrally acting opiates or narcotics, such as morphine, diamorphine and pethidine, block nerve transmission in the brain and spinal cord and decrease pain perception. There are also opiate-binding sites in the substantia gelatinosa of the dorsal horn of the spinal cord, which affect the release of neurotransmitters. Opiates increase the activity of the descending inhibitory pathways from the brain stem and act on the limbic system to elevate mood. Opiates have other physiological effects such as depressing the medullary respiratory centre, causing nausea and vomiting, sedating and affecting the heart rate. Opiates can enter the fetal circulation and may interfere with the initiation of respiratory function at birth as they cause respiratory depression.

POSITION IN LABOUR

Certain positions have advantages in optimizing uterine efficiency or increasing maternal comfort (Blackburn, 2018) (Box 13.7). Lying supine, or with legs supported and flexed 90° at hips and knees, are probably advantageous

---

BOX 13.7 Waterbirth

Over the years, delivering babies in water has become increasingly popular and is available in many hospitals, birth centres and within the home environment. Many women perceive waterbirth as a natural process without the need for analgesia. There have been concerns raised over the safety of waterbirth such as water inhalation and other complications such as hyponatremia, infection, haemorrhage associated with cord rupture, hypoxia and death (although these complications are rare). Meta-analyses of research studies have shown that there is no significant difference in infant outcomes comparing waterbirth with conventional deliveries (Vanderlaan et al., 2018). These studies show that there is a reduction in episiotomies and a reduction in the use of analgesia in women who choose waterbirth. Evidence that the newborn baby is no more at risk from infection following a waterbirth compared to a conventional delivery has been presented. The intensity of pain does not seem to be reduced by waterbirth but waterbirth does appear to reduce the use of conventional anaesthesia in the advanced stages of labour.

It is important that guidelines are referred to and followed so that safety of both mother and baby is optimized. There is also some evidence to suggest that waterbirth is effective in lowering maternal blood pressure and so may be a useful intervention in mild preeclampsia. This may be a combination of relaxation and peripheral dilation of the blood vessels due to the warming of the skin by the water. It is important to ensure the pool water temperature does not exceed 37.5°C as prolonged immersion in hot water will eventually raise the maternal core temperature and as a consequence the fetal heart rate will be affected. The buoyancy of the water provides support and reduces the stress of weightbearing so enabling the mother to move freely and change positions easily.

only to those assisting at the delivery unless medical intervention/delivery is required. Fetal monitoring and a number of procedures can usually be adapted to a variety of maternal positions. There seems to be no physiological advantage in lying supine. Fetal alignment, pelvic diameter and efficiency of contractions are not optimal. Contractions are more frequent but less intense so labour is prolonged and analgesia use seems to be increased. Many women appear to choose a supine position because they are presented with a bed and are often not encouraged to try alternative positions.

A lateral recumbent position reduces obstructive pressure on maternal blood vessels so venous return and cardiac output are optimal for uterine perfusion and fetal oxygenation. Uterine contractions are more intense but less frequent and have increased efficiency. In an upright position, the abdominal wall relaxes and the effect of gravity will augment the effect of the fetal head pressing on the cervix and the subsequent feedback to the myometrial activity. Both frequency and intensity of contractions are increased so uterine activity is enhanced and labour tends to be shorter. Squatting increases maternal pelvic diameter, through altering the angle of pelvic tilt, and enhances engagement, descent and rotation of the fetal head.

During bearing down, in the second stage of labour, directed pushing with a Valsalva manoeuvre against a closed glottis increases sympathetic discharge and catecholamine release. Minimal straining with an open glottis has fewer negative effects on maternal blood pressure, maternal and fetal oxygenation levels and is associated with reduced need for episiotomy. Therefore, active pushing in a normal labour should not be encouraged, allowing the mother to be guided by her own instinctive behavioural cues.

KEY POINTS

- Parturition in humans is poorly understood; animal studies offer limited insight into the process owing to the evolution of species-specific differences.
- Parturition is a continuous process: the defining of the various stages of labour enables clinical judgement of progress and thus intervention under the biomedical model of care.
- The fundal region of the uterus has the highest density of smooth muscle so it is responsible for the strong expelling contractions of the uterus during labour.
- Human cervical structure is complex owing to the upright stance causing an increased gravitational force as the contents of the uterus increase in mass. Structural changes within the cervix have to occur before dilation can be achieved by uterine contractions.
- Coordinated effective contractions are facilitated by the increased expression of gap junctions between myometrial cells immediately prior to parturition.
- The first stage of labour is measured from the onset of strong and regular effective contractions to full effacement and full dilation of the cervix.
- The second stage of labour is characterized by strong expulsive contractions, aided by respiratory muscle involvement, until the fetus is delivered.
- The passage of the fetus through the pelvis is described as the mechanism of labour and is achieved through the contractions forcing the presenting part to rotate against the muscle tone, structural resistance and shape of the pelvic floor within the structural confinement of the maternal true pelvic cavity.
- The third stage of labour covers the expulsion and delivery of the placenta and fetal membranes and staunching of maternal blood loss.
- Maternal blood loss immediately following separation of the placenta is limited by the myometrial fibres contracting, thus occluding the uterine vessels.
- The onset of labour is poorly understood; changes in the secretion of several hormones and in the expression and various hormone receptors subtypes, as well as inflammatory signals are involved.
- The evolution of bipedal locomotion and increasing cephalization have influenced parturition in humans so the presenting part has to negotiate, by rotational manoeuvres, rather than just pass through the pelvic girdle.
- The process of labour induces many changes within the fetus in preparation for extrauterine life, which are mediated by increasing hypoxia and catecholamine production.
- Pain in labour has a complex aetiology; there are visceral and somatic components further complicated by psychological and social factors.

APPLICATION TO PRACTICE

Midwives need to understand the physiological interactions and external factors that can affect human labour in order to underpin intrapartum care.

The development of observational skills allows the midwife not only to interpret how a woman may be coping with labour, but also to determine how the labour is progressing from observing behaviour and physical responses of the labouring woman. By ignoring, not noticing or misunderstanding certain physical cues, the midwife may inadvertently provide suboptimal support.

Intervention in labour must be justified and decisions surrounding this must be underpinned to maximize maternal and fetal well-being. Knowledge of the effects of intervention upon fetal and maternal physiology is essential so that the midwife can judge the effectiveness and quickly identify possible adverse outcomes of such interventions.

ANNOTATED FURTHER READING

Amini P, Wilson R, Koeblitz W, et al.: Mechanism by which progesterone and cAMP synergize to maintain uterine quiescence during pregnancy, *Mol Cell Endocrinol* 479:1–11, 2019.
A review of the mechanisms controlling myometrial contraction, which describes how uterine quiescence changes during pregnancy and tocolytic therapy in preterm labour.

Baskett TF: Operative vaginal delivery – an historical perspective, *Best Pract Res Clin Obstet Gynaecol*, 2018. https://doi.org/10.1016/j.bpobgyn.2018.08.002.
A fascinating history of the development and evolution of tools used in operative delivery of a live infant such as obstetric forceps and vacuum extractors.

Baston H, Hall J: ed 2, *Midwifery essentials: labour*, vol. 3. Oxford, 2017, Elsevier.
This book provides a comprehensive but easy to follow guide to women-centred care in labour including waterbirth and caesarean section.

Blackburn ST: *Maternal, fetal, & neonatal physiology: a clinical perspective*, ed 5, Oxford, 2018, Elsevier.
An excellent in-depth description of physiological adaptation to pregnancy and consequent development of the fetus and neonate that draws from physiological research studies. The chapters are clearly organized by physiological systems and link physiological concepts to clinical applications including the assessment and management of low- and high-risk pregnancies.

Chapman V, Charles C, editors: *The midwife's labour and birth handbook*, ed 3, Oxford, 2013, Wiley-Blackwell.
This book focuses on the promotion of normality through a women-centred approach to care in labour. It includes chapters on waterbirth, homebirth, breech, caesarean section and vaginal birth after caesarean section.

Cunningham FG, Leveno K, Bloom S, et al.: *Williams obstetrics*, ed 25, New York, 2018, McGraw-Hill Medical.
This classic and well-illustrated textbook is a comprehensive text for obstetrics; a particularly useful reference book for midwives interested in reproductive pathophysiology and maternal-fetal medicine.

Dick-Read G, Gaskin IM: *Childbirth without fear: the principles and practice of natural childbirth*, ed 2, London, 2013, Pinter & Martin Ltd. revised.
This classic book was first published in 1942 and has remained in print ever since. It challenges modern medical obstetric practice and is essential reading for those interested in the development of modern intrapartum care.

Dunsworth HM: There is no 'obstetrical dilemma': towards a braver medicine with fewer childbirth interventions, *Perspect Biol Med* 61:249–263, 2018.
An interesting perspective that challenges the 'obstetrical dilemma' and suggests that it creates biased thinking, which contributes to the medicalization of birth and over-implementation of interventions in childbirth.

Gruss LT, Schmitt D: The evolution of the human pelvis: changing adaptations to bipedalism, obstetrics and thermoregulation, *Phil Trans R Soc B* 370:20140063, 2015.
A discussion of findings from the fossil record of the human pelvis and comparative species, which considers the implications for childbirth, locomotion and thermoregulation.

Menon R, Bonney EA, Condon J, et al.: Novel concepts on pregnancy clocks and alarms: redundancy and synergy in human parturition, *Hum Reprod Update* 22:535–560, 2016.
Provides a recent overview of our understanding of the various factors involved in the timing of parturition.

National Collaborating Centre for Women's and Children's Health: *Intrapartum care for healthy women and babies*, 2014, updated 2017, National Institute of Clinical Excellence (Clinical guideline 190).
This guideline presents clinical based labour care from an evidenced based care perspective and is the leading 'best practice' maternity guide for standards of care within the UK NHS.

Odent M: *Childbirth and the evolution of Homo Sapiens*, ed 2, London, 2014, Pinter & Martin Ltd.
The first of a trio of books by former obstetrician, Michel Odent, that fundamentally challenge modern obstetric and midwifery practice; thought-provoking in many ways but also enabling alternative, evidence based practices to become the norm.

Odent M: *Do we need midwives*, London, 2015, Pinter & Martin Ltd.
This book is 'fearless' in the way Michel Odent argues against modern obstetric practice in childbirth. He presents evidence-based alternatives, which may challenge obstetric practice but empower midwives to move away from a stance of intervention to one of passive support and facilitation.

Odent M: *The birth of Homo, the marine chimpanzee: when the tool becomes the master*, London, 2017, Pinter & Martin Ltd.
Another challenging text exploring human birth in a way no obstetric textbook does. Michel Odent discusses many of the 'new' emerging theories explaining why the human physiology and behaviour in childbirth is unique.

Reuwer P: *Proactive support of labor: the challenge of normal childbirth*, ed 2, Cambridge, 2015, Cambridge Medicine.

Written by obstetricians, this book challenges current obstetric practice within the United States of America by focusing on the promotion of normality and presenting the arguments for natural birth to be a right; a good balance between natural birth and childbirth interventions.

Sandall J, Tribe RM, Avery L, et al.: Short-term and long-term effects of caesarean section on the health of women and children, *Lancet* 392:1349–1357, 2018.

Part of the series of papers in the Lancet reminding health practitioners that caesarean section is life-saving when medically indicated but has short- and long-term implications for maternal and infant health that are important to consider.

Smith R, Imtiaz M, Banney D, et al.: Why the heart is like an orchestra and the uterus is like a soccer crowd, *Am J Obstet Gynecol* 213:181–185, 2015.

A physiological comparison of the heart and uterus, which both demonstrate synchronous oscillatory behaviour but are organized in different ways. The heart plays (contracts) continuously under the direction of a conductor where the uterus is inactive most of the time but the contractions swell to a climax (birth of the infant) then disperse and remain quiet.

Smith R, Paul J, Maiti K: Recent advances in understanding the endocrinology of human birth, *Trends Endocrinol Metab* 23:516–523, 2012.

A good overview of the regulation of human birth and how its timing can affect the survival of the fetus; the mechanisms involved are linked to possible therapeutic targets.

Stinson LF, Payne MS, Keelan JA: A critical review of the bacterial baptism hypothesis and the impact of cesarean delivery on the infant microbiome, *Front Med (Lausanne)* 5:135, 2018.

An interesting and thoughtful challenge to the importance of the 'bacterial baptism' of vaginal birth, which points to the involvement of other factors affecting the development of the infant microbiota profile including the reason for caesarean section, use of medication and absence of labour.

Suff N, Story L, Shennan A: The prediction of preterm delivery: what is new? *Semin Fetal Neonatal Med* 24:27–32, 2019.

A succinct review of the predictive tests, which indicate a high risk of preterm delivery and emerging tests, which may be used in clinical practice in the future.

Trevathan WR, Rosenberg KR: *Costly and cute: helpless infants and human evolution*, New Mexico, 2016, University of New Mexico Press.

An anthropological view of the developmental state of the human infant at birth and the relationship between the 'helpless infant' and distinctly human characteristics.

Walsh D: *Intrapartum care: essential midwifery practice*, Oxford, 2010, Wiley-Blackwell.

This book describes how intrapartum care has evolved over the past 50 years and developed in relation to the development of midwifery practice. Its chapters explore issues such as psychology, sexuality, spirituality, feminism and complementary therapies in relation to intrapartum care.

REFERENCES

Aghaeepour A, Ganio EA, Mcilwain D, et al.: An immune clock of human pregnancy, *Sci Immunol* 2:1–11, 2017.

Amini P, Wilson R, Koeblitz W, et al.: Mechanism by which progesterone and cAMP synergize to maintain uterine quiescence during pregnancy, *Mol Cell Endocrinol* 479:1–11, 2019.

Anton O, Jordan H, Rabe H: *Strategies for implementing placental transfusion at birth: a systematic review*, Birth, in press, 2018.

Arrowsmith S, Wray S: Oxytocin: its mechanism of action and receptor signalling in the myometrium, *J Neuroendocr* 26:356–369, 2014.

Bennett VR, Brown LK: *Myles' textbook for midwives*, ed 13, Edinburgh, 1999, Churchill Livingstone, pp 393. 396 431, 451, 468, 473, 509, 993.

Besenboeck C, Cvitic S, Lang U, et al.: Going into labor and beyond: phospholipase A2 in pregnancy, *Reproduction* 151:R91–R102, 2016.

Blackburn ST: *Maternal, fetal, & neonatal physiology: a clinical perspective*, ed 5, Oxford, 2018, Elsevier.

Blencowe H, Cousens S, Oestergaard MZ, et al.: National, regional, and worldwide estimates of preterm birth rates in the year 2010 with time trends since 1990 for selected countries a systematic analysis and implications, *Lancet* 379:2162–2172, 2012.

Borsani E, Della Vedova AM, Rezzani R, et al.: Correlation between human nervous system development and acquisition of fetal skills: an overview, *Brain Dev* 41:225–233, 2018.

Brace RA, Cheung CY: Regulation of amniotic fluid volume: evolving concepts, *Adv Exp Med Biol* 814:49–68, 2014.

Chollat C, Sentilhes L, Marret S: Protection of brain development by antenatal magnesium sulphate for infants born preterm, *Dev Med Child Neurol* 61:25–30, 2019.

Fuchs AR, Romero R, Keefe D, et al.: Oxytocin secretion and human parturition: pulse frequency and duration increase during spontaneous labour in women, *Am J Obstet Gynecol* 165:1515–1522, 1991.

Geng J, Huang C, Jiang S: Roles and regulation of the matrix metalloproteinase system in parturition, *Mol Reprod Dev* 83:276–286, 2016.

Gilman-Sachs A, Dambaeva S, Salazar Garcia MD, et al.: Inflammation induced preterm labor and birth, *J Reprod Immunol* 129:53–58, 2018.

Gommers JSM, Diederen M, Wilkinson C, et al.: Risk of maternal, fetal and neonatal complications associated with the use of the transcervical balloon catheter in induction of labour: a systematic review, *Eur J Obstet Gynecol Reprod Biol* 218:73–84, 2017.

Govindaswami B, Jegatheesan P, Nudelman M, Narasimhan SR: Prevention of prematurity: advances and opportunities, *Clin Perinatol* 45:579–595, 2018.

Grammatopoulos DK: Placental corticotrophin-releasing hormone and its receptors in human pregnancy and labour: still a scientific enigma, *J Neuroendocrinol* 20:432–438, 2008.

Heck L, Clauss M, Sánchez-Villagra MR: Do domesticated mammals selected for intensive production have less variable gestation periods? *Mammal Biol* 88:151–155, 2018.

Helenius K, Sjors G, Shah PS, et al.: Survival in very preterm infants: an international comparison of 10 national neonatal networks, *Pediatrics* 140:e20171264, 2017.

Johnson SK, Groten T, Pastuschek J, et al.: Human placentophagy: Effects of dehydration and steaming on hormones, metals and bacteria in placental tissue, *Placenta* 67:8–14, 2018.

Keelan JA: Intrauterine inflammatory activation, functional progesterone withdrawal, and the timing of term and preterm birth, *J Reprod Immunol* 125:89–99, 2018.

Kidder GM, Winterhager E: Physiological roles of connexins in labour and lactation, *Reproduction* 150:R129–R136, 2015.

Kishore AH, Liang H, Kanchwala M, et al.: Prostaglandin dehydrogenase is a target for successful induction of cervical ripening, *Proc Natl Acad Sci USA* 114:E6427–E6436, 2017.

Koos BJ, Rajaee A: Fetal breathing movements and changes at birth, *Adv Exp Med Biol* 814:89–101, 2014.

Lagercrantz H, Slotkin TA: The "stress" of being born, *Sci Am* 254:100–107, 1986.

Lawn JE, Blencowe H, Oza S, et al.: Every newborn: progress, priorities, and potential beyond survival, *Lancet* 384:189–205, 2014.

Lee AC, Blencowe H, Lawn JE: Small babies, big numbers: global estimates of preterm birth, *Lancet Glob Health* 7:e2–e3, 2019.

Li XQ, Zhu P, Myatt L, et al.: Roles of glucocorticoids in human parturition: a controversial fact? *Placenta* 35:291–296, 2014.

Luu TM, Mian MOR, Nuyt AM: Long-term impact of preterm birth – neurodevelopmental and physical health outcomes, *Clin Perinatol* 44:305–314, 2017.

Man GCW, Zhang T, Chen X, et al.: The regulations and role of circadian clock and melatonin in uterine receptivity and pregnancy – an immunological perspective, *Am J Reprod Immunol* 78:e12715, 2017.

Mark PJ, Crew RC, Wharfe MD, Waddell BJ: Rhythmic three-part harmony: the complex interaction of maternal, placental and fetal circadian systems, *J Biol Rhythms* 32:534–549, 2017.

Melzack R, Wall PD: Pain mechanisms: a new theory, *Science* 150:971–979, 1965.

Mendelson CR, Montalbanoa AP, Gaoa L: Fetal-to-maternal signaling in the timing of birth, *J Steroid Biochem Mol Biol* 170:19–27, 2017.

Menon R, Bonney EA, Condon J, et al.: Novel concepts on pregnancy clocks and alarms – redundancy and synergy in human parturition, *Hum Reprod Update* 22:535–560, 2016.

Merlino AA, Welsh TN, Tan H, et al.: Nuclear progesterone receptors in the human pregnancy myometrium: evidence that parturition involves functional progesterone withdrawal mediated by increased expression of progesterone receptor-A, *J Clin Endocrinol Metab* 92:1927–1933, 2007.

Mohan S, Khan D, Moffett C, et al.: Oxytocin is present in islets and plays a role in beta-cell function and survival, *Peptides* 100:260–268, 2018.

Morton JS, Care AS, Davidge ST: Mechanisms of uterine artery dysfunction in pregnancy complications, *J Cardiovasc Pharmacol* 69:343–359, 2017.

Moser K, Macfarlane A, Dattani N: Survival rates in very preterm babies in England and Wales, *Lancet* 371:897–898, 2008.

NCCWCH: *Intrapartum care for healthy women and babies*, 2014, updated 2017, National Institute of Clinical Excellence (Clinical guideline 190).

Odent M: New reasons and new ways to study birth physiology, *Int J Gynecol Obstet* 75:S39–S45, 2001.

Peiris HN, Almughlliq VF, Koh YQ: Eicosanoids in preterm labor and delivery: potential roles of exosomes in eicosanoid functions, *Placenta* 54:e95e103, 2017.

Petraglia F, Imperatore A, Challis JRG: Neuroendocrine mechanisms in pregnancy, *Endocr Rev* 31:783–816, 2010.

Riviere D, McKinlay CJD, Bloomfield FH: Adaptation for life after birth: a review of neonatal physiology, *Anaesth Intensive Care Med* 18:59–67, 2018.

Rosenberg KR, Trevathan WR: Evolutionary obstetrics, *Evol Med Public Health* 148:2014, 2014.

Singata M, Tranmer J, Gyte GM: Restricting oral fluid and food intake during labour, *Cochrane Database Syst Rev* 8: CD003930, 2013.

Smith R, Paul J, Maiti K: Recent advances in understanding the endocrinology of human birth, *Trends Endocrinol Metab* 23:516–523, 2012.

Smyth RM, Markham C, Dowswell T: Amniotomy for shortening spontaneous labour, *Cochrane Database Syst Rev* 6: CD006167, 2013.

Sweet B, Tiran D: *Mayes' midwifery*, ed 12, London, 1996, Baillière Tindall, pp 31. 224 225, 340, 358, 993.

Trevathan W: Primate pelvic anatomy and implications for birth, *Philos Trans R Soc Lond B Biol Sci* 370:20140065, 2015.

Uldbjerg N, Malstrom A: The role of proteoglycans in cervical dilatation, *Semin Perinatol* 15:127–132, 1991.

Vain NE, Batton DG: Meconium 'aspiration' (or respiratory distress associated with meconium-stained amniotic fluid?), *Semin Fetal Neonatal Med* 22:214–219, 2017.

Vanderlaan J, Hall PJ, Lewitt M: Neonatal outcomes with water birth: A systematic review and meta-analysis, *Midwifery* 59:27–38, 2018.

Vannuccini S, Bocchi C, Severi FM, et al.: Endocrinology of human parturition, *Ann d'Endocrinol* 77:105–113, 2016.

Vogel JP, Chawanpaiboon S, Moller AB, et al.: The global epidemiology of preterm birth, *Best Pract Res Clin Obstet Gynaecol* 52:3–12, 2018.

Wray S, Burdyga T, Noble D, et al.: Progress in understanding electro-mechanical signalling in the myometrium, *Acta Physiol* 213:417–431, 2015.

Young RC, Barendse P: Linking myometrial physiology to intrauterine pressure; how tissue-level contractions create uterine contractions of labor, *PLOS Comput Biol* 10:e1003850, 2014.

Younger JD, Reitman E, Gallos G: Tocolysis: present and future treatment options, *Semin Perinatol* 41:493–504, 2017.

The Puerperium

- To describe the physiological processes that achieve haemostasis in the early puerperium, following completion of the third stage of labour.
- To discuss the timing of the physiological changes in the puerperium and how these changes are regulated.

- To discuss the aetiology of the common problems experienced within the puerperium.
- To recognize signs of pathological conditions associated with the puerperium.

INTRODUCTION

The puerperium has been traditionally defined as the period immediately following the birth of a baby and delivery of the placenta until the mother's physiology returns to her prepregnant state; it is usually considered to be about 6 weeks long. It may originate from religious traditions such as 'churching', following the 'lying-in period'. Churching was a religious ceremony where women were blessed and accepted back into the church after a period of 40 days during which time they were considered unclean. The ceremony was essentially a thanksgiving for the woman's survival; it took place whether the baby survived or died. Similar ceremonies exist in other religions and cultures. The time after childbirth is imbued with social, cultural, religious and behavioural significance and, in many cultures, puerperants (puerperal women) are given special and traditional care.

Two important physiological landmarks are often observed: the cessation of lochial discharge (women often being considered 'unclean' when lochia is present) and the shrivelling and loss of the remnants of the umbilical cord from the infant. With the rise of medical dominance, the end of the puerperium was marked by the postnatal examination of the woman by a doctor. This has structured the traditional descriptions of the puerperium as a period of maternal recovery, underpinned by the medicalization of pregnancy and childbirth rather than that of a period of adaption to parenthood. It is the midwife's responsibility to maintain careful observation and systematic checks on the physiological and anatomical changes in the puerperium and to recognize early signs of pathological conditions, while helping the mother adapt to motherhood, monitoring the neonate and ensure wellbeing of the maternal–neonatal dyad.

CHAPTER CASE STUDY

Zak was born 2 days after his expected date of delivery and was the first son born to his proud parents, Zara and James. Zak was delivered at around 04:30 hours and Zara had laboured in a birthing pool attended by her named midwife. As labour had progressed quickly without complications, the midwife followed Zara's request for no active management in the third stage of labour. The midwife was unable to accurately estimate Zara's blood loss due to the waterbirth. Once out of the bath, the midwife assessed Zara's perineal trauma, which appeared to be a first-degree tear that was not bleeding and did not require suturing.

- How can the midwife effectively assess Zara's wellbeing following the delivery, given that she has been unable to estimate Zara's total blood loss?
- What key observations would enable the midwife to assess Zara and enable the early recognition of pathological conditions common in the early postnatal period?
- What factors that have occurred during Zak's delivery will optimize Zara's transition to parenthood?
- What should the midwife do to encourage a close and effective relationship to develop between mother, baby and the father?

The puerperal period or puerperium is a vulnerable time. Most maternal and neonatal deaths occur during this time; about half of maternal deaths worldwide occur within 24 h of the infant's birth and about two-thirds occur in the first week (WHO, 2013). Neonatal deaths show a similar pattern: the first month of life is very vulnerable and the first week and day especially so. However, although the puerperium is recognized as a critical phase, it is often a neglected period and many mother–infant dyads lack the care and support they need.

The puerperium is sometimes considered to be the 'Cinderella' of maternity care as the excitement of the birth is over and, after delivery, the effects of pregnancy on maternal physiology and psychology receive little emphasis. There is not very much research into the timing or mechanisms of the changes in the puerperium. However, the puerperant woman can be very vulnerable to physiological, psychological and social stress, which can become pathological. The midwife's role is to observe and monitor the early changes and to be able to differentiate between those which are normal and abnormal and make appropriate care plans and referrals whenever the need arises.

A woman adapts to pregnancy progressively over a period of months, but, after childbirth, she suddenly no longer needs these physiological changes. During the puerperium, there is a marked decrease in the levels of oestrogen and progesterone within the maternal system. Although the placenta is the main source of progesterone in pregnancy, the corpus luteum continues to produce progesterone for several days into the puerperal period. The fall in concentrations of steroid hormones facilitates the initiation of lactation (see Chapter 16) and allows the physiological systems to regain fertility and prepare for another pregnancy. In reality, the puerperium should be described as a transitional phase. It begins at the birth of a baby and expulsion of the placenta and it ends with the re-establishment of fertility. Women do not return to the same physiological and anatomical nulligravid state. The puerperium also, within a social context, represents many transitions for the parents, infant and other members of the family. Many of the physiological changes within the puerperium, such as the establishment of parenting skills, lactation and feeding, are modified by the past and present social, cultural, educational and behavioural interactions of the individuals within the new family situation.

The puerperium is often considered in three phases: (1) the acute phase, which lasts 6–12 h after the birth; (2) the subacute postpartum phase, which lasts 2–6 weeks (and is the focus of this chapter); and (3) the delayed postpartum period, which can last up to 6 months.

PHYSIOLOGICAL AND STRUCTURAL CHANGES

Involution of the Uterus

Clinical observation and management of the puerperium is essentially based on the return of the uterus to its 'normal' prepregnant size. The puerperium begins as soon as the placenta and membranes are expelled from the uterus together with a substantial proportion of the endometrium. Oxytocin released from the posterior pituitary gland induces strong intermittent myometrial contractions, and as the uterine cavity is empty the whole uterus contracts down fully and the uterine walls become realigned in apposition to each other. The myometrial spiral fibres that occlude the uterine blood vessels (see Chapter 13) constrict the blood supply to the placental site (Fig. 14.1). Uterine vascular resistance increases soon after delivery (Guedes-Martins et al., 2015).

About an hour after delivery, the myometrium relaxes slightly but further active bleeding is prevented by the activation of the haemostatic (blood-clotting) mechanisms, which are elevated greatly during pregnancy to facilitate a swift, effective clotting response. Haemostasis is achieved in four ways:

- Pressure: apposition of the uterine walls forming the T-shaped cavity, initially augmented by uterine contractions, which compress the blood vessels
- Ligation of the blood vessels by myometrial cells within the myometrium
- Haemostatic (clotting) mechanisms
- Ischaemia

The midwife has a responsibility and duty of care to inspect the placenta and membranes to assess that they are complete and that no extraembryonic tissue remains within the uterine cavity. Retained products impede the contraction of the uterus and may be the source of abnormal bleeding and cause secondary postpartum haemorrhage (secondary PPH) as they become the focus of infection. Retained products are often spontaneously voided, usually associated with the passing of a blood clot, which facilitates the cleansing of the uterine cavity. The retention of even small remnants of placenta within the uterus can prevent lactation (see Chapters 13 and 16). Blood clots should always be checked for the presence of placental and membranous tissue. Lochia should be clot-free; the presence of blood clots indicates a risk of haemorrhage and the woman should be closely monitored.

Immediately after delivery, the uterus weighs ~1000 g and the fundus is palpable ~11–12 cm above the symphysis pubis (Blackburn, 2018) approximately at the lower edge

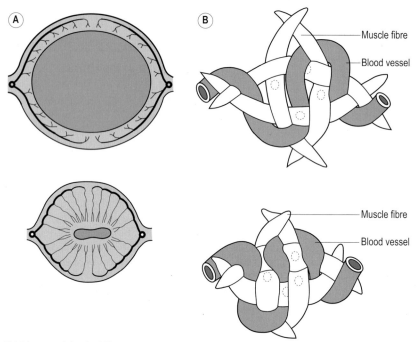

Fig. 14.1 (A) Myometrial spiral fibres around uterine blood vessels; (B) occlusion of blood supply to the placental site. (Reproduced with permission from Sweet and Tiran, 1996.)

of the maternal umbilicus (or slightly higher if the woman has a full bladder). The placental site is a raw and exposed internal wound of the endometrium layer. Initially, the uterus is continuous with the vagina with the cervix draping from the body of the uterus. Uterine involution is rapid so 50% of the total mass of the tissue is lost within a week. This physiological destruction of most of the uterine tissue is unique in adult life and the mechanisms are not clearly understood. It is suggested that 90% of uterine protein is degraded in the first 10 days of the puerperium (Hytten, 1995). There are rapid and marked changes in collagen and elastin content and protein degradation products and water are lost.

Involution involves various processes including uterine contractions, autolysis/autophagy of the myometrial cells and phagocytosis followed by epithelial regeneration and proliferation over the placental site (Chertok and Wolf, 2018). Involution starts with the withdrawal of placental hormones and is thought to be mediated by hydrolytic and proteolytic enzymes released from myometrial cells, endothelial cells of blood vessels and macrophages. Cytoplasmic organelles are autodigested, and intracellular cytoplasm and extracellular collagen are reduced. The breakdown of protein from the myometrial cells releases the amino acid components into the circulation and thence into the urine; thus, a puerperal woman is in a state of negative nitrogen

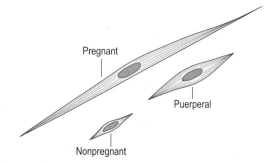

Fig. 14.2 Reduction in size of myometrial cells. (Reproduced with permission from Miller and Hanretty, 1998.)

balance (see Chapter 12). The number of myometrial cells does not decrease; they reduce in size (Fig. 14.2) rather than being destroyed and replaced, although there may be an 'overshoot' in uterine involution with rebuilding to the resting postpregnant state. The uterus ultimately returns almost to its prepregnant size (Fig. 14.3), although the proportion of fibrous tissue present in the uterus is progressively increased with successive pregnancies.

Initially, the cervix is soft, dilated and oedematous and may be bruised and lacerated following a vaginal delivery (particularly in primiparous women and those who experienced premature labour). The cervix rapidly reforms

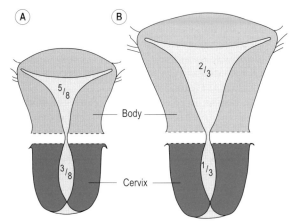

Fig. 14.3 Return of uterus to a size close to the prepregnant dimensions: (A) nulliparous uterus; (B) parous uterus. (Reproduced with permission from Miller and Hanretty, 1998.)

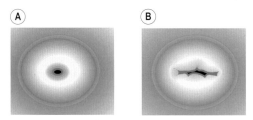

Fig. 14.4 Reformation of the external os: (A) nulliparous cervix; (B) parous cervix. (Reproduced with permission from Miller and Hanretty, 1998.)

within the first 12–18 h; it shortens and becomes firmer. It rapidly closes; by the end of the first puerperal week it is about 1 cm dilated (Chertok and Wolf, 2018). Cervical remodelling is due to the increase in fibroblasts, which synthesize collagen and proteoglycans. However, the cervix never returns to its original state and always shows evidence of parturition. The external os reforms with a slit rather than the nulliparous dimple (Fig. 14.4).

The uterus involutes quite quickly, fundal height decreases initially at about 1 cm/day; thus, by the 10th day it should no longer be palpable above the symphysis pubis. Involution is slower in women who have undergone lower-segment caesarean section (LSCS), but it can be judged by a detectable decrease in fundal height on subsequent palpation. Subinvolution (slowed, delayed or incomplete uterine involution) may be due to uterine atony, retained products of conception (RPOC), uterine inversion or lacerations and/or a secondary infection. Infection is usually found in conjunction with continued lochia rubra (high blood content, hence the red colour)

that may also have an offensive odour; abdominal tenderness and fever are also markers of infection. Subinvolution is also associated with the presence of fibroids and other uterine abnormalities.

The uterus should be well contracted, hard and central; if it is higher than the umbilicus and soft on palpation (often described as 'boggy') then this may also indicate the presence of infection. The endometrial cavity is a potential space in the nonpregnant state but gas is commonly detected in the endometrial cavity puerperally (Hytten, 1995). The rate of uterine involution is faster after a vaginal delivery. By the end of the first puerperal week, the uterus is ~500 g and by the end of the second week is ~350 g (Chertok and Wolf, 2018).

The initiation of breastfeeding and the infant suckling in the early puerperium augments stimulation of maternal oxytocin release. The oxytocin stimulates further contraction of the myometrium and so aids uterine evacuation. Involution of the uterus in breastfeeding mothers is more efficient. 'After-pains' associated with lactation are often experienced, particularly by multiparous women who often complain of increased vaginal loss while feeding. Initially, oral analgesia such as paracetamol may be offered but the intensity of the pain usually subsides after about 24 h because expression of myometrial oxytocin receptors is reduced as a result of oestrogen withdrawal. Women should be reassured that after-pains are a positive indicator in the establishment of breastfeeding but ongoing sustained pain is not normal and should be investigated further.

The superficial layer of the decidua becomes necrotic and is shed in the lochia in the first few days of the puerperium. The epithelium rapidly regenerates, re-forming an intact layer over most of the uterine surface within 7–10 days of delivery. The placental site takes ≥3 weeks to recover. The endometrium regenerates from the basal layers and grows in from the margins of the placental wound site and from glandular remnants within it.

Soft Tissue Damage, Healing and Repair

It is not uncommon for soft tissue damage to occur during the delivery of a baby. Trauma to the female genital tract is classified as follows:

- Superficial: this usually describes grazes to the skin where the epidermis has split owing to pressure of distension. These lesions do not require treatment; however, they often cause discomfort due to stinging because of the disruption of the nerve endings found within the superficial layer of the tissue. Voiding of urine can also be uncomfortable as the urine comes in contact with the grazes. Difficulty in voiding urine may initially be experienced due to oedema around the urethral opening, secondary to localized trauma.

- First degree: this describes a tear in the skin and underlying superficial tissues (excluding the muscle layer). Often the wound will heal spontaneously as the skin edges are usually in apposition (held by the intact muscle layer beneath the tear and also by localized oedema pushing the edges together). Ragged tears may result in the formation of excess scar tissue, which can cause dyspareunia (pain during intercourse). Tears on the labia minora, a well-innervated area, may also cause significant discomfort. If bilateral tears are present, suturing needs to be considered as the labia may fuse together, if the tears are in close apposition, forming a band of tissue over the vaginal opening.
- Second degree: this describes a tear involving perineal muscle damage and division. Usually these wounds are sutured to aid healing, although some small simple second-degree tears, especially in the midline, may be well apposed and therefore not require suturing. Simple second-degree tears are usually in the midline and involve one line of tearing. Some second-degree tears can be complex with more than one tear line radiating in both lateral and downward directions involving larger amounts of muscle trauma. Misalignment is more likely with the formation of excess scar tissue.
- Episiotomy: this is a surgical incision to enlarge the introitus to facilitate the delivery of the baby, which used to be thought to be beneficial and was done routinely. The resulting trauma falls into the same category as the second-degree tear. Although episiotomies can be performed in the midline, because of the increased risk of extension to a third-degree tear and anal sphincter rupture, they are usually performed to the side (mediolateral). The need for an episiotomy requires careful clinical assessment, which is made complex by so many factors, such as perineal length, presenting part, fetal size and type of delivery required, etc. Episiotomy is usually reserved for difficult complex deliveries such as a face presentation, which causes overdistension of the perineum. The main difference between an episiotomy and tear is that the surgical incision cuts across the muscle fibres whereas a tear tends to divide muscle fibres rather than dissecting them. Thus, an episiotomy is likely to avoid overstretching of the muscle layers but is more likely to form a fibrous band across the muscle at the plane of division. In a spontaneous tear, the formation of fibrous tissue is more likely to be aligned with the muscle fibres, not across them. Episiotomies tend to gape more, as the ends of the divided fibres contract away from each other whereas a tear is more likely to be loose and flappy, as the intact muscle fibres do not contract to the same degree as in an episiotomy where the fibres are dissected.
- Third degree: this describes the situation where the muscle of the external anal sphincter is involved. Obstetric repair is essential so that the sphincter activity of the muscle is restored thus avoiding complications of faecal incontinence at a later time. This type of trauma is not always easy to identify.
- Fourth degree: is when the tear is extensive, both the external and internal anal sphincter may become completely divided and the tear continues through the rectal mucosa. Specialist surgical repair by an experienced practitioner is required to ensure the resumption of normal pelvic floor and anal–rectal function; severe cases should be referred to a colorectal surgeon.
- Female genital mutilation (FGM) (also known as female circumcision; see Chapter 2). The midwife must be able to recognize all forms of female genital mutilation and act within the law of the country in which they practice. In such cases, the midwife should seek specialist help. Female genital mutilation is a safeguarding issue, not just for the mutilated woman but also if her newborn is female (who then may be at risk of FGM being performed on her) and so care should be carefully coordinated by a multiprofessional team. If FGM has been performed, then extensive genital trauma will result from a vaginal delivery and surgical intervention is necessary prior to delivery to minimize it. Following delivery, the genitalia should be restored to as near a natural form as possible to minimize further complications. It is illegal to perform re-infibulation, even if there is pressure from the woman and her relatives to have infibulation reinstated; postdelivery repair must be undertaken by an experienced practitioner.

Repair to the perineum involves the practitioner assessing and suturing the perineum. There is a wide variety of suture materials and techniques for repair; however, suturing aims to achieve the following:

- Haemostasis: to ensure that any active bleeding points are ligated to minimize blood loss and the postnatal complication of a haematoma (formation of a blood clot within the wound), which can be extremely painful.
- Alignment: to bring the tissues back into alignment to optimize healing and to achieve a near pre-tear condition. If wounds are left gaping, alignment may not occur and as healing is by granulation this can result in the formation of excess scar tissue. This can result in a rigid misshapen perineum, which can cause dyspareunia (pain during intercourse). Alignment can be difficult to achieve due to 'shortening' of the wound edges due to divided muscle fibres contracting down.

The majority of perineal traumas can be described as being deep wounds as the tissue trauma involves layers below the epidermis and the dermis. Wound healing occurs in three phases: inflammation, tissue formation and tissue

BOX 14.1 The Stages of Wound Healing

0–3 Days
- Blood clot forms, reinforced with fibrin fibres
- Acute inflammatory response occurs: polymorphs and macrophages migrate to site; high-protein exudate leads to local oedema

1 Week Later
- Eschar dries out, hardens and eventually becomes detached
- Wound contracts
- Mitotic activity occurs in epidermal cells, which migrate over living tissue
- New blood capillaries form from endothelial buds, bringing nutrients to healing tissue
- New connective tissue, formed by fibroblasts, supports capillary loops

6 Months Later
- Surface depression may still be visible at wound site; scar tissue becomes paler
- Epithelialization is complete
- Connective tissue is reorganized, less vascular and stronger

remodelling (see also Box 14.1). Some features of wound healing are common to all tissues; others are specific to the tissue involved. For instance, little granulation tissue develops in the endometrium and the wounds do not heal with scarring. In this respect, there are similarities with fetal wounds, which also heal without scarring suggesting that the process of endometrial remodelling is more a developmental mechanism than merely repair.

1. The inflammatory response is a normal reaction to tissue trauma. Perineal inflammation can initially cause great discomfort for women in the very early postnatal period. An analgesic is useful; many (like nonsteroidal antiinflammatories) also have anti-inflammatory properties. However, a degree of inflammation is beneficial to tissue healing, so analgesics should be used only when the response is severe and perineal pain restricts normal activity. Inflammation acts to isolate the damaged tissues, reducing the spread of infection and potentially pushes the wound edges together to aid alignment. White blood cells, such as neutrophils and macrophages, invade the tissue owing to the increased vasodilatation and permeability of the surrounding blood vessels. These phagocytic cells ingest invading bacteria and break down any necrotic tissue within the wound. This explains why wounds initially feel hot, however persisting redness and heat may indicate infection.

2. The migratory phase involves the infiltration of the wound by mesenchymal cells that form fibroblasts, initially creating a scab over the open wound site. Following this, blood vessels grow into the wound and the wound is gradually filled from the bottom up by new tissue growth called granulation tissue. In well-aligned wounds or wounds that have been sutured, very little granulation tissue is formed. In gaping or complex wounds, gaps will be filled by granulation tissue, which can be extensive and form tough rigid scar tissue. If the deficit to the wound is large, or if suturing is not complete, these gaps can form sinuses, which can become the foci for infections. If gaps are left between pelvic structures, fistulas can form for example vaginal–rectal fistulas, vaginal–urethral fistulas and rectal–peritoneal fistulas. This is more likely if a third or fourth degree tear is not recognized and not repaired appropriately. Any vaginal leakage of urine and or faecal material following delivery must be investigated immediately.

3. There then follows a proliferative phase where epithelial cells grow under the scab. It concludes with the maturation of the new cells and the shedding of the scab.

LOCHIA

The initial vaginal loss is termed the 'lochia rubra' and consists of blood that has collected within the reproductive tract together with autolytic products of degenerated necrotic decidua from the placental site and any trophoblastic remains. The outward flow of blood lost at delivery and the subsequent discharge of lochia are important in removing potential sources of ascending infection and protecting the placental wound site. The alkalinity of the lochia is also important in protecting the vulnerable endometrial wound site from bacteria. Lochia is the normal discharge in the puerperium; it has a characteristic sweetish smell unless there is an infection.

Lochia may be described by its visual appearance (Box 14.2); normally, the lochia lightens progressively in both volume and colour. However, at about day 7 after delivery, the fibrinous mesh deposited over the placental site may be shed as part of the normal healing process; the vaginal loss may be transiently heavier and flushed with fresh blood. By day 10, the lochia is normally scant and initially pink in colour but progressively turns a yellow to white colour (lochia alba). The discharge of lochia may persist for up to 6 weeks. Prolonged duration of lochia discharge suggests the placental wound site is not completely epithelialized or that the uterus has some retained debris, which is still disintegrating (Hytten, 1995). The duration of lochia discharge tends to be longer with the first pregnancy; it is also related to birthweight.

BOX 14.2 Lochia

- **Lochia rubra (red)**
  - decidua and frank blood loss from placental site
  - initially sterile then uterus begins to be colonized by vaginal flora
  - red colour persists for about 3 days
- **Lochia serosa (pink/brown)**
  - contains leukocytes, mucus, vaginal epithelial cells, necrotic decidua, nonpathological bacteria
  - may be blood stained for 3–4 weeks
  - characteristic sweetish odour
- **Lochia alba (yellow–white)**
  - mostly serous fluid and leukocytes
  - plus some cervical mucus and microorganisms

Heavy discharge of lochia with an offensive odour, maternal pyrexia and/or a feeling of general malaise are all indicative of intrauterine infection (endometritis). If the lochia remains abnormally heavy and further bleeding occurs, surgical intervention, dilatation and curettage (D&C) to empty the uterine cavity of any conceptual tissue may be necessary. The procedure is also termed evacuation of retained products of conception (ERPC). The cervix is progressively and artificially dilated and the retained products are gently scraped from the decidua using a curette. This procedure is not without complications; excessive scraping can scar the endometrium causing menstrual disturbance, intrauterine adhesions, infertility and placental abnormalities if conception occurs. This is known as Asherman syndrome (Conforti et al., 2013); Sildenafil (Viagra) may be an effective treatment in some women, possibly because it improves blood flow to the endometrial basal layer. Stem cell therapy has a potential role in regenerating and renovating the defective endometrial wall (Azizi et al., 2018).

Blood Loss

Excessive blood loss, defined as >500 mL or any amount that jeopardizes the wellbeing of the mother at and within 24 h of delivery, is termed a primary postpartum haemorrhage (primary PPH). It is usually caused by failure of the myometrium to contract completely, or failure of the blood-clotting mechanisms, or both (see Chapter 13); PPH can be serious (Box 14.3, Case study 14.1). Women may also lose significant amounts of blood from trauma to the genital tract and perineum. If there is excessive bleeding but the uterus is well contracted, examination of the genital tract and perineum should not be delayed to identify bleeding points and any trauma repaired as quickly as possible to minimize further blood loss.

BOX 14.3 Disseminated Intravascular Coagulation

Disseminated intravascular coagulation (DIC) is a condition caused by abnormal activation of the clotting mechanisms. The balance between coagulation and fibrinolysis is disrupted and fibrin is deposited throughout the vascular beds, so blood clots form and small blood vessels are occluded. This exhausts the clotting factors and platelets so bleeding continues unabated. Liver dysfunction in preeclampsia may be associated with DIC and microangiopathic haemolysis (erythrocyte breakdown in small blood vessels). The acronym HELLP refers to Haemolysis, Elevated Liver enzymes and Low Platelet counts.

DIC is an extremely severe condition. It is characterized by chest pain, dyspnoea, leg pain, blood in urine and faecal stools and bleeding under the skin. The affected woman may have problems moving and speaking. Although life-threatening conditions such as DIC would normally be managed by intensive care staff rather than by the midwifery unit, it is important that midwives are able to recognize the symptoms and implications of DIC, for example, the appearance of bruising on the skin not associated with trauma. In advanced cases, observation of the failure of blood to clot may indicate rapidly deteriorating DIC, which warrants immediate intervention as this indicates a critical life-threatening situation.

CASE STUDY 14.1

Lucy is a 35-year-old primigravida whose baby is delivered by emergency LSCS at 30 weeks' gestation owing to fulminating preeclampsia. Following delivery, the blood loss per vaginam is noted to be quite brisk and a Syntocinon (oxytocin) infusion is commenced in an attempt to control the bleeding. On investigation, it is discovered that Lucy's platelet count is extremely low and that the clotting time for her blood is greatly prolonged. A provisional diagnosis of disseminated intravascular coagulation secondary to HELLP syndrome is made.

- What predisposing factors may have contributed to Lucy's condition?
- What intervention would Lucy require and what care would she need following this diagnosis?
- What physiological symptoms may be present and what specific observations would the midwife be undertaking to monitor this condition.

Occasionally, there may be concealed bleeding, either into the peritoneum from ruptured blood vessels in the broad ligament or into the tissues, forming large collections of blood clots called haematomas. Therefore, even in the absence of visible blood loss, women can still be physically in shock if concealed bleeding is present. Severe shock is commonly indicated by tachycardia and hypotension.

The risk of primary PPH is lower 24–72 h following delivery but, until involution of the uterus is complete, there is a risk of a secondary PPH particularly if there is an infection within the uterine cavity. The bleeding is often due to fibrinolytic action of bacteria such as haemolytic streptococcus. These bacteria are usually anaerobic (thrive in the absence of oxygen) and so specific antibiotic treatment may be required.

Hormonal Changes

In late pregnancy, most of the steroid hormones in the maternal circulation are derived from the placenta, although the corpus luteum may continue to contribute some progesterone. Levels of progesterone and oestrogen fall to nonpregnant levels within 72 h of delivery. The placental protein hormones have a longer half-life so plasma levels fall more slowly. During pregnancy, production of the gonadotrophins is suppressed. Follicle-stimulating hormone (FSH) levels are restored to prepregnant concentrations within 3 weeks of delivery, but restoration of luteinizing hormone (LH) secretion takes longer, depending on the duration and frequency of lactation. Levels of oxytocin and prolactin also depend on lactational performance.

The Haematological System and Cardiovascular Changes

The blood lost at delivery, accepted to be about 300–500 mL normally and about 1000 mL in caesarean sections, is adequately compensated for by the increase in blood volume acquired during pregnancy (see Chapter 11). Women can lose about 1000 mL of their predelivery blood volume before postnatal haemoglobin concentration is compromised (Case study 14.2). Erythropoiesis is stimulated before and after delivery (Blackburn, 2018). Diuresis further decreases plasma volume in the first days, although as interstitial fluid is mobilized, plasma volume tends to increase transiently causing haemodilution of both haemoglobin and plasma proteins, such as clotting factors. It is this variability in blood lost at delivery and restoration of normal water balance that may result in raised concentrations of clotting factors that promote hypercoagulability. The tendency to coagulate is also affected by the loss of placental and fetal factors affecting clotting and water regulation (Blackburn, 2018). This places postnatal women at a higher risk of developing thrombolytic disorders.

CASE STUDY 14.2

Prior to delivery, Megan had a haemoglobin (Hb) concentration of 101 g/L. At delivery, her blood loss is estimated at about 1000 mL. The midwife is quite concerned over this, although Megan was asymptomatic. Prior to discharge on day 3, Megan's Hb concentration is rechecked and is 98 g/L.

- How would you account for Megan's Hb concentration being relatively stable despite her suffering a postpartum haemorrhage?
- What advice/treatment would you give to Megan following her discharge?

Haemoglobin levels return to normal prepregnant levels within 4–6 weeks and white blood cell numbers fall to normal within a week of delivery (Blackburn, 2018). Platelet number increases in the first few days following delivery, thereafter falling gradually to prepregnant levels. Fibrinolytic activity is maximal for ~48 h after delivery in response to the removal of the placenta, which produced fibrinolytic inhibitors. Clotting factors, which peaked in labour, gradually decrease reaching their lowest level about a week after delivery. The net result is that the hypercoagulable state of pregnancy is increased in the early puerperium and then slowly returns to a prepregnant state over a few weeks. This period of prolonged hypercoagulability is why women are at significantly increased risk of thromboembolic episodes in the puerperal period.

In previous eras, wealthy women were advised to rest in bed after childbirth and received indulgent cosseting (Hytten, 1995). However, early ambulation is now highly recommended as it facilitates improved blood flow and rapid dispersal of oedema, thus optimizing cardiovascular health. Mobilization is essential to optimize venous return and avoid stasis within the vascular bed, in order to minimize the risk of deep vein thrombosis (DVT) formation (see p. 432). Women who are unable to mobilize owing to obstetric complications, such as an LSCS, are given prophylactic treatment as the risks of DVT and complications are significantly increased. Women are advised to report any discomfort or swelling in the lower legs, which may indicate DVT formation (especially if one leg appears more swollen than the other, although bilateral DVTs are possible); the risks of DVT progressively diminish.

The cardiovascular system is rendered transiently unstable by delivery owing to the blood loss and the ensuing compensatory mechanisms. During the brief period of instability of fluid balance in the first week after delivery, many women experience headaches. Initially, there is a marked increase in cardiac output as the uteroplacental flow is returned to the venous system and the gravid uterus no longer impedes the vena cava blood flow. This is augmented by the mobilization of extracellular fluid. Although pregnant women are usually able to tolerate normal blood loss at delivery, those women who had decreased vascular expansion during pregnancy, such as those with preeclampsia (see Chapter 11), may be less able to tolerate blood loss. Vaginal delivery is associated with a higher haemoglobin concentration than operative deliveries because vaginal delivery tends to have less blood loss and to promote diuresis more markedly (Blackburn, 2018).

Parameters of the cardiovascular system return towards prepregnant values but remain significantly different. Resolution of ventricular hypertrophy is slow. Vascular remodelling persists for at least a year after delivery and is enhanced by second and subsequent pregnancies. Because circulating blood volume and cardiac output fall early in the puerperium and the hypertrophied left ventricle is slowly remodelled over a period of 4–6 months, the stroke volume remains relatively high for up to 12 weeks or longer (Blackburn, 2018). This means that heart rate falls in the puerperium, as the stroke volume contributes proportionately more to the cardiac output (which is lower and closer to the prepregnant value). Thus, it is normal for puerperal women to exhibit bradycardia (a reduced pulse rate of about 60–70 beats/min). A raised (or normal) pulse may indicate severe anaemia, venous thrombosis or infection.

Respiratory System

The decreased progesterone concentration following delivery of the placenta restores prepregnant sensitivity to carbon dioxide concentration promptly, so that partial pressures of carbon dioxide return to prepregnant levels. The diaphragm can increase its excursion distance once the gravid uterus no longer impedes it so full ventilation of the basal lobes of the lung is restored. Chest wall compliance, tidal volume and respiratory rate return to normal within 1–3 weeks. Changes in the elasticity of the rib cage, however, may persist for months (Blackburn, 2018).

Urinary System

It is important that bladder function is assessed in the early postnatal period. The trauma experienced by the bladder during delivery usually results in oedema and hyperaemia of the bladder, which had reduced muscle tone in pregnancy. Effects on the bladder are increased by prolonged labour, use of forceps, analgesia and anaesthetic procedures and pressure of the descending presenting part during delivery. The resulting transient loss of bladder sensation, which may result in overdistension and incomplete emptying, can last from days to weeks. Bladder changes are associated with increased risk of urinary tract infections (UTI) in the puerperium. Trauma to the sphincter of the bladder increases the frequency of stress incontinence, which is marked by urine leakage more likely to occur when coughing, laughing or with sudden movement or exercise.

If bladder function is impaired, an indwelling catheter may be inserted to enable the damaged tissue to recover; however, catheterization itself increases the risk of UTI. If the uterus can be palpated high up or is displaced over to one side following the woman voiding urine, this indicates that there may be retention of urine as the full bladder displaces the uterus, usually confirmed by postvoiding ultrasound examination of the bladder, demonstrating the presence of residual urine in the bladder. Urinary retention is compounded by the increased diuresis that occurs in the postnatal period as plasma volume acquired during pregnancy is reduced. It is normal for women to have frequent micturition as long as they are voiding large amounts of urine each time. Frequency involving just small amounts of urine being voided can also indicate a degree of urinary retention.

Pain associated with micturition may indicate a UTI. Dilation of the ureters, overdistension of the bladder, and instrumental or operative deliveries, perineal trauma and repair and use of urinary catheters increase the risk of infection. By day 10, full bladder function should be observed and assessed; there should be no evidence of unprovoked urinary incontinence.

Parameters of the renal system, such as renal plasma flow, glomerular filtration rate and plasma creatinine, are usually back to normal nonpregnant levels by the 6-week check. Urinary excretion of minerals and vitamins is normal within the first week after delivery. Plasma renin and angiotensin levels adjust to the loss of placental hormones affecting their control so levels fall and then increase before returning back to normal (Blackburn, 2018). This fluctuation in hormone levels affecting water retention, together with the redistribution of body fluid, results in rapid and sustained natriuresis and diuresis, which is particularly marked between the second and fifth day after delivery. Fluid and electrolyte balance is normal within 21 days after delivery. Oxytocin, which has antidiuretic hormone (ADH)-like activity, falls after delivery, augmenting diuresis. The voiding volume increases and many women experience night sweats in the puerperium, which also increase fluid loss. Pregnancy-induced changes in the urinary system may persist for several months. Although the dilated smooth muscle of the urinary tract appears normal within a week of delivery, it remains potentially distensible. The kidneys return to their prepregnant size within 6 months of pregnancy.

Gastrointestinal System and Defaecation

During labour, gastric motility is reduced, particularly in association with pain, fear and narcotic drugs. The reduced tone of the lower oesophageal sphincter, reduced gastric motility and increased gastric acidity result in delayed gastric emptying. The tone and pressure of the lower oesophageal sphincter are normal by 6 weeks after delivery. However, in the early puerperium, the reduced gastrointestinal muscle tone and motility and the relaxed abdomen can increase gas distension and constipation immediately after delivery. Gall bladder muscle tone and contractility are enhanced after delivery so the gallbladder may expel small gallstones that developed during pregnancy (Blackburn, 2018).

The first bowel movements usually occur within 2 or 3 days following delivery. This may become complicated by the presence of haemorrhoids, which are associated with defaecation problems. Haemorrhoids are common during late pregnancy because of the effects of progesterone on vascular smooth muscle tone. Usually haemorrhoids resolve quickly after birth and cause only minor discomfort in the postnatal period. Sometimes, particularly if they are severe owing to displacement by the passage of the presenting part through the birth canal, they can become traumatized and localized thrombosis can occur. This can be further complicated if constipation develops and the woman, because of perineal trauma, resists opening her bowels. Problems with constipation are increased by intestinal atony, lax abdominal musculature, irregular food intake, dehydration in labour and use of opioid analgesics. By day 10, the woman should have regained normal bowel function. Faecal incontinence may indicate anal sphincter damage or inadequate repair.

Weight Change

Although weight is lost at delivery of the products of conception, many women experience a weight gain in the first couple of days following delivery. This is due to a combination of increased adrenocorticotrophin (ACTH), ADH and stress, all of which increase sodium and water retention. Women who have a higher blood loss at delivery tend to gain slightly more weight during the early days of the puerperium as water is retained for compensatory expansion of their blood volume. Weight usually starts to fall from the 4th day after delivery as diuresis increases. Weight is lost steadily, usually over a period of several months. Postpartum weight retention is affected by changes in lifestyle during and after pregnancy rather than by pregnancy itself (Hollis et al., 2017). Weight loss tends to be greater with lower parity, maternal age and lower prepregnant weight. Lactation and maternal nutrition also affect the rate of weight loss (see Chapter 16).

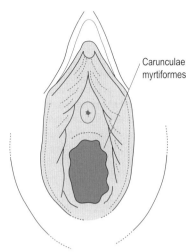

Fig. 14.5 Carunculae myrtiformes. (Reproduced with permission from Miller and Hanretty, 1998.)

Other Structural Changes

Immediately after delivery, the vagina is smooth, soft and oedematous. The elasticity of the tissue returns within a few days. As the vagina is extremely well-vascularized, episiotomies and tears usually heal well. The rugae of the vagina re-form in the third week but are less prominent than prior to pregnancy. The labia regress to a less prominent and fleshy state than in nulliparous women. The fall in oestrogen at delivery results in the vaginal epithelium becoming thinner and many women experience problems with vaginal lubrication immediately after delivery. Tags of the hymen remain and are renamed carunculae myrtiformes (Fig. 14.5). The carunculae myrtiformes are a useful landmark in restoring alignment of tissues when undertaking perineal repair.

Pelvic floor muscle strength and neuromuscular control are impaired to a greater extent in women who deliver vaginally and experience more mechanical trauma, particularly in the first week of the puerperium (Van Geelen et al., 2018); the first pregnancy can have the most significant effect on pelvic floor function. However, for many women, muscular tone and strength are normal within 2 months. Weakened circumvaginal muscles are associated with perineal outcome, episiotomy, length of second stage of labour, the weight, positioning and presentation of the baby and pushing techniques. Problems associated with a lax ineffective pelvic floor such as uterine prolapse, urinary incontinence and prolapse of the rectum are more likely as parity increases. Pelvic floor exercises help to restore the muscle tone and function of the pelvic floor; specialist advice from an obstetric physiotherapist may be required for persistent problems with incontinence. Pelvic floor disorders are a major health problem and affect 25–30% of adult women.

The abdominal wall may remain soft and flabby for several weeks. Severe stretching, for instance in a multiple pregnancy or with polyhydramnios, can result in permanently lax muscles. In severe cases, divarication (separation) of the rectus abdominis muscles (diastasis recti) can occur; the abdominal muscles become divided in the midline because the connective tissue of the linea nigra is stretched. If this occurs, a referral to an obstetric physiotherapist should be made especially if the gap between the paired muscles is >2 cm. This is more likely to occur where the stretching is more extreme (multiple birth pregnancy, excess abdominal exercise or large fetus) or is repeated (multiparous women). It is more common in older women.

The softened pelvic joints and ligaments slowly return to normal over a period of a few months. Relaxation of pelvic joints can cause or exacerbate lower backache in the puerperium. The striae gravidarum become paler and silvery rather than red over a period of several months but fade rather than completely disappear.

Pregnancy-induced changes in the skin spontaneously regress or fade, though hyperpigmentation and melasma may persist in women with darker skin and hair. Hair loss may be marked following delivery and initial regrowth may be initially less abundant. Corneal sensitivity and pressure return to normal within 2 months of delivery. Nasal congestion and effects on the ear and larynx are restored to the prepregnant state within a few days of delivery.

Body Temperature

In the first 24 h following delivery, body temperature may increase slightly (to 38°C) in response to the stress of labour, particularly dehydration. This temperature fluctuation is normally transient; a persistent raised temperature may indicate infection (see below).

SLEEP

The puerperium is associated with disrupted sleep patterns (insomnia and poor sleep quality), particularly immediately after delivery, and may affect the development of postpartum depression (Okun, 2016). The first 3 days can be extremely difficult for the mother compounded by fatigue accumulated during labour and being unable to rest comfortably due to perineal pain (see Case study 14.3). Postpartum perineal pain correlates well with the duration of the second stage of labour; certain techniques such as massage and warm compresses can reduce the trauma and pain (Aasheim et al., 2017). Euphoria, urinary, breast and

perineal discomfort combined with disturbances related to the care of the infant can all lead to reduced sleep, which may affect memory and psychomotor tasks. Theoretically, sleep patterns are close to normal within 2 or 3 weeks of delivery but breastfeeding mothers obviously have more disrupted sleep.

CASE STUDY 14.3

Sandra is a first-time mother who delivered a healthy male infant 3 days ago. She went home on the day of the birth as she appeared to be coping well with breastfeeding and caring for her infant. The community midwife visits at lunchtime on the third day to find a very distressed mother, partner and infant. They have had very little sleep and the baby has been very fractious and wakeful.

- What are the possible physiological causes that have contributed to this situation?
- What would reassure the midwife that everything was normal and what support, help and advice could the midwife give to the family during this difficult period?
- How should the midwife monitor this situation and what factors and observations would be required and if present what referrals should the midwife make?

PSYCHOLOGICAL STATE

Usually by day 10 the mother and baby have established a feeding cycle. Although fatigue is common and normal, the mother should be developing strategies to cope with this, such as daytime sleeps. The mother should be independently caring for herself and the baby and interacting fully with members of her family and other people. Offspring provide their mothers with stimuli that elicit behavioural responses and emotional reactions; these nurturing responses may be evolutionarily conserved.

Many women experience a lack of libido (sex drive) during the first few months following delivery. This may be complicated by trauma to the reproductive tract during delivery. Sexual desire, expression and satisfaction may be reduced after delivery. Sexual activity may be affected by fatigue, altered body image, marital adjustment, dyspareunia, lactation, traditional taboos, vaginal bleeding or discharge, insufficient lubrication or fear of waking the baby. Most couples resume vaginal intercourse by about eight weeks after childbirth and resume prepregnancy frequency within about a year (Jawed-Wessel and Sevick, 2017).

Return to Fertility

In pregnancy, ovarian function is suppressed by the high level of placental steroids. Women who do not breastfeed begin to menstruate, on average, about 6 weeks postpartum after delivery (Chertok and Wolf, 2018), whereas lactation can delay ovulation to 30–40 weeks after delivery and menstruation to 8–15 months, depending on the duration, extent and frequency of breastfeeding. The first menstrual cycle may be anovulatory but in about a third of cycles ovulation precedes menstruation. Although ovarian activity is almost invariably suspended in the early postpartum period, there have been reported cases of women who conceive within 2 weeks of giving birth (Hytten, 1995). The return to fertility exhibits similar hormonal profiles as puberty with a circadian pattern of LH secretion. A proportion of women become pregnant during lactational amenorrhoea but the degree of suppression of fertility depends on infant-feeding patterns and perhaps on maternal nutrition. Lactational effects on fertility are reduced as the spaces between the feeds increase and as the baby receives supplementary feeding. Where the number of sucking episodes is 10–20 per day, as is normal in many developing countries, resumption of ovarian activity is unlikely. With 5–6 feeds per day, the duration of feeds is important in suppressing ovulation. However, the lactational amenorrhoea method of contraception is unpredictable since it only reduces the likelihood of conception (Van der Wijden and Manion, 2015).

Many women choose to limit the number of children they have. There are many economic, social and cultural issues that impinge on this; however, it is important to recognize that there are some women for whom certain (or all) methods of contraception are not acceptable on cultural, religious, moral and/or ethical grounds. The return of fertility is very difficult to assess as factors such as breastfeeding, cultural and religious practice, genetic variation and disease may all compound the reliable identification of a return of fertility. It is important to emphasize that ovulation may precede menstruation so amenorrhoea does not guarantee the absence of fertility.

THE ROLE OF THE MIDWIFE

In the UK, most women are discharged from midwifery care by postnatal day 10; however, the midwife may visit up to day 28 in the postnatal period if required. In many countries, the postnatal input from a midwife varies. Once the midwife is satisfied that the physiological transition for both mother and baby is progressing normally, then the discharge can be completed. The health visitor and general practitioner (GP) continue to provide ongoing care of the mother and baby. The responsibilities of the midwife in the puerperium and at discharge include giving advice to women on a number of issues including infant feeding, parentcraft, pelvic floor exercises, contraception and sources of psychological and emotional support.

COMPLICATIONS OF THE PUERPERIUM

Two of the most common and most serious problems in the puerperium are PPH and hypercoagulability. It is suggested that human vulnerability to PPH is a consequence of the very invasive nature of human placental development and the extensive remodelling of the spiral arteries in order to supply the intervillous spaces with an efficient supply of oxygen and nutrients to promote fetal growth (Abrams and Rutherford, 2011). If the delicate balance between the invasive nature of the trophoblasts and remodelling of the maternal blood vessels and their limitation by the maternal immune system is disrupted, it leads to an adverse outcome. For example, in preeclampsia, one of the significant contributors to maternal mortality, placental invasion is shallow and the maternal blood vessels are incompletely remodelled. Preeclampsia seems to be a disease unique to humans and other large-brained New World primates such as gorillas and chimpanzees (Carter, 2011), which also have characteristically deep trophoblastic invasion and a high rate of blood flow, particularly in late gestation, to support fetal brain development. (Note that deep trophoblastic placental invasion is not the only mechanism to support the growth of a large fetal brain; dolphin neonates have brains twice the size of human neonates but do not have an invasive placenta; Martin, 2007).

Haemostasis, the balance between coagulation and fibrinolysis (see Chapter 1), is extremely efficient in vertebrates; blood loss is quickly staunched after an injury by the formation of a fibrin mesh, which entraps platelets. In placental mammals, the coagulation system shifts to a hypercoagulability state in later pregnancy; there is an increase in clotting factors and a decrease in anticoagulants (Ribeiro et al., 2015). All three elements of the haemostatic system are affected: vascular-endothelial components, platelet-thrombin interaction and plasma proteins as well as the inflammation and complement pathways that they interact with (see p. 313 for details of Virchow's Triad of factors, which predispose to thrombosis.)

The intricate complexity of mammalian haemostasis has evolved over the last 450 million years and is particularly marked in those placental mammals with deeper placental invasion. This is a mechanism to limit blood lost at delivery or abortion and also to efficiently repair any small blood vessel ruptures associated with the placenta that develop during pregnancy. This comes with a cost; a significantly higher risk of thromboembolic disorders during pregnancy particularly if the protective hypercoagulable state is exacerbated by endothelial injury, activation of the coagulation pathway or altered blood flow (Struble et al., 2015).

Thromboembolic Disorders

The increase in potential clot formation can be a physiological disadvantage both in pregnancy and following delivery because thrombi (blood clots) can form more readily within the venous system. During the third trimester, the pregnant woman develops a pronounced state of hypercoagulation, such that her blood is more likely to clot than it would in the nonpregnant state and the effects of progesterone relaxing venous muscle tone increase stasis of flow and decrease venous capacitance. In addition, mechanical obstruction by the uterus can decrease venous outflow and women may become less mobile. Metabolic syndrome and the related changes of gestational diabetes also enhance both coagulopathy and haemodynamic changes, which increase the risk for thrombosis as well as preeclampsia and pregnancy-associated hypertension. The risk of thromboembolic disorders in pregnancy is about six times higher than it is before pregnancy, and increases further in the puerperium, made worse if obesity and/or an underlying clotting disorder is also present (thrombophilia). This is enhanced by a decrease in fibrinolytic activity (the breakdown of fibrin forming a blood clot) and a raised concentration of many clotting factors such as fibrinogen and thrombin. Vascular trauma during delivery and haemoconcentration (an increase in the proportion of red blood cells relative to the plasma) of the blood from physiological diuresis following delivery further augments the increase in clotting factors. Some women may suffer from protein C and protein S deficiencies. These proteins are anticoagulants so that, in pregnancy and the postnatal period, these women are at greater risk of developing DVT (Villani et al., 2017). The risk of thrombosis persists for at least 8 weeks following delivery (Fogerty, 2018).

Thrombophlebitis

Pregnancy affects the lower extremity venous system; blood volume and venous pressure are increased and flow rate in the deep veins is decreased (Taylor et al., 2018). Thrombophlebitis is vascular inflammation, due to the formation of a thrombus (clot), in a superficial vein. It can occur in different locations but the commonest site of thrombus formation is in the saphenous vein supplying the calf of the leg. Symptoms include a tender reddened area over the thrombosed vein, which is often warm and painful, and possibly a small increase in pulse and temperature. Motility, fluid intake and elevating the legs at rest will all reduce the risk of thrombus formation; a warm compress or compression stockings may also be

helpful whereas immobility and smoking increase the risk. Thrombophlebitis is unlikely to progress to pulmonary embolism (PE).

Deep Vein Thrombosis

Venous thromboembolism (VTE) includes PE and DVT; VTE is five times more likely to occur in pregnancy and the puerperium compared to the rate in women of a similar age who are not pregnant. The risk of VTE disorders increases with gestation and peaks immediately after delivery.

DVT is less common than thrombophlebitis but carries the added risk of a clot, or part of a clot dislodging, which can cause PE. Hypercoagulability is increased with increased maternal age, parity, dehydration following delivery and delivery by caesarean section. Risk factors include maternal age >35 years, immobility, pelvic or leg trauma, obesity, preeclampsia, caesarean section, operative delivery, haemorrhage, multiparity, varicose veins, a previous history of a thromboembolic event and hereditary or acquired thrombophilia (RCOG, 2015). In pregnancy, 85% of DVT affects the left leg, especially after a caesarean section, because blood flow velocity is reduced to a greater extent in the left leg, because compression of the left common iliac artery by the right common iliac artery is increased by the enlarging uterus (McLean and James, 2018). DVT may be asymptomatic, the symptoms may be nonspecific or the woman may experience pain and swelling over the affected area and possibly pyrexia or difficulty walking. There may be marked differences in calf size or, in extreme cases, circulation to the leg below the thrombosis may be affected so the leg appears cold and white and possibly oedematous. DVT is confirmed by imaging techniques such as Doppler ultrasound or impedance plethysmography.

Pulmonary Embolism

PE is an obstetric medical emergency that may follow DVT or occur without warning. PE is a major cause of maternal deaths (Lim et al., 2016). If a thrombus (a fragment of the blood clot) breaks away and enters the venous system, it is then carried by the systemic veins to the right side of the heart and can enter the pulmonary circulation. As the pulmonary arteries reduce in size as they approach the alveolar capillaries, the thrombus may occlude arterial vessels within the lungs, causing major hypoxic then anoxic damage. PE is usually the consequence of a DVT in the leg or pelvic veins. Symptoms of PE include low blood oxygen, tachycardia, acute severe chest pain (which is worsened by breathing), dyspnoea, cough, cyanosis, haemoptysis (coughing up blood), sudden collapse, shock and, in severe cases, sudden death. Smaller pulmonary emboli can lodge in peripheral vessels causing infarctions and effusions; while these usually cause pleuritic pain and are less likely to cause as much damage as a large fragmented embolism, they can indicate potential risk of more significant damage developing.

A PE is more common in the postnatal period compared with the antepartum period. This may be due to the physiological reversal of haemodilution happening much faster (usually by day 3) than the physiological reversal of increased clotting factors, which may take up to 6–8 weeks to return to prepregnancy values. Risk of PE is assessed by medical history, haemostatic activation (measurement of biomarkers in blood) and scoring tools (such as the Wells score). Diagnosis may be confirmed by imaging, usually CT pulmonary angiography, or a ventilation-perfusion (V/Q) scan.

A woman with a PE requires intensive treatment and care. Women assessed to be at increased risk of thrombus formation may be treated with prophylactic anticoagulants, but there is then a risk of maternal bleeding complications. DVT may be treated with low molecular weight or unfractionated heparin and, if required, long-term anticoagulation therapy with drugs such as warfarin. The use of warfarin in pregnancy is contraindicated as it is transported across the placenta but postnatal women who choose to breastfeed can have warfarin treatment as it not secreted in significant levels into the breast milk.

Postpartum Thyroid Disorders

Transient thyroid disorders are common during the postpartum period and may indicate a risk of permanent hypothyroidism developing in the next year or so (Weetman, 2011). Postpartum women, especially if older than 35, are at increased risk of developing postpartum thyroiditis (PPT; inflammation of the thyroid gland) and Graves disease (the most common cause of hyperthyroidism during pregnancy), at least transiently. The 12-month period following parturition is a peak time for exacerbation of existing autoimmune diseases or the development of them *de novo*.

The initial effects of PPT are thyrotoxicosis with thyroid cell destruction and excessive release of stored thyroid hormone from the damaged thyroid tissue causing mild hyperthyroidism for 2–4 weeks (thyrotoxic phase). This is followed by a period of hypothyroidism as the damage to the thyroid progresses, which usually lasts 2–4 months (hypothyroid phase). Typical symptoms are mild and include fatigue, cold intolerance, hair damage and weight gain with high TSH and low free T4 levels. Normal thyroid function is re-established in most women with PPT within a year (euthyroid phase) but almost 50% of affected women will have permanent hypothyroidism (Di Bari et al., 2017). PPT may recur in subsequent pregnancies

(Weetman, 2011) and the risk of developing permanent hypothyroidism is increased.

Postpartum Graves disease is an autoimmune disorder, which affects fewer women than PPT (Nguyen et al., 2018). Thyroid hormones normally feedback to limit their own production by inhibiting the production of TSH by the pituitary gland. In Graves disease, autoantibodies are produced, which are agonists for the TSH receptor and therefore stimulate excess production of thyroid-stimulating immunoglobulin (TSI), which binds to the receptors for TSH and stimulates the thyroid gland to secrete thyroid hormones. Graves disease often starts in the puerperium and is the most common cause of hyperthyroidism. Graves disease usually causes marked hypertrophy of the thyroid gland (goitre), signs of increased metabolic rate (such as tachycardia, weight loss, fatigue) and exophthalmos (protruding eyes).

Postpartum Pituitary Disorders

Hypopituitarism or Sheehan syndrome, decreased functioning of the pituitary gland, is a rare complication of the puerperium. It is due to excessive blood loss after delivery and hypovolaemic shock, which causes ischaemic necrosis of the pituitary gland, affecting the secretion of some or all of the hormones it normally produces. The onset may be gradual; it may affect lactation and the resumption of menstrual cycles.

Risk of Infection

In the puerperium, the woman is at increased risk of infection, particularly that associated with the genital tract, urinary system, breast and any site of thrombophlebitis. The placental wound site, lacerations and incisions of the perineum and the lax urinary system are especially vulnerable. The lochia provides ideal culture conditions for some microorganisms. Other predisposing factors include anaemia, fatigue, malnutrition, traumatic delivery and the presence of retained tissue in the uterus. Both maternal and neonatal infection (see Chapter 15) may be caused by endogenous or exogenous organisms (Box 14.4).

Common symptoms of infection include:
- pyrexia (up to 40°C)
- tachycardia (up to 140 b.p.m.)
- subinvolution of the uterus
- headache
- malaise, lower abdominal pain and back pain
- heavy offensive-smelling lochia

Less common symptoms usually associated with severe sepsis, which remains a leading cause of maternal mortality (Burlinson et al., 2018) are:
- hypothermia (may be severe)
- tachypnoea

- hypotension
- rigor
- altered mental state (drowsiness and confusion, unconsciousness)
- marked oedema and positive fluid balance with acute oliguria (indicating acute kidney damage)
- hyperglycaemia in the absence of diabetes
- markers of inflammation such as high WBC count, high plasma C-reactive protein or procalcitonin levels
- haemodynamic variables such as arterial hypotension or hypoxia, signs of organ dysfunction, coagulation abnormalities and/or thrombocytopenia, high creatinine, ileus (absent bowel sounds)
- markers of impaired tissue perfusion such as hyperlactataemia or decreased capillary refill (or mottling)

Infection in the acute phase can inhibit lactation. When choosing antibiotics to treat infection in the puerperium, one needs to take into consideration whether the woman is breastfeeding and the potential effect of the transfer of the drug into breast milk.

Breast Discomfort and After-pains

The establishment of lactation is covered in detail in Chapter 16; however, it is important to include two common problems in this chapter that can occur in the puerperal period in relation to breastfeeding.
- If the baby has been incorrectly positioned, often because it is fractious or hungry and wanting to feed constantly, the nipple may become sore, cracked and bleed as a consequence. A break in the integrity of the nipple skin increases the risk of mastitis (localized and ascending infection usually caused by *Staphylococcus aureus*). Women experiencing early feeding problems need a lot of help and support. The baby needs to 'fix' or 'latch on' properly in order to provide adequate nipple stimulation to establish the feeding cycle.

- The breasts become engorged or extended. Initially, this may be a venous cause due to the increased vascularization of the breast (venous engorgement). However, when milk production increases (described as the milk 'coming in'), the breast may initially be overproductive. The breasts may overfill with milk causing them to become distended and hardened, which may be uncomfortable or painful (lactational engorgement). The baby may need help in achieving an appropriate position; however, once the feeding cycle is established the demand/supply balance is achieved and the breast engorgement problems will resolve.

Pharmacological Effects

Many deliveries within the UK have the third stage actively managed as opposed to passive or physiological management, where the women deliver the placenta naturally (see Chapter 13). However, the administration of an antitocolytic (or 'uterotonic') drug such as Syntometrine, which combines ergometrine (an α-adrenergic, dopaminergic and serotonin receptor agonist) and Syntocinon (synthetic oxytocin), may cause side-effects following completion of the third stage; for example:
- nausea and vomiting
- transient rise in blood pressure
- palpitations and tachycardia
- chest pain
- headache

Most of these side-effects are strongly associated with ergometrine, so it is recommended that administration by intramuscular injection of syntocinon is used instead (NCCWCH, 2014). Also, during the early puerperium, women may suffer side-effects from pharmacological methods of pain relief administered during labour. Pethidine may induce drowsiness, fatigue and nausea within the mother and reduce the suckling instinct of the infant, thus interfering with feeding. The effects of an epidural anaesthetic may take several hours to wear off, which affects maternal mobility and the ability to void urine.

Psychological Problems

During pregnancy and the puerperium, the dramatic changes in steroid and peptide hormone levels influence the hypothalamic–pituitary–gonadal (HPG) and hypothalamic–pituitary–adrenal (HPA) axes; perturbation of these axes is associated with mood disorders. The puerperal period is often a challenging transition period. The 5th edition of the definitive *Diagnostic and Statistical Manual of Mental Disorders* (DSM5) (American Psychiatric Association, 2013) added a peripartum onset to the psychiatric mood disorder category.

Women in the postpartum period have increased vulnerability to affective or mood disorders; these are classified

BOX 14.5 Classic Signs of Postnatal Depression

- Depressed mood: hopelessness, sadness, crying and swings of mood
- Sleep disturbance not related to discomfort and infant wakening
- Unable to cope: guilt, irritability, feeling of being overwhelmed
- Inability to make decisions or concentrate
- Loss of interest in usual or pleasurable activities
- Anxiety
- Rejection of baby or disinterest in caring for the baby
- Altered libido, difficulty in maintaining relationships
- Unexplained physical pain and muscle aches
- Thoughts of harming self or baby

on the basis of severity: postpartum or baby 'blues' or mood disturbance, postpartum depression and anxiety (PPD) and postpartum psychosis. It is estimated that 50–80% of women experience fluctuations in mood, mostly transient emotional disorders, in the first few days after delivery, described as 'the blues' (Shorey et al., 2018). Approximately 10–20% of puerperal women develop true depressive illness, PPD, which may have a later onset (or referral) and delayed recovery. There is no consensus about the time-frame for diagnosis of PPD. It persists for several weeks or months and usually results in functional impairment. A few women (0.1–0.2%) develop severe prolonged psychotic illness following childbirth. This is a psychiatric emergency that requires urgent medical attention because there is a risk of suicide and infanticide. Although many of these cases in the spectrum of psychiatric syndromes may be recognized in the early postnatal period, some become evident much later and depression is frequently underreported and not always recognized. Certain symptoms are recognized to be important in the diagnosis of postnatal depression (Box 14.5). Overall, these figures mean that postnatal depression is the most common disorder of the puerperium.

The aetiology of puerperal mood and affective disorders is complex and not well understood. Immediately after delivery, the infant may feed often and this may be increased at night adding to maternal fatigue. Initially, the mother's fatigue may be overcome by intense feelings of relief and excitement at the birth of her baby. First time mothers are often more vulnerable because they may have unreasonable expectations. By about days 2–4, however, the woman may become overwhelmed, emotional, irritable, tearful and tired and in need of a lot of support and comfort during this period. This low ebb of hormonal withdrawal is physiologically marked by the commencement of full lactogenesis, following the initial production of small volumes of colostrum (see Chapter 16). The 'blues' coincide with lactation, breast engorgement, perineal pain and wound discomfort and usually resolve within 2 weeks.

Hormonal changes are implicated in the aetiology of puerperal depressive disorders such as the withdrawal of steroid hormones. Oestrogen is associated with psychological wellbeing; the abrupt change in oestrogen levels in the puerperium may affect release of neurotransmitters, such as serotonin, and the metabolism of tryptophan (Duan et al., 2018). Cortisol, β-endorphin and oxytocin are also associated with postnatal depression (Brummelte and Galea, 2016). The HPA axis is very active in the third trimester as placental corticotrophin-releasing hormone (CRH) production increases and CRH-binding protein (CRH-BP) levels fall (see Chapter 13). Loss of placental CRH, suppression of hypothalamic CRH secretion and the resulting decreases in cortisol levels are implicated in the aetiology of postnatal depression (Seth et al., 2016).

The relationship between breastfeeding and postnatal depression is controversial; the direction and nature of the relationship is not clear (Pope and Mazmanian, 2016). Some studies suggest breastfeeding is positively associated with depression, others suggest it may be protective. Possibly, postpartum depression reduces the rate of breastfeeding and not engaging in breastfeeding or having problems establishing breastfeeding may increase the risk of depression. Hormones involved in lactation affect cortisol levels and lactation often predisposes the breastfeeding mother to depression by isolating her and increasing her levels of fatigue. There is also an association between PPD and perturbed thyroid function (Le Donne et al., 2017).

There are a number of tools to assess maternal mood such as the Edinburgh Postnatal Depression Scale and the Beck Depression Inventory (for a review, see Ukatu et al., 2018). Women who develop postnatal depression make a good recovery with specialist treatment and support. Exercise and physical activity interventions have been found to be effective in preventing and decreasing anxiety and depression in the puerperium (Carter et al., 2018). The recurrence of postnatal depression is high in subsequent pregnancies and women who have antenatal depression or depression in pregnancy are also at increased risk.

The nutritional demands of pregnancy and lactation are high (see Chapters 12 and 16); the high requirements can result in depletion of nutrients essential for the nervous system and increase the risk for perinatal depression. Several nutrient deficiencies have been implicated as having a possible role in the aetiology of postnatal depression; these include B vitamins including folate, vitamin D, iron, selenium, zinc and certain fatty acids (Sparling et al., 2017). Many of the results of studies investigating this field are inconsistent and inconclusive, particularly in preventing PPD rather than treating it. Women who have a low intake of fish (and therefore omega-3 fatty acids) are at higher risk of suffering PPD (Ellsworth-Bowers and Corwin, 2012). The high docosahexaenoic acid (DHA) requirements of the fetus and for breast milk may deplete the levels remaining in women. Several studies have identified a relationship between low serum vitamin D levels and PPD (Trujillo et al., 2018). Nutritional solutions are important because the current mainstay of treatment for PPD is antidepressant drugs; there are concerns about these entering the breastmilk and affecting infant neurodevelopment.

Case study 14.4 describes an example of a woman with a rare hormonal complication of the puerperium.

CASE STUDY 14.4

At delivery, Sarah suffered a large haemorrhage that was difficult to control; she finally underwent a hysterectomy following a total blood loss of over 4 L. Her recovery was uneventful but within 6 months she was diagnosed as suffering from Sheehan syndrome (necrosis of the pituitary gland).

- What would her symptoms be?
- Which endocrine functions would be affected by this condition?
- How would this affect Sarah in the early postnatal period and how could these problems be overcome?
- What long-term treatment and care is Sarah likely to require?

KEY POINTS

- Maternal physiology and anatomy adapt rapidly to the withdrawal of steroid hormones, following the delivery of the placenta. These dramatic physiological changes increase the risk of infection, haemorrhage and psychological and emotional problems.
- The uterus rapidly involutes after delivery; normal involution can be monitored by assessment of fundal height, characteristics of the lochia and general wellbeing of the mother.
- After delivery, there is a dramatic and rapid decrease in circulating blood volume followed by a return to normal cardiovascular parameters. As stroke volume initially remains high, bradycardia is usual, particularly in the first 2 weeks following delivery.

- The postpartum physiological changes allow the woman to tolerate considerable blood loss at delivery, but alteration in clotting factor concentration and venous stasis predispose the woman to thromboembolic disorders; the risk is enhanced by immobility, obesity and sepsis.
- Marked diuresis is normal in the puerperium but overdistension, or decreased sensitivity, of the bladder can predispose the woman to short and long-term urinary problems.
- Ovulation returns, before menstruation, but is delayed by breastfeeding; lactational amenorrhoea is useful in birth spacing rather than being a reliable method of contraception.

APPLICATION TO PRACTICE

In comparison to pregnancy, when the changes induced by endocrine effects are at a relatively slow pace, the reversal of this in the puerperium is much more dramatic. These rapid changes occur at the same time as another endocrine-induced change resulting in the initiation of lactation.

Fatigue from labour and delivery (including assisted and surgical), perineal pain from trauma and the demands of a newborn infant can also complicate the situation.

The midwife needs to use her skills and knowledge of the puerperium to support women through this often-difficult period of adaptation.

A useful rough reckoner of whether changes in heart rate and blood pressure might indicate shock is to compare the *number* of the heart beats per minute with the *number* of mmHg of the systolic blood pressure; the difference will be greater in severe shock because it is characterized by a fast pulse (tachycardia) and low blood pressure (hypotension).

Knowledge of mental health issues in the postnatal period is essential in differentiating between mild depressive states and recognizing severe psychotic disorders.

ANNOTATED FURTHER READING

Baston H, Hall J: *Midwifery essentials: postnatal*, vol. 4. Oxford, 2017, Elsevier.

The fourth title in the Midwifery Essentials series, which includes the postnatal examination of the woman and neonate, hospital postnatal care and caesarean section, emotional well-being, postnatal fertility issues and lactational support.

Jordan RG, Farley CL, Grace KT: *Prenatal and postnatal care: a woman-centred approach*, ed 2, Oxford, 2018, Wiley-Blackwell.

This comprehensive and authoritative text has been updated and covers all aspects of antenatal and postnatal care including complementary therapies and the management of common health issues.

National Collaborating Centre for Mental Health (UK): *Antenatal and postnatal mental health: clinical management and service guidance (NICE clinical guideline CG192)*, British Psychological Society and the Royal College of Psychiatrists, 2014. updated 2017, NICE.

This is an extensive to a wide range of mental health issues in pregnancy, childbirth and the postnatal period.

Royal College of Obstetricians and Gynaecologists: *Reducing the risk of venous thromboembolism during pregnancy and the puerperium. (Green-top Guideline No. 37a)*, London, 2015, RCOG.

Royal College of Obstetricians and Gynaecologists: *Thromboembolic disease in pregnancy and the puerperium: acute management. (Green-top guideline No. 37b)*, London, 2015, RCOG.

This guideline covers the risk factors for venous thromboembolism and provides clinical guidance for management to prevent of venous thromboembolism.

Stone L, editor: *Perinatal depression: detection and treatment*, New York, 2017, Hayle Medical.

This book provides an in-depth exploration and explanation of perinatal and postpartum depression and treatment.

Sutter-Dalley AL, Glangeaud-Freudenthal NM-C, Guedeney A, Riecher-Rossler A, editors: *Joint care of parents and infants in perinatal psychiatry*, New York, 2016, Springer.

This book presents the key issues in perinatal mental health and discusses the different approaches of psychiatric care for pregnant women, parents, and infants, with emphasis on the need for multiprofessional care within the pregnancy and postnatal continuum.

Taub RL, Jensen JT: Advances in contraception: new options for postpartum women, *Expert Opin Pharmacother* 18:677–688, 2017.

A review, which covers the return of postpartum ovulation, the optimal timing of advice to reduce unintended pregnancy and promote optimal birth spacing, and different methods of contraception including long acting reversible contraception (LARC).

Vaught AJ: Maternal sepsis, *Semin Perinatol* 42(1):9–12, 2018.

A short summary of risk factors for maternal sepsis, the implications of infection and the steps to aid recovery.

REFERENCES

Aasheim V, Nilsen ABV, Reinar LM, Lukasse M: Perineal techniques during the second stage of labour for reducing perineal trauma, *Cochrane Database Syst Rev* 6:CD006672, 2017.

Abrams ET, Rutherford JN: Framing postpartum hemorrhage as a consequence of human placental biology: an evolutionary and comparative perspective, *Am Anthropol* 113:417–430, 2011.

American Psychiatric Association: *Diagnostic and statistical manual of mental disorders (DMS5)*, ed 5, Washington, DC, 2013, American Psychiatric Publishing.

Azizi R, Aghebati-Maleki L, Nouri M, et al.: Stem cell therapy in Asherman syndrome and thin endometrium: stem cell-based therapy, *Biomed Pharmacother* 102:333–343, 2018.

Blackburn ST: *Maternal, fetal, & neonatal physiology: a clinical perspective*, ed 4, Philadelphia, 2018, Elsevier.

Brummelte S, Galea LA: Postpartum depression: etiology, treatment and consequences for maternal care, *Horm Behav* 77:153–166, 2016.

Burlinson CEG, Sirounis D, Walley KR, Chau A: Sepsis in pregnancy and the puerperium, *Int J Obstet Anesth* 36:96–107, 2018.

Carter AM: Comparative studies of placentation and immunology in non-human primates suggest a scenario for the evolution of deep trophoblast invasion and an explanation for human pregnancy disorders, *Reproduction* 141:391–396, 2011.

Carter T, Bastounis A, Guo B, Jane MC: The effectiveness of exercise-based interventions for preventing or treating postpartum depression: a systematic review and meta-analysis, *Arch Womens Ment Health* 22:37-53, 2018.

Chertok IRA, Wolf JH: Postpartum period and lactation physiology. In Blackburn ST, editor: *Maternal, fetal & neonatal physiology: a clinical perspective*, ed 4, Philadelphia, 2018, Elsevier, pp 142–161.

Conforti A, Alviggi C, Mollo A, et al.: The management of Asherman syndrome: a review of literature, *Reprod Biol Endocrinol* 11:118, 2013.

Di Bari F, Granese R, Le DM, et al.: Autoimmune abnormalities of postpartum thyroid diseases, *Front Endocrinol (Lausanne)* 8:166, 2017.

Duan KM, Ma JH, Wang SY, et al.: The role of tryptophan metabolism in postpartum depression, *Metab Brain Dis* 33:647–660, 2018.

Ellsworth-Bowers ER, Corwin EJ: Nutrition and the psychoneuroimmunology of postpartum depression, *Nutr Res Rev* 25:180–192, 2012.

Fogerty AE: Management of venous thromboembolism in pregnancy, *Curr Treat Options Cardiovasc Med* 20:69, 2018.

Guedes-Martins L, Gaio AR, Saraiva J, et al.: Uterine artery impedance during the first eight postpartum weeks, *Sci Rep* 5:8786, 2015.

Hollis JL, Crozier SR, Inskip HM, et al.: Modifiable risk factors of maternal postpartum weight retention: an analysis of their combined impact and potential opportunities for prevention, *Int J Obesity* 41:1091, 2017.

Hytten F: *The clinical physiology of the puerperium*, London, 1995, Farand Press.

Jawed-Wessel S, Sevick E: The impact of pregnancy and childbirth on sexual behaviors: a systematic review, *Journal Sex Res* 54:411–423, 2017.

Le Donne M, Mento C, Settineri S, et al.: Postpartum mood disorders and thyroid autoimmunity, *Front Endocrinol (Lausanne)* 8:91, 2017.

Lim A, Samarage A, Lim BH: Venous thromboembolism in pregnancy, *Obstet, Gynaecol Reprode Med* 26:133–139, 2016.

Martin RD: The evolution of human reproduction: a primatological perspective, *Am J Phys Anthropol* 45:59–84, 2007.

McLean KC, James AH: Diagnosis and management of VTE in pregnancy, *Clin Obstet Gynecol* 61:206–218, 2018.

Miller AWF, Hanretty KP: *Obstetrics illustrated*, ed 5, New York, 1998, Churchill Livingstone, p 336.

NCCWCH: National Collaborating Centre for Women and Children's Health: *Intrapartum care for healthy women and babies: clinical guideline (Cg190)*, London, 2014, National Institute for Health and Care Excellence (NICE).

Nguyen CT, Sasso EB, Barton L, Mestman JH: Graves' hyperthyroidism in pregnancy: a clinical review, *Clin Diabetes Endocrinol* 4:4, 2018.

Okun ML: Disturbed sleep and postpartum depression, *Curr Psychiatry Rep* 18:66, 2016.

Pope CJ, Mazmanian D: Breastfeeding and postpartum depression: an overview and methodological recommendations for future research, *Depress Res Treat* 2016:4765310, 2016.

RCOG. Royal College of Obstetricians and Gynaecologists: *Thromboembolic disease in pregnancy and the puerperium: acute management.* (Green-top guideline No. 37b), London, 2015, RCOG.

Ribeiro AM, Zepeda-Mendoza ML, Bertelsen MF, et al.: A refined model of the genomic basis for phenotypic variation in vertebrate hemostasis, *BMC Evol Biol* 15:124, 2015.

Seth S, Lewis AJ, Galbally M: Perinatal maternal depression and cortisol function in pregnancy and the postpartum period: a systematic literature review, *BMC Pregnancy Childbirth* 16:124, 2016.

Shorey S, Chee CYI, Ng ED, et al.: Prevalence and incidence of postpartum depression among healthy mothers: a systematic review and meta-analysis, *J Psychiatr Res* 104:235–248, 2018.

Sparling TM, Nesbitt RC, Henschke N, Gabrysch S: Nutrients and perinatal depression: a systematic review, *J Nutr Sci* 6:e61, 2017.

Struble E, Harrouk W, DeFelice A, Tesfamariam B: Nonclinical aspects of venous thrombosis in pregnancy, *Birth Defects Res C Embryo Today* 105:190–200, 2015.

Sweet B, Tiran D: *Mayes' midwifery*, ed 12, London, 1996, Baillière Tindall. 405, 406.

Taylor PN, Zouras S, Min T, et al.: Thyroid screening in early pregnancy: pros and cons, *Front Endocrinol (Lausanne)* 9:626, 2018.

Trujillo J, Vieira MC, Lepsch J, et al.: A systematic review of the associations between maternal nutritional biomarkers and depression and/or anxiety during pregnancy and postpartum, *J Affect Disord* 232:185–203, 2018.

Ukatu N, Clare CA, Brulja M: Postpartum depression screening tools: a review, *Psychosomatics* 59:211–219, 2018.

Van der Wijden C, Manion C: Lactational amenorrhoea method for family planning, *Cochrane Database Syst Rev* 10: CD001329, 2015.

Van Geelen H, Ostergard D, Sand P: A review of the impact of pregnancy and childbirth on pelvic floor function as assessed by objective measurement techniques, *Int Urogynecol J* 29:327–338, 2018.

Villani M, Ageno W, Grandone E, Dentali F: The prevention and treatment of venous thromboembolism in pregnancy, *Expert Rev Cardiovasc Ther* 15:397–402, 2017.

Weetman AP: Thyroid function–effects on mother and baby unraveled, *Nat Rev Endocrinol* 8:69–70, 2011.

WHO: *Postnatal care of the mother and newborn*, Geneva, 2013, World Health Organization.

The Transition to Neonatal Life

LEARNING OBJECTIVES

- To identify the key steps in the transition to successful neonatal life and the role of glucocorticoids.
- To describe the maturation of the fetal physiological systems in preparation for birth.
- To outline the principles of thermoregulation in the newborn.
- To compare the fetal and neonatal circulatory and respiratory systems, describing the transition stages in adapting to extrauterine life.

- To describe factors relating to the neonatal gastrointestinal, immune, renal and nervous systems that make breast milk the ideal source of nutrients.
- To describe normal physiological fetal to neonatal transition and to recognize signs of a neonate experiencing compromised transition.
- To describe the vulnerability of the neonate, with particular reference to the potential risks of respiratory problems, hypothermia, hypoglycaemia and jaundice.

INTRODUCTION

During fetal life, the placenta carries out the crucial physiological roles of gas exchange, nutrition, elimination of waste products and additional aspects of circulation. Within minutes of birth, the placental support ceases so the baby's own cardiovascular, respiratory, gastrointestinal, renal and metabolic systems must function independently. The transition from fetal to neonatal life is the most complex and challenging adaptation in life; it needs to be smooth, swift and successful. The majority of infant deaths occur within the neonatal period (first 28 days) and most of these are linked to inadequate progression to neonatal physiological functions. All physiological systems are involved in neonatal transition but changes within the cardiovascular and respiratory systems need to be immediate. The Sustainable Development Goals (SDG), a collection of 17 global goals, were proposed by the United Nations General Assembly in 2015 as targets for 2030. One of the main targets of SDG3 'Ensure healthy lives and promote wellbeing for all at all ages' is to reduce the worldwide under-5 mortality rate to <25 per 1000 live births. This is one of the most challenging SDGs and it seems that a significant number of countries will not meet this target (Kharas et al., 2018). The SDG follow and build on the Millennium Development Goals (MDG). MDG4 aimed to reduce child mortality (deaths under 5 years of age) by two-thirds between 1990 and 2015. Although under-5 mortality rates fell from 78 to 41 deaths per 1000, the neonatal death rate increased (Akseer et al., 2015). The leading causes of both neonatal mortality (death within the first year of life) and for children under 5 years of age are related to complications of preterm birth and compromised transition to neonatal life, severe infections and asphyxia.

The transition to extrauterine life depends on the degree of maturation in late gestation, the process of delivery itself and establishment of independent physiological processes for regulating homeostasis after placental separation. These physiological processes include establishing continuous respiration, changing from a parallel to a serial circulatory organization and ceasing the right-to-left shunting across the heart so oxygenated blood can be delivered to the tissues and establishing oral intermittent feeding. Independent thermoregulation and glucose homeostasis also have to be established. These complex physiological changes must occur within a relatively short timeframe. Monitoring and reviewing neonatal transition are important in order to recognize delayed or compromised adaptation or the warning signs of more serious conditions such as birth injury, congenital abnormality or disease (Michel and Lowe, 2017). It is essential that health professionals involved in the care of neonates are able to recognize deviations from normal transition to extrauterine life.

CHAPTER CASE STUDY

The midwife officially recorded Zak as having an Apgar score of 9 at ~1 min of age. Following the delivery, James was surprised how alert his son Zak was, that he seemed to be aware of his surroundings and appeared to be actively looking around.

- What factors could have contributed to Zak's behaviour and what are the possible explanations for Zak being so alert following his delivery?
- What observational information would the midwife record to demonstrate that Zak's transition to independent life was progressing normally.
- What should the midwife do to encourage Zak to suckle?

The process of birth is physiologically stressful with fluctuations in placental blood flow resulting in varying and transient hypoxia and respiratory acidosis. The primary mediators orchestrating the transition from intrauterine to extrauterine life are cortisol and catecholamines. Cortisol is the major hormone controlling the maturation of the fetal physiological systems. Increased secretion of adrenal catecholamines, stimulation of the sympathetic nervous system and the subsequent mobilization of glycogen and lipid stores are fundamental in the activation of essential physiological mechanisms that result in an alert and active baby at birth. However, a prolonged or difficult delivery, excessive or inappropriate use of opioid-based analgesia and marked hypoxia/anoxia and acidosis can result in an overstressed or seriously asphyxiated baby (Box 15.1).

Both the fetus and the neonate can tolerate degrees of hypoxia and intermittent periods of anoxia that would result in serious morbidity or mortality in an adult. The neonate retains the capability to divert a significant proportion of its cardiac output to the brain thus protecting it, possibly at the expense of the other organs. Although the brain is vulnerable to hypoxia, the compensatory mechanisms can increase tolerance to hypoxic states (Rei et al., 2016). However, severe asphyxia can cause cerebral or intraventricular haemorrhage resulting in a spectrum of damage from delayed development, neurological disorders (such as spasticity and cerebral palsy), seizures, hypoxic-ischaemic encephalopathy (HIE) to irreversible brain damage and perinatal death (Yli and Kjellmer, 2016). Intervention strategies to reduce the risk of cerebral palsy developing include therapeutic hypothermia, prophylactic methylxanthine (caffeine) and magnesium sulphate treatment (Shepherd et al., 2018). Neonates are also vulnerable to infection and hypoglycaemia especially if their oxygenation is compromised.

BOX 15.1　Fetal Hypoxaemia, Hypoxia and Asphyxia

Reduced oxygen supply to the fetus can be classified as hypoxaemia, hypoxia or asphyxia. Hypoxaemia is due to a slightly decreased oxygen level in the arterial blood but cells and organs are normally not affected. Hypoxia is more significant because the reduced level of oxygen results in anaerobic metabolism in the peripheral tissues. Fetal asphyxia is due to a significant reduction in the amount of oxygen available via the placenta from the maternal circulation. Fetal asphyxia affects the function of the central organs such as the heart and brain; widespread anaerobic metabolism can lead to metabolic acidosis.

There are many possible causes for asphyxia, for example placental abruption, rapid deterioration in the maternal condition, such as eclampsia, uterine hyperstimulation in response to syntocinon augmentation. Whatever the reason, prolonged fetal hypoxia can result in asphyxia (low oxygen levels and raised carbon dioxide levels). Fetal hypoxia, if suspected during labour, can be assessed by obtaining a small sample of blood from the fetal scalp, from which the pH and base excess can be measured. Acidaemia is diagnosed if the pH of the fetal blood is <7.2, however many babies can tolerate moderate acidaemia without long-term problems. A base excess above 12 mmol indicates chronic or prolonged acidaemia. The risk of asphyxia rises with lower pH and higher base excess. Babies born with asphyxia require active resuscitation to restore pH and base excess. In extreme cases, severe asphyxia results in irreversible brain damage.

Although there is usually a good correlation between gestational length and degree of maturity, infants affected by intrauterine growth restriction (IUGR) may have precocious organ development because undernutrition and the resulting fetal stress promote increased fetal cortisol secretion thus accelerating fetal organ maturation. In humans, fetal cortisol appears not to have the same role in inducing labour as has been demonstrated in other species (see Chapter 13) but it is the major hormone controlling maturation of the fetal systems in preparation for extrauterine life (Box 15.2). The major problems of premature infants can be attributed to a shorter duration of glucocorticoid (GC) exposure (even though fetal stress results in actual levels being higher); this results in an increased risk of persistent fetal-type circulation, increased likelihood of lung immaturity and respiratory distress syndrome (RDS) and immaturity of thermoregulatory responses, the

BOX 15.2 Glucocorticoids

Glucocorticoids are physiological stress hormones. In humans, the predominant glucocorticoid is cortisol synthesized from the cortex of the adrenal gland (in other species the predominant glucocorticoid is corticosterone). Cortisone is a metabolite of cortisol, which is far less active. The placenta expresses 11β-hydroxysteroid dehydrogenase II, which reversibly inactivates cortisol from the maternal circulation so the developing fetus is exposed to the less active cortisone and is protected from excess cortisol in early gestation. The placenta also activates cortisone from the fetal circulation forming cortisol via the alternative isoform 11β-hydroxysteroid dehydrogenase I. For most of gestation, the primary source of cortisol is the mother's adrenal gland. Glucocorticoids diffuse across the placenta because maternal levels are higher so there is a concentration gradient, which is maintained by placental activity. As the fetal adrenal gland matures, the fetus produces its own cortisol, which has an important role in physiological maturation. Note that the expression of placental 11β-hydroxysteroid dehydrogenases is affected by maternal factors such as excessive stress and poor nutrition; this results in exposure of the developing fetus to high levels of cortisol, which can negatively affect fetal development and growth. The effects of glucocorticoids depend on the circulating level of the hormones, the relative abundance of the glucocorticoid and mineralocorticoid receptors and the expression of the isoforms of 11β-hydroxysteroid dehydrogenase.

The nomenclature is complicated by the common use of 'cortisone' for synthetic glucocorticoids, which have anti-inflammatory properties and are used therapeutically.

gastrointestinal system and enzymes involved in maintaining glucose homeostasis. The preterm infant is more likely to be functionally immature, to have poorer viability and to fail to thrive (Fowden et al., 2016).

Fetal preparation for birth includes storing glycogen, producing catecholamines and increasing brown and white fat deposits; this is greatly reduced in IUGR babies resulting in reduced energy reserves. Cortisol from the fetal adrenal gland is pivotal in the fetal preparation for birth (see Chapter 13). Initially, fetal cortisol levels are low (5–10 μg/mL); it is during this time that raised glucocorticoids in the fetal compartment (either due to increased maternal levels and/or because of less placental inactivation) (see Box 15.2) acts to signal less than optimal environmental conditions, influencing tissue differentiation and affecting fetal and placental growth and development (Fowden et al., 2016). The effects

of raised glucocorticoids on the placenta include reducing placental transport of glucose and amino acids. The outcome depends on the time of the exposure to GC (organogenesis is a particularly sensitive period) and the gender of the fetus. As the fetal adrenal gland matures, glucocorticoid levels increase independently of maternal levels and rise progressively from ~28–30 weeks' gestation with levels reaching ~20 μg/mL by 36 weeks and 45 μg/mL just before labour (Hillman et al., 2012). This increase in fetal cortisol is the driving force for maturation of the physiological systems and preparation for birth. The physiological stress of labour results in cortisol levels reaching a peak of ~200 μg/mL within a few hours. Synthetic glucocorticoids such as dexamethasone and betamethasone are used clinically to promote fetal maturation and promote viability when a preterm delivery is planned or appears imminent. The synthetic glucocorticoids are more potent and have a significantly longer half-life in the circulation than natural glucocorticoids (Fowden et al., 2016) because they are poorly inactivated by 11β-hydroxysteroid dehydrogenases and bind only to the glucocorticoid receptors (whereas natural glucocorticoids also bind to the mineralocorticoid receptors).

Glucocorticoids cause the natural decrease in growth that occurs towards term and are also thought to be responsible for the growth retardation associated with physiological stress *in utero* such as that due to prolonged hypoxia and undernutrition. Glucocorticoids are responsible for important changes in many biochemical pathways, affecting gene expression of enzymes, ion channels, growth factors and other proteins, resulting in changes in hormone sensitivity, morphology, biochemistry and tissue structure (Fowden et al., 2016). Fetal cortisol stimulates surfactant production and maturation of the alveoli and other respiratory tissues, thus promoting lung maturation. Together with increased thyroid hormones, cortisol stimulates the sodium pump, which is involved with the clearance of fetal lung fluid at birth. In late gestation, cortisol affects the fetal heart and blood vessels and increases fetal blood pressure. Cortisol stimulates glycogen deposition in the fetal liver and skeletal muscle and increases the fetal potential for gluconeogenesis by inducing the expression of hepatic gluconeogenic enzymes. Fetal cortisol also promotes adrenaline synthesis, induces hormone receptors and increases the production of the active form of thyroid hormone, (tri-iodothyronine T_3, and also leptin. Cortisol induces increased expression of phenylethanolamine-*N*-methyltransferase (PNMT) in the adrenal gland. PNMT is the enzyme that catalyses the final methylation step in the synthesis of adrenaline from noradrenaline. The increased activity of adrenaline together with increased expression of β-adrenoceptors, particularly in the liver, means the neonate responds to stress (e.g. hypoglycaemia or cold) by producing adrenaline, which stimulates gluconeogenesis and mobilization of glucose from hepatic glycogen. Cortisol also enhances proteolysis so fetal protein accretion and growth rate are reduced at the end of gestation. Fetal corticotrophin-releasing hormone (CRH), together with maternal and placental CRH, stimulates the secretion of adrenocorticotrophic hormone (ACTH) from the both the maternal and fetal anterior pituitary. The increase in plasma ACTH then increases cortisol secretion from both the maternal and fetal adrenal cortex. As mentioned in Chapter 13, both hypothalamic CRH and pituitary ACTH secretion are inhibited by raised plasma cortisol levels in a negative feedback loop. Placental secretion of CRH is different, however, in that plasma cortisol further stimulates CRH release (positive feedback).

At birth, there are also changes in the regulation of growth. Fetal growth is substrate limited and actively constrained to optimize successful delivery (see Chapter 9). The rise in glucocorticoids towards term suppresses growth and is responsible for the natural decrease in the rate of growth that occurs at this time (Fowden et al., 2016). The increase in glucocorticoids also induces growth hormone receptors and changes in expression of insulin-like growth factor I (IGF-I).

THE CARDIOVASCULAR SYSTEM

Blood

Before Birth

Haemoglobin changes at different stages of life to meet the changing oxygen requirements during development. This haemoglobin 'switching' results in three distinctly different haemoglobins: embryonic, fetal and adult. The general structure of haemoglobin is a tetramer comprising two α- and two β-like globin subunits or chains. In the early stages of embryonic development, haemoglobin contains two ζ- (zeta) and two ε- (epsilon) globin subunits. In the first trimester, the genes for the ζ-globin subunit are silenced and genes for the α-globin subunit are expressed; these will persist throughout the rest of in utero (fetal) and postnatal life. Haemoglobin switching for the β-like globin subunit is more complex. In the first trimester, the genes for the ε-globin subunit are silenced and genes for the γ-globin subunit are expressed, which results in the main form of fetal haemoglobin (HbF) being produced: $\alpha_2\gamma_2$. The second haemoglobin switch of the β-like subunit is completed shortly after birth when γ-globin subunit expression is silenced and replaced by production of the adult-type β-globin subunit so adult haemoglobin (HbA; $\alpha_2\beta_2$) is formed. (There is also another type of β-like globin subunit produced in postnatal life: δ-globin. However, $\alpha_2\delta_2$ represents a tiny proportion of haemoglobin so is insignificant.)

Fetal haemoglobin has a higher affinity for oxygen in the fetal circulation, which is slightly more acidic compared with adult haemoglobin.

Therefore, fetal blood (Table 15.1) is structurally and functionally different to adult blood; it contains larger and more numerous erythrocytes (red blood cells) with a higher haemoglobin content, which maximizes their uptake of oxygen (Morton and Brodsky, 2016). Less-effective binding of 2,3-bisphosphoglycerate (or 2,3-diphosphoglycerate) to the fetal γ-globin subunits means that the oxygen–haemoglobin dissociation curve of the fetus and neonate is shifted to the left (Fig. 15.1). Shifts of pH in the placenta further increase both dissociation of oxygen from

TABLE 15.1 Fetal and Adult Blood		
	Fetal/Neonatal	Adult
Blood volume	80–100 mL/kg 90–105 mL/kg (preterm)	75 mL/kg
Red blood cell number	6–7×10⁶/µL	Female: 4.8×10⁶/µL Male: 5.4×10⁶/µL
Haemoglobin content	207 g/L	Female: 140 g/L Male: 160 g/L
Oxygen content of 100 mL saturated blood	21 mL (theory) 13 mL (practice)	16 mL (theory) 15.7 mL (practice)
Red blood cell lifespan	80–100 days 60–80 days (preterm)	120 days
Haemoglobin type	HbF: $\alpha_2\gamma_2$	HbA: $\alpha_2\beta_2$

Note: the theoretical value is the amount of oxygen the blood can be saturated with, whereas in practice, the blood is saturated to a lesser degree because the transfer of oxygen across the placenta is less efficient than the transfer of oxygen across the alveoli.

maternal haemoglobin and its uptake by fetal haemoglobin. This means that, although fetal haemoglobin has an increased oxygen uptake, it is less efficient at releasing oxygen to the tissues. This is mitigated by the higher concentration of haemoglobin and higher erythrocyte number in fetal than in adult blood.

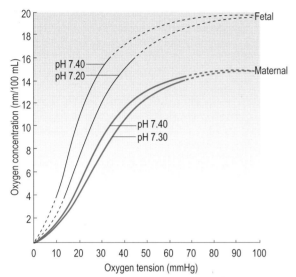

Fig. 15.1 The maternal and fetal oxyhaemoglobin dissociation curves.

At birth of the term infant, the ratio of fetal haemoglobin to adult haemoglobin (HbF:HbA) is 80:20; by 6 months production of the β-globin subunit replaces the γ-globin subunit so the ratio is 1:99 (Fig. 15.2). Preterm infants tend to have an even higher HbF level and a decreased 2,3-bisphosphoglycerate concentration; therefore oxygen unloading at the tissue level is even less efficient. The raised levels of HbF in the neonate mean that haemoglobinopathies caused by altered synthesis of β-globin subunit (such as β-thalassaemia) or altered structure of β-globin subunit (such as sickle cell disease; SCD) are not always evident immediately at birth, because some HbF is still present in the neonatal blood but become obvious as the child ages. The observations that residual HbF in the blood of young children with SCD was protective against sickling and that some adults with SCD have a milder form of the disease because natural mutations have resulted in the continued expression high levels of HbF (hereditary persistence of fetal haemoglobin; HPFH) throughout life has led to the development of therapies that induce the formation of HbF (Wienert et al., 2018). Hydroxyurea and/or recombinant erythropoietin (rEPO) are an effective treatment for haemoglobinopathies affecting the β-globin subunit as they induce the formation of HbF. Current research aims to reactivate the fetal γ-globin genes through gene-editing technologies such as CRISPR (see Chapter 7).

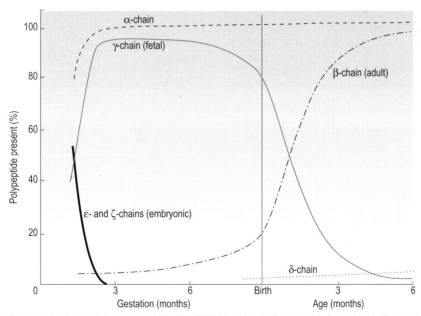

Fig. 15.2 Changes in fetal:adult haemoglobin (HbF:HbA) ratios in fetal and infant blood. (Reproduced with permission from Begley et al., 1978.)

BOX 15.3 Fetal Microchimerism (FMc)

Fetal microchimerism was originally identified by chance after Y-chromosome material was repeatedly found in the blood of women who had previously given birth to a son (Bianchi, 2018). Microchimerism is a common finding in placental mammals and is more marked with highly invasive placentation such as that of the human (Boddy et al., 2015). More fetal cells are transferred to the mother than maternal cells are transferred to the fetus. After parturition, most, but not all, of the fetal cells are destroyed by the maternal immune system; some fetal cells can be detected decades after the birth (Bianchi, 2018). The residual fetal cells may have no effect on maternal health or may be harmful (such as contributing to maternal tissue damage and disease) or beneficial (helping to maintain and repair maternal tissue). Several theories are postulated. The fetal microchimeric cells might affect the immune system and increase the risk of autoimmune diseases, which are significantly more prevalent in women with higher numbers of fetal microchimeric cells; this led to the hypothesis that the fetal cells may promote a graft-versus-host response. As the fetal cells evade the maternal immune system and induce angiogenesis, they could contribute to the development and progression of cancer. However, women with evidence of microchimerism have a lower risk of death from cancer and also from developing Alzheimer's disease. The fetal cells appear to retain characteristics of stem cells and have been described as pregnancy-associated progenitor cells (PAPCs), which can differentiate into functional cells and contribute to the repair of maternal organs. The fetal cells may benefit the offspring by enhancing maternal milk production, maternal thermogenesis and maternal attachment and bonding; the fetal cells appear to accumulate in breast, thyroid and brain tissue.

Fetal microchimerism may be more marked following caesarean section than after a vaginal delivery (Shree et al., 2019).

BOX 15.4 Physiological Anaemia of Infancy

Haemopoiesis (red blood cell production) is controlled by the hormone erythropoietin, which increases when oxygen delivery to the kidney is reduced; it stimulates red blood cell production by the bone marrow. The increased oxygen levels inhibit erythropoietin levels in the neonate postnatally. Levels remain low for 2–3 months (longer in preterm infants) and then increase, resulting in increased bone marrow activity and red blood cell production. As the neonate appears to tolerate the fall in haemoglobin concentration without ill-effects, it is deemed to be physiological. The haemodilution effects are increased by rapid growth being matched by total blood volume, which precedes any change in red blood cell number.

and trisomies (e.g. Down syndrome) (see p. 194) or determine fetal Rhesus-D genotype (see Chapter 10) or test for paternity during pregnancy (Gerson and O'Brien, 2018).

After Birth

At birth, the infant's blood has the high fetal number of nucleated erythrocytes (even more so if the baby has been subjected to increased stress, is immature or has Trisomy 21 (Down syndrome)). For the first 3 months of life, the erythrocytes are more fragile, have an increased metabolism and a shorter half-life (Box 15.4). Erythropoietin (EPO) production is initially suppressed, until the high number of erythrocytes from fetal life has reduced and bone marrow activity resumes under the influence of hypoxia to increase production of red blood cells.

In fetal life, EPO is both a haemopoietic growth factor (increases red blood cell production) and also promotes the development of other systems such as the brain, cardiovascular system and gut. The higher level of EPO in infants that have been exposed to hypoxia reflects the role of EPO protecting the fetal tissues; EPO has anti-inflammatory, antioxidant, antiapoptotic and neurotrophic effects (Teramo et al., 2018). rEPO has been used to treat neonatal anaemia, HIE and necrotizing enterocolitis (NEC) in preterm neonates (Ananthan et al., 2018).

Once respiration in the neonate is established, the excess red blood cell number, which compensated for the lower oxygen saturation within the uterine environment, becomes physiologically redundant. These red blood cells are broken down and so physiological jaundice (hyperbilirubinaemia) may result, usually manifesting around day 3 of life as the neonatal liver is immature and initially cannot keep up with the rate of bilirubin production from red blood cell breakdown.

During pregnancy there is a natural bidirectional transfer of a very small number of fetal and maternal cells (but note the fetal and maternal circulations do not mix); this is 'microchimerism' (Box 15.3), which describes the acquisition and persistence of a genetically distinct population of allogeneic cells (from the fetus) inside another organism (the mother). The bidirectional cell trafficking in pregnancy means it is possible to detect cell-free fetal DNA (cffDNA) from fetal blood cells in the maternal circulation prenatally and noninvasively screen for single cell disorders (e.g. Huntington disease, cystic fibrosis, achondroplasia)

Haemostasis

Neonates, particularly those born prematurely, have significantly lower levels of components of the fibrinolytic system including procoagulant proteins and anticoagulants, and less effective platelet function (Jaffray et al., 2016). Concentrations of vitamin K-dependent coagulation factors are lower in preterm infants. The coagulation system undergoes developmental haemostasis (rapid maturation of the coagulation system) in the first 6 months of life. Deficiencies in components of the coagulation and fibrinolytic system tend to be balanced; the lower levels of procoagulants are offset by lower levels of anticoagulants so whole blood clotting times tend to be slightly shorter than adult values (Blackburn, 2018). The healthy term neonate does not usually have thrombotic or haemorrhagic problems unless there is a predisposing factor such as an inherited condition or inappropriate maternal medication.

One of the most common examples of a neonatal haemostatic problem is disseminated intravascular coagulation (DIC), a consumptive coagulopathy (VanVooren et al., 2018). DIC results in blood clots forming throughout the body; it depletes the body's supply of platelets and clotting factors and so paradoxically increases the risk of haemorrhage. Susceptibility is increased because, first, the immature neonatal reticuloendothelial system has a decreased capacity to remove intermediary products of coagulation so they can further stimulate coagulation and consumption of clotting factors and, second, synthesis of clotting factors by the immature liver is inefficient. Vitamin K levels in the neonate are ~50% of adult values, which affect the efficiency of the clotting cascade. Vitamin K levels are low because placental transport of the vitamin is poor, colonization of the gut by bacteria that synthesize vitamin K takes time to be established and breastmilk has low levels of vitamin K. The consequent reduced level of all vitamin K-dependent clotting factors is associated with an increased bleeding tendency, which can predispose to vitamin K deficiency bleeding (VKDB) (previously known as haemorrhagic disease of the newborn) (Box 15.5). Neonatal platelets exhibit decreased aggregation and adhesiveness because their production of thromboxane A_2 (TxA_2) is impaired. This appears to protect the term neonate against thrombosis, but to increase the vulnerability to bleeding in the preterm, IUGR and/or sick baby. Placental transfer of maternal anticoagulant drugs such as aspirin can also affect coagulation in the neonate.

The Circulation
Before Birth

As the fetal oxygen source is the placenta rather than the lungs, blood in the fetal circulation flows in a circuit that perfuses the placenta and largely bypasses the lungs

---

> **BOX 15.5   Vitamin K Deficiency Bleeding (VKDB)**
>
> - Also known as haemorrhagic disease of the newborn (HDNB) but renamed because it can also occur in the postnatal period
> - Causes bleeding from the gut, umbilicus, circumcision wounds and oozing from puncture sites because vitamin K is required as a cofactor for the activation of clotting factors (II, VII, IX and X)
> - Severe late VKBD can result in neurological defects such as developmental delay, epilepsy, encephalopathy, hydrocephalus, cerebral atrophy
> - Three forms:
>   - Early form: evident within 24 h of birth, usually a result of maternal medication, which affects recycling of vitamin K (such anticonvulsants, antituberculosis drugs, some types of antibiotic and vitamin K antagonists, e.g. warfarin)
>   - Classic form: evident 2–7 days after birth, related to low placental transfer of vitamin K, lack of gut microbiota, low concentration of vitamin K in breast milk and poor oral intake as breastfeeding is being established
>   - Late form: occurs between 2nd week and 6th month of life, typically in breastfed infants with fat malabsorption problems; significant morbidity and mortality rate
> - Associated with antibiotics, which affect colonization of the gut with vitamin K-synthesizing bacteria
> - Associated with anticonvulsant drugs (e.g. phenobarbital, diphenylhydantoin), which concentrate in the fetal liver and antagonize the effect of vitamin K
> - Associated with maternal warfarin treatment, which decreases levels of vitamin K-dependent clotting factors and prolongs prolonged clotting times
> - In many countries, prophylactic vitamin K (usual dose is 1 mg, which is about 1000 times the daily requirement) is routinely administered intramuscularly to all babies
> - Term babies respond well to vitamin K therapy but synthesis of clotting factors is further limited in preterm babies by inadequate hepatic synthesis of precursor proteins

(Fig. 15.3), although oxygen and nutrients are required for lung growth and maturity. In order to do this, the ventricles of the fetal heart pump in parallel, and the fetal circulation has several additional structures, which divert blood to the placenta and away from the lungs. These include the umbilical vein, which carries blood rich in oxygen and nutrients to the underside of the liver, the ductus venosus (a venosus

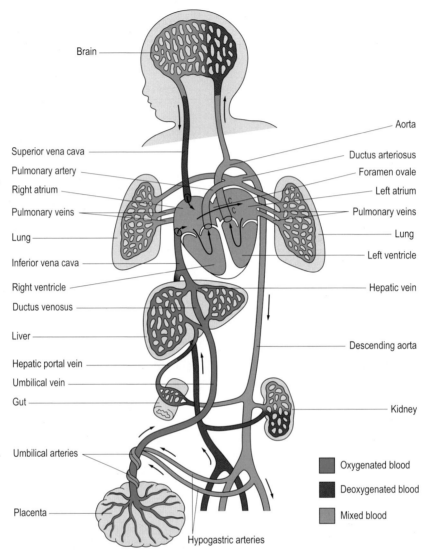

Fig. 15.3 The fetal circulation. (Reproduced with permission from Goodwin, 1997.)

is a shunt that connects a vein to a vein), which bypasses the liver taking blood from the umbilical vein to the inferior umbilical vein en route to the right side of the heart. With increasing gestational age, more blood goes directly to the liver rather than bypassing it via the ductus venosus (Finnemore and Groves, 2015). The hypogastric arteries, which branch off the internal iliac arteries, are contiguous with the umbilical arteries of the umbilical cord, returning blood to the placenta. The lungs are bypassed by two structures: the foramen ovale (a small oval hole or opening in the atrial septal wall), which allows blood to move directly from the right atrium to the left atrium, and the ductus arteriosus (DA), which connects the pulmonary arterial

trunk to the descending aorta (an arteriosus is a vascular shunt that connects an artery to an artery).

The oxygenated and nutrient-enriched blood flows away from the placenta in the umbilical vein that goes through the fetal abdominal wall to the underside of the liver. This is the only unmixed blood and is about 80–90% saturated with oxygen; most of the blood is shunted away from the hepatic circulation and goes through the ductus venosus to the inferior vena cava where it mixes with oxygen-depleted blood (~20% saturated with oxygen) returning to the heart from the lower body (Fig. 15.4A) so the oxygen saturation in this mixed blood reaching the right atrium is ~67%. A small proportion of blood

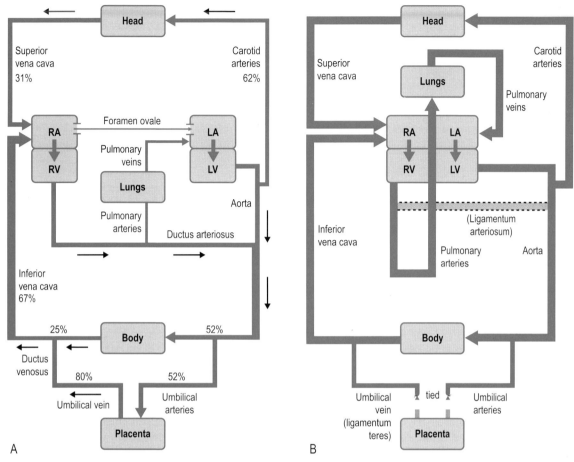

Fig. 15.4 Changes in circulation at birth: (A) fetal circulation showing oxygen saturation of blood; (B) neonatal circulation. (Reproduced with permission from Chamberlain et al., 1991.)

perfuses the liver and then is transported from the liver to the inferior vena cava via the hepatic veins. In humans, the fraction of blood perfusing the liver is higher than in other mammalian species and increases from about 12% in mid-gestation to about 20% close to term (Kessler et al., 2011) reflecting the increasing physiological role of the fetal liver. The higher fetal blood flow to the liver is associated with the greater fat deposition in human fetal life; the fat is important for neonatal thermoregulation and provides an energy buffer for the brain development if the neonate experiences periods of limited nutrient supply. Fetal liver perfusion is affected by maternal body composition, gestational weight gain and maternal diet; it increases more, particularly in the third trimester, in macrosomic fetuses (Godfrey et al., 2012). The inferior cava carries the oxygenated blood to the right atrium, which also receives oxygen-depleted blood from the head and upper body via the superior vena cava. The inflows of blood from the

inferior and superior venae cavae do not mix thoroughly because of their angle of entry and the shape of the right atrium and because the free edge of the interatrial septum, the crista dividens, projects from the foramen ovale and maintains the incoming blood into two streams. This means that ~60% of the blood entering the right atrium (predominantly the oxygenated blood arriving from the inferior vena cava) travels across the posterior aspect of the right atrium and through the foramen ovale into the left atrium and then to the left ventricle and the ascending aorta. The foramen ovale is kept open because the high pulmonary vascular resistance (PVR) means that the pressure in the right atrium is higher than in the left atrium and so blood passes through the foramen ovale, which is the pathway with least resistance. The small proportion of blood perfusing the pulmonary circulation is returned to the left atrium so the mixed blood leaving the left side of the heart is ~62% saturated with oxygen.

Most of the poorly oxygenated blood entering the right atrium from the from head and upper body of the fetus via the superior vena cava passes through the tricuspid valve into the right ventricle and to the pulmonary arterial trunk. The DA is inserted into the vessel at the bifurcation of the right and left pulmonary arteries (taking blood to the right and left lung, respectively); it shunts most of the blood from the pulmonary arterial route into the descending aorta. The fetal pulmonary circulation is vasoconstricted and has a high PVR because the pulmonary environment is relatively hypoxic; the partial pressure of oxygen in the fetal blood reaching the lungs is ~20–25 mmHg compared with 80–100 mmHg in adults. Systemic vascular resistance (SVR) is low. Only about 10% of the output of the right ventricle continues into the pulmonary circulation for the growth and metabolic needs of the lungs; the rest is diverted through the DA, which has a low resistance; its patency is maintained by the low fetal PO_2 and by high levels of prostaglandins produced by the placenta. Towards the end of gestation, the proportion of blood perfusing the lungs tends to increase. From the descending aorta, the blood supplies the remaining organs and the lower body. The hypogastric arteries branch off the internal iliac arteries (that supply the fetal legs) and return blood to the placenta via the umbilical arteries. The blood in the umbilical arteries is relatively depleted in oxygen but still contains some nutrients and oxygen.

The upper body and head are fed from arteries, which branch off from the aortic arch before the insertion of the DA and the subsequent mixing of slightly less-well-oxygenated blood. The early branching of the coronary and carotid arteries means the heart and brain receive slightly better oxygenated blood (~62% saturated with oxygen). In comparison, the blood from the DA has a lower saturation of about 52%. The advantages conferred by the early branching of the subclavian arteries, which supply the upper limbs, can be illustrated by the enhanced development of arms compared to the legs (and the forelimbs of four-legged neonates).

After Birth

One of the most important transitional stages in the adaptation to extrauterine life is the establishment of the neonatal circulation. In fetal life, the source of oxygen is the placenta so most of the blood flow bypasses the fetal lungs. At birth, blood has to fully perfuse the lungs and so flow through the fetal vascular structures ceases. At birth, these changes that mark the transition from the fetal into the adult-type circulation (Fig. 15.4B) are not rapid or immediate. They are initiated within 60 s of delivery but may not be fully completed for a few weeks. The two determining events that initiate the closure of the fetal shunts are the arrest of the umbilical circulation, and therefore placental perfusion, and lung inflation and expansion, which results in a markedly decreased PVR and

therefore increased pulmonary blood flow. The first breath results in lung expansion and vasodilatation of the pulmonary vessels in response to the increased partial pressure of oxygen so blood flow to the lungs increases. The tortuosity of the capillaries is reduced and the pulmonary circulation changes from a high-resistance to a low-resistance pathway so 90% of the blood flows from the right ventricle through the pulmonary vascular bed and then to the left atrium. There is a brief reversal of blood flow through the DA. Closure of the DA involves two phases: functional closure within hours of birth and structural closure by vascular remodelling. The DA vasoconstricts in response to the elevated oxygen tension and decreased level of prostaglandin PGE_2 (Hung et al., 2018). PGE_2 falls because the placenta and fetal membranes no longer contribute to prostaglandin production and prostaglandin breakdown is markedly increased in the lungs, which receive more blood so increased prostaglandin metabolism and clearance occur. Other factors that contribution to the vascular smooth muscle contraction include glutamate, osmolality, nitric oxide and carbon monoxide. Anatomic and permanent closure of the DA involves changes in the endothelial cells, disruption of the internal elastic lamina, production of extracellular matrix, proliferation and migration of smooth muscle cells and interaction with blood cells. A patent ductus arteriosus (PDA) is a leading cause of mortality in preterm infants (Box 15.6).

Unlike most blood vessels, the umbilical blood vessels are not innervated. The umbilical arteries are physiologically irritable; their tone is modulated by vasoactive substances that regulate contraction (and relaxation in fetal life) of the vessels (Lorigo et al., 2018). Vasoconstriction is stimulated by stretching and handling the cord, by cooling and in response to stress-related catecholamine release. The most potent vasoconstrictive agent promoting physiological closure of the umbilical arteries after birth is serotonin (also called 5-hydroxytrptamine or 5HT); this is augmented by other vasoconstrictors such as bradykinin, histamine, thromboxane, endothelin 1 and $PGF_{2\alpha}$. Human umbilical artery smooth muscle cells can be harvested from the discarded umbilical cord after delivery and used to investigate cellular mechanisms; inappropriate vasoconstriction of the umbilical arteries occurs in disorders such as preeclampsia and gestational hypertension.

The thicker walls of the umbilical arteries are able to generate high intraluminal pressure, which arrests the placental circulation, preventing blood from flowing from the infant back to the placenta. This is augmented by the increased synthesis of $PGF_{2\alpha}$ and thromboxane in response to the raised oxygen level due to the infant breathing air, which increases vessel irritability and vasoconstriction.

The umbilical vein initially remains dilated; blood may continue to flow from the placenta to the infant. This

BOX 15.6   Congenital Cardiovascular Disorders

Disease (% of Congenital Heart Anomalies)	Causes
Septal Defects ('holes in the heart')	
Atrial septal defect (ASD) (5–10%)	An opening in the interatrial septum, which allows a left to right shunt of blood
Patent foramen ovale (PFO)	Failure of the foramen ovale to close, or it becomes functionally closed and can leak or re-open. Present in 25% of adults and 40–50% of patients with strokes of unknown cause
Ventricular septal defect (VSD) (2nd most common, ~20%)	A hole in the septum, which separates the ventricles
Valve Defects	
Bicuspid aortic valve (BAV) (Most common)	Fusion during fetal development of two of the three leaflets (bicuspid) of the aortic valve. Can become narrow causing aortic valve stenosis. Present in ~1.5% of adults
Pulmonary stenosis	Obstructed blood flow from the right ventricle to the pulmonary artery
Patent ductus arteriosus (PDA) (5–10% of term neonates; incidence increases with prematurity)	Retention of the fetal vessel (ductus arteriosus) between the aorta and pulmonary artery, after birth. Blood from the left ventricle passes via the aorta into the lungs via the pulmonary arteries. Can cause lungs to become congested and also damage to blood vessels in the lungs
Tetralogy of Fallot (7–10%)	A combination of pulmonary stenosis, a large ventricular septal defect, a displaced aorta directly overlying the ventricular septal defect and right ventricular hypertrophy. Deoxygenated blood from the right ventricle can flow directly into the aorta instead of via the pulmonary artery to the lungs
Patent ductus venosus	Extremely rare

Heart disease is the most common congenital anomaly occurring in ~1% of live births with both genetic and environmental components. Common symptoms of these disorders include cyanosis (blue tinge of skin due to hypoxaemia), acute or chronic fatigue, heart murmurs, poor circulation, decreased or nonpalpable pulse and hyperventilation (rapid breathing).

potentially acts as a placental transfusion of blood to the infant and could affect the neonate's blood volume, haemoglobin level and iron status. Blood flow to the infant is thought to be affected by uterine contractions until the placental expulsion in the third stage of labour and possibly by gravity. Initial neonatal blood volume is affected by the timing of clamping of the umbilical cord, type of management of the third stage, and by the relative positions of the infant and placenta at the time of clamping. The current recommendations are to delay umbilical cord clamping for at least 30 s and possibly until the cord has ceased pulsing unless there is interrupted placental circulation or the infant requires resuscitation (Katheria et al., 2018). In addition, the practice is often to clamp the umbilical cord earlier if the baby is subject to fluid overload (hydropic), or if the baby is polycythaemic (has an abnormally high haematocrit, which is more likely in infants of diabetic mothers, IUGR infants or a the 'recipient' twin of twin-to-twin transfusion syndrome), to limit the transfer of maternal analgesic agents or known

antibody incompatibilities or to avoid possible baby-to-baby transfusions in the cases of multiple births at birth or if there is maternal haemorrhage. However, recently assumptions about the benefits of delayed cord clamping have been challenged (Hooper et al., 2016a) because the duration of the delay in clamping is not a major determinant of net placental-to-infant blood transfer, gravity appears to have little effect and uterine contractions generate partial cord occlusion (like clamping) rather than facilitating infant blood transfusion.

The flap of the foramen ovale (Fig. 15.5) is pushed closed because the decreased umbilical flow results in a decreased venous return from the inferior vena cava so the pressure in the right atrium and PVR falls in response to changes in oxygenation. The increased pulmonary blood flow results in an increased return to the left atrium and consequent increase in pressure. Thus, the pressure gradient across the foramen ovale is reversed forcing the flap of the foramen ovale to obstruct the flow from the right atrium to the left atrium. So at birth, PVR falls and SVR

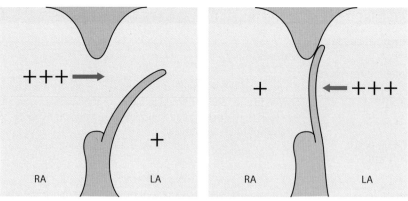

Fig. 15.5 Initiation of neonatal circulation and closure of the foramen ovale between the right atrium (RA) and left atrium (LA).

increases. The relatively thick layer of smooth muscle in the pulmonary blood vessels begins to thin from birth.

The closure of the fetal structures may not be immediate or permanent and may never be fully completed. The closure of the foramen ovale is reversible at first; interruption of ventilation or a drop in alveolar oxygenation results in constriction of the pulmonary capillaries and consequent reversal of pressure across the atria and reversion to fetal circulation as the flap is forced open again by the reversal of pressures. The incomplete closure can result in intermittent and reversible cyanotic episodes, which if detected, will require that the neonate should be observed closely. After a few days of functional closure, the tissue associated with the foramen ovale fuses and closure becomes permanent. Therefore, ongoing periods of cyanosis need to be fully investigated to exclude underlying congenital heart disease. Patent foramen ovale (PFO) or 'a hole in the heart' is a nonpermanent closure of the foramen ovale and the most common atrial septal defect. PFO is present in ~25% of adults and for most people it causes no health problems and most affected individuals are unaware of the condition. It can be demonstrated (a probe can be passed through) although the pressure gradient maintains effective functional closure. The prevalence of PFO is ~25% in adults but ~50% in sufferers of migraine with aura or in subjects who suffer a stroke of unknown cause (cryptogenic stroke). The bypassing of the lungs by a thrombus passing into the aorta may account for some cases of cryptogenic stroke and a similar shunting of gas bubbles triggered by a too rapid ascent of scuba divers can cause a brain embolism, with no prior indication that their foramen ovale was patent.

Intermittent flow through the DA may initially occur during each cardiac cycle when aortic pressure is maximal following ventricular contraction. Bradykinin released from the newly inflated lungs mediates the constriction of the DA. Production of prostaglandins, which had maintained the open DA in the fetus, is decreased as oxygenation increases. Most neonates have some degree of patency of the DA in the first 8 h of life but it becomes functionally closed within the first or second day (Riviere et al., 2017). Fibrolysis and obliteration of the lumen of the DA are usually complete within 3 weeks; continued patency of the DA can be serious (see Box 15.6).

The internal component of the umbilical vein remains patent for the first week of life; it can offer a route for blood transfusion if required. The ductus venosus remains open for the first few hours of life and can be used as a means of access to the neonatal circulation, for instance to administer intravenous fluids or medication. This is particularly useful in premature babies where it is difficult to achieve peripheral venous access. Access to arterial blood via the umbilical vessels can be used to measure blood pressure and blood gases to monitor respiratory effectiveness, which is important if mechanical respiratory support is being utilized.

The ductus venosus begins to constrict as the blood flow in the umbilical vein dwindles. but the mechanisms involved and the timing are less well characterized than for the other fetal structures. The obliterated vessels remain as vestigial anatomical ligaments; the slow closure of the umbilical vein results in its degeneration into the ligamentum teres.

The nervous control of the cardiovascular system is well developed in the neonate with mature physiological control of blood pressure and cardiac output demonstrable. The systemic arterial blood pressure is relatively low in the first few weeks as vascular tone develops, which increases vascular resistance. Pulmonary arterial blood pressure is initially high but falls to mature values as pulmonary resistance falls. The neonate's heart rate is fast, as in the fetus. Also like the fetus, neonatal control of cardiac output is largely achieved by changing heart rate because the heart is small and noncompliant and has a relatively thick wall so stroke volume remains relatively unchanged. At birth, the wall of the right ventricle is thicker than the left, which hypertrophies in response to the changed pressure and workload of the postnatal circulation.

THE RESPIRATORY SYSTEM

The primitive air sacs are developed by the 20th week of gestation, and by 26 weeks respiratory bronchioles with a rich capillary supply are evident. Although the enzymes for synthesis of phospholipid/lipoprotein components of surfactant are present from week 18, the type II pneumocytes secrete surfactant only from week 26 with a surge in production after week 30. Surfactant, a detergent-like wetting agent, increases pulmonary compliance by decreasing surface tension, so the force required to inflate the alveoli is greatly reduced and the alveoli do not collapse at the end of expiration. A lack of surfactant causes infant RDS (also known as surfactant deficiency disorder) (see below). Historically, the maturity of the respiratory system was determined by measuring the lecithin:sphingomyelin (L:S) ratio of the surfactant in amniotic fluid samples from amniocentesis (Fig. 15.6). By week 35, the L:S ratio in a healthily developing fetus is 2:1. This ratio is decreased in preeclampsia, prematurity, maternal narcotic addiction, maternal diabetes and other problems in pregnancy. Administration of cortisol (dexamethasone) to the mother prior to delivery of a baby born from 24 to 34 weeks' gestation increases fetal surfactant production within 24 h and can be used to decrease the risk and or severity of RDS.

Variations (polymorphisms) in the genes for pulmonary surfactant proteins are associated with a range of inherited neonatal and lifelong respiratory problems including bronchopulmonary dysplasia (BPD), RDS and respiratory syncytial virus (RSV) bronchiolitis and may influence susceptibility to influenza virus and other respiratory problems (Jo, 2014). Premature infants, particularly those born before 28 weeks, have immature alveoli with fewer type II cells so they are vulnerable to RDS, which is the major cause of morbidity and mortality in this group. The incidence of RDS is inversely associated with gestational age but is also influenced by ethnicity, gender (premature male infants are more vulnerable) and maternal health. Preterm infants developing respiratory distress may be given animal-derived or synthetic surfactant via an endotracheal tube to reduce the risk of RDS. Poor ventilation suppresses surfactant secretion so the severity of hypoxia, hypercapnia

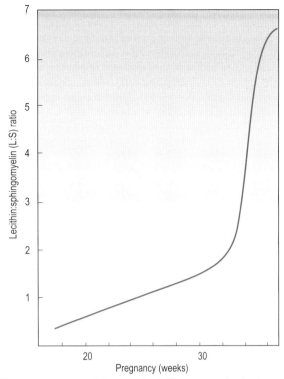

Fig. 15.6 Lecithin:sphingomyelin (L:S) concentration in the amniotic fluid; the concentration rises very sharply after 30 weeks' gestation. (Reproduced with permission from Chamberlain et al., 1991.)

and acidosis is worsened and respiratory muscle activity is compromised, which further compromises surfactant production. Maternal obesity is associated with increased respiratory problems at birth (McGillick et al., 2017).

The Lungs
Before Birth

In fetal life, the lungs are filled by fluid secreted by the lung epithelium; the lung fluid is essential for growth and development of the lungs and this fluid exchanges with amniotic fluid.

Fetal breathing movements (FBM), defined as an inward chest movement coinciding with an outward abdominal movement and movement of the diaphragm, which moves abdominal fluid in and out of the lungs, are observed on ultrasound from the first trimester. Initially, the FBM are intermittent, rapid and irregular; they are normal and essential for development of the fetal lungs. As gestation progresses, FBM increase in strength and frequency, occurring up to 80% of the time in an organized episodic pattern in periods of ~30 min coinciding with rapid eye movement

(REM) sleep (Koos and Rajaee, 2014). The lung fluid is 'breathed' out by the fetus into the amniotic fluid. Patterns of FBM dominate during the daytime and are correlated with fetal behavioural states. Fetal wakefulness and arousal are associated with sustained vigorous respiratory patterns. Quiet or slow wave sleep and wakefulness stages are associated with an absence of FBM. Adrenergic and cholinergic compounds, prostaglandin synthesis inhibitors and raised maternal carbon dioxide levels stimulate FBM. They are inhibited by hypoglycaemia, cigarette smoking, alcohol consumption and accelerated labour.

Despite the relatively low partial pressure of oxygen and high partial pressure of carbon dioxide, the fetus makes only shallow respiratory movements although severe hypoxia and acidosis may stimulate gasping. Severe hypoxia increases the likelihood of the fetus passing of meconium into the amniotic fluid so the risk of meconium aspiration is increased by intrauterine hypoxic induced gasping. Meconium stained amniotic fluid (MSAF) together with fetal distress in preterm and term labour warrants careful observation of the newborn infant to enable the early detection of respiratory complications. Mild hypoxia leads to quiet sleep and reduced energy expenditure and oxygen consumption, which may be protective.

After Birth

The most urgent need, immediately after delivery, is the initiation and establishment of independent ventilation; the neonate has to clear its lungs of fluid, establish regular breathing and increase pulmonary blood flow to match pulmonary perfusion to ventilation. At birth, the neonate has to rapidly clear fluid from its air spaces. About 10–25 mL/kg fluid will be expelled or resorbed; some will be redistributed as the alveoli expand creating a greater surface area for the fluid to spread over thus increasing reabsorption and facilitating gaseous exchange.

Many factors interact to stimulate the first breath, including changes in ambient temperature and environmental state. The mild asphyxia (decreased oxygen concentration, raised carbon dioxide concentration) and acidosis (decreased pH) due to flow in the cord ceasing sensitize the fetal aortic, carotid and central (medullary) chemoreceptors that increase ventilatory drive. Tactile stimulation, such as that which occurs during delivery, also promotes respiration. In addition, it is thought that the placental prostaglandins may inhibit breathing (decreased oxygen concentration, raised carbon dioxide concentration). The surge of endogenous steroids and catecholamines associated with labour also contributes; infants who do not experience labour, for example those born by lower (uterine) segment caesarean section (LSCS), are more likely to retain residual lung fluid in their lungs and have less efficient respiratory performance. Transient tachypnoea of the newborn (TTN) is the most common respiratory problem of term neonates; it usually resolves within a few days.

The fluid-filled lung with collapsed alveoli and undispersed surfactant proffers a high resistance to inflation requiring a very high negative intrapleural pressure (>50 cm H_2O or 35 mmHg) to open the alveoli for the first time. The diaphragm contracts strongly, and the compliant flexible ribs and sternum of the newborn baby are pulled concave in the effort of the first breath. Similarly, a considerable positive pressure is also needed to deflate the lungs due to viscous resistance of fluid in bronchioles. Once the lungs are inflated, the lung fluid is forced into the alveoli where it aids dispersal of surfactant and is rapidly resorbed into the pulmonary lymphatic vessels. The first inspirations of neonate are therefore extremely strong but the pressure changes required for inspiration and expiration (which can be plotted as the lung compliance curve) rapidly decrease to near-adult values within the first hour. The thoracic compression of a vaginal delivery contributes to fluid loss from the upper respiratory tract; the compression of the chest (known as the 'vaginal squeeze') creates negative pressure, which draws air into the lungs and they re-expand through recoiling of the rib cage. Most of the fluid clearance is due to a change in the lung epithelium from being a predominantly chloride and fluid secreting epithelium before birth to being predominantly a sodium and fluid absorbing epithelium after birth. Increased expression of epithelial Na^+ channels (ENac) near to term increases the passive absorption of Na^+ across the apical membrane of alveolar epithelial cells, so that water uptake from the lumen follows by osmosis. Intracellular Na^+ levels are kept low by the active transport of Na^+ across the basal membrane and out of the cells, so that water also moves into the interstitial tissue and then into the lung vasculature. This directional absorption of water from the alveolar lumen driven by Na^+ transport is vital to the establishment of normal breathing in the neonate and, when disrupted, is implicated in several disease states, including TTN.

Most babies gasp within 6 s of birth and have patterns of normal neonatal breathing and gas exchange within 15 min. Initially, the newborn infant has metabolic and respiratory acidosis due to decreased oxygen concentrations (resulting in increased lactic acid) and increased carbon dioxide levels, respectively; this acid–base imbalance is corrected as ventilation improves, further aided by vigorous crying. The risk of TTN is increased in babies who are delivered by caesarean section or those who experience perinatal hypoxia.

The respiratory rate of the newborn is high compared with an adult but is similar when relative size is taken into account. Ventilation is often irregular with the baby exhibiting periods of fetal-like shallow breathing. The reflexes associated with lung inflation also appear to be different. As well as the Hering–Breuer reflex (where filling of the lungs is detected by pulmonary stretch receptors to inhibit inspiration and increases expiratory centre activity to prevent over-inflation), the newborn infant demonstrates Head's paradoxical reflex (also known as the inspiratory augmenting reflex; where filling the lungs excites the inspiratory centre thus stimulating further inspiration) (Hillman and Lam, 2019). For the first few weeks, babies breathe via the nose facilitating suckling via the mouth. 'Snuffley' babies usually have nasal mucous build-up affecting their ability to nose breathe, which is often a cause of poor feeding. Control of ventilation by chemoreceptors is functional but qualitatively different in that hypoxia tends to increase depth of respiration (rather than respiratory rate) and that the response is temperature-dependent and is abolished in cold temperatures. The chemoreceptors seem to be more sensitive to raised carbon dioxide levels.

Babies have a relatively large oxygen demand, which reflects their heat generation and that their more metabolically active tissues (e.g. liver and brain) are a larger proportion of the total body mass. The higher airway resistance means that the energy cost of respiration is initially greater. PVR drops 6–8 weeks after birth when the diameter of the small arterioles increases. The relatively high requirement for oxygen means that neonates are more susceptible to asphyxia than other age groups. Neonatal resuscitation aims to prevent mortality and morbidity. Hypothermic neonates are predisposed to hypoglycaemia and acidosis. Acidosis compromises respiration because it increases PVR and suppresses both respiratory drive and surfactant production. The aims of neonatal resuscitation are to promote and maintain adequate ventilation and oxygenation, to initiate and maintain adequate cardiac output and perfusion and to maintain body temperature and adequate blood glucose levels.

Respiratory Distress Syndrome

RDS is caused by a deficiency in surfactant, which results in alveolar collapse and increased airway resistance. Surfactant deficiency is usually inversely related to gestational age and lung maturity. Abnormal pH, stress and inadequate pulmonary perfusion also inhibit surfactant synthesis and recycling. RDS is exacerbated by asphyxia and is the most common cause of respiratory failure in the preterm infant. The high surface tension in RDS hinders alveolar expansion. Small alveoli tend to recollapse and normal alveoli are overdistended following expiration. Segments of the lung close and hypoxaemia and carbon dioxide retention (hypercapnia) progressively increase. The resulting metabolic and respiratory acidosis further limits the production of surfactant from the type II pneumocytes. Hypoxaemia causes vasoconstriction of the pulmonary arteries thus compromising pulmonary perfusion and increasing the likelihood of right-to-left shunting through the foramen ovale and DA. Local ischaemic damage affects the alveolar tissue and the capillary endothelium. Changes in pulmonary pressure brought about by the infant attempting to maintain adequate air flow, together with the low plasma protein level common in preterm infants, tend to cause displacement of fluid into the alveoli. Fibrinogen in the exudate is converted into fibrin and lines the alveoli thickening the membrane. The thickened membrane and excess fluid increase the diffusion distance and impair gas transfer.

The infant responds to the respiratory difficulties by increasing respiratory rate and effort. The clinical signs appear early and increase in severity over 2 or 3 days. The infant may 'grunt', has nasal flaring and exhibits oedema and cyanosis. Cyanosis tends to be progressive and is due to high levels of deoxygenated haemoglobin in the capillaries. Mild-to-moderate RDS may cause peripheral cyanosis. Cyanosis is worsened by right-to-left shunting, alveolar hypoventilation and impaired gas diffusion across the alveolar membranes. The baby grunts because expiration is against a partially closed glottis, which increases pressure and retards expiratory flow, therefore increasing gas exchange. RDS risk is increased in prematurity, babies of diabetic mothers (because insulin is antagonistic to cortisol), antepartum haemorrhage and second-born twins. RDS is also associated with high circulating levels of PGF2α in the neonate (see Chapter 13). Male babies are twice as susceptible to RDS. Chronic hypertension, maternal heroin addiction, preeclampsia and growth retardation appear to protect against RDS.

TEMPERATURE REGULATION

Before Birth

In utero, the fetus depends on its mother for temperature regulation. It loses heat via the placenta and via conduction (from skin to amniotic fluid to uterus). The fetus is a net heat producer although raised maternal temperature may compromise it. Brown fat metabolism is actively inhibited and fetal oxygen consumption is ~30% of postnatal levels. Fetal temperature is maintained at about 0.5°C above maternal temperature and so the fetus does not expend energy in keeping warm. Research has focused on raised maternal temperature due to fever, exercise and external raised temperature (such as hot baths and saunas). The results are inconclusive. However, maternal fever has effects not only on temperature gradients but also on oxygen consumption and haemodynamics and may be associated with teratogenesis in embryonic development and preterm labour.

After Birth

The infant is born wet in a relatively cold environment. As environmental temperature is usually lower than maternal body temperature, the baby will experience a temperature loss at birth. Heat transfer is affected by two gradients: the internal gradient involving transfer from the core to the surface of the baby and the external gradient involving heat transfer from the body surface to the environment. Cooling is usually rapid at a rate of 0.2–1.0°C/min depending on the environmental factors, gestational age and size of the infant (e.g. IUGR, which affects body composition). Transfer of heat through the internal gradient depends on insulation and blood flow. Neonates are predisposed to heat loss; they have less subcutaneous fat than adults do (~16% body fat compared with 30%), a higher surface area:mass ratio (about three times the ratio of an adult) and a lower ability to shiver. Should the baby be born small, it will not only have an even larger surface area:mass ratio but also the insulation provided by its subcutaneous fat will be further compromised and skin permeability will be increased. Small-for-dates babies have proportionately bigger heads and higher metabolism and are disadvantaged, in that their heat losses are also higher. Changes in peripheral circulation affect heat loss via conduction. Heat loss across the external gradient depends on the temperature difference between the body and the environment. Conduction, convection, evaporation and radiation transfer heat from the baby. Warming objects that will come into contact with the neonate, and increasing insulation by wrapping, limit heat loss by conduction. Evaporation offers the greatest route for heat loss immediately after delivery but drying the baby, especially the head, immediately after delivery is effective at reducing the loss. Skin keratinization is inadequate in immature infants so evaporative heat losses are higher. Evaporative insensible heat loss increases with respiratory problems, activity, the use of radiant heaters or phototherapy and low relative humidity. Convective losses are related to draughts and are affected by ambient temperature and humidity. Higher air temperatures, minimal air circulation, swaddling and baby hats reduce heat loss by convection. Radiation is the major form of heat loss from babies in incubators. It involves the transfer of radiant energy to surrounding objects not directly in contact with the baby. Consideration therefore has to be given to the temperature of objects in the local environment including the incubator, walls and windows. Skin-to-skin contact with the mother immediately following birth is a very efficient way of reducing heat loss from the neonate. The large skin area and the softness of the breasts enable a large amount of maternal skin to come into direct contact with the baby's skin surface.

The mechanisms of heat conservation and generation mediated by the peripheral nervous system are insufficient in the neonate. Infants can produce heat from metabolic processes and by increasing activity. Postural changes are also important in conserving heat; for example, a baby laid in an outstretched position will lose more heat than a baby in the curled up 'fetal' position. Shivering does not contribute significantly to heat generation in the newborn infant but heat generation by nonshivering thermogenesis (NST) is important. NST takes place in brown adipose tissue (BAT), a specialized type of adipose tissue that is well vascularized, particularly by sympathetic nerves, and has cells densely packed with mitochondria, the brown pigments that give the tissue its colour and description (Fig. 15.7). In humans, BAT is mostly replaced by white adipose tissue (WAT); adults have very few BAT cells, which are interspersed with WAT (Chondronikola and Sidossis, 2019). However, BAT has a major role in heat production in the neonate. BAT is formed from ~30 weeks' gestation until about 4 weeks' postbirth. Fat mass is significantly altered by maternal nutrition and gestational length; stores of BAT (and white fat) are lower in preterm infants. BAT comprises ~2–7% of birthweight and is predominantly located around the core organs (Fig. 15.8). It generates heat by uncoupling electron transport from oxidative phosphorylation in the mitochondria so the energy generated by electron transport will not be used to synthesize ATP but will be liberated as heat instead (Fig. 15.9). Fifty percent of cellular respiration is uncoupled from ATP formation in BAT (Chondronikola and Sidossis, 2019). The unique uncoupling protein (UCP1) is a proton transporter located in the inner mitochondrial membrane. UCP-1 allows the re-entry of protons into the mitochondrial matrix that were pumped into inter-membrane space by the electron transport. This 'futile cycle' results in the energy being liberated as heat instead of being used for ATP synthesis. When UCP1 is maximally activated, it allows the production of at least 100 times as much heat from BAT compared with other tissues. UCP1 is synthesized during the maturation of fetal fat (Carobbio et al., 2019). At birth, the activation of BAT is accompanied by mobilization of the small droplets of stored fat and a marked increase in lipolysis. The very high level of circulating fetal catecholamines following birth (significantly higher than ever found in adults) acts via β_3-adrenoceptors on BAT cells via the sympathetic nervous system in response to cold exposure. Interference with this surge leads to cardiorespiratory collapse. Thermogenesis by BAT is inhibited in the fetus

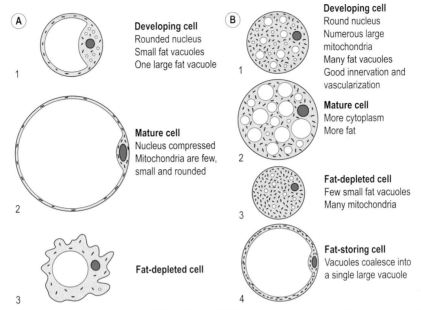

Developing cell
Rounded nucleus
Small fat vacuoles
One large fat vacuole

Mature cell
Nucleus compressed
Mitochondria are few,
small and rounded

Fat-depleted cell

Developing cell
Round nucleus
Numerous large
mitochondria
Many fat vacuoles
Good innervation and
vascularization

Mature cell
More cytoplasm
More fat

Fat-depleted cell
Few small fat vacuoles
Many mitochondria

Fat-storing cell
Vacuoles coalesce into
a single large vacuole

Fig. 15.7 Structures and development of (A) white and (B) brown adipose tissue. (Reproduced with permission from Hull, 1966.)

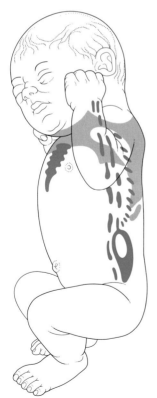

Fig. 15.8 Location of brown adipose tissue in the human infant.

by PGE_2 and prostacyclin (PGI_2) produced by the placenta. The placenta also suppresses formation of active T_3 (triiodothyronine) from T_4 (thyroxine) (see below).

Heat production per unit mass of the neonate is higher than that of an adult; thermogenesis begins when a critical temperature difference of 12°C between the environment and the skin is exceeded. At birth, catecholamines from the adrenal medulla and rise in T_3 production by the thyroid gland augment the effect of noradrenaline. Inhibition of BAT by the placenta ceases following delivery of the infant. Oxygen consumption and metabolic rate increase markedly in response to a reduction in core temperature. Heat generation involves lipolysis of BAT, which depends on the availability of oxygen, ATP and glucose. There is a strong interrelationship between ventilation, feeding and temperature regulation, which means that hypoglycaemia, hypoxia or acidosis can affect the ability of the neonate to produce heat (thermogenesis) (Fig. 15.10). Persistent hypothermia can therefore result in metabolic acidosis (due to increased lactic acid production), decreased surfactant production and, if it is chronic, compromised growth. Cold stress or hypothermia will increase metabolic rate and peripheral and pulmonary vasoconstriction. The increased metabolic rate will increase oxygen demand. Peripheral and pulmonary vasoconstriction can compromise oxygenation and perfusion efficiency. Tissue hypoxia may increase acidosis because anaerobic metabolism increases lactic acid production as the oxygen deficit increases. Hypoxia inhibits

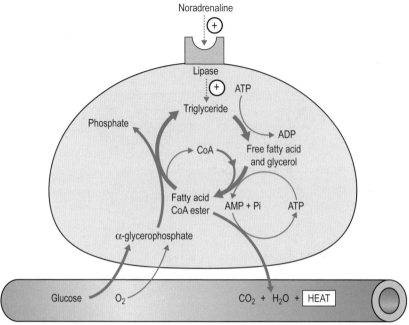

Fig. 15.9 Metabolic pathways in brown adipose tissue: triglycerides break down to yield useful heat (about 160 kcal/mol are produced during each turn of the cycle). (Reproduced with permission from Begley et al., 1978.)

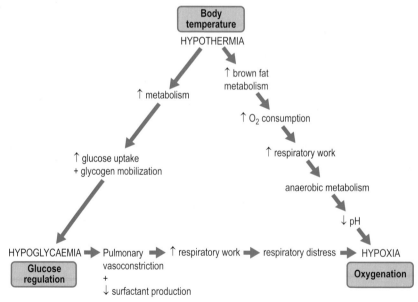

Fig. 15.10 Interrelationship between temperature regulation, glucose concentration and respiration.

metabolic rate and compromises the thermal response; it also affects surfactant production.

Mechanisms for losing heat are not well developed in the neonate (Hillman et al., 2012). The neonate can lose some heat by sweating (which increases evaporation) but peripheral vasodilatation is the main source of heat loss. Although the density of neonatal sweat glands is high in some areas, they are less responsive and less efficient at sweat production. Phototherapy, if required, will further increase water loss. Sweating is more inefficient in preterm babies and those with central nervous system dysfunction. Neonates are also at risk from hyperthermia (over-heating), which may be a contributing factor towards sudden infant death syndrome (SIDS). As the baby gets older and can rely on physical methods of generating and dissipating heat, NST becomes less important. BAT gradually diminishes in the first year.

WAT provides both insulation and an energy reserve. Development of body fat in the fetus is under nutritional constraint whereas postnatal growth is controlled by genetic potential. Compared with other mammals, human infants are not only extremely fat at birth but they also continue to increase in adiposity during early postnatal life. Although it has been suggested that the role of the fat is insulation required as compensation for human hairlessness, evidence to support this is weak. A more likely explanation is that the adipose tissue acts as an energy reserve both to support the demands of a large brain and to protect the infant from nutritional disruption at birth and weaning or during infection (Burini and Leonard, 2018).

THE NEONATAL LIVER

Bilirubin

The functions of the neonatal liver are similar to those of an adult but are relatively immature at birth. The ability to synthesize plasma proteins such as albumin and to metabolize foreign substances is inefficient. Neonates produce more bilirubin because of the high turnover of red blood cells and this, together with immature intestinal processes, means the neonate is at increased risk of developing hyperbilirubinaemia. Before birth, bilirubin is cleared by the placenta and then handled by maternal metabolism. If bilirubin accumulates in the serum of the neonate, jaundice (or icterus) can occur; yellow staining of the skin and sclera. In pigmented skin, jaundice is harder to detect and may only be obvious from discolouring of the sclera. Neonatal jaundice is common, affecting over 60% of healthy term and up to 80% of preterm infants (Pan and Rivas, 2017) and will usually disappear spontaneously over the first

few days postpartum without the need for phototherapy or other treatments. However, markedly elevated levels of bilirubin can cause severe jaundice and potentially cause brain damage. As the blood–brain barrier of the neonate is more permeable, free bilirubin can access the brain easily and in sufficient concentrations can deposit in the basal ganglia causing kernicterus (brain tissue is heavily stained with bilirubin, which is fat soluble so it is deposited within the lipid structures). Bilirubin encephalopathy, damage to the brain by bilirubin deposits, results in a range of symptoms from convulsions and abnormal behaviour such as lethargy, hypotonia and poor suck to cerebral palsy, deafness or death.

Physiological jaundice is a result of normal breakdown of red blood cells and neonatal immaturity; it is usually mild and resolves relatively quickly. Severe jaundice may result from increased production of bilirubin and/or decreased excretion. Risk factors include sepsis (which both compromises the liver's ability to breakdown excess haemoglobin and increases haemolysis), excessive trauma and interstitial bleeding (e.g. haematomas, excess bruising, etc.), polycythaemia, AB-Rhesus incompatibility (neonatal blood cells are destroyed by maternal antibodies) and liver abnormalities. In such cases, kernicterus is more likely to occur and so careful monitoring of serum bilirubin levels is required.

Iron from red blood cells is recycled. Haem, the pigment, is degraded by macrophages of the reticuloendothelial system to biliverdin and then to bilirubin (Fig. 15.11). Unconjugated (indirect) bilirubin is insoluble and cannot be excreted. It is transported bound to plasma albumin to the liver to be metabolized into conjugated (direct) bilirubin, which is soluble. Conjugation involves binding of glucuronide sugars to bilirubin forming bilirubin diglucuronate. Conjugated bilirubin is excreted into bile and so into the duodenum. It is a major component of bile and faeces. In the intestine, conjugated bilirubin is further metabolized by bacterial flora to produce urobilin and stercobilin (which give the characteristic colour of faeces). Some of the breakdown products of bacterial metabolism of bilirubin are deconjugated and absorbed across the gut wall to be recirculated. Small amounts of bilirubin are also excreted via the kidneys in the form of urobilins, which give the yellowish colour to urine. As urine becomes more concentrated then the colour darkens due to the concentration of the urobilins increasing.

Decreased production of plasma proteins can result in raised unconjugated bilirubin levels. The pathways in the liver that deconjugate bilirubin to its water soluble, and therefore excretable, metabolite may also be compromised. As meconium is rich in bilirubin, delayed passage

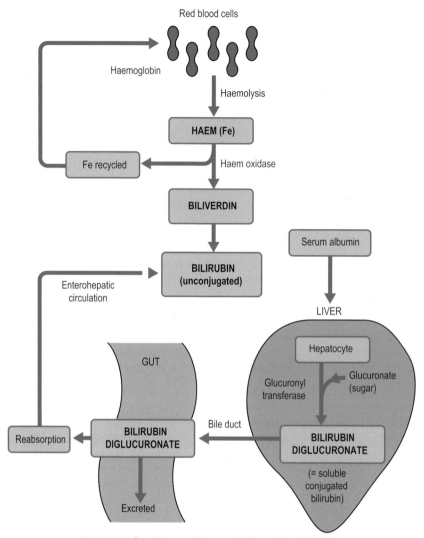

Fig. 15.11 Breakdown of haemoglobin to form bilirubin.

of meconium increases the possibility that bilirubin will be deconjugated, absorbed and re-enter the circulating pool. Production of bilirubin in neonates is inversely correlated to gestational age and remains high for a few weeks (Pan and Rivas, 2017). This is partly due to higher numbers and size of red blood cells in fetal blood, which are then removed in the neonate, and also to having more fragile red blood cells with a shorter lifespan (see Table 15.1). The risk of hyperbilirubinaemia is further increased by other conditions that stress this pathway such as excess blood cell breakdown (as in excessive trauma at birth or due to infection) or increased red blood cell breakdown (as in polycythaemia due to maternal diabetes).

Infants are vulnerable to a number of diseases associated with oxidative injury, including retinopathy of prematurity, NEC, intraventricular haemorrhage and BPD. It has been suggested that as bilirubin has antioxidant properties, there may be a potential benefit of raised levels of bilirubin in early infancy to help protect infants from oxidative damage.

Fuel Storage

Fetal metabolism is dominated by anabolic pathways, whereas the neonate has to catabolize fuel stores to provide nutrients between periodic neonatal feeds. The last weeks of gestation are an important time for laying down fetal adipose tissue and glycogen. During fetal life, glycogen is stored in the liver and skeletal muscle. Hepatic glycogen provides the substrate for energy metabolism during delivery and the first few hours of postnatal life. Fat stores serve as an alternative energy source; the neonate markedly increases fatty acid oxidation and uses ketone bodies for energy production. In the first few days of life, the respiratory quotient falls from 1.0 (as glucose sources are exhausted) to about 0.7 (a value similar to that seen in adult diabetics) as fat and protein are mobilized until adequate milk is consumed.

Glucose Regulation

Thyroxine (T_4) is relatively inactive and is usually converted to active tri-iodothyronine (T_3). Fetal T_3 levels are low because fetal liver levels of outer-ring deiodinase are low and placental levels of inner-ring deiodinase are high, both of which drive preferential production of inactive reverse T_3. The resulting low level of the active thyroid hormone T_3 can support brain development but suppresses oxygen consumption by non-neural tissues and inhibits thermogenesis. In late gestation, the rise in glucocorticoids induces expression of outer-ring deiodinase in the fetal liver so production of fetal T_3 increases markedly. The rise in T_3 plays a role not only in hepatic enzyme activity but also in tissue maturation and lung and bone development. At birth, the T_3 levels increase further as the inner-ring deiodinase is reduced on placental separation, and evaporative cooling induces a rise in thyroid-stimulating hormone (TSH, thyrotrophin), which further stimulates hormone production by the thyroid gland. Adipose tissue significantly contributes to the conversion of T_4 to T_3 after delivery; smaller fat depots result in less thyroid hormone production, potentially further compromising thermogenesis in premature infants.

Blood glucose levels in the neonate tend to fall after delivery because of detachment from the placental supply, the greater ability of the immature liver to synthesize glycogen than to break it down to glucose (glycogenolysis), and because the baby has increased activity and metabolism at birth. At birth, neonatal plasma glucose concentrations are ~70% of adult levels and fall to their lowest point 1–2 h later. The neonate has a high requirement for glucose because it has a relatively large brain and more and larger red blood cells. The stress of delivery and cooling at birth stimulate the release of catecholamines, which stimulate glucagon release and suppress insulin release and are important in activating the metabolic pathways in the liver. The neonate is unable to regulate blood glucose levels efficiently and is usually hypoglycaemic (glucose levels can be ~2 mmol/L) (Box 15.7). The enzymes involving

---

BOX 15.7 Risk Factors for and Symptoms of Hypoglycaemia

Risk Factors

- Hypothermia, evaporation, draughts, cold room
- Babies who do not feed or have a poor response to feeding in the early postnatal period
- Intrauterine growth retardation (IUGR)
- Prematurity
- Maternal diabetes
- Stress (hypoxia and anoxia)

Symptoms

- Lethargy: 'floppy baby' (normal muscle tone is reduced to conserve glucose usage of skeletal muscle)
- Drowsiness: difficult to rouse, indicating neurological function is impaired by lack of glucose
- Jitteriness: an adverse tremor in response to stimulation such as loud noise or touch, indicating neurological inhibition of reflexes is affected
- Coldness: may be a cause or consequence of hypoglycaemia

Note: many babies may be hypoglycaemic without clinical symptoms, indicating that they are maintaining normal neurological function by other metabolic pathways. The clinical symptoms indicate these pathways are failing and the infant is at risk. Hypoglycaemic screening of the neonate involves measuring the level of glucose in the infant's blood by analysis of a small amount obtained from a heel prick.

---

glucose metabolism do not reach optimal levels in the liver for 2–3 weeks, so glycogenolysis (mobilization of glycogen stores) and gluconeogenesis (hepatic synthesis of glucose from substrates) are relatively slow in correcting falls in blood glucose. Lipolysis generates ketones, which are used as alternative sources of energy for brain metabolism. If fetal delivery is protracted, the neonate may deplete its glycogen stores. The response to raised levels of glucose is also slow; although adequate concentrations of insulin are present in the pancreas, the β-cells initially lack sensitivity to glucose, responding better to amino acids. Thus, neonatal blood glucose levels fluctuate and hypoglycaemia may occur because hepatic glucose production is inadequate or there is excess insulin secretion (common in the infants of mothers with gestational diabetes). Hypoxia and hypothermia can exacerbate hypoglycaemia because of the energetic costs of respiration and heat production, respectively. Blood glucose values lower than 1.0 mmol/L have been recorded. In an adult, such a level of hypoglycaemia would cause convulsions, hypoglycaemic coma and probable neurological damage, whereas in the newborn they might cause an apnoeic attack. The central nervous system of the neonate exhibits a degree of plasticity and is partially protected as it can utilize fatty acids and ketones efficiently. Physiological responses to hypoglycaemia activate the sympathetic nervous system and cause neuroglycopenia (reduced glucose in the brain). Clinical signs of hypoglycaemia can include changes in level of consciousness (such as lethargy and drowsiness), changes in behaviour (such as irritability and jitteriness, hypotonia and poor feeding) and changes in vital signs (such as apnoea, hypothermia, bradycardia, bounding pulse and sweating).

THE GASTROINTESTINAL SYSTEM AT BIRTH

The gut completes anatomical development by week 24 and the term neonate is able to digest and absorb milk from birth. The fetus swallows amniotic fluid, which passes through the gut. Water, electrolytes and glucose are absorbed in the small intestine. Species-specific growth factors in milk are important in promoting postnatal development of the gut. The neonatal gut has immature digestive and absorptive capacities but there are a number of compensatory mechanisms, particularly for babies who are breastfed and receive both digestive enzymes and growth factors from the milk that stimulate gut development (Haschke et al., 2016).

Feeding Reflexes

From birth, a normal infant can suck from the breast, convey milk to the back of the mouth and swallow it for a period of 5–10 min while breathing normally. There is an innate programme of reflexes and behaviour, which become evident within an hour or so following delivery, including the ability to move from the mother's abdomen to her breast, coordinated hand–mouth activity, rooting for the nipple, attaching to the breast and feeding vigorously before falling asleep. Touching the palate triggers the sucking reflex. The neonate exhibits rhythmic jaw action, which creates a negative pressure, and the peristaltic action of the tongue and jaw strips milk from the breast and moves it to the throat thus triggering the swallowing reflex. These breastfeeding reflexes are strong at birth in the normal neonate and are evident in preterm babies from about 32 weeks (~1200 g). Extremely preterm babies and those that are sick or have a very low birthweight have markedly decreased or absent reflexes. Other babies who experience feeding problems include those with physical problems such as

cleft lip or palate, trisomies and other genetic defects and those subjected to obstetric sedation, analgesia or extreme stress at birth.

The sucking and swallowing reflexes are aided by the particular morphological configuration of the neonate's mouth, which has a proportionately longer soft palate. The neonate also has an extrusion reflex in response to the presence of solid or semisolid material in the mouth. This reflex is lost at 4–6 months and is replaced by a pattern of rhythmic biting movements coinciding with the development of the first teeth at 7–9 months.

Hormone and Enzyme Production

Gastric secretion is developed but low; responses to gut regulatory hormones also appear to be low. The effect is that the gastric juice has a pH close to neutral (compared with a pH of 2 in an adult's stomach). The higher gastric pH means that salivary amylase is not inactivated in the stomach so starch digestion can continue. Reflux of gastric contents is common, as the lower oesophageal sphincter is immature in both musculature and neurological control. Less-acidic gastric juice does not cause painful tissue damage to the oesophageal mucosa but also it is less effective at denaturing proteins including microorganisms. It has been suggested that a reflux of human milk is advantageous as very small amounts of milk may reach the upper part of the respiratory tract conferring an immunological benefit there. Breastfed babies have a lower incidence of respiratory problems. Decreased acid production in the stomach means that the activation of pepsinogen to pepsin is restricted, limiting protein digestion in the stomach. The decreased acidity and protein digestion may enhance the defence mechanism by maintaining the activity of immunoglobulins and antigen recognition in the gastrointestinal tract as these proteins survive the gentler gastric environment.

Pancreatic amylase levels are low in the newborn but breast milk contains mammary amylase, which can augment starch digestion. Colostrum is particularly rich in mammary amylase. Lactase activity is relatively late in developing, reaching adequate levels after 36 weeks' gestation. However, many preterm babies can digest lactose satisfactorily as unabsorbed lactose can be metabolized by colonic bacteria to form short-chain fatty acids, which can then be absorbed thus salvaging the energy. The low pancreatic lipase levels are compensated for by lingual and gastric lipase produced by the neonate (stimulated by suckling) and by bile salt-stimulated lipase in human milk. Bile acid formation is low but human milk is rich in taurine, which is used for neonatal conjugation of bile salts.

Bowel Movements

Passage of meconium, a mix of mucus, epithelial and gut cells, larger molecules and skin cell debris from the amniotic fluid, fatty acids and bile pigments (which gives it the characteristic greenish-black colour) confirms that the lower bowel is patent. (Usually defaecation does not occur *in utero* unless the fetus is stressed.) Passage of a changing stool (meconium and food residue), usually within 24 h, indicates the whole gut is patent and motile. Slow (>48 h after birth) or absent passage of meconium can indicate Hirschsprung disease, impaired motility of the colon due to the absence of ganglion cells; diagnosis is usually made following biopsy of the bowel wall. At birth, the stomach capacity is 10–20 mL, which rapidly increases to 200 mL by 1 year.

THE KIDNEYS

Before Birth

In utero, from 9 to 10 weeks' gestation, the fetus produces large volumes of hypotonic (dilute) urine, which is an important contributor to amniotic fluid (Box 15.8). However, the regulatory and excretory functions of the kidneys are minimal before birth. The placenta corrects any osmotic imbalance. Mature kidney function is not developed until about 1 month; until then the urine is fetal-like. The neonatal kidneys, weighing ~12.5 g each, have a low glomerular filtration rate (GFR) and relatively low surface area. The ability to reabsorb or excrete sodium (Na^+) is poor so water reabsorption is also poor and the urine produced is of low specific gravity and hypotonic, reaching 1.5 times plasma concentration (700–800 mOsm)

compared to adult values of three to five times plasma concentration (1200–1400 mOsm).

After Birth

At birth, the normal obligatory water loss means the baby loses 5–10% of its birthweight in the first 4 days as a result of the loss of water and Na^+. Neonatal renal function can efficiently prevent dehydration and eliminate the lower level of metabolic waste products of the breastfed infant. Because the newborn infant does not retain Na^+ efficiently, it is vulnerable to dehydration. Changing fluid intake (or increasing the solute load) can result in osmotic imbalance, acidosis or dehydration. The risks are lower if the baby is feeding on demand; however, the very immature renal function of preterm babies requires careful calculation of fluid and electrolyte balance as Na^+-rich urine may be produced despite low plasma Na^+ levels. This can be crucial if there is high extrarenal water loss, for instance in the presence of fever or high ambient temperature.

The ability to excrete protons (hydrogen ions, H^+) is also limited, thus increasing the neonate's susceptibility to acidosis. Elimination of drugs such as antibiotics cleared by the renal system is decreased so the half-life of the drug in the circulation is increased necessitating a requirement for decreased frequency of administration. The neonate should urinate within 24 h of delivery. Initially, 15–30 mL/kg of urine is produced per day increasing to 100–200 mL/kg by day 7 as the fluid intake increases. Mature renal function is not achieved until 12 months to 2 years old.

THE NERVOUS SYSTEM

Before Birth

The fetus responds to noises, intense light, noxious stimulation of the skin and decreased temperature by changing autonomic responses such as heart rate and by moving. Fetal movements can be felt from about week 14; the 'exercise' is thought to aid muscle growth and limb development. By term, the nervous system is prepared to process and receive information. Human cortical function is relatively immature compared with that of some other mammalian species. Complete myelination of the long motor pathways occurs after birth, therefore fine movements of the fingers, for instance, are not evident until several months after birth.

After Birth

After birth, the nervous system undergoes accelerated development in response to increased sensory input. Reflexes may be slightly depressed for the first 24 h, particularly if there has been transplacental transfer of narcotic analgesia, after which several reflexes can be elicited. In cases of severe asphyxia, low Apgar scores (see p. 465) or neurological damage, reflexes are depressed, abnormal and may take longer to appear. The grasping reflex and the Moro embrace are used to assess CNS development of the newborn. Babies also demonstrate a strong palmar grasp and a rhythmic stepping movement. Many reflexes common to the neonate disappear unless there is pathological interference, in which case they may be exhibited in the adult, for example Babinski's reflex. The baby exhibits general awareness to its surroundings and reacts to sound and light.

Babies are born with active sensory pathways. Studies have demonstrated that neonates can recognize the smell of their mother's milk. They can differentiate between tastes and appear to have a preference for sweet tastes. Although babies can see at birth, there are big postnatal developments in visual capability, particularly in the first 6 months. The neonate has limited visual acuity but appears to focus at a distance of 20 cm. From birth, babies can discriminate between contrast and contours and can follow movement. The neonate is able to hear and discriminate between sounds particularly those of low- to middle-range frequency. Studies have demonstrated a neonate's ability to recognize the characteristics of their mother's voice and to demonstrate a preference for rhythmic sing-song intonation. Neonates are reassured by the rhythmic sounds of breathing, heart beat and gut peristalsis, which they hear, for instance, while being held, even more so with direct skin to skin contact. Newborn infants can be trained to activate a tape recorder by sucking non-nutritively on a modified nipple; they demonstrate that they recognize not only their mother's voice but also particular passages of a book that they were read *in utero* (Lipsitt and Rovee-Collier, 2001). The development of motor function is described by the 'Jacksonian principle', a hierarchical model whereby the last reflexes to develop are the first to be lost when the organism degenerates and dies.

SLEEP AND BEHAVIOURAL STATES

The fetus exhibits slow-wave and REM sleep between patterns of wakefulness. The neonate sleeps about 16 h per day, 40% in REM sleep, compared with a total of 12 h asleep at 2 years of age (20% in REM sleep). Sleep patterns are not diurnal and do not follow a light–dark cycle. Six sleep–wake states are recognized: quiet (deep) sleep, active (light) sleep, drowsy state, awake (quiet) alert, active alert and crying. The proportion of time in each state varies with postconceptual age. Quiet deep sleep is restful and the baby is in an anabolic state when growth hormone secretion is high, mitotic rate is high, oxygen consumption is low and there is little movement. In active sleep, the eyes are closed but the baby moves its face and extremities. Respiration and heart rate are irregular. The baby exhibits 'paradoxical' REM sleep, in which the brain activity is similar to awake states. This state is associated with learning and synapse development. The drowsy state is transitional between being awake and asleep. The eyes are open, and the baby is alert but has little movement. The baby appears to focus on visual stimuli and appears to be processing sensory information. In the active alert state, respiration rate is increased and is irregular. There are skin colour changes, much activity and the baby has increased sensitivity to stimuli. Crying is the method of communication usually in response to unpleasant stimuli. Characteristically, neonates close their eyes, grimace and make sounds. However, preterm infants may not be capable of making a noise.

At one time, it was believed that the immature degree of myelination and lack of experience meant that neonates were unable to perceive pain. In fact, not only do the anatomical and functional requirements for pain perception develop early and the fetus, preterm and term infants demonstrate similar physiological responses to the adult, but there is also evidence that pain perception is more intense and that early experience of pain has long-term developmental and behavioural consequences. Neonates are more sensitive to painful stimuli because their nervous system is immature and less able to inhibit nociceptive pain (Perry et al., 2018). Abundant sensory fibres, a functional spinal reflex, connections to the thalamus and connections to subplate neurons are evident by 20 weeks of fetal development but mature thalamocortical projections, which are involved in localization of pain, are not present until about 24 weeks. It is obviously difficult to measure and interpret pain in the fetus during gestation but many countries are introducing legislation to require consideration of possible fetal pain during intentional termination of pregnancy. In the neonate, procedures likely to cause pain cause increased levels of catecholamines and cortisol, increased heart rate and respiratory rate, metabolic rate, oxygen consumption and blood glucose levels. The rate of transmission may be slower but a probable shorter distance between the pain receptor and brain compensates for this. Assessment of pain can be difficult as pain may be expressed differently in neonates; facial expressions may be used but some babies tend to withdraw and increase passivity and sleep more in response to pain.

THE SKIN AND IMMUNE SYSTEM

The skin is the largest organ of the body; it acts as a physical barrier and is colonized by commensal (beneficial) microorganisms. The surface of the skin is covered with an 'acid mantle', a slightly acidic film derived from the mixture of sebum and sweat. The skin of a neonate initially appears relatively transparent and soft and velvety. It is important in temperature regulation, as a protective layer and as a sensory organ. Part of the appearance is due to the lack of large skin folds and localized oedema. Melanin production and pigmentation are low in the newborn so the skin is vulnerable to damage by ultraviolet rays. However, residual levels of maternal and placental hormones can produce transient pigmentation of certain skin areas, for example the genitalia. During delivery, the skin is subject to changes in blood flow and mechanical stress from the pressure of contractions and from maternal structures, which can result in abrasions and ischaemia, most commonly seen on the scalp after a cephalic presentation and delivery. Obstetric interventions, for example, fetal monitoring using scalp electrodes, scalp sampling and use of amniohooks, forceps and vacuum extraction, also compromise the integrity of the skin. Immediately after birth, most fair-skinned babies have characteristic pink coloration with blue but warm extremities.

Vernix caseosa is a superficial fatty 'cheesy' substance that coats the fetal skin from the middle of gestation and subsequently decreases as gestation progresses. Lanugo is the first generation of downy body hair that is fine and unpigmented; it appears from the 12th week and is mostly shed before birth. Vernix caseosa tends to accumulate at the sites of dense lanugo growth and is more evident on the preterm baby on the face, ears and shoulders and in folds. At term, traces of vernix are present on the brow, ears and in the skin creases. Vernix caseosa is composed of sebaceous gland secretions (sebum) and skin cells and is rich in lipids, cholesterol and protein. Its role is to protect the fetus from the amniotic fluid and to prevent loss of water and electrolytes. It provides insulation for the skin and helps to reduce friction at delivery; it is an effective antimicrobial (contains lysozyme and lactoferrin) and has proven antibacterial and antifungal properties (Taieb, 2018). It may have a growth promoting effect on the gut *in utero*. Vernix retention is associated with significantly higher skin hydration and lower skin pH. Longer exposure of the neonatal skin to vernix enhances development of the stratum corneum (outermost and most protective layer of the skin), protects the skin and enhances wound healing and favourable colonization with microorganisms. Since 2009, the WHO has recommended vernix retention for at least 6 h after birth (WHO, 2009) but this guidance is not always implemented. Humans are the only primates who produce vernix caseosa; it is rare in other mammalian species apart from semiaquatic mammals such as seals.

The barrier properties of the stratum corneum of the skin increase with increased gestational age, especially after 24 weeks. The epidermis of a preterm baby might be only five layers thick compared with ~15 layers in a term infant. A thinner epidermal layer results in increased transepidermal water loss, decreased ability to cope with friction, thermal instability because of the increased blood supply to the surface and increased permeability to microorganisms and chemicals (such as topically applied substances and reagents on clothes). Premature babies have translucent shiny red skin that becomes pinker through to the white thick skin of term infants. Drying out of the skin is a normal maturation process. Substances that interfere with the keratinization process, such as emollients, can delay the development of the skin becoming effective as a barrier. The transepidermal water loss can be limited by use of a thermal blanket, altering the air flow and maintaining an insulating layer of saturated air in contact with the skin.

The neonate is a compromised host, vulnerable to nosocomial infection (acquired from the hospital or healthcare facility). Host defence mechanisms are immature, partly because of lack of previous exposure to common organisms and partly because the neonate has limited cellular responses (see Chapter 10). Breaks in the delicate mucosa and skin from delivery and invasive obstetric procedures provide opportunities for the entry of pathogenic bacteria. In relation to formula or artificial feeding, neonates are at increased risk of developing gastrointestinal infections, which may be associated with later development of allergies and autoimmune diseases. Preterm infants, especially those of <34 weeks' gestation, are very vulnerable as they have received less maternal IgG transfer *in utero*.

At birth, the neonate leaves the more sterile fetal environment for one laden with microorganisms. The initial colonization of the skin depends on mode of delivery (Byrd et al., 2018). The skin of infants born vaginally will be colonized by bacteria from their mother's vagina, whereas the skin of those born by caesarean section will be initially colonized by microorganisms from their mother's skin. Subsequently, ingestion and inhalation provide routes for microbial colonization after birth. There is a close relationship between the profile of microorganisms colonizing the skin and the profile on the gut. The neonate's skin, umbilical cord and genitalia are colonized first, followed by the face, respiratory system and gut. The establishment of skin microbiota is affected by the amount and retention of vernix and the use of antiseptic agents and alkaline soaps. The use of detergents may affect the integrity of the skin and cause dermatitis by interfering with the acid mantle; therefore, the use of water only to clean neonatal skin is advocated. If heavy soiling is present, then the use of pH neutral products may minimize skin irritation (Taieb, 2018). Skin microbial colonization is also affected by skin-to-skin contact following birth.

CASE STUDY 15.1

During a routine visit, the midwife examines Tracy, a 3-day-old baby, who was delivered in hospital and discharged the day before. Her umbilicus appears moist and sticky so the midwife takes a swab for culture and sensitivity. Two days later it is revealed that Tracy's umbilicus has been colonized with methicillin-resistant *Staphylococcus aureus* (MRSA). The infant appears well, has been exclusively breastfed and has regained her birthweight.

- What treatment, if any, would Tracy require and what reasons could be applied to argue against the use of antibiotic therapy?
- Do you think it is necessary to try to identify the source of the infection and, if identified, what other action should be taken?
- What should the midwife do to ensure that further cross-infections do not occur?
- What factors may put Tracy and other individuals at risk?

Initially, gut colonization is with organisms that the infant comes into contact with, at and immediately after delivery (see Chapter 16). The profile of organisms is affected by the diet; breastmilk provides growth factors for the protective lactobacilli and bifidobacterium. Different patterns of colonization are seen in babies of very low birthweight and those who require feeding or ventilatory assistance or are given antibiotics. Meconium *in vivo* is usually sterile but when excreted after birth provides rich culture conditions for microorganisms. The use of antibiotics changes the pattern of bacterial colonization of the neonate and can promote the growth of resistant bacteria and, in severe cases, result in NEC.

Case study 15.1 describes an infant with a neonatal infection.

NORMAL NEONATAL TRANSITION

Much of the physiological adaptation to extrauterine life takes place during the first few hours following birth but final cardiovascular changes may take up to 6 weeks. During the first few hours, most of the fetal lung fluid is absorbed, normal lung function is established and the normal neonatal blood flow to the lungs and tissues is initiated and maintained. This results in a pattern of predictable changes, which can be monitored as changes in heart rate, respiratory pattern, gastrointestinal function and body temperature.

Neonatal transition can be considered as three discrete phases based on the respiratory changes, which underpin

neonatal adaptation (Hooper et al., 2016b). The first phase (0–30 min) is a period of reactivity; heart rate increases, respiration is irregular and fine crackles in the chest are sometimes accompanied by nasal flaring and grunting. This is followed by a phase of decreased responsiveness (30 min to 3 h), in which respiration is shallower, heart rate decreases and muscle activity is decreased but jerks, twitches and sleep may occur. The third phase is another phase of reactivity (3–8 h after birth) in which tachycardia and a labile heart rate are common, tone and colour may change and retching and vomiting may occur. Healthy infants may continue to exhibit normal signs of transition in the first 24 h of life; these may include lung crackles, a benign soft heart murmur (due to turbulent blood flow following the closure of fetal vascular shunts), tachypnoea, tachycardia and acrocyanosis. Some infants may also exhibit mild-to-moderate respiratory distress, slight temperature instability and slightly low blood sugar levels. Immediately following delivery, it is considered normal for infants to exhibit transient acrocyanosis during episodes of crying.

Delayed or suboptimal adaptation or increased signs of distress in the neonate must be identified and assessed quickly to ensure appropriate interventions are initiated. Risk factors for abnormal transition include maternal factors such as diabetes, hypertension, prolonged anaemia and maternal shock predelivery. Prenatal risk factors including growth restriction, placental problems, multiple gestation, malpresentation, drug exposure and congenital abnormalities also affect neonatal transition. Intrapartum factors such as infection, instrumental delivery, MSAF and fetal distress or factors affecting the neonate directly such as prematurity, postmaturity or birth trauma can also hinder appropriate adaptation.

Moderate-to-severe respiratory distress is indicated by intermittent grunting, nasal flaring, marked retractions of the chest wall with sternal recession, tachypnoea (respiratory rates of 100–120 breaths per min) and a prolonged need for supplemental oxygen. Persistent pulmonary hypertension of the newborn (PPHN) is due to the normal drop in PVR not occurring so there is continued shunting of blood away from the lungs in a fetal circulatory pattern. The resulting hypoxia causes further constriction of the pulmonary vessels and ongoing shunting. Mild respiratory problems such as TTN may result in acrocyanosis (dusky blue-purple skin colour), whereas more severe problems can be indicated by central cyanosis, pallor or greyness. Cyanosis is due to the presence of desaturated haemoglobin (deoxyhaemoglobin) so hypoxia can be masked by anaemia and polycythaemic babies can look cyanotic at higher oxygen saturation levels because they have more haemoglobin. Pallor might indicate anaemia. Although a soft heart murmur is common in the first 24 h

TABLE 15.2   Apgar Scores

	0	1	2
Heart rate	Absent	Slow (<100 b.p.m.)	Fast (>100 b.p.m.)
Respiratory effort	Absent	Irregular, slow	Regular, cry
Muscle tone	Limp	Some flexion in limbs	Well-flexed limbs
Reflex irritability	Nil	Grimace	Cough, cry
Colour	White, blue	Body pink, extremities blue	Completely pink

The APGAR mnemonic: Appearance, Pulse, Grimace, Activity and Respiration.

after birth, a cardiac murmur accompanied by respiratory distress, cyanosis or signs of congestive heart failure needs further investigation. Abnormal heart rate and rhythm might indicate compromised cardiovascular function. Persistent bradycardia (heart rate <80 b.p.m.) can be due to heart block associated with maternal systemic lupus erythematosus (SLE) and bradycardia during rest and sleep can indicate hypoxia and sepsis.

INITIAL EXAMINATION OF THE NEWBORN

After delivery, the baby is always examined by a midwife who, in accordance with professional legislative requirements, must refer any deviation from the normal to a medical practitioner. There is a statutory requirement to document findings, any actions and referrals made. It is good practice to perform the examination in the presence of the parents and discuss the findings with them.

The Apgar Score

The baby's condition, including mental and physical development and level of alertness, is assessed using the Apgar score (Table 15.2). 'Apgar' is named after Virginia Apgar, the doctor who developed the scoring system in 1953; the mnemonic: **A**ppearance, **P**ulse, **G**rimace, **A**ctivity and **R**espiration, can be useful in facilitating a structured assessment of extrauterine adaptation following birth. The combined Apgar score includes the five original items of the scoring system and adds points for interventions that may be required to achieve the described condition (Rüdiger, 2017). The Apgar score assesses the infant's physiological state at a specified point in time and is useful in gauging response to intervention but immediate resuscitation, if required, should always take precedent over calculating a clinical score.

Although the interpretative value of the Apgar score has been questioned mostly because of interobserver and intraobserver variability and the subjective nature of some of the components, it is a useful means of assessing a baby for the absence or presence and degree of birth asphyxia. It is quick and simple and no other test has been routinely adopted. The Apgar score assesses the baby's heart rate, respiratory effort, colour (of the skin in pale-skinned infants and of the mucous membrane in dark-skinned babies), muscle tone and reflex responses at 1 and 5 min following birth. It is repeated at 5-min intervals when active resuscitation measures are undertaken. The 1-min score may be low as the baby has been subjected to physical stress including a drop in temperature. Measurement of heart rate should be done by auscultating the heart with a stethoscope although palpating and counting the heart rate via the anterior chest wall can also be used to assess cardiac activity quickly. A heart rate of 110–150 b.p.m. is considered normal. A heart rate persistently >160 may be due to respiratory problems secondary to prolonged acidosis or sepsis. A heart rate of ≤90 may be indicative of congenital heart block, for example, associated with antiphospholipid syndrome or maternal SLE. A baby who is crying is obviously breathing in order to produce sound. Breathing can be seen easily, even on quiet babies. The respiratory rate of a healthy newborn baby is about 40–60 breaths per minute and should not be punctuated by grunting. A high-pitched or irritable cry may indicate brain damage or cerebral irritation due to oedema or haemorrhage. Rapid respirations in conjunction with chest retractions should be observed closely – early resolution is common in TTN but if prolonged may indicate sepsis and/or meconium aspiration.

The colour of the mucous membranes inside the mouth and the eyelids is assessed. If the blood flow is good, as in a healthy baby, these areas will be pink and moist. If the tissues are being deprived of oxygen, they appear purplish or navy blue if the deprivation is severe resulting in central cyanosis. Extreme pallor, when the baby has complete peripheral shutdown, is a sign of prolonged and severe oxygen deprivation. Healthy babies often appear bluish at the extremities but this may be due to cold rather than poor circulation. The face may appear congested if the cord was around the neck or if pressure from the delivery was prolonged. Pale babies may be anaemic, and polycythaemic babies (with an excess of red blood cells) tend to look very red.

The rooting reflex, turning of the head towards a touch on the cheek, is noted. Alternative reflexes include the baby curling the toes if the sole of the foot is stroked or responding with a grabbing movement if the palm of the hand is stroked (palmar grasp reflex). Abnormal responses such as the toes curling upwards (Babinski's sign) are often associated with congenital abnormalities. The Moro reflex is looked for by startling the baby. If the head is allowed to drop back a few centimetres, the baby responds by flinging the arms outwards, usually accompanied by crying.

Muscle tone is more difficult to assess. All newborn babies have poorly developed musculature and seem fairly floppy, but babies who are especially floppy because they have immature coordination do not resist limb movement. Healthy babies have flexed limbs and respond to handling; the normal procedure is to lay the baby on the midwife's hand resting on its stomach and to observe position of the limbs. In a healthy baby, the limbs are usually still and slightly outstretched whereas in a baby with poor muscle tone the limbs tend to dangle and swing freely.

A baby that needs urgent resuscitation is pale and floppy, has a sluggish, possibly absent pulse and makes no respiratory effort. This is apparent and needs an immediate response without having to calculate the Apgar score first. The Apgar score indicates the baby's capability to survive without intervention. If the Apgar score is above 7, little intervention is required, but a baby with an Apgar score of 5–7 will often need cutaneous stimulation and oxygen via a facemask. A score of 3–5 usually requires administration of oxygen via a manual resuscitation bag or equipment that allows facial oxygen to be delivered, primarily at least 5 inflation breaths are required to initially expand the alveoli, once initial inflation is achieved then cycles of positive pressure to ventilate the lungs can be performed until spontaneous respiratory effort is present. A persistent low score requires immediate active treatment usually requiring ventilation via an endotracheal tube. If no pulse is detected once inflation of the lungs has commenced, auscultation of the heart must be prompt to identify extreme bradycardia or asystole. If this is the case, cardiac massage must be commenced in conjunction with manual ventilation until cardiac rate has improved in the presence of spontaneous respiration.

Case study 15.2 describes an example of a baby possibly in need of resuscitation.

Body Measurements and Inspection

Once initial assessment is completed, further examination of the newborn can take place. The initial development and external physical check should be followed by a fuller examination about 24 h later. It is becoming more common

---

CASE STUDY 15.2

Paul is only a few seconds old. He appears blue, not moving and limp and does not respond to touch. The midwife summons help and a paediatrician is called. The paediatrician arrives 4 min later to find a healthy, well-perfused infant, crying while being held by his mother.

- Was the midwife justified in being cautious by summoning a paediatrician early?
- How many midwives in practice wait a full minute before their initial assessment of the newborn?
- What actions do you think the midwife took prior to the arrival of the paediatrician?
- What care will Paul require in the first few hours of his life and are there any specific observations that the midwives should be carrying out during this period?

---

for midwives to undertake this more detailed examination of the newborn, which traditionally was always undertaken by a paediatrician or general practitioner. This examination includes screening for common conditions such as congenital cataracts, cardiac and circulatory abnormalities, and congenital hip dysplasia (CHD). Minor physical anomalies and variations can be found in 15–20% of newborns but most are not significant; some specific anomalies may indicate an underlying medical condition or genetic syndrome. Major congenital anomalies are structural defects, such as cleft palate, gastroschisis and spina bifida, present at birth that significantly affect function or social acceptability. Minor congenital anomalies, such as birthmarks and skintags, have minimal effect on function but may have social significance particularly if they predominantly occur on the face or hands. Developmental or normal variations are found in ~4% of the population and have no functional or social significance. Chromosomal investigation may be recommended if three or more congenital anomalies are present.

The baby's weight, length and head circumference are measured and recorded; however, it is important to note that head circumference and length may change as moulding of the fetal skull and oedema in the scalp resolve following birth. Babies with birthweights above the 90th centile or below the 10th centile are at increased risk of becoming hypoglycaemic.

Examination of the genitalia allows assignation of the sex of the baby (see Chapter 5). Small genitalia may indicate underlying endocrine disorders or genetic syndromes. In male infants, the scrotum is felt for the presence of both testes and the position of the urethral exit on the penis is checked. In female babies, the vaginal and urethral orifices are inspected. Presence of meconium demonstrates patency of the anus; this may become evident on rectal temperature measurement although rectal temperature recording should be avoided, unless the baby is very cold and the core temperature needs assessing, due to the increased risk of developing NEC.

Moulding of the head, oedema of the scalp and distortion of the face are common at birth because of intrauterine pressure, the pressure imposed by the birth canal (see Chapter 13) and birth trauma. Microcephaly or macrocephaly feature in a number of syndromes and may indicate intrauterine infection such as Zika virus. The normal term infant is well endowed with subcutaneous fat and usually has vernix caseosa in the skin folds. Postmature babies may have dry and peeling skin. The fontanelles and suture lines are observed. Bulging fontanelles may indicate an increased intracranial pressure and sunken fontanelles usually indicate that the baby is dehydrated. An abnormal-shaped head indicates abnormal moulding (see Chapter 13). Eyes and ears are checked for abnormalities; the eyes should be clear and free from discharge; the eyes should be opened to observe the ocular structures including the cornea for the presence of congenital cataracts. Low-set, absent or deformed ears may be associated with chromosomal abnormalities. The baby's mouth is inspected for the presence of teeth, which can be removed, or other extraneous material. Both the soft and hard palates are checked to ensure completeness; the baby should also demonstrate a sucking reflex. Minor skin blemishes are common. Hypertrophic sebaceous glands or milia present as white spots on ~40% babies. Both these spots and 'stork marks' – minor capillary haemangiomas – usually on the nose or eyelids, disappear within a few months of delivery.

The overall morphology of the baby should be symmetrical. The insertion of the umbilicus should be central, and is checked for swellings and herniation. The nipples, of either male or female babies, may be swollen and transiently producing milk in response to circulating maternal hormones. Respiratory movement of the chest of a healthy baby should be symmetrical and the abdomen appearance rounded. The limbs are checked for equal length and free movement; short limbs can indicate achondroplasia. A single crease across the hand (Simian crease) is a common variant but occurs with higher incidence in Down syndrome. The digits are counted; extra digits (polydactyly), a curved fifth finger (clinodactyly), fused fingers (syndactyly) and webbing between the digits (partial syndactyly) are relatively common. The feet and ankles are examined for talipes and other abnormalities.

Visible signs of congenital dislocation of the hips (CDH; also known as congenital hip dislocation, CHD) are asymmetry of the pelvis, asymmetrical creases in the groin and apparent differences in leg length. Midwives may be discouraged from undertaking manipulative tests of the hips as there is a danger of malpositioning the head of the femur into the acetabular cup, which can trap the femoral blood flow resulting in necrosis of the head of the femur. Midwifery units usually have local policies, protocols and training procedures for screening the hips for congenital dislocation.

The neck is observed for shortness, webbing or folds of skin on the back of the neck; these characteristics are associated with chromosomal abnormalities, such as Turner syndrome. The spine is checked for swellings or defects and for pilonidal dimples or hairy patches, which may indicate occult spina bifida, and abnormal curvature of the spine. Before the baby is discharged from the postnatal ward, there should be confirmation that the baby is feeding normally; excretion of urine and meconium normally occurs within 24 and 48 h of delivery, respectively. Early screening is important both to reassure the parents and to detect any abnormality or problem requiring further investigation.

KEY POINTS

- Many changes must occur at birth for successful transition to neonatal life, including initiation of breathing, conversion from fetal to neonatal circulation and physiological homeostatic control of thermoregulation and metabolism.
- The transition to neonatal circulation requires closure of the fetal shunts and vasodilatation of the pulmonary circulation; oxygen is a major stimulant.
- Successful breathing requires adequate maturation of the lungs, particularly the presence of adequate surfactant and neuromuscular control, and clearance of lung fluid.

- The relatively large surface area of neonates means they are vulnerable to excessive heat loss; body temperature is maintained by heat production by brown adipose tissue (nonshivering thermogenesis). Efforts to reduce heat loss at birth are essential.
- Normal newborn infants are able to maintain adequate blood glucose levels but this may be compromised by a long or stressful labour, abnormal maternal metabolism, restricted fetal growth, prematurity and congenital abnormalities.
- Human milk compensates for the immature development of the neonatal gut (see Chapter 16).

APPLICATION TO PRACTICE

An understanding of the transition to neonatal life is important for the following reasons. Many infants require some degree of intervention to support establishment of respiration after birth. An infant who does not appear to adapt fully at birth (i.e. is cyanotic) may, for example, have an underlying cardiac defect or be suffering from sepsis.

The midwife should use her or his assessment of adaptation as part of the neonatal check and not check solely for visible abnormalities; therefore assessment of factors such as alertness, movement, muscle tone, vital signs and feeding, in the context of maternal, family and antenatal/perinatal history, is an important component of the initial and 24-h detailed examinations.

Many parents are distressed at the appearance of a baby that has just been born and need reassurance that the transition is not always completely spontaneous and that this is quite normal. An understanding of the effects of hypoxia and anoxia during labour is important in planning the subsequent care of an affected neonate following delivery.

ANNOTATED FURTHER READING

Baston H, Durward H: *Examination of the newborn: a practical guide*, ed 3, London, 2016, Routledge.
For practitioners wanting to develop their skills in undertaking examination of the newborn, this book is a comprehensive text intended for midwives, covering all aspects of the physical examination, which takes a structured step-by-step approach.

Blackburn S: *Maternal, fetal, & neonatal physiology: a clinical perspective*, ed 5, Oxford, 2018, Elsevier.
An in-depth and well-illustrated description of physiological adaptation to pregnancy and development of the fetus and neonate that draws from physiological research studies. The chapters are clearly organized by physiological systems and link physiological concepts to clinical applications, including the assessment and management of low- and high-risk pregnancies.

Campbell D, Dolby L: *Physical examination of the newborn at a glance*, Oxford, 2018, Wiley-Blackwell.
A comprehensive guide, written by midwives, to the routine examination of the neonate and subsequent full physical assessment, produced in the double-page spread format of the 'At a Glance' series with copious diagrams and succinct explanations.

Hansmann G: *Neonatal emergencies*, ed 1, Cambridge, 2009, Cambridge University Press.
This book provides a useful and easy to use reference guide to neonatal emergencies common in the first 72 h of life. It provides a multidisciplinary approach in such emergency situations including the role of the midwife.

Hooper SB, Kitchen MJ, Polglase GR, et al.: The physiology of neonatal resuscitation, *Curr Opin Pediatr* 30:187–191, 2018.
An excellent summary of the dramatic physiological changes at birth and how the stage of adaptation affects approaches to care and resuscitation in order to optimize the chances of recovery and avoid lung injury.

Johnson MH: *Essential reproduction*, ed 8, Oxford, 2018, Wiley-Blackwell.
An excellent, well-organized research-based textbook that explores comparative reproductive physiology of mammals including a chapter on the fetus and its preparations for birth.

Kenner C, Lott J: *Neonatal nursing care handbook: an evidence-based approach to conditions and procedures*, ed 2, New York, 2016, Springer.
This book is a useful reference guide providing care and guidance of the common pathological conditions seen in the neonatal unit; includes useful patient management tools and templates.

Rennie JM: *Rennie & Roberton's textbook of neonatology*, ed 5, Edinburgh, 2012, Churchill Livingstone.
This book is invaluable for practitioners who require information on congenital disorders and pathological conditions in the neonate. It covers a wide range of conditions but it is especially useful for the rarer conditions not commonly observed in clinical practice.

Sankar MJ, Chandrasekaran A, Kumar P, et al.: Vitamin K prophylaxis for prevention of vitamin K deficiency bleeding: a systematic review, *J Perinatol* 36(Suppl 1):S29–S35, 2016.
A recent systematic review, which begins with an overview of VKDB and critically evaluates the research studies giving intramuscular prophylactic vitamin K. While it raises several issues about the optimal dose and timing, the overall conclusion is that it is appropriate to administer vitamin K prophylaxis to all neonates at birth given the risks and possible outcomes of VKBD.

Schump EA: Neonatal encephalopathy: current management and future trends, *Crit Care Nurs Clin North Am* 30:509–521, 2018.
An overview of the causes and consequences of hypoxic ischaemic encephalopathy, how it is assessed and scored, and approaches to management and treatment including emerging therapies.

Shane AL, Sáinchez PJ, Stoll BJ: Neonatal sepsis, *Lancet* 390:1770–1780, 2017.
A review of the current knowledge about the pathophysiology of neonatal sepsis and the relationship with the immunological maturity and other risk factors; includes an overview of the steps in diagnosis and management.

Tappero EP, Honeyfield ME: *Physical assessment of the newborn: a comprehensive approach to the art of physical examination*, ed 6, New York, 2018, Springer.
This book gives very detailed guidance on how to systematically perform the physical examination of newborn infants. Midwives undertaking this role will find this an excellent reference book.

REFERENCES

Akseer N, Lawn JE, Keenan W, et al.: Ending preventable newborn deaths in a generation, *Int J Gynaecol Obstet* 131(Suppl 1):S43–S48, 2015.

Ananthan A, Balasubramanian H, Rao S, Patole S: Clinical outcomes related to the gastrointestinal trophic effects of erythropoietin in preterm neonates: a systematic review and meta-analysis, *Adv Nutr* 9:238–246, 2018.

Begley DJ, Firth JA, Hoult JRS: *Human reproduction and developmental biology*, 160. New York, 1978, Macmillan, p 199.

Bianchi DW: The inadvertent discovery of human fetal cell microchimerism, *Clin Chem* 64:1400–1401, 2018.

Blackburn S: *Maternal, fetal, & neonatal physiology: a clinical perspective*, ed 5, Oxford, 2018, Elsevier.

Boddy AM, Fortunato A, Wilson SM, Aktipis A: Fetal microchimerism and maternal health: a review and evolutionary analysis of cooperation and conflict beyond the womb, *Bioessays* 37:1106–1118, 2015.

Burini RC, Leonard WR: The evolutionary roles of nutrition selection and dietary quality in the human brain size and encephalization, *Nutrire* 43:19, 2018.

Byrd AL, Belkaid Y, Segre JA: The human skin microbiome, *Nat Rev Microbiol* 16:143–155, 2018.

Carobbio S, Guénantin AC, Samuelson I, et al.: Brown and beige fat: from molecules to physiology and pathophysiology, *Biochim Biophys Acta Mol Cell Biol Lipids* 1864:37–50, 2019.

Chamberlain G, Dewhurst J, Harvey D: *Illustrated textbook of obstetrics*, London, 1991, Gower Medical (Mosby), pp 14–16.

Chondronikola M, Sidossis LS: Brown and beige fat: from molecules to physiology, *Biochim Biophys Acta Mol Cell Biol Lipids* 1864:91–103, 2019.

Finnemore A, Groves A: Physiology of the fetal and transitional circulation, *Semin Fetal Neonatal Med* 20:210–216, 2015.

Fowden AL, Valenzuela OA, Vaughan OR, et al.: Glucocorticoid programming of intrauterine development, *Domest Anim Endocrinol* 56:S121–S132, 2016.

Gerson KD, O'Brien BM: Cell-free DNA: screening for single-gene disorders and determination of fetal Rhesus D genotype, *Obstet Gynecol Clin North Am* 45:27–39, 2018.

Godfrey KM, Haugen G, Kiserud T, et al.: Fetal liver blood flow distribution: role in human developmental strategy to prioritize fat deposition versus brain development, *PLoS One* 7:e41759, 2012.

Goodwin B: *Health and development: conceptions to birth*, Milton Keynes, 1997, Open University, p 259.

Haschke F, Haiden N, Thakkar SK: Nutritive and bioactive proteins in breastmilk, *Ann Nutr Metab* 69(Suppl 2):17–26, 2016.

Hillman NH, Kallapur SG, Jobe AH: Physiology of transition from intrauterine to extrauterine life, *Clin Perinatol* 39:769–783, 2012.

Hillman NH, Lam HS: Respiratory disorders in the newborn. In Wilmott R, Bush A, Deterding R, Ratjen F, editors: *Kendig's disorders of the respiratory tract in children*, ed 9, Oxford, 2019, Elsevier, pp 338–366.

Hooper SB, Binder-Heschl C, Polglase GR, et al.: The timing of umbilical cord clamping at birth: physiological considerations, *Matern Health Neonatol Perinatol* 2:4, 2016a.

Hooper SB, Te Pas AB, Kitchen MJ: Respiratory transition in the newborn: a three-phase process, *Arch Dis Child Fetal Neonatal Ed* 101:F266–F271, 2016b.

Hull D: The structure and function of brown adipose tissue, *Br Med Bull* 22:92–93, 1966.

Hung YC, Yeh JL, Hsu JH: Molecular mechanisms for regulating postnatal ductus arteriosus closure, *Int J Mol Sci* 19, 2018.

Jaffray J, Young G, Ko RH: The bleeding newborn: a review of presentation, diagnosis, and management, *Semin Fetal Neonatal Med* 21:44–49, 2016.

Jo HS: Genetic risk factors associated with respiratory distress syndrome, *Korean J Pediatr* 57:157–163, 2014.

Katheria A, Hosono S, El-Naggar W: A new wrinkle: umbilical cord management (how, when, who), *Semin Fetal Neonatal Med* 23:321–326, 2018.

Kessler J, Rasmussen S, Godfrey K, et al.: Venous liver blood flow and regulation of human fetal growth: evidence from macrosomic fetuses, *Am J Obstet Gynecol* 204:429, 2011.

Kharas H, McArthur JW, Rasmussen K: *How many people will the world leave behind? Assessing current trajectories on the Sustainable Development Goals*, Global Economy and Development at Brookings, 2018.

Koos BJ, Rajaee A: Fetal breathing movements and changes at birth, *Adv Exp Med Biol* 814:89–101, 2014.

Lipsitt LP, Rovee-Collier C: Prenatal and infant development. In Smelser NJ, Baltes PB, editors: *International encyclopedia of the social and behavioral sciences*, London, 2001, Elsevier, pp 11994–11997.

Lorigo M, Mariana M, Feiteiro J, Cairrao E: How is the human umbilical artery regulated? *J Obstet Gynaecol Res* 44:1193–1201, 2018.

McGillick EV, Orgeig S, Giussani DA, Morrison JL: Chronic hypoxaemia as a molecular regulator of fetal lung development: implications for risk of respiratory complications at birth, *Paediatr Respir Rev* 21:3–10, 2017.

Michel A, Lowe NK: The successful immediate neonatal transition to extrauterine life, *Biol Res Nurs* 19:287–294, 2017.

Morton SU, Brodsky D: Fetal physiology and the transition to extrauterine life, *Clin Perinatol* 43:395–407, 2016.

Pan DH, Rivas Y: Jaundice: newborn to age 2 months, *Pediatr Rev* 38:499–510, 2017.

Perry M, Tan Z, Chen J, et al.: Neonatal pain: perceptions and current practice, *Crit Care Nurs Clin North Am* 30:549–561, 2018.

Rei M, Ayres-de-Campos D, Bernardes J: Neurological damage arising from intrapartum hypoxia/acidosis, *Best Pract Res Clin Obstet Gynaecol* 30:79–86, 2016.

Riviere D, McKinlay CJD, Bloomfield FH: Adaptation for life after birth: a review of neonatal physiology, *Anaesth Intensive Care Med* 18:59–67, 2017.

Rüdiger M: Resuscitating neonates: 65 years after Virginia Apgar, *BMJ Paediatr Open* 1:e000195, 2017.

Shepherd E, Salam RA, Middleton P, et al.: Neonatal interventions for preventing cerebral palsy: an overview of cochrane systematic reviews, *Cochrane Database Syst Rev* 6:CD012409, 2018.

Shree R, Harrington WE, Kanaan SB, et al.: Fetal microchimerism by mode of delivery: a prospective cohort study, *BJOG* 126:24–31, 2019.

Taieb A: Skin barrier in the neonate, *Pediatr Dermatol* 35(Suppl 1):s5–s9, 2018.

Teramo KA, Klemetti MM, Widness JA: Robust increases in erythropoietin production by the hypoxic fetus is a response to protect the brain and other vital organs, *Pediatr Res* 84:807–812, 2018.

VanVooren DM, Bradshaw WT, Blake SM: Disseminated intravascular coagulation in the neonate, *Neonatal Netw* 37:205–211, 2018.

WHO: *Newborn care until the first week of life: clinical practice pocket guide*, Manila, 2009, WHO Regional Office for the Western Pacific, World Health Organization.

Wienert B, Martyn GE, Funnell APW, et al.: Wake-up sleepy gene: reactivating fetal globin for beta-hemoglobinopathies, *Trends Genet* 34:927–940, 2018.

Yli BM, Kjellmer I: Pathophysiology of foetal oxygenation and cell damage during labour, *Best Prac Res Clin Obstet Gynaecol* 30:9–21, 2016.

Lactation and Infant Nutrition

INTRODUCTION

Infant feeding is the result of multifaceted interactions between infant nutritional demand and maternal physiology and behaviour. The physiological basis of lactation is important in understanding and facilitating successful breastfeeding. Successful lactation depends on extensive breast tissue growth and differentiation in pregnancy. Despite increased awareness of the health benefits of human milk, many women discontinue breastfeeding because they perceive that they have an insufficient milk supply and/or the baby is not satisfied. Most breastfeeding problems have identifiable physiological, rather than pathological, causes and should be addressed by considering the interactions between the mother and the baby. Successful breastfeeding has nutritional, emotional, behavioural developmental and economic benefits. It can be argued that the nutrient requirement of the infant is one of the best understood areas of nutrition; it is the only time when it is possible to absolutely determine optimal nutritional requirements. Human milk, however, does not just provide the optimal balance of nutrients in a form appropriate to the developmental needs of the infant, it also compensates for the immature digestive capability, the vulnerable immune status of the neonate, and promotes the colonization of the gut by beneficial microbiota, which may have life-long positive effects on health.

Breast milk is a complex biological fluid that provides for the optimal growth, development, and protection of the neonate. Short-term benefits are a result of the immunological properties of breast milk and protection against infectious diseases. Medium-term benefits are that breastfeeding is associated with a lower incidence of inflammatory bowel diseases (IBD), type 1 diabetes and childhood cancers. In addition, there are long-term benefits; health in later life appears to be improved in those individuals who were breastfed as infants. There are also benefits for the mother (see Box 16.9).

Breastfeeding is universally agreed to be one of the most effective preventative measures of reducing the morbidity and mortality rate of children under 5 years of age.

CHAPTER CASE STUDY

Almost immediately following his birth, Zara placed Zak in her arms and he instinctively latched onto the breast and started feeding before his cord was cut. Zak fed on the breast for over 45 min before detaching himself.
- What are the advantages of offering the baby the breast as soon as possible after delivery for both mother and baby?
- What factors could have a negative influence on the early establishment of breastfeeding and how can the midwife optimize breastfeeding?
- What factors during labour and delivery may have affected Zak's ability to breastfeed; how would the midwife identify these factors and what potential interventions might mediate against them.

As mentioned in Chapter 3, it was recently estimated that if breastfeeding could be increased worldwide to near-universal levels, >800,000 lives could be saved each year, mostly of children under 5 years of age, as well as >20,000 deaths prevented per annum from breast cancer in mothers (Victora et al., 2016). Breastfeeding also contributes to birth spacing.

ANATOMY OF THE BREAST

Mammary glands are unique to mammals; they synthesize, secrete and deliver milk to the neonate. Milk is species-specific and uniquely appropriate to provide for the different nutritional, protection and developmental needs of the offspring that it is produced for. Both the biochemical and cellular composition of milk and the lactational strategies employed have evolved to be optimal for the specific species.

The adult human breast is a complex mammary gland, made up of 15–20 irregular lobes separated by connective tissue. The tissue of each breast overlie the pectoralis major muscles, extending from about the second to the sixth rib (depending on posture). The breasts are roughly symmetrical. Most of the variation in size and shape of breasts is due to differences in the amount of adipose and connective tissue content; there is less variation in the proportions of glandular or lactational tissue.

The breast tissue is tear-shaped. The extension of the tail of the tissue into the axilla (Fig. 16.1) can result in discomfort in the early puerperium when it may become swollen. The mammary gland is made up of a branching network of ducts ending in lobular–alveolar clusters, which are the sites of milk synthesis and secretion. Each breast is divided into sections or lobes by fibrous septae, which run from behind the nipple towards the pectoralis muscle. These septae are important in localizing infections, which are often visually evident as a wedge of red inflamed skin on the surface of the breast. Each of the 15–20 lobes, separated by connective tissue, contains glandular tissue composed of clusters of alveoli and small ducts (Fig. 16.2). The alveolar secretory cells are grouped in grape-like lobules around an extensive branching system of small ducts, which lead to the nipple. Adipose tissue is located between the lobes. The widely held view that milk ducts swell under the areola to form engorged lactiferous sinuses where milk is stored was revised by seminal research studies, which used ultrasound imaging of the breast during feeding; this showed no discernible lactiferous sinuses in the human breast and that the ducts, even close to the nipple, can branch and be very small and compressible (Ramsay et al., 2005). It is thought that the misconception that

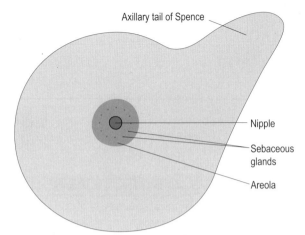

Fig. 16.1 The position of the breast.

the ducts formed storage sinuses came from the techniques used by anatomists in the 1800s; hot coloured wax was injected into the breasts of cadavers of lactating women and, retrospectively, it seems very likely that the wax damaged and distorted the delicate duct structure. The nipple is central to and surrounded by the areola, a roughly circular area of pigmented skin varying in size, which becomes increasingly pigmented during pregnancy (see Chapter 11). It has a rich vascular supply and sensory innervation from mechanoreceptors. Surrounding the nipple are Montgomery's tubercles (or Montgomery's glands), which are sebaceous glands that hypertrophy and become prominent during pregnancy, providing lubrication and protection. Heavy use of soap can increase the risk of nipple damage, particularly drying and cracking as it can strip the skin of natural emollients. The sensitivity of the nipple and surrounding area increases markedly immediately after delivery. Suckling results in an influx of afferent nerve impulses to the hypothalamus controlling lactation and maternal behaviour through the pulsatile release of prolactin and oxytocin.

Each lobe consists of 20–40 lobules, each containing 10–100 alveoli, the glandular secretory units. The mammary epithelial cells (MECs) that surround the alveolar lumen are cuboidal in the resting nonpregnant breast and change remarkably to develop complex secretory features during lactation. These cells secrete milk into the lumen and are surrounded by oxytocin-sensitive myoepithelial (contractile) cells, which are important in milk ejection. The ducts are also surrounded by myoepithelial cells that relax to allow the ducts to open and then contract to increase the flow of milk towards the nipple during the milk ejection reflex.

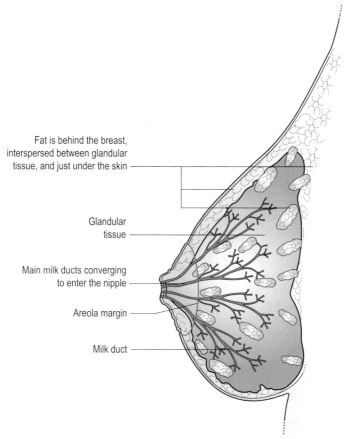

Fat is behind the breast, interspersed between glandular tissue, and just under the skin

Glandular tissue

Main milk ducts converging to enter the nipple

Areola margin

Milk duct

Fig. 16.2 Anatomy of the human breast. (Reproduced with permission from Ramsay et al., 2005.)

BREAST GROWTH AND DEVELOPMENT

Mammary growth and development can be divided into four phases: resting, development (pregnancy), milk secreting (lactation) and involution. At birth, breast structures in the neonate are simply the nipple and a few small rudimentary ducts, with few or no alveoli, reflecting their evolutionary origin as modified apocrine or sweat glands. Until puberty, the only degree of development may be a little branching of the ducts.

The human is unusual, even compared with other primates, in having extensive breast development at puberty, rather than solely during pregnancy, which has been assumed to have an erotic significance, though it is also suggested that it hides the presence of early pregnancy (see Chapter 5). The increase in oestrogen secretion by the ovaries at puberty triggers a proliferation of the milk ducts, which elongate, sprout and branch with further contributions from growth hormone (GH) and adrenal hormones.

The modest alveolar development at this stage is stimulated by progesterone, providing the tissue has been primed by oestrogen. Prolactin may also play a role although the interaction between the adrenal and pituitary glands and the ovaries is not fully understood. The hormonal fluctuations of the menstrual cycle give repeated exposure of the tissue to oestrogen and progesterone, which allow additional but limited growth. Many nonpregnant women experience cyclical changes, especially premenstrually, in breast volume, which is associated with water retention. Occasionally, some secretory activity may occur within the alveoli and a mammary secretion may be expressed premenstrually.

The human mammary gland does not reach a physiologically and functionally mature state until it is exposed to a pregnancy–lactation cycle (PLC) and undergoes extensive remodelling into a milk-secretory unit (Hassiotou and Geddes, 2013). This cycle will be repeated with each pregnancy but once the breast tissue has been through a PLC, minimal stimulation in the future is required to begin milk secretion even if there is no pregnancy. Lactation can be induced, usually with pharmacological and physical support, in women who are not the biological mothers and relactation (a return to lactation in women who have ceased breastfeeding) can be stimulated (Box 16.1). It is thought that this is an evolutionary advantage, particularly for a strongly social species or where there might be high risks of maternal mortality. Allomaternal nursing (breastfeeding by women other than the natural mother) is common in some human cultures (Burkart et al., 2017); humans are cooperative breeders and engage in cooperative childcare.

Growth in breast size is most marked in early pregnancy (see Chapter 11). Fewer hormonal stimuli are required for human breast development during pregnancy than in other species with neither human placental lactogen (hPL) nor GH being essential.

In early pregnancy, breast size and areolar pigmentation increase. The tubercles of Montgomery enlarge and the nipples become more erect. Blood flow to the breast doubles so blood vessels become more prominent and the skin may appear to have a translucent marbled appearance and feel warmer to the touch. There is a sharp increase in ductal and glandular elements so the breasts often feel slightly lumpy in early pregnancy. This initial increase in cell number (hyperplasia) is followed by an increase in alveolar cell size (hypertrophy) and initiation of secretory activity in later pregnancy.

BOX 16.1   Relactation

Relactation, or induced lactation, is the process whereby lactation is initiated at a time not associated with birth. For instance, an adoptive mother who has not borne a child may wish to breastfeed her adopted baby or a mother may want to resume feeding her own child. Relactation is easier if the woman has previously lactated or been pregnant and if the infant is young. Hormonal support such as oxytocin nasal sprays may be used. The woman is usually advised to eat well and rest, and to stimulate the nipple and breast often, either by hand or with a breast pump. Supplementary formula milk can be given to the baby by spoon or dropper; bottle teats and dummies are avoided. Use of a 'Lact-Aid' device may be found helpful. This device allows the baby to feed on formula milk from a tube attached to the mother's nipple. As the baby feeds, it stimulates the nipple and increases endogenous prolactin secretion. The formula milk is in a bag maintained at body temperature because it is in contact with the mother's body. As breast milk production increases, the amount of supplementary formula milk can be reduced.

Oestrogen plays the dominant role in development of the ducts and progesterone in the development of glandular tissue, although insulin and other growth factors, such as epidermal growth factor (EGF) and transforming growth factor alpha (TGFα), have a role in regulation. Changes in pregnancy depend on the lactogenic hormones, prolactin and hPL, with placental oestrogen and progesterone playing important modulatory roles. Under these hormonal influences, proliferation of alveolar and ductal cells gives rise to prominent lobules, resembling bunches of grapes. The lumens of the alveoli become dilated by mid-pregnancy and the secretory cells become fully differentiated (Box 16.2). The areola becomes pigmented and a secondary patchily and often darkly pigmented areola may also develop. The nipple enlarges and becomes more mobile and protractile, as the connective tissue anchorages soften and become more stretchable with the oestrogen-driven increase in hydration (see Chapter 11). By the 4th month of pregnancy, the alveolar cells have begun to accumulate substantial amounts of secretory material and the mammary glands are morphologically developed. Subsequently, the alveolar cells undergo secretory differentiation, as lactogenic genes are expressed, to become secretory MECs (also known as lactocytes). Prolactin levels progressively increase throughout the pregnancy and are maximal at term.

Although it is possible to express some breast secretions throughout pregnancy, this is not true colostrum. Full colostrum and milk production are inhibited by high progesterone levels so copious milk production is not established until after parturition. Placental hPL may also contribute to blocking of prolactin responses in pregnancy. It is becoming increasingly common for women to 'harvest' or express colostrum antenatally, usually after 37 weeks of pregnancy, and freeze it, so it can be used postnatally as a

---

BOX 16.2   Changes to the Breasts in Pregnancy

- Increased vascularization – may cause tingling
- Dilatation of superficial veins – fair skin appears 'marbled' and warmer to touch
- Hypertrophy – full development of lobules
- Dilatation of alveoli and ducts – may feel nodular
- Thickening of nipple skin
- Pigmentation of nipple and areolar – persists after pregnancy
- Secondary areola may appear in dark-skinned women
- Montgomery's tubercles become prominent
- Small quantity of clear colostrum can be expressed in latter half of pregnancy

supplement to feeding. While in normal healthy straightforward pregnancies this should not be necessary, there may be some advantages for the neonates of diabetic mothers, multiple births, or infants with gestational abnormalities diagnosed *in utero*.

The increase in glucocorticoids that occurs in association with the raised levels of free placental corticotrophin releasing hormone prior to the onset of labour (see Chapter 13) is also important for the breast secretory activity and milk synthesis and secretion (Napso et al., 2018). Glucocorticoids play a significant role in cell maturation such as the formation of rough endoplasmic reticulum and tight junctions, which are required for milk synthesis and secretion. They are also involved in the regulation of milk protein gene expression and the maintenance of secretory cell differentiation and lactation by preventing the second phase of involution.

PHYSIOLOGY OF LACTATION

Mammary differentiation and milk secretion are coordinated by the endocrine system and involve three categories of hormones: reproductive hormones, which change during reproductive development and affect mammary gland development and coordinated milk delivery; metabolic hormones, which regulate metabolic responses to nutrient intake or stress; and mammary hormones produced by the lactating mammary gland (Neville et al., 2002).

Lactation can be considered as two phases: lactogenesis, the initiation of lactation; and galactopoiesis (sometimes referred to as lactogenesis stage 3), the maintenance of milk secretion. Lactogenesis itself has two stages. Stage 1 may begin up to 12 weeks before parturition and is the enzymatic and cellular differentiation of the MECs. This results in colostrum formation, and uptake of immunoglobulins prior to parturition but very little milk synthesis and secretion. Lactogenesis stage 2 is the onset of copious secretion of all milk components about 2–4 days after parturition, following detachment from placental

progesterone at parturition and concurrent stimulation by prolactin and cortisol. These orchestrated changes result in breast engorgement and increased blood flow to the breast to support secretory activity. Even if very small amounts of the placenta or fetal membranes are retained after delivery, lactation is inhibited (see Chapters 13 and 14) until these are surgically removed by dilation and curettage. Stage 2 lactogenesis is normally robust but may be delayed with stressful deliveries, in poorly controlled diabetes and in obese women (Nommsen-Rivers, 2016). Overweight and obese women have delayed milk secretory activity, possibly related to prolactin resistance and decreased insulin sensitivity. Studies in obese rodents have identified abnormal mammary gland structure, impaired mammary gland development during puberty, defects in areolar development, accumulation of lipids in MECs (consistent with secretory inactivation) and inflammation (Lee and Kelleher, 2016). Obesity is associated with leptin resistance and therefore higher leptin levels than normal; leptin inhibits the effect of oxytocin on myoepithelial cell contraction. The increased adipocyte number can increase local production of oestrogen, which may suppress lactation (as it does in pregnancy) by downregulating the prolactin signalling pathways. Maternal obesity is associated with a lower breastfeeding rates; obesity affects breastfeeding intention, time taken to initiate lactation and duration of exclusive and any breastfeeding (Marshall et al., 2019).

Other factors associated with delayed lactogenesis are increasing maternal age, large infant birthweight (>3.6 kg), use of formula milk (especially >60 mL in the first 48 h of life), lower maternal educational status, low Apgar scores (see Chapter 15) and caesarean section.

Once lactation commenced, removal of milk is essential to its maintenance. This is orchestrated by prolactin, which stimulates milk production and oxytocin, and which is involved in the milk ejection reflex (Table 16.1, see Fig. 16.4). Starting breastfeeding within 1 h from birth, and the frequency of breastfeeding in the first 2–3 days postpartum, are essential to establishing optimal lactation. Maternal

TABLE 16.1	**Prolactin and Oxytocin**	
Source	**Anterior Pituitary Gland**	**Posterior Pituitary Gland (but Synthesized in Hypothalamus)**
Primary control	Lifting of dopamine inhibition	Neural pathway
Modulating factors	Positively stimulated by oestrogen, TSH, VIP	Neurotransmitters
Peak response	30 min	30 s
Stimulus	Suckling	Suckling, sound, sight and thought of baby
Target cell	Alveolar cell	Myoepithelial cell
Effect	Milk synthesis	Milk ejection

TSH, thyroid-stimulating hormone; *VIP*, vasoactive intestinal peptide.

perception of inadequate milk supply may influence mothers to augment breastfeeding with formula milk, which interferes with the establishment of lactogenesis and galactopoiesis and the demand-feed production cycle of breastfeeding. Offering supplementary food or liquids other than breast milk in the first days of life can have adverse effects on establishing lactation. This is a common occurrence and should be discouraged unless there are recognized pathological features in the mother–baby dyad. Women at risk of lactational failure need careful support and encouragement in the initiation of breastfeeding. Women whose babies suckle frequently should be reassured that this is an important component in establishing lactation and does not mean their milk supply is adequate. If it is the case, it is important to ensure that correct positioning is used to optimize suckling and reduce nipple soreness and trauma from friction due to suboptimal latching on. One of the most important strategies to optimize successful breastfeeding is for it to be initiated well within the first hour after delivery (UNICEF-WHO, 2018). This is also beneficial to the mother as it is associated with less blood loss. Skin-to-skin contact immediately after birth has been found to be positively associated with successful breastfeeding.

Prolactin

Prolactin (PRL) is a pleiotropic hormone with different isoforms and complex functionality, which includes important roles in both breast development during pregnancy and in stimulating milk production and MEC function during lactation. Suckling results in the firing of afferent impulses from the nipple via the anterolateral columns of the spinal cord to the brain stem and hypothalamus. The hypothalamus subsequently decreases release of dopamine (formerly described as prolactin inhibitory factor) into the portal circulation to the pituitary gland. It was postulated that a dopamine-stimulating factor existed but, although several hormones positively modulate prolactin secretion, control is largely by the lifting of the tonic inhibition from dopamine. The abrogation of the dopamine inhibition stimulates the release of prolactin from the lactotroph cells of the anterior pituitary. Secretion of prolactin by lactotrophs is modified by oestrogen and thyroid-stimulating hormone (TSH). Studies in rats have demonstrated that vasoactive intestinal peptide (VIP), released from the pituitary gland, is an extremely potent prolactin-releasing factor and affects mammary blood flow. The number of signals affecting prolactin release indicates a complex neuroendocrine axis. β-Endorphin and melanocyte-stimulating hormone (MSH), which are co-released from the intermediate lobe of the pituitary gland, also seem to have a role. β-Endorphin stimulates prolactin secretion and blocks dopamine inhibition of prolactin release (Crowley, 2015),

and MSH stimulates the release of prolactin by lowering the threshold of the lactotrophs (Seoane et al., 2018).

Levels of prolactin begin to rise within 10 min of suckling, peak about 30 min after initial stimulation and then progressively fall back to basal levels within a further 3 h. This delay in prolactin secretion following suckling led to the concept that the rise in prolactin was the 'order for the next meal'. This also fits with the mode of action of prolactin to stimulate milk protein gene transcription; this would necessitate a delay while new proteins are synthesized and processed by the MECs. Prolactin in also internalized after binding to receptors on the basolateral surface of these cells and transcytosed into the lumen, with the secreted milk. Areolar stimulation is essential for prolactin release; negative pressure alone is not adequate and denervation of the nipple prevents prolactin release in response to nipple stimulation.

Prolactin levels fall abruptly about 2 h before delivery then dramatically rebound. These fluctuations in prolactin level probably relate to changing oestrogen concentrations. The level of prolactin seems to be important in establishing lactation but levels are much diminished after 6 weeks at a rate dependent on suckling frequency and duration. The peak prolactin levels in response to suckling also fall progressively.

Prolactin has a pulsatile pattern of release and a diurnal rhythm of secretion with higher circulating levels during sleep. Prolactin is critical for lactation but the exact quantitative relationship between prolactin levels and milk produced is not clear (Powe et al., 2010a). The dopamine D_2 receptor agonist, bromocriptine, will inhibit prolactin secretion and abolish milk secretion at any stage of lactation, even when prepregnant prolactin levels have been re-established after prolonged breastfeeding. Dopamine-receptor blockers (such as metoclopramide, haloperidol, domperidone and sulpiride) increase prolactin levels and milk production. The use of drugs that stimulate prolactin should be the last resort after excluding all the other factors that might negatively affect milk supply such as checking the positioning of the infant. All the drugs have a risk of side-effects. Domperidone, a selective D_2 dopamine receptor antagonist used as a prescription antiemetic drug, is usually preferred because it has a lower risk of toxicity since its transfer into the breast milk is extremely low and it does not cross the blood–brain barrier (it has a large molecular weight, is less soluble and is usually bound to proteins). However, it has been recommended that pharmaceutical galactagogue medications should only be considered for mothers who have received full lactation support and still have insufficient breast milk 14 days after delivery (Donovan and Buchanan, 2012). Domperidone causes hyperprolactinaemia by blocking the receptors for dopamine, which acts to inhibit prolactin release by the pituitary gland.

Prolactin binds to receptors on the MEC to increase the expression of genes for milk proteins, stimulate the synthesis of lactose and have other effects, including the maintenance of tight junction integrity. During pregnancy, MECs proliferate and acquire the characteristics of highly active secretory cells including numerous mitochondria, an extensive endoplasmic reticulum, well-developed Golgi apparatus and many secretory vesicles.

Early suckling is important to stimulate prolactin to ensure that milk production is optimal and sustained. This is the underlying physiological reason why breast-feeding soon after birth and certainly within the first 45–60 min has such a positive impact. The first hour of life is called the 'Golden Hour'. There are a number of initiatives, which aim to increase the number of babies fed in the first hour of life such as the annual World Breastfeeding Week (WBW), which adopts a theme such as 'Breastfeeding: the foundation of life' or 'Breastfeeding: a key to sustainable development', the Baby-friendly Hospital Initiative (BFHI) focusing on 'Ten Steps to Successful Breastfeeding' (Box 16.3) and UNICEF's global campaign 'Every Child ALIVE'. Despite this, three in five babies worldwide are not breastfed in the first hour, increasing the risk that they will not be breastfed at all and putting them at higher risk of death and disease (UNICEF-WHO, 2018). Breastfeeding protects against the three preventable conditions that account for >80% of newborn deaths: complications that arise during labour, complications related to prematurity and infections such as sepsis, pneumonia and meningitis. As the UNICEF poignantly expresses it: 'We are failing the world's youngest citizens'.

Successful breastfeeding in the first hour is more likely in low- and middle-income countries. One in five babies in high-income countries are never breastfed, compared with one in 25 in low- and middle-income countries. Waiting between 2 and 23 h after birth to start breastfeeding increases the risk of infant death by 30%; waiting >24 h more than doubles the risk of infant death. Babies are born physiologically ready to breastfeed. Initiating breastfeeding is best accomplished with good support (the presence of skilled birth attendants) and guidance on positioning and feeding. Mothers who give birth to preterm infants or have a caesarean section are particularly in need of good support.

Infrequent and/or poor suckling in the early postnatal period may significantly reduce the optimal long-term milk production, as less prolactin receptor complexes are formed so stimulation of the acinar cells is suboptimal and the potential for milk production is reduced.

> ### BOX 16.3 Ten Steps to Successful Breastfeeding (WHO, 2018)
>
> **Critical Management Procedures**
> 1a. Comply fully with the *International Code of Marketing of Breast-milk Substitutes* and relevant World Health Assembly resolutions.
> 1b. Have a written infant feeding policy that is routinely communicated to staff and parents.
> 1c. Establish ongoing monitoring and data-management systems.
> 2. Ensure that staff have sufficient knowledge, competence and skills to support breastfeeding.
>
> **Key Clinical Practices**
> 3. Discuss the importance and management of breastfeeding with pregnant women and their families.
> 4. Facilitate immediate and uninterrupted skin-to-skin contact and support mothers to initiate breastfeeding as soon as possible after birth.
> 5. Support mothers to initiate and maintain breastfeeding and manage common difficulties.
> 6. Do not provide breastfed newborns any food or fluids other than breast milk, unless medically indicated.
> 7. Enable mothers and their infants to remain together and to practise rooming-in 24 h a day.
> 8. Support mothers to recognize and respond to their infants' cues for feeding.
> 9. Counsel mothers on the use and risks of feeding bottles, teats and pacifiers.
> 10. Coordinate discharge so that parents and their infants have timely access to ongoing support and care.

It is important to support and reassure mothers whose infants frequently suckle in the early postnatal period that this is a positive process that promotes prolactin release and establishes long-term breastfeeding, rather than reflecting an inadequate milk supply (see Case study 16.1). Introduction of formula feeds, in the belief that the infant may be too hungry to wait for breastfeeding to be initiated, significantly interferes with the establishment of lactation. Initiation of breastfeeding is affected by the duration of labour, mode of delivery, Apgar score at 1 min, skin-to-skin contact (SSC or S2S) and whether the infant is admitted into neonatal intensive care facilities (Lau et al., 2018). In the first few hours after birth, spontaneous suckling is facilitated by maternal–neonatal skin-to-skin contact, which also shortens the duration of the third stage of labour and reduces the prevalence of hypothermia (Safari et al., 2018).

Lactation insufficiency can result from several causes and may affect up to 15% of first-time mothers. A minority of such cases are due to very low prolactin production resulting in very low levels of milk production. In mothers where prolactin deficiency is due to low lactotroph numbers such as in postpartum pituitary gland necrosis (Sheehan syndrome), dopamine antagonists such as domperidone will not function. A possible future treatment for these mothers is exogenous prolactin administration using recombinant human prolactin. In very premature deliveries where neonates are unable to suckle, removal of milk via manual expression and/or with a breast pump is recommended but often results in decreased milk production in the longer term because the milk expression does not replicate the physiological impact of the infant feeding.

Dysphoric milk ejection reflex (D-MER) is a condition where the breastfeeding woman experiences recurrent and transient dysphoria (negative feelings and loneliness, ranging from wistfulness to intense self-loathing) when she breastfeeds; it is thought to be due to the sudden fall in dopamine levels when suckling starts (Heise and Wiessinger, 2011). Women who experience this condition need a lot of support; it is possible that failure to recognize D-MER may be a major contribution to the women abandoning breastfeeding in the early postnatal period. This condition may also contribute to postpartum 'baby blues' and mood disturbance (see Chapter 14). Little research has been carried out in D-MER but it may be much more common than conditions such as Sheehan syndrome and galactosaemia. As well as the dopamine-antagonist drugs, there are a number of herbal galactagogues that have been traditionally used to promote milk production; these include fenugreek (*Trigonella foenumgraecum*) seeds; fennel (*Foeniculum vulgare*); brewer's yeast; alfalfa; shatavi (*Asparagus racemosus*); garlic (*Allium sativum*); milk thistle (*Silbum marianum* or *silymarin*); malunggay (*Moringa oleifera*); chasteberry (*Vitx agnus castus*); goat's rue (*Galega officinalis*); rescue remedy and Ignatia 6x (Bazzano et al., 2016). There is a lack of scientific evidence, such as randomized placebo-controlled trials, for the effectiveness of these herbal galactagogues (Mortel and Mehta, 2013), and being herbal does not mean they are harmless. Some volatile components of herbal galactagogues enter the breast milk and may have a sedating effect on the infant. Poor quality control means that herbal galactagogues may be contaminated with heavy metals or microorganisms. Brewer's yeast, which is easily available in most supermarkets and is often recommended as an ingredient in lactation cookies, is often contaminated with ochratoxin A (OTA), which is a possible human carcinogen and nephrotoxin (Munoz et al.,

2014). Interest in herbal galactagogues has increased, possibly because of the current trends related to maternal health such as increased prevalence of obesity, high rates of caesarean section and older age of pregnancy. Smoking may also affect prolactin production.

Biosynthesis of Milk

The secretory cells of the alveoli (Fig. 16.3) synthesize, or extract from maternal blood, the components of milk, which are then secreted into the alveolar lumen (Truchet and Honvo-Houeto, 2017) These MECs or lactocytes form a strong epithelium, resistant to the stretching that accompanies milk accumulation, with anchoring junctions on their lateral surfaces connecting the cytoskeletons of adjacent cells and tight junctions near to their apical surface, restricting the flow of solutes through the paracellular space between adjacent cells. The apical plasma membrane has a smooth surface with microvilli, in contrast to the tightly folded basal membrane, which facilitates uptake of substrates such as amino acids, glucose, acetate and fatty acids from the extracellular space. Proteins, lactose and triglycerides are synthesized in the cell and packaged, respectively into secretory vesicles or lipid droplets, which are transported to the apical membrane of the cell where they are secreted into the alveolar lumen. Milk proteins include casein and α-lactalbumin, which are specific to milk, with an estimated 976 different proteins being present in the milk proteome (Molinari et al., 2012). Many of these proteins have important roles in immune protection of the neonate. For example, lactoferrin, an iron-binding glycoprotein, also has important antimicrobial properties.

The MECs have a unique mechanism for lipid secretion, whereby the small lipid droplets released from the endoplasmic reticulum coalesce to form progressively larger lipid droplets and finally milk fat globules (MFGs). These MFGs are enclosed in a specialized milk fat globule membrane (MFGM), prior to release across the apical membrane into the lumen by a process of 'budding'. The MFGM prevents the fat globules from coalescing into large fat droplets that would be difficult to secrete and very difficult for the infant to digest. For example, it is the disruption of these MFGMs that allows milk to be churned into butter suggesting that without the MFGM, the neonate would be tasked with digesting a butter-like fat content. Another important function of the MFGM is that it is the primary dietary source of phospholipids and cholesterol for the breastfed infant.

The composition of the maternal diet can influence the components of breast milk, especially those components passing directly from the maternal blood to the milk, with little modification by the MEC such as lipids,

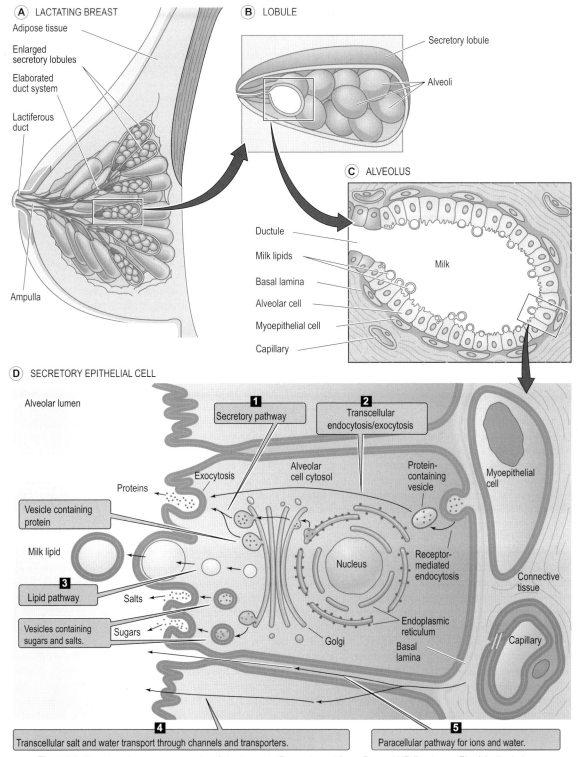

Fig. 16.3 The alveolar secretory cells of the breast. (Reproduced from Boron WF, Boulpaep EL, *Medical physiology: a cellular and molecular approach*, updated 2 ed, Elsevier 2012, Fig. 56.11.)

most of which are triglycerides. Aqueous solutes including proteins, oligosaccharides, lactose, citrate, phosphate and calcium are secreted into the milk by exocytosis after being packaged into secretory vesicles by the Golgi apparatus. Macromolecular substances derived from maternal serum, such as serum proteins (IgA, albumin and transferrin), endocrine hormones (insulin, prolactin and oestrogen), cytokines and lipoprotein lipase, are transported by a transcytosis pathway. Various membrane transport pathways transfer small molecules and ions, such as glucose transporters, amino acid transporters and the water transporter aquaporin. Blood cells and serum follow a paracellular route, squeezing between the cells of the alveoli through the paracellular pathway via the tight junctions.

The milk-specific disaccharide, lactose, is produced in the lumen of the Golgi apparatus of the MEC and trapped within, since it is membrane impermeable. The resulting increase in osmolarity draws water into the Golgi vesicles, which contributes to fluidity of the milk. In addition to free calcium and calcium salts, secretory vesicles containing casein micelles also transport calcium into the alveolar lumen to provide a concentration of up to 8 mM calcium in milk, which is important for neonatal bone development.

Oxytocin

Oxytocin levels control the milk ejection reflex, which is responsible for the transfer of the milk from the breast to the baby. Suckling by the neonate is rapidly detected by mechanoreceptors in the areola of the nipple. Neural signals are sent via cholinergic afferent neurons to the hypothalamus, which triggers the secretion of oxytocin from the posterior pituitary. Oxytocin acts via G-protein-coupled receptors on the myoepithelial cells that surround each alveolus to stimulate their contraction (see Fig. 16.3), so that milk can be ejected into the ducts that also shorten and widen. Oxytocin receptors are also present in MECs and uterine myocytes (Chapter 13). Although secretion of oxytocin is under a similar neuroendocrine reflex to prolactin, it is physiologically independent. Oxytocin synthesis in the hypothalamus, and its release from the posterior lobe of the pituitary gland, is also increased in response to handling the baby, hearing cries or thinking about feeding as well as by tactile stimulation at the nipple. Oxytocin release is pulsatile, with short-lived bursts of less than a minute immediately in response to stimuli. Frequently, the largest response is to the baby crying before feeding, so maximum release of oxytocin may occur before suckling even starts. Between feeds, isolated pulses of oxytocin

are released possibly in response to other babies' cries or fleeting images of the baby. Unlike prolactin secretion, the milk ejection reflex can be conditioned, as demonstrated by dairy farmers who clang their buckets to stimulate oxytocin and a good milk yield. Similarly, a baby's cry can often trigger oxytocin secretion, which is why the practice of babies 'rooming-in' with their mothers (sleeping close to their mother's bed) is often associated with successful breastfeeding.

The milk ejection reflex is very sensitive to inhibition by physical and psychological stresses such as pain and discomfort, anxiety, emotional swings, tiredness, embarrassment, worry and alcohol. Women who have had long labours, high levels of intervention and traumatic deliveries may be particularly at risk of impaired oxytocin production. In addition, the use of oxytocin to augment labour and actively manage the third stage of labour may reduce endogenous oxytocin levels in the early postnatal period and also affect the milk ejection reflex (Sriraman, 2017). The limbic system, which coordinates the body's responses to emotions, is involved in oxytocin release. The likely mechanism is catecholamine inhibition of oxytocin release and adrenergic vasoconstriction of mammary blood vessels limiting access of the oxytocin to the myoepithelial cells. Women experiencing problems in establishing milk flow are often helped by covering their breasts with warm flannels, which appears to aid blood flow and oxytocin access. Women may be embarrassed by exposing their breasts or being touched by practitioners helping them to establish breastfeeding and so a 'hands-off' approach must be adopted while focusing on maintaining privacy and dignity and minimizing inhibition. Psychological distress can adversely affect the success of lactation and affect milk ejection and subsequently milk synthesis so stress reducing interventions such as relaxation therapy might improve milk yield and infant outcome (Mohd Shukri et al., 2018).

Surprisingly, denervation of mammary glands in experimental animals appears to have little effect on milk production (Sriraman, 2017). This suggests that the afferent nerve pathway may not be as important as the interactions of neurotransmitters. Transmitters that have been implicated in the control of the milk ejection reflex include noradrenaline, β-endorphin, serotonin and dopamine. As with control of prolactin secretion, the number of factors influencing oxytocin secretion suggests that the pathway is much more complicated than originally thought. Stimulation of the female reproductive tract, especially the vagina and cervix, increases oxytocin release so milk may be ejected from the breasts during coitus.

Oxytocin also binds to receptors on the longitudinal cells in the duct walls. Contraction of the myoepithelial cells results in milk being expelled into the ducts, which shorten as the longitudinal cells contract causing an increase in pressure in the ducts and a faster flow rate towards the nipple. Oxytocin-induced contraction generates pressure waves within the breasts and is responsible for the prickly sensations associated with breastfeeding. When the milk ejection reflex is well established, milk may be spontaneously ejected from both breasts.

Oxytocin pulses increase in amplitude during labour and are involved in the positive-feedback amplification in labour (see Chapter 1). Oxytocin is associated with changes in maternal behaviour promoting the bonding of the maternal–baby dyad and increased alertness at delivery. The pulses of oxytocin induced by feeding have an effect on the uterus, stimulating uterine contractions and involution in the early postnatal period. Multiparous women tend to feel these contractions or 'after-pains' with increased intensity. Women who do not want to breastfeed may find the physiological changes in the breasts at delivery uncomfortable; various techniques are recommended to inhibit lactation (Box 16.4).

SUCKLING AND MILK TRANSFER

Breastfeeding involves the synchronization of the breast milk ejection reflex and the movements of the infant's jaw and tongue. The baby latches into the breast and nipple so the nipple, areolar, some underlying mammary tissue and the lactiferous ducts are drawn into the baby's mouth with the tip of the nipple extended to the junction of the hard-soft palate (Elad et al., 2014). Initially, the milk ejection reflex causes milk to be ejected straight into the baby's mouth. Mouthing (i.e. the movement of the baby's jaw) means that the areola and lactiferous ducts are rhythmically compressed by the baby's gums. The suckling creates a negative pressure, which extracts the milk into the baby's mouth. The baby's tongue undulates and channels the milk into the back of the mouth, which triggers the swallowing reflex.

Babies exhibit two distinct patterns of suckling. Nutritive suckling is a continuous stream of strong slow sucks, which efficiently allows milk transfer. This occurs predominantly in the early part of the feed following the initial milk ejection reflex. Non-nutritive suckling increasingly replaces nutritive suckling during the progression of the feed. It is characterized by alternation of rapid shallow bursts of suckling and rests. It is thought that patterns of thumb sucking may reflect these two conducts. Breastfed

> ### BOX 16.4   Methods for Suppression of Lactation
>
> **Passive**
> - If lactation is established and baby is no longer feeding – gradual reduction of manual expression over a period of time rather than an abrupt stop is less likely to cause discomfort and problems
> - Avoid breast stimulation
> - Wear a well-supporting bra
> - Frequently change breast pads until milk stops leaking
> - Analgesia only if required
> - Drink when thirsty – restricting fluids makes no difference
>
> **Interventional**
> - Dopamine agonists such as Bromocriptine – use with great caution
> - Treatment with sex steroids to antagonize prolactin effects – there is very little empirical evidence to support this
> - Breast-binding – this is a traditional practice but it is extremely uncomfortable for women and may not be effective
> - Application of ice-packs – may give short-term relief but use with caution to avoid ice 'burns'

babies have two distinct rhythms of thumb sucking and tend to put more of the root of the thumb into their mouths. Although non-nutritive suckling is associated with a decreased transfer of milk, it is still very effective in stimulating prolactin release and so may be important in establishing and maintaining successful lactation. Olfactory signals from volatile compounds in the secretions from the Montgomery's tubercles may promote arousal and alignment of the neonate and positive feeding behaviour, such as rooting, also contribute to the establishment of effective milk production and transfer (Schaal, 2010). The use of perfume, soap and body lotions may interfere with this interaction.

The amount of milk produced is extremely variable; that mothers can feed multiple babies and produce additional milk for banking or storage suggests that the mammary synthetic capacity exceeds the normal requirement of a single infant. A demand-fed baby consumes irregular quantities of milk at irregular times. The suggestion that the baby determines milk yield by local control is supported by the strong correlation between degree of breast emptying and rate of milk synthesis. Some women feed exclusively from one breast (and not at all from the other). An autocrine factor capable of overriding the central hormone control was first implicated from research in goats and named feedback inhibitor of lactation (FIL) (Wilde et al., 1995). FIL was suggested to be a 10–30 kDa protein secreted as a component of the whey protein fraction. Definitive identification is still lacking and several other milk components are contenders for this autocrine inhibition of milk secretion when milk accumulates in the alveolar lumen. Milk component(s) inhibit secretion of lactose, probably by blocking the action of prolactin, and therefore provide the mechanism to adjust supply to demand. When milk is not removed from the breast, the concentration of the factor or factors increases and blocks the action of prolactin thus reducing the rate of milk synthesis. It helps to explain why maternal dietary intake has relatively little influence on the amount of milk produced. Women in traditional societies have a much greater frequency and longevity of breastfeeding, so their production of FIL is probably not enough to have an autocrine effect on lactation; milk synthesis is most likely to be influenced solely by metabolic and endocrine mechanisms (Hartmann et al., 1998). Ankyloglossia or tongue-tie may interfere with the suckling reflex and surgical division of the tie (frenulotomy) was thought to be effective in improving breastfeeding but this is now controversial (Walsh and Tunkel, 2017). Many babies with ankyloglossia are able to breastfeed successfully so other factors may also be involved such as the size and length of the maternal nipple affecting ability to suckle. The degree to which tongue mobility is restricted varies greatly in infants and is difficult to assess.

INVOLUTION

After cessation of lactation, involution of the breast takes about 3 months. Regular breastfeeding or removal of milk is essential for the maintenance of lactation. When milk removal stops, the process of involution is triggered. Involution is a 2-step process. Initially, involution is reversible if suckling is restarted but becomes irreversible with a more prolonged absence of milk removal together with a lack of stimulation of prolactin and glucocorticoid levels that suckling provides. After cessation of lactation, milk accumulates in the alveoli and small lactiferous ducts and this inhibits further milk secretion, causes distension and mechanical atrophy of the epithelial cells and stimulates disruption of the secretory lobules. Massive programmed cell death (apoptosis) and autophagy together with breakdown of tight junctions disrupts the alveolar

units. Phagocytosis of apoptotic cells and glandular debris results in fewer and smaller lobular–acinar structures. The alveolar lumens decrease in size and may disappear. The alveolar lining changes from a single secretory layer to a nonsecretory double layer. Together, these processes essentially reverse the developmental changes in the breast, which made lactation possible. Complete involution takes about 3 months but if breastfeeding is stopped suddenly, the process described above is more intense and painful. The breasts remain larger after lactation as the deposits of fat and connective tissue are increased. Involution after lactation is different to the structural atrophy and loss of adipose tissue, which occur in postmenopausal mammary glands deprived of oestrogen.

PROBLEMS ASSOCIATED WITH LACTATION

Milk Insufficiency

Most problems have an identifiable physiological basis; breast milk insufficiency is frequently suspected and so may be overdiagnosed; it can often be solved with adequate support. The majority of women with apparently insufficient milk supply have unsubstantiated worries and require confidence, improved technique (especially positioning), encouragement or advice. This can be supported by physiological strategies such as electric breast pumps and pharmacological (anti-dopamine) agents, which are ideally used as temporary solutions until the natural feedback mechanisms between mother and baby allow the establishment of a robust milk supply. Avoiding pressure on the breasts (such as that due to wearing a tight bra or other tight clothing or sleeping prone) is important as it can negatively affect milk supply.

Iatrogenic low milk supply can be a result of excessive downregulation of the milk supply during the calibration period, which is often due to the infant receiving formula milk soon after birth and not consuming enough breast milk, effectively sending a physiological signal that little milk is required. It can also occur if the mother or infant is unwell and cannot feed properly. The time immediately after birth is a critical period for the establishment of successful breastfeeding; the physiological pathways involved in milk production and ejection are particularly responsive. Breast stimulation from the infant is important in effective initiation of lactation; it starts a cascade of maternal hormonal responses that trigger the synthesis and ejection of milk. Newborn infants placed skin-to-skin with their mothers demonstrate a cascade of innate behaviours to seek and attach to their mother's breast. The behaviours, which include licking, mouth opening, massaging the breast with their hands and hand-to-mouth movements, are effective in stimulating maternal oxytocin release. The newborn sucking pattern, characterized by higher suction pressure, is distinctly different at this time (Kent et al., 2016). This interaction between the mother and infant is affected by interruption (e.g. related to assisted delivery, resuscitation of a preterm, low birthweight or ill baby, or another cause of mother–infant separation) and by medication associated with pain relief.

It is well established that breast milk has important advantages over infant formula for health of the neonate, including passive immunological protection against infectious diseases, particularly in less hygienic environments. It is also well established that some infant formula manufacturers have intentionally exploited the importance of the calibration period by offering free samples of breast milk substitutes or other inducements to mothers to use infant formula early in lactation. If the initial calibrated volume cannot be increased, the mother will then be unable to increase her milk supply later and will be forced to purchase infant formula. Use of these practices in low and middle-income countries has compound effects; infant formula is expensive and is often diluted to save costs, lacks the passive immune protection of breast milk and can actually infect the neonate if water supplies are contaminated. In regions without access to clean water, using formula milk increases infant mortality because the water used to make up the formula increases the transmission of water-borne parasites (Anttila-Hughes et al., 2018). As well as potentially interrupting the important synergy between the mother and infant in the sensitive period immediately after birth described above, some infants also have difficulty attaching to the breast after being bottle fed (known as 'nipple confusion').

Behavioural problems acquired by the baby as coping strategies to avoid aversive events may also induce a low milk supply. These problems include discomfort during positioning at the breast and problems with breathing. Infants with craniofacial anomalies (such as cleft palate), certain genetic syndromes and neurological problems (including prematurity) may have breastfeeding difficulties. Infants who have had surgery related to the mouth or that required prolonged tracheal or orogastric intubation may develop hypersensitivity, usually a hyperactive gag reflex or a complete feeding aversion, which affects feeding. Ankyloglossia can affect feeding and, if the criteria for diagnosis are met (such as poor latching, long feeds, restlessness and signs of hunger, poor weight gain and clinical evidence of tongue-tie), may be resolved by frenotomy. Self-limitation of intake

and lack of persistence may account for the condition often described as 'contented underfed babies'.

Pathophysiological lactational failure is rare and probably affects <2% of women with apparent milk insufficiency. Rare causes include mammary hypoplasia or absence of normal breast development at puberty or in pregnancy. Cosmetic breast surgery, especially reduction or augmentation mammoplasty, involving extensive excision or remodelling of breast tissue may increase rate of lactation failure. Retained placental products may inhibit lactation, at least transiently until the placental tissue is spontaneously shed or surgically removed. Sheehan syndrome (autoimmune related necrosis of the anterior pituitary gland due to acute hypovolaemic shock; see Chapter 14) is rare in developed countries but is serious and requires specific management. The usual presenting signs of Sheehan syndrome after pregnancy are agalactorrhoea (no lactation) or problems with lactation. Women who are unable to breastfeed as planned need support; not meeting expectations can predispose to postnatal depression (see Chapter 14).

Infants not receiving adequate milk may develop hypernatraemia (raised sodium in blood; electrolyte imbalance), nutritional deficiency and failure to thrive (poor weight gain). Nearly half of all infants demonstrate gastro-oesophageal reflux (GOR) or regurgitation of milk feeds (sometimes called 'posseting' or 'spilling') to some extent (NICE, 2015). This is a physiological phenomenon in infants, which starts from about 2 months of age and is usually resolved by 12 months. About 5% of the affected infants have more than six episodes of regurgitation a day, possibly with every feed. Frequent regurgitation where there are more serious complications, such as oesophagitis, and failure to gain weight may indicate gastro-oesophageal reflux disease (GORD). It is sometimes difficult to discriminate between these conditions particularly when the parents are distressed. The best indicator is the observation of adequate weight gain and signs of an otherwise healthy infant. Gastrointestinal symptoms of GORD include projectile vomiting (which may indicate pyloric stenosis and problems with the milk leaving the stomach – the enlarged or tender pylorus or 'olive' may be palpated in the abdomen), blood-stained vomit (possible upper gastrointestinal damage), bile-stained vomit (possible intestinal obstruction), chronic diarrhoea and late onset or persistence of regurgitation (starting after 6 months or continuing after 12 months, which may indicate causes unrelated to the gut) (Davies et al., 2015). There are also systemic conditions with a range of signs and symptoms, including vomiting. Cows' milk protein allergy is often suggested but, unless temporary removal (for 2–4 weeks) of dairy products from the mother's diet demonstrates a positive improvement, it is not likely. Lactating women on self-imposed restrictive diets are likely to compromise their own nutritional status during the period when their nutritional requirements are at their highest. Overfeeding is easier to assess in a formula-fed infant but is a possible reason for excessive regurgitation.

Drugs

Many drugs are secreted into breast milk, but the data on the effects of specific drugs on the breastfed infant are often not available. Of particular concern are those drugs with central nervous system (CNS) activity as the postnatal development of the infant's nervous system is vulnerable. The benefits of maternal treatment and the advantages of breastfeeding have to be balanced against the risk of exposure of the neonate to the medication. Passive diffusion of the unbound, unionized form of the drug into the breast milk is the major mechanism of transfer. Therefore, it is affected by maternal compartmentalization and molecular properties and the composition of the breast milk. There is a lack of information about the safety of many drugs during lactation and the use of rodent models presents problems because of the marked differences in milk composition between species and different transporters in mammary tissue (Anderson, 2018). Assessment of adverse drug reactions in infants is also difficult. Drugs that are minimally transported into the breast milk and are not associated with adverse effects are obviously the preferred choice.

Socially used drugs such as alcohol, nicotine and illicit drugs, such as heroin and cocaine, also cross into the milk. Inhaled cannabis also transfers into breast milk. How much these affect the baby is not clear and the topic is sensitive to research. Women who smoke are less likely to want to breastfeed, or initiate breastfeeding, and more likely to breastfeed for a shorter duration. Drug metabolism and elimination by the neonate is often limited, so exposure to apparently low doses of the drug in milk can have a cumulative effect, particularly in premature babies and those who have prolonged or frequent exposure. Drugs tend not to accumulate in milk but have a bidirectional transfer to and from the breast and maternal circulation. Therefore, the amount of drug received by the infant will be reduced if the mother takes the drug immediately after a feed so the baby does not feed when the drug is at peak concentration in the maternal plasma and milk.

Production of breast milk is also a method of excretion and contains drugs, viruses, food additives, chemical contamination (such as lead), volatile solvents, pesticides and radioactivity. Chemical residues of pollutants are detected in most human milk throughout the world. Heavy metals are of concern because of the susceptibility of the infant's nervous system. Mammals do not have a mechanism to excrete pesticide residues such as polychlorinated

biphenyls and dichlorodiphenyltrichloroethane (DDT). However, the pesticide residues cross the blood–breast barrier so lactation is the only way to reduce the body load. The burden of persistent organic pollutants or environmental contaminants is then transferred to the breastfed infant. Breastfeeding is not contraindicated but a slow and steady rate of maternal weight loss during lactation is important to limit the mobilization of maternal fat and release of lipid-soluble environmental contaminants stored in it, which can then partition in the breast milk.

Psychological Stress and Breast Diseases

Women often cease breastfeeding prematurely in the first 6 months after birth because they experience breastfeeding-related problems such as pain, cracked nipples, which may have a local infection, milk stasis, mastitis and possibly breast abscess formation. These conditions may occur in isolation or may be compounded by anxiety about milk insufficiency and lack of confidence in ability to breastfeed. It is estimated that a significant proportion of breastfeeding women will experience some difficulty in the first few days of feeding. Women experiencing breastfeeding problems are likely to have a higher level of psychological stress and, if prolonged, increased anxiety. Although lactation may be protective against stress in the short-term, longer lasting psychological stress may negatively affect the endocrine, immune and nervous systems. Early identification of lactation problems can prevent longer-term complications.

Viruses

Viruses present in the lactating mother may enter the breast milk. Vertical transmission and subsequent infection of the infant via breast milk have been confirmed for a number of viruses including human immunodeficiency virus (HIV), tuberculosis (TB), cytomegalovirus (CMV), herpes simplex and hepatitis B. It is probably inadvisable for mothers with active, untreated TB to breastfeed as the infection can be reactivated by maternal tiredness and stress (Box 16.5).

BOX 16.5 Contraindications to Breastfeeding

- Maternal illness
- Maternal drug consumption
- Congenital abnormalities, e.g. cleft palate (however, mothers can express milk to feed their babies by various artificial methods; if the baby cannot take oral fluids, the mother can express and freeze her milk for feeding when problems have resolved)
- TB infection (depending on strain and treatment and compliance of the mother in taking the medication)

If the TB-positive mother is compliant with treatment regimens and the baby is given the BCG vaccination as soon as possible after birth, breastfeeding is possible with careful monitoring of both mother and baby.

Advice for HIV-positive mothers is unclear. Women with low HIV viral loads who are compliant with treatment can safely breastfeed but mixed feeding with formula milk supplementation should be avoided because the milk protein can interact the gut wall rendering it more permeable to HIV increasing the risk of transmission. The WHO currently recommends exclusive breastfeeding for at least 6 months and breastfeeding concurrently with complementary feeding for the first 2 years of life because the benefits of the infant receiving human milk outweigh the risk of increased infant morbidity and mortality associated with formula feeding. The rationale for this is the protective effect of breastfeeding on infection rate. However, in developed countries where the water supply is clean and good quality, alternatives to breast milk are feasible and affordable, it may be preferable for mothers with serious infections not to breastfeed to reduce risk of vertical transmission.

Advice for HIV-positive mothers is that for those women receiving antiretroviral therapy (ART) who are adherent to treatment, the risk of transmission of HIV to a breastfeeding baby is very low (~1%) so the health benefits of breastfeeding remain positive, particularly in less hygienic environments. The immunological properties of breast milk are important in protecting against illnesses that accelerate the development of AIDS, particularly in areas of the world where it is endemic. The risk of HIV transmission is affected by maternal viral load, the volume of the milk consumed, the duration of breastfeeding, inflammation of the breast (e.g. caused by cracked nipples), the presence of neonatal oral candidiasis infection ('thrush') and the introduction of formula milk. (Note that several medications used in HIV prophylaxis can transfer to the breast milk and have potentially serious side-effects on the neonate, including anaemia, seizures, hepatitis and feeding difficulties.)

Case study 16.2 is an example of a woman's concerns about breastfeeding.

INHIBITION OF FERTILITY

Breast milk is also important to the infant because suppression of fertility is an advantage. An adequate birth interval is important for both maternal and child health. Lactational amenorrhoea may last from 2 months to over 4 years. It is particularly important in developing countries where breastfeeding prevents more pregnancies than all the other methods of contraception combined. The

---

CASE STUDY 16.2

Elma expressed concerns about breastfeeding throughout her pregnancy. She complained that the midwives running the antenatal classes were biased towards breastfeeding and unsupportive of mothers who did not want to breastfeed. Elma argued that bottle feeding was just as good. Elma described her own family as an example; she is the oldest of five children all of whom were bottle-fed by her mother and were well and healthy. Two days after delivery, Elma experienced breast discomfort and tentatively asked a midwife whether it was too late to try breastfeeding.

- How would you, as the midwife, respond to Elma's feelings about breastfeeding, during the antenatal classes?
- What are the health advantages to the woman and her baby if the mother chooses to breastfeed?
- Do you think a woman should be informed of the risks of infection for the baby if she decides to feed her baby with formula milk? If so, remember it is not just about sterilization of feeding equipment that is important but also that formula milk lacks many of the components of breast milk that actively protect the newborn infant from infection.
- What factors would increase Elma's chances of succeeding to breastfeed for the recommended 6+ months?
- What support would she require from the midwives?
- Would breastfeeding or anything else help to relieve the breast discomfort?

---

variability in duration of suppressed fertility seems to be related to a number of factors; the most important seems to be frequency of suckling. At the end of pregnancy, levels of gonadotrophins are very low because high levels of oestrogen continue to impose a negative feedback. At delivery, the placental hormones begin to disappear at different rates depending on their half-life. hPL disappears from the plasma within hours. Oestrogen and progesterone levels fall to prepregnant levels within a week of the placental loss. Levels of human chorionic gonadotrophin (hCG) are negligible about 3 weeks after delivery. There is a gradual recovery of the pituitary-ovarian axis over the first 4 months after delivery; this recovery is delayed by regular frequent suckling.

In nonlactating women, body temperature measurements and the first menstrual bleeding suggest that the earliest ovulation may occur at 4 weeks after delivery but is usually delayed until 8–10 weeks (McNeilly, 2001). Most women have resumed their normal menstrual patterns by 15 weeks. The first menstrual cycle is often anovulatory or associated with an inadequate luteal phase but most women ovulate by the third cycle and 50% of nonlactating women who do not use contraception conceive within 6–7 months.

Menstruation and ovulation return more slowly in a lactating woman. Ovarian activity usually returns before the end of lactational amenorrhoea. Therefore, menstruation is a poor indicator of fertility; conception can occur before the resumption of menstrual cycles. Neither ovulation nor menstruation normally occur within 6 weeks, but about half of all contraceptive-unprotected breastfeeding mothers conceive within 9 months of lactation and 1–10% during lactational amenorrhoea. Between 30% and 70% of first cycles are ovulatory; the longer the period of lactational amenorrhoea, the more likely the woman is to ovulate prior to the first menstruation.

The precise mechanisms involved in lactational amenorrhoea are not clear. High prolactin levels abolish the pulsatile luteinizing hormone (LH) secretion and decrease the pituitary response to gonadotrophin-releasing hormone. The mid-cycle positive feedback in response to oestrogen is absent. The sensitivity to negative feedback is enhanced and that to positive feedback is decreased. So, even if enough LH and follicle-stimulating hormone (FSH) are present to stimulate follicular development, the inhibitory effect of oestrogen results in an inadequate luteal phase. Prolactin is inhibitory at the level of the ovary, blocking the effects of LH and FSH. It also has a direct effect on the brain, possibly affecting libido.

As prolactin secretion has a pulsatile and circadian rhythm with larger amounts being released at night, the frequency of stimulation by suckling and the night-time feeds are particularly important in maintaining prolactin levels high enough to suppress fertility (McNeilly, 2001). Both the duration and number of feeds are important because the prolactin levels are augmented before they return completely to the basal secretory level. Prolonged amenorrhoea is also associated with maternal malnutrition. Poor nutrition is associated with suppression of fertility in nonlactating women (see Chapter 12). The extra nutrient requirement for milk production can increase the degree of maternal malnutrition, although women receiving less than optimal nutrition can breastfeed their babies adequately, they secrete milk more slowly so the infants feed more often and for longer, which raises their circulating prolactin levels.

MATERNAL BEHAVIOUR

Maternal commitment to reproduction is more than pregnancy; it involves the establishment of lactation and appropriate maternal behaviour. The demands of the parents and offspring during lactation may conflict. It is suggested that parents will tend to maximize the survival of their young but not to the extent that would limit investment in other offspring, including those as yet unborn. This theory suggests that, although mothers will try to recoup the investment of pregnancy by favouring the offspring's survival, should this cost compromise their future reproductive ability there are definite advantages in discontinuing this investment in favour of future offspring. There may be genetic components affecting the time course of lactation or the upper limit of milk production. The rate of milk secretion and duration of lactation vary with nutritional state. Some mammals respond to decreased food supply in ways that favour the succeeding pregnancies, such as killing some or all of the litter. Species with long gestation and long-term commitment to the offspring, such as humans, usually favour the wellbeing of live offspring.

Behavioural changes include preparatory behaviour such as nest building and increased aggression. Care and protection are associated with lactation, particularly with the maternal level of oxytocin (Gordon et al., 2010). These behavioural patterns are associated with the progressive independence of the young. In humans, this behaviour is more difficult to observe than in other species. In many human groupings, such as extended families and very small close communities, sharing childcare is common. In contrast, in many modern societies, social isolation may contribute to the psychological difficulties experienced by women.

The nutritional status of the mother may affect feeding and interaction with her infant so that maternal malnutrition can affect infant development, depending on its duration and timing. Infants malnourished *in utero* may have decreased capacity to respond to appropriate cues and therefore an increased likelihood of social and further nutritional deprivation. Malnourished infants have poorer muscle tone, increased lethargy, irritability and frequency of illness, decreased attention and responsiveness and altered sleep–wake states. Malnourished mothers experience more fatigue, which can affect their own sensitivity to cues from the baby, such as responses to stress and attention–behavioural patterns.

NUTRITION OF THE LACTATING MOTHER

Lactation os one of the most nutritionally demanding times of a woman's life; the requirements for almost all nutrients markedly increase above those of pregnancy and prepregnancy. Human growth rate is much slower than that of other animals. Neurological development is relatively late and the duration of human lactation is long. Breastfeeding supports the development of the neonatal brain both directly and via its impact upon the establishment of the gut microbiota and the gut–brain axis. The milk composition and the nutritional requirements of the mother reflect the relatively slow growth rate of the human neonate and its high demand for nutrients for brain growth.

During lactation, daily nutrient intake is supplemented by mobilization of nutrient reserves laid down in pregnancy. The ability of the lactating female to mobilize these nutrient reserves for milk production is a powerful way to protect both the mother and offspring from fluctuations of food supply. It is a ubiquitous feature of all mammals and is thought to be a critical survival advantage and therefore an evolutionary pressure in the rise of the class Mammalia and lactation (Dall and Boyd, 2004). There is increasing evidence that lactational performance, milk volume and composition are modified by maternal factors such as genetic variation, maternal diet and exposure to environmental influences. Research into milk production in the dairy industry is better funded than health-related research in human lactation but some of the findings are applicable to lactating women. Genetic variation is known to have a significant effect on the composition and volume of milk produced by domesticated animals but little is known about genes affecting lactational physiology in humans. However, single nucleotide polymorphisms (SNPs or mutations) of various genes have been identified in humans including those for oxytocin, prolactin, the prolactin receptor and α-lactalbumin (Lee and Kelleher, 2016).

Nutritional requirements for lactation are increased significantly to maintain optimal milk production and maternal energy balance; they are higher in lactation than during or before pregnancy (though lower in humans compared to other species, which provide for neonates with faster growth rates). Substrates required for milk synthesis are not flexible. Mammary glands are not able to synthesize essential amino acids nor long-chain polyunsaturated fatty acids (LC-PUFAs); they also require nonessential amino acids for protein synthesis and glucose or glucose precursors for lactose and oligosaccharide synthesis. These have to be provided from the maternal diet or from maternal body reserves.

Energy Requirements for Milk Production

The energy content of milk is a significant proportion of the total energy output of the lactating woman; it is suggested that peak lactation requires an increase of energy intake above prepregnant intake of ~20–25%. In dairy animals, the level of food intake strongly correlates with milk yield. It may not be valid to apply knowledge of nutrition and physiology of dairy animals, which are completely milked twice a day, to mammals that suckle their young according to natural patterns of behaviour.

Anthropological studies on human hunter–gatherer communities suggest that babies feeding on true demand, because they are held close to their mother's breasts, choose to feed very frequently, e.g. every half hour at 2 weeks and every 4 h at 4 months. The characteristics of mammalian milk relate directly to the interaction between the mother and child. Marsupials and animals that bear their young during hibernation are always present and produce milk that is dilute with a lower fat content. In contrast, in animals where the mother nurses her young at widely spaced intervals, for instance a hunting lioness, the milk is very concentrated and high in fat. Human milk has most resemblance to the former; it is dilute with a low-fat content, suggesting that humans have evolved as a species where the young have unlimited access to milk and there is high attentiveness shown by a constantly present mother. This may be facilitated by the use of a papoose-type carrier where the naked infant is strapped in direct contact with the naked breast. The stress of human lactation is relatively low compared with species that have faster growing or multiple young, but this is countered by the high cost of maintaining a dependent infant for a prolonged period. The high level of maternal investment in pregnancy and slow reproductive cycle mean that humans are committed to sustain a conception.

There is a discrepancy between the theoretical calculated energy requirement for milk production and the observed intake of lactating women, even taking into account the fat reserves laid down in pregnancy. The theoretical requirements are based on the energy calculated for milk synthesis and secretion and the increased maternal energy costs. It is assumed that the woman resumes her usual level of physical activity soon after the birth of her infant and does not make energy savings from adopting a more sedentary lifestyle. Dewey (2004) calculated that an exclusively breastfeeding woman requires an additional 1850 kJ (440 kcal) per day for the first 2 months of lactation, increasing to 2170 kJ (515 kcal) per day for 3–8 months of lactation when the infant's milk intake is higher. This assumes an energy contribution from maternal fat mobilization at a rate of ~500 g fat per month or 17 g per day, which is equivalent to about 630 kJ (150 kcal). In practice, these requirements are much higher than the observed intakes in successfully lactating women even when offered unlimited access to food. This has led to a range of recommendations: the UK and USA dietary reference values suggest the additional energy requirements for lactation are 1390 kJ (330 kcal) per day for the first 6 months of lactation and WHO recommends an additional 2120 kJ (505 kcal) per day for well-nourished women with adequate gestational weight gain and 2830 kJ (675 kcal) per day for undernourished women and/or those with insufficient gestational weight gain.

Lactational performance is particularly resilient in humans as demonstrated by the efficiency of lactation in undernourished and impoverished communities. Even when the mother is nutritionally deprived, she is able to produce breast milk of sufficient quality and quantity to support the growth of the infant. The mammary gland appears to have metabolic priority of nutrients so milk production could have a negative impact on maternal nutrient status and body composition; this may have implications for subsequent pregnancies, particularly if interbirth spacing is short. In some communities, infant feeding may be augmented by 'wet nursing', for example involving grandmothers or other female relatives breastfeeding infants.

In animals, a decrease in heat production by brown adipose tissue (nonshivering thermogenesis; NST) and therefore the provision of extra energy for milk production are suggested to account for this difference. The mechanism in humans is not thought to be mediated by changes in NST but the lactating woman has increased sensitivity to insulin. This energy-sparing effect and efficient energy utilization by lactating women may have a particularly big implication in developing countries where women's normal activity and energy expenditure are high.

Increased incidence of obesity in Western societies is of concern; the WHO global estimates for 2016 were that 40% of women aged 18 or over were overweight (BMI >25 kg/m^2) and a further 15% of women were obese (and that the prevalence will increase). Pregnancy is a risk factor for the development of obesity; it is suggested that postpartum weight loss may not be inevitable and gestational weight gain may not all be lost postpartum (see Chapter 12). Possibly, the changes in energy metabolism associated with pregnancy and lactation may persist after weaning. If so, lactation could contribute to the problem. Different species of mammal lay down body fat during pregnancy to different degrees. In lactation, mammals rely on the deposited fat to different extents. Whales and seals, for instance, rely entirely on body fat and protein reserves to sustain lactation, whereas dairy cows and laboratory rats are very dependent on increased food intake to provide the substrates and energy for milk production. Pregnant women deposit fat and have a changed hormonal environment. The reported studies tend to conflict and do not show significant differences in weight loss with different patterns of infant feeding. However, interpretation of the studies is confused by confounding factors such as different duration and extent of feeding, and the increased tendency of women who are not breastfeeding to reduce their food intake and weight deliberately.

There is also a large variation in the energy content of the milk produced (see below). Lactating women produce adequate to abundant quantities of milk of sufficient quality to promote growth of healthy infants, even when maternal nutrition is not adequate. Whereas the health of the breastfeeding infant is apparently protected should maternal nutrition be compromised, it is probably at the cost of depletion of maternal nutrient stores and potentially negative effects on subsequent pregnancies.

Deliberate weight loss in well-nourished healthy breastfeeding women appears to have no effect on the yield or composition of breast milk. However, it is recommended that weight loss should not be more than 1–2 kg per month (Moran, 2018). Although reduction in energy intake does not affect milk synthesis, lower intakes of food mean that micronutrient intake, particularly calcium, vitamin D and iron, might be compromised unless nutrient density is deliberately increased. As energy intake falls, the likelihood of a number of nutrients failing to reach the recommended intake progressively increases. In order of vulnerability, the nutrients most likely to be affected are calcium, zinc, magnesium, thiamin, vitamin B$_6$, vitamin E, riboflavin, folate, phosphorus and iron. Overweight lactating women are advised to restrict their energy intake by decreasing consumption of foods high in simple sugars (refined) and fat and by increasing their intake of calcium-rich foods, vegetables and fruit.

Minerals

Both pregnancy and lactation present a tremendous challenge to maternal calcium status. The average fetal skeleton contains 30 g of calcium (Kovacs, 2016), 80% of which is accrued in the third trimester, which is equivalent to ~300–350 mg of calcium per day during the final 6 weeks of pregnancy. The lactational demand for calcium is greater; average daily production of ~800 mL milk requires (and provides) about an additional 200–210 mg of calcium per day but this will continue for at least 180 days if the mother exclusively breastfeeds for at least 6 months as recommended. Nursing twins or triplets will double or triple the calcium transfer from mother to infants. Pregnant adolescents who are still completing their own bone mineral accrual may also have higher requirements for calcium.

It is estimated that about 10% of total maternal calcium stores (~105 g) is transferred to the fetus/neonate in total, predominantly during lactation. There are several possible physiological adaptations that can contribute to meeting the lactational demand for calcium: increased intake of calcium from the diet, increased absorption, decreased excretion or increased bone demineralization (net loss of bone). In the third trimester of pregnancy, absorption of calcium increases together with a modest increase in bone resorption (mobilization of calcium from bone). Calcium demands of lactation are met by an increase in the rate of bone resorption and a decrease in renal calcium excretion, which are speculated to have evolved from the adaptations in bone and mineral metabolism that supply calcium for egg production in lower vertebrates. The oestrogen level during lactation is relatively low so the bone mass is not protected to the same extent.

The maternal mobilization of calcium from skeletal reserves has been described as 'plundering' the skeleton (Kovacs, 2017); the average intake of calcium in most women is not adequate to maintain calcium in the bone and produce breast milk. This means that lactation is the period of most rapid bone loss in a woman's life; there is a net drain of calcium from the body, with a selective decrease in trabecular bone. This reduction is independent of parathyroid hormone and vitamin D levels. Lactation may contribute to an increased future risk of osteoporosis, but risk factors shown to be associated with fractures do not necessarily include breastfeeding. When breastfeeding is ceased, an imbalance between bone resorption and bone formation results in a rapid and complete recovery of bone mass within 6–12 months. The duration of breastfeeding does not appear to have an adverse effect on later bone mineral density but short interpregnancy intervals of <12 months are associated with increased risk of later osteoporosis, presumably because the recovery time is compromised. Modern practices of delaying childbearing resulting in decreased time for skeletal recovery before menopause may be countered by the cumulative effect of having fewer children. Prolonged lactational amenorrhoea may also help to restore maternal iron status.

There is no consensus for recommendations for iron requirements in lactation. Iron deficiency is the most common micronutrient deficiency worldwide. The mammary gland expresses transferrin receptors and imports holo-transferrin bearing ferric iron (see Chapter 12) but little is known about the molecular mechanisms involved between iron uptake into the cells and secretion of iron into the milk. Iron is required for ATP production and because milk synthesis is energetically demanding, iron deficiency might compromise mammary gland function and milk production (Lee and Kelleher, 2016). Breast milk is not rich in iron; the recycling of red blood cells after birth (see Chapter 15) contributes to the iron requirements of the neonate. However, preterm infants, those born to mothers with iron deficiency, and infants who do not receive appropriate complementary sources of iron when their stores are depleted after about 6 months of breastfeeding may be at risk of iron deficiency.

The mammary gland homeostatically controls the concentrations of essential nutrients in milk; levels of major minerals including calcium, sodium, potassium, phosphorus and magnesium in milk are not affected by the dietary intake. The mammary gland can adapt to some degree of maternal deficiency (or excess) of iron, zinc and copper because there are active transport mechanisms for these nutrients in the mammary gland (Lönnerdal, 2007). When milk production falls with the consumption of complementary foods by the infant, milk iron levels decrease and milk zinc levels increase.

Maternal intakes of iodine and selenium affect levels in breast milk. As iodine is so important for fetal and neonatal neurodevelopment and many women do not have an optimal intake of iodine (partly because salt use is decreasing and fewer iodine-containing cleaning agents are used in the dairy industry), iodine supplements are widely recommended and often routinely prescribed for pregnant and lactating women and for women considering pregnancy (Dold et al., 2018). This is particularly important in countries where there is no mandatory iodization of table salt. The demands of lactation can precipitate goitre in women with marginal iodine status. Iodine deficiency remains a significant health problem worldwide.

Zinc is a cofactor for many enzymes. Studies in rodent models have identified that zinc deficiency impairs mammary gland development and affects lactation performance. Marginal zinc deficiency is relatively common in woman of reproductive age and exclusively breastfed infants of mothers with poor zinc status may be vulnerable.

Water and Fluids

The volume of milk produced is robust; only very severe dehydration and extreme malnutrition affect the volume of milk produced. There is no evidence that increasing fluid intake increases the volume of milk produced or that reducing fluid intake prevents engorgement. When fluids are restricted, urine output decreases and the woman is at risk of dehydration. Breastfeeding women should be advised to drink when they are thirsty and to be aware that they will need more fluid than normal.

INFANT NUTRITION AND THE COMPOSITION OF HUMAN MILK

Human milk optimally fulfils the nutritional requirements of the human neonate. It has a unique composition that is particularly suitable for the rapid growth and development of the infant born with immature digestive, renal and hepatic systems. Unique features of human milk are able to compensate for the underdeveloped neonatal capabilities. Human milk contains not only the macronutrients, vitamins and minerals but also non-nutrient growth factors, hormones and protective factors.

There are at least 1000 components in human milk, including over 900 milk proteins (Gao et al., 2012); many of these components have yet to be identified and their roles elucidated. In the Koran, breast milk is described as 'white blood'. This is a particularly apt description, because the early milk has more white blood cells than blood itself. Milk is a solution in which other substances are dissolved, emulsified or colloidally dispersed. The value of breast milk is undisputed; rarely should breastfeeding be discouraged.

Both the volume and composition of human milk are extremely variable. Some of this variability is genetic (any genetic mutation leading to inadequate mammary development in humans would no longer be eliminated by natural selection as alternatives to human milk are available). Postponing childbearing until long after sexual maturity has an effect on breast development, as advancing age causes some atrophy of the mammary tissue. However, there is little relationship between the overall size of the breast and milk output.

The unique characteristic of humans is the large complex brain, which undergoes much development in the first 2 years of life. Human milk provides levels of lactose, cysteine, cholesterol and thromboplastin, which are required for CNS tissue synthesis. However, as breast milk provides a model of optimum nutrition, analysis of its composition has allowed good (but not perfect or identical) substitutes to be produced as formula feeds. Infant formula milk will never completely mimic human milk, however, as the quality of the nutrients is not reproducible and the immunological aspects of breast milk make it superior to formula feeding.

Although breast milk may be considered to be optimal nutrition for the neonate, its composition is variable. It varies from woman to woman, hourly through the day and from one period of lactation to another, the latter of which allows the composition to reflect the changing requirements of the developing neonate. Milk composition is also related to the timing and frequency of the feeds, how much is produced and parameters relating to the last feed; it has also been suggested that maternal age, parity, health and social class affect the composition of the milk. Mothers of premature infants produce milk that has a higher concentration of some nutrients, but this probably reflects the small volumes produced for small infants. Except for vitamin and fat content, the composition is largely independent of maternal nutrition unless the mother experiences severe malnutrition. Supplementation of the maternal diet may improve maternal health rather than affect milk composition and volume.

There are many difficulties encountered in the estimation of the volume of milk produced. Weighing either the mother or baby before and after the feed is fraught with problems. Although double-labelled water measurements have allowed more accurate estimations, the variability within a feed and from feed to feed makes it very difficult to ascertain precisely the nutrient consumption of a healthy growing baby. These estimates of ~60 kcal per 100 mL are lower than UK food composition tables (69 kcal per 100 mL). The volume of daily milk intake by healthy infants has a wide range. Factors that influence frequency, intensity or duration of feeds will affect volume consumed.

Breastfed infants appear to self-regulate their energy intake and consume more milk if it has a lower energy level; there is a lower incidence of obesity in individuals who were breastfed as infants. Breastfeeding allows infants to learn self-regulation of energy intake, whereas bottle-fed infants may be encouraged to finish the bottle, which suppresses their autoregulatory mechanism. Breast milk may also contain appetite inhibitors and stimulators. It is suggested that different modes of infant feeding have different metabolic programming effects. Formula-fed infants tend to receive more protein, which results in an increased insulin response. Insulin stimulates adipose tissue deposition (increased number and fat content of adipocytes), which is associated with weight gain and obesity. Alternatively, breastfeeding may affect leptin metabolism; the higher level of fatness in formula-fed infants may programme reduced sensitivity to leptin in later life. However, it should be noted that this issue is confounded parental attributes and the family environment. Parents who choose to breastfeed tend to have a healthier lifestyle with more optimal dietary habits and higher levels of physical activity; they also exert less parental control over child-feeding practices.

The low levels of gastric secretion and other immature digestive characteristics of the neonatal gut confer a number of immunological advantages, which were described in Chapter 15 (p. 460).

Colostrum

In the first 3 days postdelivery, the mother produces about 2–10 mL of colostrum per day. More colostrum is produced sooner if the woman has had previous pregnancies, particularly if she has breastfed before. In some cultures, colostrum is thought to be old milk or 'pus' and is discarded rather than fed to infants.

Colostrum is translucent and is yellow from the high β-carotene content. Mature milk in contrast looks less viscous and slightly bluish. Colostrum has more protein and vitamins A and K and less carbohydrate and fat than mature milk. It is easily digested and well absorbed. It has a lower energy content of 58 kcal per 100 mL compared with 70 kcal per 100 mL in mature milk. Levels of sodium, potassium, chloride and zinc are high in colostrum but these reflect the low volume produced rather than the infant's requirements for a bolus dose of certain nutrients. The composition is extremely variable, which reflects its unstable secretory pattern.

Colostrum facilitates the colonization of the gut with *Lactobacillus bifidus* and meconium also contains growth factors for *L. bifidus*. Colostrum seems to have a laxative effect, stimulating the passage of meconium. The high protein content is largely due to the abundant antibodies, which protect against gastrointestinal tract infection.

Secretory immunoglobulin A (sIgA), which accounts for ~90% of the total immunoglobulin content of human milk and 35% of the protein content of colostrum, falls rapidly from its peak level at day 3 to 15% of total protein content by 2–4 weeks postpartum (Lönnerdal et al., 2017). sIgA is mostly resistant to the proteolytic enzymes in the infant gut, conferring specific resistance to pathogens from the maternal acquired immune system. In the first few days of life, priming and maturation of the mucosal immune system is maximal and the gut is permeable and able to absorb macromolecules; colostrum contains many immunomodulatory molecules particularly anti-inflammatory agents, which help to protect the vulnerable immature gut from mucosal damage.

During the first 30 h or so, the secreted colostrum has a high protein:lactose ratio. In the following days, as the baby suckles more and stimulates milk production, the resulting increase in prolactin secretion stimulates production of the major whey protein α-lactalbumin, which is a specific component of the enzyme lactose synthetase and so regulates lactose production. The effect of increasing lactose production is that water is drawn into the secretion to maintain osmotic equilibrium so the volume increases thus diluting the protein content. The absolute amounts of protein secreted into the milk are maintained or increased even though the concentration falls.

The composition of the milk becomes relatively stable from about day 5 but it is variable in volume. The amount of breast milk produced is related to the weight and requirement of the infant; there is a steady increase in volume in the first few weeks. Milk production appears to get underway regardless of the size and requirements of the baby, although hPL levels may play a role in the increased production of milk in mothers of twins. The early weeks of lactation can be considered to be a time of calibration between maternal production and the infant's demand. The volume of milk produced is usually increased to match demand. Downregulation may be irreversible. It is suggested that mothers of small or preterm babies should hand express as much milk as they can to maximize increasing milk flow (i.e. reach milk peak yield early in lactation rather than only enough for the baby's transiently limited requirement).

Milk secretion in women who do not suckle their baby may persist scantily for 3 or 4 weeks while prolactin levels are still high. The effect of suckling is to stimulate the release of prolactin and oxytocin, which are essential for the maintenance of lactation (Fig. 16.4). Provided breastfeeding is regular, lactation can continue for several years; in some women the ability to lactate is not lost, including following the menopause. Most studies suggest that the average daily volume of milk produced is ~800 mL. However, measurement of the milk produced is notoriously difficult but it is clear that there is much variation depending on demand: mothers of twins produce about twice as much milk (Box 16.6).

Energy

The energy requirements of infants can be estimated from total energy expenditure and the energetic cost of tissue deposition during growth. Energy expenditure also includes basal metabolism, thermic effect of feeding, thermoregulation and physical activity. The energy requirement to maintain the tissue takes precedence over the energy requirements to synthesize new tissue. Satisfactory growth is a sensitive indicator of whether energy needs are being met. Infectious diseases increase energy requirement because there is an increased protein turnover, production of cytokines and phagocytic cells and raised body temperature; the repair of tissue is costly and lipids are metabolized less efficiently. Originally, infant energy requirements and recommendations were based on a compilation of energy intakes of well-nourished infants. Measurement of infant energy expenditure using doubly labelled water was subsequently used as the basis for revised energy requirements, which were lower than the original recommendations.

Total energy requirements increase with age. Energy requirements are higher in male infants because male infants tend to be larger. This has an influence on lactation; increased energy content of milk is associated with a male infant. It is proposed that this increased nutritional investment may account for the often-observed greater growth rates in male infants (Powe et al., 2010b).

Protein

Protein is the limiting nutrient for tissue growth and development. It provides nitrogen, and the amino acids required for biosynthesis of membrane and transport proteins, hormones, enzymes, growth factors, neurotransmitters and immunoglobulins. Human neonates have a slow growth rate compared with other species, which is reflected in the low protein concentrations (0.7–0.9 g protein per 100 mL compared with 3.5 g per 100 mL in cow's milk). (Note that early estimates of protein neglected the high concentration of nonprotein nitrogen (NPN) thus significantly

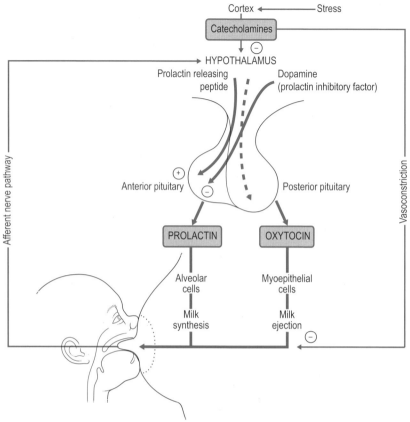

Fig. 16.4 Suckling stimulates the release of prolactin and oxytocin.

overestimating protein level; see below.) Excess protein intake can present an excessive solute load to the immature kidneys, which results in acid–base imbalance and metabolic acidosis.

The growth and body composition changes of infants is affected by the mode of feeding. Breastfed infants grow faster in the first 2–3 months then their rate of growth slows down. Formula-fed infants continue to grow more rapidly. Breastfed infants tend to be leaner. The faster growth rates of formula-fed infants are probably related to the higher level of protein and different ratio of amino acids in formula milks compared to breast milk; as appropriate infant growth has short- and long-term health implications, reducing the protein content and improving the protein quality of formula milks may be desirable. The growth rate of infants fed formula milk or breast milk is different from the first days of life and diverges markedly after 2–3 months. Breastfed infants have lower weight-for-length (Nommsen-Rivers and Dewey, 2009) but it is evident that this is not related to insufficient breast milk.

Breastfed infants are also taller as adults (Schack-Nielsen and Michaelsen, 2007).

Chronic maternal protein undernutrition or prolonged lactation may result in changes in the protein composition of milk. Protein supplementation of the mother's diet tends to increase milk volume rather than affecting protein concentration but has an important role in supplementing maternal health.

When milk proteins are exposed to the relatively acidic environment of the neonatal stomach, they separate into casein (proteins that precipitate, forming curds) and whey (those proteins that remain soluble). This means that there is a continuous flow of nutrients, initially as soluble lactose and whey proteins, and later from digested curd. Whey proteins include serum albumin, α-lactalbumin, lactoferrin, secretory IgA and some enzymes and protein hormones transported from the maternal circulation. Whey proteins are easy to digest by a human neonatal gut, which has particularly low levels of trypsin and pepsin. The whey-dominant content of milk reduces the risk of

BOX 16.6 Breastfeeding Twins and Multiples

Human milk is nutritionally and immunologically superior to formula milks, which is particularly important for twins as multiple pregnancies have a relatively high incidence of prematurity and low birthweight infants. There is no physiological reason for not breastfeeding multiple infants; milk supply will increase in response to increased demand. Mothers feeding multiple infants are advised to increase their nutrient intake and to rest more. Advice about simultaneous feeding or feeding the infants individually will need to be given. Simultaneous feeding saves time and can mean that a more vigorous infant on one breast can stimulate the let-down reflex for the other infant. There are three commonly used positions for feeding twins: 'double cradle' (where the two infants' bodies cross on the mother's abdomen); 'double football' (where the infants' bodies are tucked under the mother's arms); and a cradle-football combination. Mothers feeding triplets or quadruplets choose between the various combinations; these mothers often intend to provide their infants with some exposure to human milk rather than feeding them exclusively.

Many women now practice tandem feeding; the women continue to feed one infant while pregnant and will breastfeed both siblings concurrently.

---

lactobezoars (obstructive milk curd balls) forming in the stomach. Also, human α-lactalbumin is easier to digest than bovine β-lactalbumin.

The ratio of whey to casein in human milk is 60:40 (1.5). The β-casein in human milk forms curds that are soft and flocculent with a low curd tension, which are easily digested. Bioactive peptides formed from partial hydrolysis of human milk casein may be important in stimulating the neonatal immune system. In contrast, cow's milk has a whey to casein ratio of 20:80 (0.25). Bovine casein is predominantly α-casein, which forms a tough rubbery precipitate unless heat-treated, which is more difficult for human infants to digest and decreases the bioavailability of calcium and other cations. Human β-casein tends to form smaller micelles incorporating minerals that are easier for the neonate to digest. κ-Casein in cow's milk has a marked effect on the development of the bovine gastrointestinal physiology, stimulating the secretion of chymosin, which is the dominant protease of the fourth stomach. Casein associates with calcium, phosphate and magnesium in the micelles.

Colonization of the Neonatal Gut

Over recent years the vital importance of the commensal microbiota to human health has become increasingly clear. These microorganisms colonize our gastrointestinal, respiratory, renal and reproductive tracts, outnumber our own body cells by at least 10-fold and live in mutualism with body tissues. Dysbiosis of the major population of these microorganisms, the gut microbiota, has been extensively implicated in a large and growing number of human diseases. The long-held belief that the fetus *in utero* is sterile and acquires its microbiota during delivery and postbirth has recently been challenged and it is now well established that the fetal microbiome originates *in utero*, long before parturition (Stinson et al., 2017). Microbiota, with a high degree of similarity to those found in the mother's gut, can be isolated from the umbilical cord blood of healthy neonates born by caesarean section (before the infant is exposed to the mother's body) and bacteria can be detected in the meconium of preterm infants. The infant at birth is exposed to additional microorganisms from the mother's vagina, skin and faeces and subsequently to environmental microbiota from the 'outside world'. Infants born by caesarean section have a reduced number of bacteria and are more likely to receive medication. Breast milk also provides a source of bacteria; there are up to 10^9 microbial cells per litre of human milk.

Initially the composition of the infant microbiota has low diversity (limited number of different species). The species depend on a range of factors including the mode of delivery, environment (hospitalization), prematurity, geography (country of birth) and use of antibiotics. Infants born by vaginal delivery are initially colonized by bacteria from their mother's vaginal and perineum such as *Lactobacillus* and *Prevotella*, whereas infants born by caesarean section are colonized by *Staphylococcus*, *Corynebacterium* and *Propionibacterium* from their mother's skin. Initially, the gut microbiota are dominated by facultative aerobes (*Enterobacteria*, *Streptococcus* and *Staphylococcus*), which are then replaced by obligate anaerobes (*Bacteriodes* and *Clostridium*) because there is little oxygen available (Strzepa et al., 2018). There is a marked second shift in the profile of gut microbiota when solid foods are introduced at weaning. Between 2 and 5 years, the child's gut microbiota become more stable and more like adult gut microbiota. Until this stability is reached, the gut microbiota are not stable and are easily perturbed, e.g. by the use of antibiotics. The administration of antibiotics in infants during development of the gut immune system has been associated with an increased risk of Crohn's disease, one of the two major types of IBD.

The gut microbiota have many important functions including roles in the postbirth establishment of the infant immune system and the protection of the gut, the major portal of infective pathogen entry, from pathogenic colonization (colonization resistance). The importance of breastfeeding is further supported by the demonstration that the microbiota of breastfed and formula-fed infants are distinctively different. Exclusively breastfed infants have more microbiota from the protective Actinobacteria class and formula-fed infants have more γ-Proteobacteria, which is proinflammatory. Breastfed infants have a high preponderance of lactobacilli (especially *Bifidobacterium bifidum* formerly known as *L. bifidus*), which generates a lower pH and inhibits growth of enteric pathogens. The microbiota of breastfed infants is less diverse because there is an enrichment of genes that code for enzymes required to degrade and utilize human milk oligosaccharides (HMO). Supplementation of breastfed infants with even small amounts of formula milk changes the composition of the gut microbiota towards a broader spectrum of bacteria.

Human milk contains large amounts of a variety of complex carbohydrates such as glycans and oligosaccharides. Some glycans inhibit pathogens binding to the gut; there is structural homology between the milk glycan and gut cell surface molecules so the pathogen binds to the glycan, which effectively acts as a decoy binding site. The glycans are indigestible and so arrive in the colon in an undigested state where they have a prebiotic effect and influence the composition of the intestinal microbiota. This may be particularly important as modern-day hygiene practices limit exposure of the neonatal gut to environmental microbiota. Optimizing gut colonization is thought to be important in developing a stable microbial ecosystem, which promotes the growth of symbiotic microorganisms and colonization by enteric pathogens. There is an increasing practice of 'seeding' the neonatal gut by placing a maternal vaginal swab in the newborn's mouth to promote colonization of the neonatal gut but the research suggesting this is beneficial is limited.

The establishment of the optimal profile of gut microbiota in a time-restricted period in early postnatal life may influence health throughout life. During this period, the composition of the microbiota colonizing the gut is unstable and vulnerable to perturbation (and manipulation); this time coincides with the development of the immune system. The gut microbiota affect host susceptibility to disease and the development of allergies (Gensollen and Blumberg, 2017). The microbiota affect the transition of the infant's immune response from a type 2 immune response, which favours allergy, towards a type 1 immune response required for the elimination of pathogens. An imbalance between the responses can cause increased prevalence of allergy and autoimmunity. The 'hygiene hypothesis' suggested that the decreased incidence of infections (i.e. lower number of pathogens associated with a cleaner environment and the use of antibiotics) led to the increased prevalence of allergic disorders (such as asthma) and autoimmune disorders (such as type 1 diabetes, multiple sclerosis and IBD). However, this is a little misleading; it is not cleanliness per se that is the issue. It is more that the diversity of microbiota is reduced by modern living conditions, which affects the optimal signalling between the microbiota and the immune system at a critical period of life (Bjorksten, 2009).

Protein

Proteins are formed of chains of amino acids. Some of the 20 amino acids involved cannot be made in the body and these are termed essential or indispensable amino acids (see Table 12.1). Nonessential amino acids can be synthesized from glucose and ammonia via the Krebs cycle or from free amino acids by transamination. Some amino acids are conditionally essential for the neonate because the neonate has limited synthetic capability. The amounts and proportions of essential amino acids determine the quality of a protein. A protein that is rich in all essential amino acids has a high biological value or net protein utilization, which means all the amino acids supplied are converted into proteins. A food with a deficiency of an amino acid has a low biological value. Human milk has a very high biological value because it is fully utilized by the neonate as its amino acids are exactly in proportion to requirement. Few other foods have such a high value. By the end of the 2nd week of life, 90% of the ingested nitrogen-containing substances in milk are absorbed, suggesting that milk contains the optimal pattern of amino acids.

The amino acid content of human milk, especially whey proteins, is ideal for the growth requirements of the human infant. Neonatal metabolism of certain amino acids (e.g. phenylalanine, tyrosine and methionine) is initially limited because the enzymes involved in their metabolism are expressed late in development. If these amino acids reach high concentrations, they can cause damaging effects. Human milk is relatively low in tyrosine, phenylalanine and methionine but high in amino acids that the infant cannot synthesize in adequate amounts. The inability to synthesize adequate quantities of histidine, cysteine and taurine means that these amino acids become conditionally essential for infants and need to be provided in the diet. The enzyme that converts methionine to cysteine, cystathionase, is low or undetectable in the neonate. Cysteine is required for growth and development. Infants, especially preterm infants, fed unmodified cow's milk may develop hyperphenylalaninaemia and hypertyrosinaemia, which can increase the net acid load and adversely affect development of the CNS.

Taurine is the second most abundant free amino acid in human milk. Infants use taurine for bile acid conjugation (in contrast to adult conjugation by glycine) so this amino acid is important in the digestion and metabolism of cholesterol and fats. There are also high levels of taurine in fetal brain tissue where it may act as a neurotransmitter or neuromodulator and be involved in myelination of nerves and the optimal maintenance of retinal integrity. The absolute requirement for taurine is unknown but it is added to formula milk at the levels found in human milk.

Aspartame is a sweetener composed of aspartic acid and phenylalanine. If maternal consumption of foods containing aspartame is increased, there is an increase in plasma levels of phenylalanine but levels in milk only increase marginally suggesting that the mammary gland regulates the transfer of amino acids into the milk.

Nonprotein Nitrogen

More than 25% of the nitrogen found in human milk comes from sources other than protein. This is the NPN fraction (Box 16.7). Methods for protein determination usually rely on measuring the total nitrogen in a foodstuff and calculating the average amount of protein that would

---

BOX 16.7   Nonprotein Nitrogen

The protein content of human milk was initially overestimated because it was based on the assumption that the nitrogen fractions within the milk would all be components of protein. In fact, about 25% of the nitrogen-containing components in the milk are not within proteins. This is high compared with other species; for instance, cow's milk contains only 5% of the total nitrogen as NPN.

NPN includes:

- Amino sugars: which promote the growth of *Lactobacillus bifidus* and are also incorporated into neural tissue and gut epithelial membrane
- Taurine: a free amino acid that is a component of bile salts and therefore contributes to fat digestion
- Peptides: these have roles as growth factors and hormones
- Cysteine: a free amino acid that is conditionally essential in the infant because the conversion of methionine to cysteine is limited
- Binding factors: these facilitate absorption of other nutrients
- Urea
- Creatine
- Creatinine
- Uric acid

---

contain that much nitrogen. Therefore, the protein content of human milk was overestimated before it became clear how large the proportion of NPN was. Each mammalian species has a characteristic amount and profile of NPN, which is of nutritional significance. The NPN of human milk includes a variety of compounds such as peptides and free amino acids (such as those that are conditionally essential), nucleotides, traces of inorganic compounds, urea, creatinine, *N*-acetyl sugars and glycosylated amines. Some of the NPN compounds are of developmental importance but the biological significance of others is uncertain. Urea is high in early milk, reflecting high plasma levels due to uterine involution (see Chapter 14).

Fat

Fat is the main energy source in breast milk. The nutritional status of the mother can affect the fat concentration of the milk and therefore the energy content, fatty acid composition and immunological properties. Of all the macronutrients in milk, fat is the most variable component; it is influenced by the maternal diet, parity, the season of the year and amount of milk removed at the last and current feed, the length of the time between feeds and the fat content of the last feed (Innis, 2014). The fat content of human milk averages 38–39 g/L in mature milk (Koletzko et al., 2001), compared with 20 g/L in colostrum. The sampling method used to collect milk is important as hindmilk has three to five times the fat content of foremilk. Averaging foremilk and hindmilk is unlikely to produce a good estimate of the overall composition. The fat content of milk is lowest in the early morning (~6 a.m.) and then rises to a peak mid-morning (~10 a.m.) before falling during the day. There is also a progressive decline in the average fat content with increasing maternal age but with much individual variability. The diurnal rhythm of milk composition is related to GH secretion. The fatty acid pattern is variable, reflecting maternal energy intake and dietary fat consumption. It is possible to discriminate between the milk of vegetarian and nonvegetarian mothers.

Before birth, the fetus accumulates substantial amounts of palmitic acid (16:0) much of which is synthesized by the fetal liver. After birth, human milk provides substantial amounts of palmitic acid (a saturated fatty acid). About 50% of the energy in milk comes from fat, of which about 20% is palmitic acid so 10% of milk energy is derived from palmitic acid. Whereas the composition of fat within human milk tends to reflect maternal dietary fat intake, the palmitic acid content is remarkably constant and independent of maternal diet (Innis, 2016). This level is maintained by the mammary gland, which increases elongation of myristic acid (14:0) to compensate if maternal intake decreases. Palmitic acid is a component of membrane phospholipids and can be oxidized to form ATP. The human infant is one of the fattest known newborns and is born well-endowed with adipose tissue; fat accounts for 13–15% of body weight (whereas the fat content of nonhuman primates at birth is ~2–3%). A 3 kg human infant has about 450 g fat, which is significantly more than the 122 g predicted for its body size. After birth, the infant adipose tissue reserve continues to expand, gaining ~400 g of fat per month, to reach ~25% of body weight by 4–5 months old. It has been hypothesized that the large human brain requires a good energy buffer, which the fat provides (Kuzawa, 1998). The body fat can be mobilized to meet the energy demands of the brain; the infant is vulnerable to negative energy balance when lactation is being established, if there are infections related to the immunological immaturity and there may be transient negative energy balance as solid foods are introduced. Human infants quickly become ketotic if energy intake decreases and body fat is mobilized. The body fat is not only extraordinary in amount but it is also composed of 45–50% palmitic acid (16:0) and a further 13–15% for the palmitic acid-derived palmitoleic acid (16:1, ω7). These two fatty acids can be oxidized very efficiently to ketones, which the brain can use as an energy source.

The other notable characteristic of palmitic acid in human milk is that it is esterified to the glycerol backbone in position 2 of the triacylglyceride (TAG), which is unusual. This means that it is likely to be absorbed across the gut in the monoacylglycerol form (see Chapter 12), which means that it is absorbed efficiently because there is less free palmitic acid, which tends to form insoluble complexes (soaps) with divalent cations like Ca^{2+} and Mg^{2+} at the alkaline pH of the small intestine. Bovine TAGs usually have palmitic acid at position 1 or 3 of the TAG so digestion of cow's milk fat in formula milk can release free palmitic acid, which is precipitated by calcium as soap. This can result in the loss of absorption of both fat and calcium.

As fat concentration affects the energy content of the milk, these variations in fat content make it particularly difficult to arrive at the average fat content and therefore energy content of human milk. Previous overestimation of energy levels in breast milk resulted in formula milk providing too high an energy level, which may have led to overfeeding and potential obesity problems of previous generations.

Of the lipid present in human milk, 98% is TAGs and 90% of the TAG molecule is fatty acids. The remaining 2% of the lipid fraction is made up of phospholipids, glycolipids cholesterol, cholesterol esters, diacylglycerides and monoacylglycerides. Fat provides the vehicle for fat-soluble vitamins and essential fatty acids required for brain development. Phospholipids are critical components of cell membranes and of surfactant and are precursors for

important signalling molecules. The fatty acid composition of human milk is very different to that of cow's milk. Human milk has more essential fatty acids (linoleic and α-linolenic acids), has a higher proportion of unsaturated fatty acids and is rich in long-chain fatty acids. Cow's milk has more short-chain fatty acids (SCFAs) (C_4–C_8) and a higher content of saturated fatty acids. The products of lipase digestion are predominantly 2-monoacylglycerides and free fatty acids, which can be absorbed. Free fatty acids, such as linoleic and lauric acid, and monoacylglycerides at the concentrations found in the stomachs of breast-fed babies are toxic to many pathogens including viruses and some parasites. Monoacylglycerides have bactericidal properties and can act as detergents to damage the membrane of pathogens. Free oleic acid can form a protein–lipid complex with the α-lactalbumin in human milk known as HAMLET (Human Alpha-lactalbumin Made LEthal to Tumour cells), which induces apoptosis in tumour cells (Ho et al., 2017).

Human milk and vegetable oil fats are better absorbed than is the saturated fat of cow's milk. Long-chain fatty acids require bile salt micelle formation and lipase activity whereas short- and medium-chain fatty acids can be absorbed intact.

Human milk has a high content of cholesterol, which is required for myelin synthesis (important for the CNS development). The cholesterol content of breast milk is not affected by maternal diet. There may be a connection between cholesterol exposure early in life and the development of enzymes for cholesterol degradation and amounts of endogenous cholesterol synthesized (Innis, 2016), which results in lower cholesterol levels in adults who were breastfed as infants.

As lactation progresses, TAG levels increase and cholesterol levels fall but phospholipid content remains stable. Usually, 20% of the available milk remains in the breast after feeding; this contains about half of the initial fat content. This effect may be due to absorption of MFGs on the surface of the alveolar cells in the secretory and ductal surfaces of the breast. Babies suck in longer bursts and decrease the rest intervals when they are feeding on hindmilk.

Essential Fatty Acids

Human milk provides all the dietary essential fatty acids (see Chapter 12) (Table 16.2), which are required for cell proliferation, retinal development and myelination of neurons in the CNS. The LC-PUFAs, docosahexaenoic acid (DHA) and arachidonic acid (ARA) are essential constituents of cell membranes, particularly of the nervous system, occurring at notably high concentrations in the brain and retina. The brain undergoes a growth spurt in late gestation and early neonatal life when the brain weight increases

TABLE 16.2 Long-chain Polyunsaturated Fatty Acids

	Omega-6 ($N-6$)	Omega-3 ($N-3$)
Predominant source	Vegetable oils	Marine oils (fish)
Essential fatty acid	Linoleic	α-Linolenic
Converted to	Arachidonic acid	Docosahexaenoic acid

about 60-fold from 20 g in the second trimester to ~1200 g by the age of 2 years. The neonate has a limited ability to desaturate and elongate fatty acid chains thus limiting the conversion of linoleic acid into ARA and α-linolenic acid into DHA, so these PUFAs may be conditionally essential in the neonatal diet. Infants acquire PUFAs prenatally via the placenta and postnatally in milk. Human milk is particularly rich in ARA and DHA. DHA levels in human milk seem closely related to maternal fish intake (Fu et al., 2016), whereas ARA is less related to maternal diet. The human brain undergoes dramatic growth from the last trimester of pregnancy through the first years of life. During this time, cerebral levels of ARA and DHA increase. The concentrations of these LC-PUFAs in human milk are associated with the markers of brain development such as the raised IQ levels and better visual perception of breastfed infants This has led to the supplementation of formula milk particularly that intended for preterm infants (Lien et al., 2018).

Maternal PUFA status, and therefore milk levels, varies with fish and fatty acid intake but despite the demonstrated beneficial effects, there is a lack of consistent and specific dietary fat recommendations for pregnancy and lactation. As the raised levels of oestrogen in pregnancy would increase the conversion of dietary essential fatty acids to long-chain fatty acids, the more vulnerable time is lactation when oestrogen levels are low. It is suggested that lactating women who do not consume the currently recommended intakes of oily fish (two portions per week) should take a supplement (1–2 g fish oil per day) to achieve the optimal breast milk levels of 1% by weight of DHA and eicosapentaenoic acid (EPA), which is marked by the maternal erythrocyte DHA+EPA being about 8% of total membrane lipid (Stoutjesdijk et al., 2018).

LC-PUFAs are important for synaptogenesis in the visual system, which is assessed by measuring visual acuity and speed of processing in infants. Breastfed infants appear to have a slight neurodevelopmental advantage, which is attributed to the high PUFA level of human milk. However, it should be noted that there are a number of selection biases, as women who choose to breastfeed tend to have higher IQ, level of education and socioeconomic status. Patterns of parent–child interactions may also be different.

The concentration of the LC-PUFAs (such as DHA, a component of membrane phospholipids of the brain and retina) in human milk is related to maternal intake and status. High fish oil intake or DHA supplementation of lactating women to optimize their status may confer neurodevelopmental and immunological benefits to the breastfed infants and, in addition, may possibly affect postnatal depression and cognitive function of the mothers. If maternal energy and fat intake fall, the fat composition of the milk resembles maternal adipose fat composition as fat stores are mobilized. If the maternal diet is high in energy but low in fat, milk triglycerides are higher in medium-length fatty acids (lauric acid, C_{12}, and myristic acid, C_{14}) indicating synthesis of fatty acids from carbohydrates is increased. Women of high parity (>10) may have decreased capacity for milk synthesis and therefore produce milk of lower fat (and energy) content.

The variation in milk fat reflects the variation in maternal diet. A low-fat maternal diet may maximize *de novo* synthesis of fatty acids for milk TAGs but should contain adequate quantities of LC-PUFAs. As a species, humans have a uniquely large brain, which is composed of ~60% lipid. The essential dietary requirement for LC-PUFAs required for the development of the human cerebral cortex has some interesting evolutionary aspects. It has been proposed that the freshwater lakes of the Rift Valley in East Africa provided the optimal environment to promote development of *Homo sapiens* (Broadhurst et al., 1998). Freshwater fish and shellfish are particularly rich in LC-PUFAs and have an ARA:DHA ratio similar to that of the human brain.

The importance of the long-chain fatty acid ratios may explain some of the observed benefits of breastfeeding such as the decreased incidence of multiple sclerosis and neurodegenerative diseases in later life (Echeverría et al., 2017). Animal fats, including human milk, tend to be rich in omega-6 fatty acids. Formula milks are supplemented with fat derived from vegetable sources so tend to be far richer in the omega-6 fatty acid, linoleic acid, than the omega-3 family of long-chain polyunsaturated fats. Milk intended for preterm babies is now supplemented with ARA and DHA because premature babies have a very limited capability in elongating and desaturating fatty acids and have not experienced as much placental transfer of fatty acids in the third trimester. As premature infants have a high requirement for neurodevelopment, optimal levels of these LC-PUFAs in breast milk of mothers of preterm infants can be achieved by giving the mothers a supplement or by adding DHA directly to expressed milk.

Lipases

The lipids present in human milk provide 40–60% of the infant's energy requirements during exclusive breast-feeding. The transition to extrauterine life at parturition places new demands on the neonatal gut for macronutrient digestion and absorption and this necessitates a different sequence of lipid degradation from that found in mature gut. These differences are difficult to study in healthy term neonates, where the invasive methods required would not be ethical, so our understanding of them is incomplete.

The key enzymes involved in lipid digestion are a family of lipases, which differ in their location and action. The neonatal GI tract has low levels of pancreatic TAG lipase and utilizes gastric lipase (GL), bile salt-dependent lipase (BSDL) from the pancreas and pancreatic lipase-related protein 2 (PLRP2) (Abrahamse et al., 2012). Breast milk itself also contains a high activity of bile salt-stimulated lipase (BSSL), which supplements the action of the neonatal lipases. BSSL breaks down TAGs including those with palmitic acid in the sn-2 position, which is common in breast milk. BSSL is a major component of TAG digestion in the neonate as demonstrated in preterm infants where faecal fat loss was greater (and therefore fat absorption was lower) with pasteurized breast milk consumption, which inactivates BSSL (Andersson et al., 2007). This enzyme, which is stable and active in the gut, has a significant effect on hydrolysis of milk TAGs and is activated by concentrations of bile salts even lower than those required for micelle formation.

Lipid digestion begins in the stomach and may be catalysed by both GL and lingual lipase that has been secreted into saliva. Digestion by these enzymes continues in the small intestine and together these may account for 60% of TAG digestion in the infant. Lingual lipase is stimulated by the presence of milk in the mouth and by suckling, even non-nutritive suckling. Human milk fat digestion is 85–90% efficient compared with the <70% efficiency of the fat digestion of cow milk-derived formulas. Lipoprotein lipase (serum-stimulated lipase) is also present in milk as a result of transcytosis from mammary tissue. Refrigerated and frozen milk undergo lipolysis resulting from their innate lipase activities.

As discussed above, human MFGs are enclosed in a trilaminar phospholipid layer, which maintains an optimal surface area for emulsification and absorption, protects the fat from lipolysis and oxidation, and prevents the fat globules from coalescing into large fat droplets that would be difficult to secrete and very difficult for the infant to digest. These factors mean that human milk stores well.

Carnitine

Human milk contains carnitine, which has an important role in facilitating the entry of long-chain fatty acids into mitochondria where they are oxidized. Carnitine is synthesized from the essential amino acids, lysine and methionine, but neonates may have limited synthetic capacity. Carnitine is also involved in the initiation of ketogenesis and in the regulation of heat generation by brown adipose tissue. As infants use fat as a major source of energy and have limited ability to synthesize carnitine, they have an increased need for carnitine, which is provided by breast milk.

Carbohydrate

Lactose, which is unique to mammalian milk (and probably therefore important in the development of the mammalian order), is the principal carbohydrate of milk, present at about 70 g/L and the main source of carbohydrate until weaning occurs. The lactose concentration of mature human milk is thought to be related to the size of the adult brain. Levels of lactose in milk are stable because, as described above, lactose transport drives the osmotic movement of water into milk and therefore the volume of milk produced. There is no evidence that maternal nutrition affects lactose concentration. As well as lactose, milk contains another 130 sugars, the most prevalent of which are glucose, galactose, glucosamine and other oligosaccharides (see below). Some of the nonlactose sugars contribute to favourable gut colonization. Some oligosaccharides, including the complex sugar L-fucose, promote the growth of *L. bifidus* resulting in increased gut acidity, which suppresses the growth of pathogenic bacteria and may also facilitate calcium absorption.

Lactose is digested by the enzyme lactase into its component monosaccharides, glucose and galactose. Lactase levels develop rapidly in late gestation and should be adequate for lactose digestion from 36 weeks in preterm infants but its activity cannot be prematurely induced by exposure to lactose. Although most babies are born with the ability to digest lactose, 75% of the world's population lose this ability at some stage after weaning. This loss reflects differences in genotype in different ethnic groups, not of the lactose gene itself, but of so-called 'lactase-persistence' genes that are inherited in different populations. The ability to produce lactase throughout life seems to be related to continual exposure to lactose in communities that have a strong economic dependence on dairy farming.

Lactose is relatively insoluble and is slowly digested and absorbed in the small intestine. It promotes the growth of microorganisms that produce organic acids and synthesize many B vitamins. The acidic environment is inhospitable to many pathogenic bacteria. Lactose forms soluble salts so the absorption of calcium, phosphorus, magnesium and other metals is increased in the presence of lactose.

Loss of lactase activity can result in lactose intolerance, a condition in which undigested lactose reaches the colonic microbiota, which ferment it to produce SCFAs, hydrogen, carbon dioxide and methane. The gases can cause bloating, flatulence and abdominal pain. SCFAs acidify the colon and increase the osmotic load, resulting in loose stools and diarrhoea.

Clinical Application: Nutritional Problems of Preterm Infants

Human milk is nutritionally inadequate for preterm infants, leading to poor growth rates and osteopenia. However, it does have clear advantages over formula feeds. It has valuable immunological properties, protecting against necrotizing enterocolitis (NEC; Box 16.8); 90% of infants affected by NEC have not been exposed to any human milk. Human milk is associated with improved cognition and it stimulates gut maturity and immunomodulation. The ideal food for a preterm infant able to tolerate lactose is the baby's own mother's milk fortified with additional calories, protein and minerals. Babies requiring parenteral feeding benefit from receiving some colostrum/milk in the gut. One of the problems of tube feeding is the loss of energy, as the fat tends to stick to the tubes. If the mother has a good supply of milk, fractionating the milk and feeding the baby the fat-rich hindmilk can increase the

---

BOX 16.8   Necrotizing Enterocolitis

- Due to a section of the gut dying from ischaemia and infection; most prominent in jejunum, ileum and colon
- Seen predominantly in premature infants (inversely related to gestational age at birth)
- Associated with infection, hypertonic feeds, hypovolaemia, perinatal asphyxia, congenital heart disease, premature/prolonged rupture of membranes, antibiotic therapy
- Clinical signs usually appear at 3–10 days old
- Symptoms may include abdominal distension, blood in stools, vomiting, lethargy, respiratory distress and poor thermoregulation
- Human milk (mother's own or donor) fed enterally is protective, possibly by stimulating gut maturity and integrity, providing substrates for enzymes and increasing perfusion. Probiotics may be protective
- Treatment may include bowel rest, enteral or parenteral feeding, intravenous antibiotics, fluid and electrolyte repletion.

---

energy content. Skin-to-skin contact has also been found to be important for premature babies and it helps to stimulate the mother's lactational capabilities. It also increases the maternal IgA in the milk, which might protect against pathogens encountered in hospital, which are potentially antibiotic resistant (nosocomial flora) or another environment that the mother and infant have been exposed to.

In preterm babies, with low lactase activity, a large proportion of lactose reaches the large intestine in an undigested form. SCFAs are absorbed across the intestinal mucosa and a proportion of the energy is recovered. This means that preterm babies are able to utilize a large proportion of the energy contributed from lactose. The extent of colonic salvage can be determined by measuring the amount of hydrogen in the baby's breath and can be severely compromised by antibiotics or surgery disrupting the gut microbiota. It is suggested that overaccumulation of organic acids in the lower gut may be a factor in the initiation of NEC (see Box 16.8).

Although galactose is directly involved in the synthesis of glycoproteins and glycolipids of the CNS, it is not essential in the diet. Galactose can be synthesized from glucose in the liver so glucose can substitute for lactose in a lactose-free diet. Alternatively, lactase can be added directly to bottles or milk can be fermented prior to ingestion.

Table 16.3 compares the composition of human colostrum, mature human milk and cow's milk.

Starch

Starch digestion in young babies is possible. Infant saliva contains some amylase activity but levels rapidly increase from 3 to 6 months. Pancreatic amylase activity is minimal in the first 3 months and remains low until about 6 months. Mammary amylase in human milk has a high activity in colostrum, and is retained for about 6 weeks. Intestinal mucosa has both disaccharidase and glucoamylase, which hydrolyse oligosaccharides and disaccharides. Glucoamylase is a brush-border enzyme that can hydrolyse glucose polymers in formula milk. Formula feeds derived from cow's milk often contain maltodextrin, a polymer of maltose and glucose. This has the advantages of being easily digested and increasing the viscosity and mineral content of the formula. Babies are born with relatively high levels of glucoamylase activity, which further increases after birth. Glucoamylase is less susceptible to being affected by intestinal mucosal damage and is distributed along the length of the small intestine, which increases the efficiency of hydrolysis and uptake of its products.

There is evidence that the ability to digest starch can be induced if starch is present in the diet. Adaptation is not quick and may take days to weeks. Undigested starch causes gastrointestinal disturbances, such as diarrhoea, interfering with the absorption of other nutrients, so affected infants

TABLE 16.3 Comparison of the Composition of Human Colostrum, Mature Human Milk and Cow's Milk

	Colostrum (100 mL)	Mature Human Milk (100 mL)	Cow's Milk (100mL)	Comments
Energy	243 kJ (58 kcal)	293 kJ (70 kcal)	276 kJ (66 kcal)	Colostrum is produced in small but easily digested amounts – produced during first 3 days of life; neonate may feed frequently as metabolic process adapts from the constant feed environment of the uterus to an extra-uterine fast/feed cycle
Protein	1.5-2.0 g Immu-noglobulins account for increased pro-tein content	0.8-1.1 g (mostly whey); lact-albumin; immuno-globulins; lactoferrin; lysozyme; enzymes; hormones [Note: old data derived protein content from total nitrogen so included nonprotein nitrogen and over-estimated total protein]	3.7 g (high casein content)	Colostrum is rich in passive immune factors to provide initial protection to the infant. Cow's is milk harder to digest owing to increased casein, it also contains lactoglobulin not found in breast milk (may be responsible for cow's milk allergy). The higher cow's milk protein concentration supports the faster growth trajectory of the calf.
Lactose	2.0-5.0 g	6.7-7.2 g provides 37% of energy requirement	4.5 g	Breast milk tastes sweeter than cow's milk
Fat	1.5-2.0 g	3.5-4.8 g (98% tri-glycerides) provides ~50% of energy requirements	3.7 g	All mammalian milks are rich in fats which provides a high yield of energy. Hind milk has more fat and energy than fore milk.
Sodium	40 mg	18 mg	44 mg	Higher concentrations of organic ions in cow's milk; the human neonatal kidney may be unable to regulate higher ion concentrations owing to immaturity
Potassium		52.5 mg	174.2 mg	
Chloride		43 mg	29 mg	
Calcium		28 mg	120 mg	
Phosphorus		14 mg	91 mg	
Magnesium		3.1 mg	11.6 mg	
Vitamin A	Increased level	65 µg	43 µg	
Vitamin D		0.05 µg		
Vitamin E	0.8 mg	0.23 mg	0.09 mg	
Vitamin K	2x higher	0.2 µg		
Thiamin	16 µg	20 µg		
Riboflavin	30 µg	35 µg		
Vitamin B_{12}	0.01 µg	0.4 µg		
Vitamin B_6	5-20 µg	10 µg	20 µg	
Folate	5.2 µg	5.2 µg		
Pantothenic acid	0.26 mg	0.26 mg	0.31 mg	
Biotin		0.73 µg		
Vitamin C	3.5 mg	4.2 mg	0.37 mg	
Iron	0.12 µg	0.04-0.08 mg	0.02-0.06 mg	Breast milk has low levels of iron; however, iron from breast milk is absorbed much more efficiently than from iron supplements or for-tified infant formula derived from cows milk

TABLE 16.3 Comparison of the Composition of Human Colostrum, Mature Human Milk and Cow's Milk

	Colostrum (100 mL)	Mature Human Milk (100 mL)	Cow's Milk (100mL)	Comments
Copper	0.13 mg	0.025 mg		
Zinc	1.3 mg	0.15 mg	0.34 mg	
Iodine	30 µg	5-15 µg		Breast milk iodine depends on the mother's iodine status so it is higher in countries where there are salt iodization programmes.

may exhibit symptoms of failure to thrive. Hypoxia and ischaemia result in decreased intestinal perfusion, which alters the structure of the epithelial cells affecting uptake of monosaccharides.

Human Milk Oligosaccharides

HMOs are a diverse group of structurally complex unconjugated glycans; about 200 different HMOs have been identified, which have a lactose backbone with additions of galactose, fucose, N-acetylglucosamine or sialic acid molecules. Compared with other mammals, human milk seems to have a particularly diverse profile of oligosaccharides, which vary genetically and with the duration of lactation and the time of day. The concentration of HMOs is ~5–15 g/L (making it the third most abundant component after lipids and lactose; Triantis et al., 2018). The role of oligosaccharides in milk is protective and facilitative. HMOs are minimally absorbed and act as substrates (prebiotics) for the gut microbiota. HMOs also act as soluble decoy receptors and to bind pathogens, so the pathogens do not bind to the infant gut cells. A small proportion of the total HMOs is absorbed and enters the circulation; the urine contains excreted HMOs, which act as decoy receptors for urinary pathogens and thus protect against urinary infections

HMOs promote a beneficial profile of gut microbiota in the colon of breastfed babies, which results in a characteristic pH; effectively they make human breast milk (HBM) a functional food. HMOs interact with cells of the immune system both via the gut and systemically, protecting breastfed infants against allergies, NEC and other inflammatory diseases, and enhancing cognitive function. Breast milk also has high concentrations of gangliosides, which are found in high concentrations in the brain; they are deposited in the developing brain in fetal and early neonatal life and play a role in the development and maturation of the brain such as neuronal growth and myelination. They may influence cognitive function and development of the gut.

Vitamins

A plentiful supply of breast milk from a well-nourished woman contains all the vitamins required by the term neonate, with the possible exceptions of vitamins D and K. Dietary taboos practised during lactation in some cultures may affect the vitamin content of breast milk. As fat is the most variable constituent of the milk, the level of fat-soluble vitamins is relatively unstable. There is a seasonal variation in the vitamin A content of cow's milk. Water-soluble vitamins in breast milk fluctuate with maternal intake as they move readily from maternal serum to milk. Human milk has a high level of vitamin C but there may be a seasonal variation in vitamin C content and both infant and maternal requirements for vitamin C increase with stress (including lactation). B vitamin levels in milk are acutely affected by maternal diet. Vitamin B_{12}, which is found in animal protein, is likely to be deficient in the milk from strict vegetarian or vegan women who should be advised to take vitamin B_{12} supplements during pregnancy and lactation. Breastfed infants of mothers who are vitamin B_{12} deficient may develop clinical signs of deficiency even if their mothers have not reached that stage. Transfer of folate from maternal plasma into milk occurs against a steep concentration gradient so the nursing infant is well protected against maternal folate deficiency. However, maternal folate reserves may be depleted during lactation, which would have important consequences for the mother and her own folate status, especially if the interpregnancy interval is short.

Vitamin D

Breastfed babies rarely develop rickets although the level of vitamin D in breast milk is low. The vitamin D content of foods is measured by assessing the vitamin D content of the fat fraction. However, breast milk may contain an aqueous vitamin D sulphate, which is not included in the fat fraction, so the vitamin D content of breast milk may be underestimated. Although the vitamin D level in breast milk has been reported to be low, it is not low if the mothers have had optimal vitamin D status themselves throughout pregnancy and lactation (though there is no consensus about what that level is). Neonates have stores of all fat-soluble vitamins, including vitamin D, and although they have the physiological capability of synthesizing vitamin D on exposure to sunlight from an early age, it is recommended that infants <6 months old are protected from direct sunlight. Vitamin D-deficient milk is associated with low exposure of the lactating mother to sun, long winters, Northern climes, use of sun screen, pigmented skins and cultural practices such as covering the skin, all factors that compromise maternal vitamin D status. Increased levels of pollution may also affect vitamin D synthesis in the skin. Certain ethnic groups, who cover up for cultural and religious reasons, have an increased risk of vitamin D deficiency. Supplementing breastfeeding mothers ensures the breastfeeding infant receives adequate vitamin D.

Vitamin E

Vitamin E, mostly in the form of α-tocopherol, is an antioxidant. Deficiency compromises the integrity of the red blood cell membrane and can lead to microhaemorrhages if severe. In formula feeds, the α-tocopherol:PUFA ratio is held constant (1 IU vitamin E per gram of linoleic acid).

Vitamin K

Vitamin K deficiency may be associated with vitamin K deficiency bleeding (see Chapter 15), usually due to low stores of vitamin K rather than low levels in the milk. There is a critical need for vitamin K during birth and in the first days of life when the risk of bleeding, particularly intracranially, is high. Vitamin K is not efficiently transferred across the placenta. The major source of vitamin K in postnatal life is from the byproducts of bacterial metabolism, but the baby is born with a low level of gut microbiota, and gut colonization capable of producing vitamin K is not adequate until the baby is at least 6 weeks old as lactobacilli do not synthesize menaquinones (vitamin K_2 homologues). Concentrations of vitamin K are higher in colostrum and early milk, particularly the hindmilk as vitamin K is fat soluble. Breast milk stimulates colonization of the gut by vitamin K-producing bacteria. A prophylactic dose of vitamin K is routinely given at birth to protect against vitamin K deficiency bleeding (VKDB).

Vitamin A

Vitamin A requirement is increased if stores accrued in fetal life are inadequate or there are problems with fat absorption. A deficiency of vitamin A in infancy is associated with bronchopulmonary dysplasia. This may result from a low intake or increased requirement for the vitamin in healing the damaged lung epithelium. Breastfeeding women are advised to select plenty of vegetables and fruit rich in provitamin A (see Chapter 12). Breastfed infants of mothers with adequate vitamin A status are protected from deficiency but the milk content is sensitive to maternal diet.

Minerals

The mineral content of milk is slightly affected by maternal diet but milk provides all the major minerals and trace elements required by the normal term infant. Usually the mother's dietary deficiency or excess intake of minerals does not affect the composition of her milk very much as maternal homeostasis protects the infant against fluctuations of most minerals in the maternal diet. Parenteral feeding of infants, rather than frank deficiencies, has elicited most information about mineral requirements. Deficiencies are usually associated with short gestation or severe placental insufficiency.

The concentration of most minerals remains generally low but the bioavailability is high. Human milk has a number of binding proteins, notably for iron, calcium and zinc. Although the level of iron in breast milk is low, absorption of iron from human milk is particularly efficient, aided by the lactoferrin and transferrin content of milk and its low pH. Iron requirements in infants are relatively low for the first few months of life because there is recycling of the iron from red blood cells as their higher number in fetal blood is reduced in the neonate and the iron is recycled. Lactoferrin binds to the iron in milk and makes it unavailable for pathogens in the neonatal gut.

The sodium content of human milk is inversely related to the volume of milk produced so it is higher initially and at weaning. Cow's milk has four times the sodium content of human milk. Hypernatraemia, caused for instance by hot weather, mild infection or overconcentrated formula reconstitution, can result in dehydration.

Calcium absorption is affected by vitamin D, calcium and phosphorus concentrations, fatty acids and lactose. It is particularly enhanced by the acid environment and low phosphorus content of human milk. The concentration of calcium in blood is tightly regulated; there seems to be similar homeostatic mechanisms ensuring a relatively constant concentration of calcium in breast milk (Kent et al., 2009). The calcium:phosphorus ratio of human milk is 2:4 (compared with 1:3 in cow's milk). If phosphorus levels are high, there is increased phosphorus absorption at the expense of calcium absorption as they compete for the same mechanism of transfer across the gut wall. The resulting fall in plasma calcium concentration can cause hypocalcaemia with symptoms of jitteriness, tetany and convulsions.

The iodine content of breast milk is determined by the mother's intake, which depends on the iodine in the food supply (i.e. soil). The physiological demands of lactation can precipitate thyroid hypertrophy (goitre). Adequate infant iodine intake is crucial for optimal neurodevelopment so in many countries lactating women are advised to take a daily iodine supplement.

Milk-borne Trophic Factors

As well as nutritive and immunological factors, human milk contains a group of biologically active factors that affect nutritional status and somatic growth. The immature neonatal mucosa can allow potentially immunogenic molecules to cross the gut wall; human milk accelerates maturation of the gut barrier function. Human milk contains products of the maternal adaptive immune system such as antibodies and components of the innate immune system; in addition, components in human milk attenuate early inappropriate inflammatory responses. The biologically active factors in human milk can be classified into four groups: hormones and peptide growth factors, nucleotides and nucleosides, polyamines and digestive enzymes. The hormone group includes insulin, GH, insulin-like growth factors (IGF-I and IGF-II), somatostatin, EGF, prolactin, erythropoietin and GH-releasing factor. Some of these hormones and growth factors are absorbed across the permeable neonatal gut into the body where they affect metabolism and promote growth and differentiation of organs and tissues. Other hormones, such as somatostatin, appear not to be absorbed but resist proteolysis, having an effect directly on the wall of the gut. The growth factors in human milk may modulate the development of the infant gut, protecting gastrointestinal cells and therefore reducing the risk of NEC.

Both human and bovine colostrum are rich in nucleotides, which are precursors of nucleic acids. Nucleotides appear to have a role in enhancing growth and differentiation. They are particularly involved in liver cell function, lipid metabolism and lipoprotein synthesis. They also affect the development of the gut-associated lymphoid tissue (GALT). Unlike cow's milk, mature human milk maintains high levels of nucleotides.

The polyamines, spermine and spermidine, are present in all cells but human milk has about 10 times as much polyamine content as cow's milk. Levels of polyamines are particularly high in the first days of lactation. They may have mitogenic, metabolic and immunological effects promoting gut development of the newborn. Enzymes present in milk include amylase, lipase and proteases to aid digestion.

Case study 16.3 is an example of concerns about newborn nutrition.

Special Considerations

Breast milk can vary in taste and colour and may contain components that can affect the infant's digestive system. Some components of the mother's diet such as artichokes, asparagus, peppers, legumes, brassica (vegetables from the cabbage family) and alliums (vegetables from the onion family) may occasionally result in a reaction from the infant though the evidence that maternal diet is the cause of infant colic is inconsistent. The taste and flavour or odour of breast milk can be altered by components in the maternal diet such as garlic, blueberries or carrots (Mennella, 2014) and are thought to be related to flavours

of the amniotic fluid. When the breastfeeding mother consumes garlic, the infant consumes more milk. These early flavour and odour experiences may programme later food preferences including those at weaning. The weanling seeks and prefers flavours encountered in gestation and breastfeeding; effectively breast milk offers an early learning experience about what is safe to eat.

Rarely, breast milk colour has been reported to be affected by excessive maternal consumption of food colouring (usually from soft and sports drinks) and drug therapy (Lawrence and Lawrence, 2015).

It has been suggested that susceptible infants might be exposed to environmental allergens and dietary antigens via their mother's breast milk. Previously, women with a history of allergy were advised to avoid potential allergens, such as nuts, eggs, cow's milk, berries and tropical foods, while breastfeeding. However, the previously advocated advice to avoid common food allergens in pregnancy and while breastfeeding appears to have been detrimental and caused increased prevalence of allergies and potential nutritional deficiencies in women following very restrictive diets. The current advice is that early exposure to allergens and increased dietary diversity decreases the risk of allergy. Women are recommended to follow a normal diet and to avoid delaying the introduction of solid foods including potentially allergenic foods. Breastfeeding while introducing new foods is beneficial (Julia et al., 2015).

Caffeine and alcohol both pass into breast milk. Caffeine is the most commonly consumed psychoactive drug in the

---

CASE STUDY 16.3

Isla is 11 days old and has just regained her birthweight. She has been breastfed since birth and appears to be very healthy and alert. Julia, her mother, contacts the midwife because she is concerned about Isla who is sleeping 12 h at night and feeds only four times a day. Julia's elder sister also gave birth recently and her 21-day-old baby feeds every 2 h, day and night, and has been progressively gaining weight. Julia's sister reported that her midwife told her that this is how a newborn baby normally behaves and advises Julia to stop breastfeeding because her baby is not growing properly.

- How can the midwife reassure Julia that Isla is well, feeding normally and gaining adequate nutrition?
- What concerns, if any, would you have for Julia's niece or how would you reassure Julia that all was normal?
- Why do some babies have different patterns of feeding and weight gain?

world and is derived from coffee, tea, cocoa, chocolate and many sugar- and artificially-sweetened beverages including sports and energy drinks.

With all substances including caffeine, nicotine, alcohol and drugs, the levels are reduced in the milk if maternal consumption is timed immediately after a feed with the longest possible time before the next feed. There are differences in individual metabolism of caffeine so caffeine levels in breast milk may be high if the mother is a slow metabolizer. Not surprisingly, there is no consensus about the safe intake, though some authorities such as the UK NHS and European Food Safety Authority suggest 200 mg/day (half the prepregnant maximum guideline), despite insufficient evidence (McCreedy et al., 2018). The effects of caffeine on the neonate include agitation and jitteriness, being unsettled and having sleeping difficulties, and having gut problems including constipation and colic. Given the importance of the first 1000 days in an individual's life and that breastfeeding is promoted, caffeine avoidance is the best option until more robust evidence about the safety of caffeine for neonates is available.

Breastfeeding women are encouraged to exercise and many are motivated by the desire to lose weight. It is recommended that women resume normal physical activity as soon after delivery as it is medically and physically safe to do so. Moderate exercise and short-term weight loss do not affect milk composition or production or affect the infant's growth; they have positive effects on the mother's physical and psychological health. More intense or exhaustive exercise (and fasting, e.g. for religious reasons) can affect milk composition and may also affect infant growth. Intense exercise transiently increases blood lactic acid levels but it returns to normal within about an hour. There may be some transfer of lactic acid into breast milk. Human milk is characteristically sweet, whereas the addition of lactic acid, which has a sour or bitter taste, may result in infants displaying puckering facial expressions and even rejecting milk if they are offered it close to exercise. However, not all infants are sensitive to the taste of lactic acid and discarding the first few millilitres of milk by manual expression often remedies the situation (Lawrence and Lawrence, 2015). Physical activity and energy intake must be balanced. Severe energy restriction and rapid weight loss can result in fat-soluble environmental contaminants, such as pesticide residues, being mobilized and secreted in milk.

IMMUNOLOGICAL PROPERTIES OF HUMAN MILK

Human milk provides a broad range of non-nutritive components as well as nutrients. Neonates are particularly

---

BOX 16.9   Advantages of Breastfeeding

- Improved survival, health, growth and development of all infants
- Optimal infant nutrition
- Convenience, cost and lack of contamination, low environmental impact
- Reduced risk of mortality from necrotizing enterocolitis and sudden infant death syndrome
- Reduced infection: gastrointestinal, respiratory, urinary tract, ear, meningitis, intractable diarrhoea
- Reduced atopic disease and allergy (eczema, asthma)
- Increased intelligence
- Reduced overweight and obesity in childhood and adulthood
- Reduced risk of autoimmune disease
- Enhanced immunity
- Reduced risk of maternal cancer: breast, ovarian
- Increased maternal oxytocin levels: promote expulsion of placenta, minimize postpartum blood loss, and facilitates rapid uterine involution (see Chapter 14)
- The promotion of exclusive breastfeeding for at least the first 6 months of life:
  - may significantly reduce the healthcare costs within the population both in the short- and long term
  - may reduce the incidence and severity of mental health problems for the neonate in later life
  - may reduce the risk of maternal late onset diabetes

---

susceptible to infection (see Chapter 15) because of the immaturity of their immune system. There is limited exposure to antigens in the relatively sterile environment of the uterus and the cells responsible for adaptive immunity are lower in number and less responsive to infectious threats. Some of the nutrient components of human milk can be multifunctional in that either in their native or partially digested state, they are immunologically active. Human milk hinders bacterial growth in the proximal small intestine, whereas cow's milk promotes bacterial growth, which is optimal for ruminants. Breastfed infants have fewer infections (Box 16.9), but some of this effect may be due to a decreased exposure to other foods bearing microorganisms. Breastfeeding appears to protect against sudden infant death syndrome (SIDS). (Note that there are several significant risk factors for SIDS including not being breastfed, sleeping face down, overheating and exposure to smoke.) The immune properties of milk are also important in protecting the breasts themselves from infection. Many cultures use breast milk topically, for instance to treat eye infections. Immunological properties of human milk are increased with better maternal nutrition. Human milk has a high antioxidant capacity because it is rich in ascorbic acid, uric acid, α-tocopherol and β-carotene; this may be particularly important for preterm infants who have an immature antioxidant defence system and so are more prone to oxidative stress.

Immunoglobulins

The immunoglobulins (antibodies) in milk are distinct from those found in maternal serum. The major immunoglobulin is secretory IgA, which is produced from plasma cells in the breast; milk also contains minor amounts of monomeric IgA, IgG and IgM. Secretory IgA is at very high concentrations in the colostrum but declines to lower levels over the first 1–2 weeks as milk volume increases. The mother will produce specific immunoglobulins to every pathogen she encounters. The transfer of IgA into the milk is a form of passive immunity, whereby antibodies to antigens in the mother's environment are transferred to the neonate (see Chapter 10), augmenting the placental transfer of IgG to the fetus. The baby's own immune system is further stimulated by factors in the milk. Breastfed babies have superior responses to vaccination programmes and have higher IgA in their saliva, nasal secretions and urine.

IgA is stable at low pH and resistant to proteolytic enzymes (because its structure is 2 molecules of IgA linked together by a joining chain and a secretory component that confers resistance to digestion by trypsin and chymotrypsin) so its activity is maintained in the gastrointestinal tract. IgA has an important role in the defence against infection, slowing bacterial and viral invasion of the mucosa by neutralizing toxins. It adheres to the gastric mucosa and binds to antigens on the pathogen so preventing adhesion of microorganisms to the gut wall. IgA promotes closure of the gut and so decreases its permeability to allergens such as cow's milk β-lactoglobulin and serum bovine albumin. The type of IgA secreted into breast milk will depend on the antigens the mother has been exposed to; the infant receives IgA antibodies against the same antigens (this is known as the enteromammary link; Lönnerdal, 2016).

Binding Proteins

Lactoferrin is the predominant whey protein in HBM (1–7 g/L) and has multiple bacteriostatic, antimicrobial and anti-infective functions (Telang, 2018). It is a member of the transferrin family of iron-binding glycoproteins that facilitates the absorption of iron from milk. In binding iron, it reduces the amount of free iron available for microorganisms in the gut, thus inhibiting the growth of certain pathogenic bacteria. Lactoferrin in breast milk helps to reduce the incidence of gastrointestinal tract infections, whereas excess free iron is associated with increased bacterial pathogens in the gut. These bacteria have a high iron requirement and can cause gut damage and microhaemorrhages; oral iron therapy in infants can enhance the growth of these iron-requiring pathogens and cause further gut damage and exacerbate the iron deficiency. Lactoferrin also inhibits the pathological activity of several bacteria, stimulates macrophage phagocytotic activity and inhibits viruses such as HIV, CMV and herpes virus. Partial digestion of lactoferrin produces lactoferricin B, a peptide that has antibacterial activity against Gram-positive and Gram-negative bacteria. Some lactoferrin and its pepsin-mediated breakdown product, lactoferricin, are absorbed and excreted in the urine where they probably also protect against urinary tract infections. Lactoferrin also promotes the maturation of the neonatal immune system, stimulates intestinal growth and proliferation of enterocytes and promotes the growth of intestinal bifidobacteria.

Lactoferrin is damaged by heat treatment (in pasteurization) and is sensitive to cold (damaged by freezing). This is why fresh breast milk has a greater protective effect against sepsis and NEC compared with donor milk.

Haptocorrin (transcobalamin-1), the binding protein for vitamin B_{12}, is similarly resistant to digestion; haptocorrin inhibits the enterotoxigenic bacterium *Escherichia coli* (*E. coli*).

Other Protective Properties

Breast milk contains high levels of lysozyme, an antimicrobial enzyme protective against Gram-positive bacteria because it breaks down peptidoglycan, which is the major component of Gram-positive bacterial cell walls. It is produced in many body secretions, including breast milk, and protects the mucosal surfaces of the gut and respiratory tract in later life but levels are very low in infancy. Lysozyme has a bacteriostatic effect against *E. coli* and can also inhibit growth of fungi such as *Candida albicans*. Breast milk contains prebiotic substances, called bifidogenic or bifidus factors, which together with lactose stimulate the growth of lactobacilli that produce organic acids, thus promoting an acidic and protective environment. Bifidus factors are human milk glycans (glycopeptides and glycoproteins). Fibronectin, which is present in high concentrations in human milk, is a nonspecific opsonin (see Chapter 10) that increases phagocytosis of bacteria. Milk also contains other protective factors (Table 16.4).

Milk is not sterile but contains about 4×10^9 maternal cells per litre including lymphocytes from maternal Peyer's

TABLE 16.4 Protective Factors in Milk

Factor	Function
Immune and stem cells	Respond to infections and differentiate into functional cells in infant
B lymphocytes	Produce antibodies against specific microbes
T lymphocytes	Kill infected cells
Macrophages	Produce lysozyme and activate parts of the immune system
Neutrophils	Phagocytose bacteria
Lacto bifidus factor	Promotes an acidic environment favourable for the growth of *Lactobacillus bifidus* and inhibits the growth of pathogenic microorganisms
Immunoglobulins (antibodies IgA, IgG, IgM, IgD and IgE)	Active against specific organisms, that is, poliomyelitis, salmonella
Immunoglobulin A (IgA)	Lines the gut to discourage adhesion of pathogenic microorganisms and limits allergen entry
Lactoferrin	Decreases iron available by binding to iron for bacterial growth
	Acts as a bacteriostatic agent
Lysozyme Lactoperoxidase	Act in a nonspecific way by damaging the cell walls of microorganisms
Complement	Contributes to immune responses
Lipids	Inhibit growth of staphylococcus and viruses by disrupting cell membranes
Fibronectin	Promotes macrophage activity and aids repair to damaged gut tissue
γ-Interferon	Promotes activity of immune cells
Mucins	Adhere to microorganisms inhibiting attachment to the gut wall
Oligosaccharides	Inhibit attachment of microorganisms to mucosal surfaces, promotion of optimal profile of microbiota in colon
Bile salt-stimulated lipase	Acts as an antiprotozoal
	Promotes fat digestion
Lipoprotein lipase, α-amylase	Promotes fat digestion
α_1-Antitrypsin α_1-Antichymotrypsin	Prevent breakdown of protective factors
Epidermal growth factor	Promotes maturation of the gut wall
Binding proteins B12-binding protein (haptocorrin) Lactoferrin Transferrin Folate-binding protein Somatomedin C	Increase absorption of nutrients and limit availability of nutrients utilized by bacteria

patches, epithelial cells, and scavenger macrophages and neutrophils. Levels of maternal cells are particularly high in the colostrum. In addition, milk contains 10^4–10^6 commensal and beneficial bacterial cells (Ojo-Okunola et al., 2018) and other microbes per litre. The HBM bacterial cells, predominantly lactic acid bacteria, serve as probiotic species, which are delivered and function in the infant's gut. The stable 'core' human milk bacteriome of nine bacterial genera is not observed in colostrum but becomes established

as lactation progresses (Hunt et al., 2011). Some of the bacterial species may come from the mother's skin or infant's mouth and enter the mammary tissue by retrograde flow (Ramsay et al., 2005) but others are obligate anaerobes, which would not survive in the skin. An enteromammary pathway is suggested, whereby bacteria from the mother's gut are transported to the mother's lymphatic system and then to the mammary gland (Rodriguez, 2014). HBM bacteria are thought to protect the breastfed infant from infections by producing antimicrobial substances and competitively excluding pathogens. They may also improve the intestinal barrier function by decreasing permeability and increasing mucus production. They may also have anti-allergy and immune-modulatory properties. The HBM bacteria have the capability of digesting HMO and enhancing the production of SCFAs in the infant's gut. In addition, they have a role in protection of the mammary gland from short-term infection or mastitis (dysbiosis of the HBM bacteriome), which may protect against breast cancer in the future. Breast milk also contains stem cells, which have the capability to differentiate into neural cell lines and may be involved in the development of the infant's enteric nervous system (Witkowska-Zimny and Kaminska-El-Hassan, 2017).

Proteins and mucins of the MFGM itself may confer immunological advantages (Lönnerdal, 2016). The milk fat TAGs are surrounded by three membranes, which contain a range of proteins (e.g. lactadherin, butyrophilin and MUC1) and which have antimicrobial properties. Other factors in human milk with anti-infective or immunological properties include anti-proteases, which inhibit the breakdown of anti-infective immunoglobulins and enzymes, free fatty acids, which have antiviral properties and cytokines, which stimulate an inflammatory response from the immune cells.

FORMULA FEEDING

Human milk substitutes existed before the modern age of infant formulas. There were two approaches, either using a surrogate mother or wet nurse, or feeding milk from another mammal. In Western countries, where dairy farming is established, cow's milk is modified and processed into the formula feeds, which are the basis of bottle feeding. Children in other cultures are reared on buffalo, goat, horse, camel and yak milk. Mammalian milks may be quantitatively similar but the quality is variable, being species-specific and the subtypes of antibodies present, for example, might be very different.

Cow's milk is supplemented with carbohydrate, either lactose or maltodextrin, which dilutes the higher mineral and protein content. Cow's milk fat (which has a high commercial value as butter and cream) is substituted with vegetable oil-fat blends. This increases the absorption efficiency; unabsorbed fat decreases the energy content, lowers calcium absorption and produces steatorrhoea.

For whey-dominant formulas, demineralized whey (which is expensive) is blended with skimmed milk to increase the whey:casein ratio and decrease the electrolyte content. The profit margin of whey-dominant formulas is lower than that of casein-dominant formulas. Casein-dominant formulas are marketed for the 'hungrier baby' and, although the energy content is constant, are considered to be a progressive step in feeding. Mothers often demonstrate a strong brand loyalty when choosing formula milk. Many formula milks for term infants, particularly the prestige or 'gold' versions, are supplemented with LC-PUFAs, DHA and ARA, to benefit brain growth and optimize the immune system. The source of these fatty acids is often algae rather than marine oils, which may result in fishy odour.

Hydrolysed protein formula milks are produced for infants with gastrointestinal or allergy problems; the hydrolysis of the bovine milk proteins into smaller protein fragments appears to facilitate absorption and the smaller particles are less allergenic. Soy-based formulas were originally designed for infants intolerant of cow's milk protein-based formula milks. The early problems of loose malodorous stools, nappy rash and stained clothing associated with soy milk have been remedied by the use of isolated soy protein rather than soy flour. Concerns have been raised about the high levels of aluminium and phytoestrogens in soy formula milk; phytoestrogens may affect sexual development, immune and thyroid functions and neurobehavioural development. Soy-based formula milks are suitable for infants with the rare inborn errors of metabolism such as galactosaemia and hereditary lactase deficiency or where a vegetarian diet is preferred. Many infants with diagnosed allergy to cows' milk protein also have an allergy to soy so the extensively hydrolysed protein formula is usually the preferred option. Soy-based formula milks are not appropriate for preterm infants.

Trace minerals and vitamins are added according to legal limits. Taurine is added to formula milk and, more recently, nucleotides have been added; they probably act as growth factors and may have immune effects, strengthening responses to immunization and reducing diarrhoea. Carnitine may also be added to formula milks. Carnitine is required for the transport of long-chain fatty acids from cytosol into the mitochondrial matrix for oxidation; levels in unsupplemented soy-based and protein hydrolysate formula milks are particularly low.

Packaging of formula feed is important. Anaerobic storage and copper supplementation help to reduce fatty acid oxidation. Scoop and granule size are carefully designed to optimize precision in reconstitution. Current research into the optimal (and most profitable) formulations includes adding specific proteins such as α-lactalbumin, adjusting the ratio of amino acids such as glycine, leucine, arginine, cysteine and tryptophan, and adding probiotics and prebiotics such as synthetic HMO.

Breastfed infants grow faster in the first 2 months of life and then more slowly (in weight gain and length) in the first year and have a different body composition than formula-fed infants. Some of the differences in body composition may be related to leptin and adiponectin in breast milk, which affect appetite and growth (Larsson et al., 2018). Breastfed infants consume less milk (~85% of that consumed by formula-fed infants) and have lower energy expenditure. Breastfed infants have a lower risk for obesity, insulin resistance and type 2 diabetes in later life. Gastric emptying is faster in breastfed infants and there is less gastro-oesophageal reflux and loss of food intake in breastfed infants. They also have less infectious disease (see below) and a lower rate of NEC. Concerns have been raised about rapid rates of weight gain in infancy, particularly in formula-fed infants, being associated with later obesity. Breastfed infants self-regulate their appetite, whereas formula-fed infants are often encouraged to 'finish their bottle'. In addition, there may be factors in breast milk that affect satiety. Breastfed infants are often introduced to complementary feeding at a slightly older age, which may protect against later weight gain. Growth charts derived from data from formula-fed infants are not appropriate to assess growth of breastfed infants.

COMPLEMENTARY FEEDING (WEANING)

Weaning can be defined as the progressive transition from milk to 'solid food' or 'a normal family diet'. The WHO recommendations, which are almost universally adopted, are that the best options are to exclusively breastfeed for at least 6 months, then to offer nutritious complementary foods and continue breastfeeding up to the age of 2 years or until mutually agreed by the mother and child. These recommendations are often not followed. Early cessation of breastfeeding is considered inadvisable, because it is associated with an increased incidence of diarrhoea and interference with the maintenance of breastfeeding (the nutritional value of most complementary foods is usually lower than that of breast milk). An increase in dietary cereals and vegetables tends to affect the absorption of iron, which can be delicately balanced in younger infants. By 6 months, many babies may require complementary feeding and will have sufficiently developed to cope with it. Deciduous teeth erupt at about 6 months. Incisors, which cut food, are the first teeth to appear, followed by molars at about 12 months, which allow grinding of food. Although it is not the current practice in many developed and developing countries, there is a call for meat to be introduced as an early complementary food, as it provides essential micronutrients.

Determination of the appropriate time to introduce foods other than milk is not just by age but should also take into consideration the food available, conditions to prepare it, the growth velocity and the neuromuscular development of the infant. It is not clear which pattern of growth is optimal. Growth charts are based on weight and height data from clinical surveillance. Ethnicity, environmental and genetic factors all affect growth. Practically, the high weight velocity, which is seen in the first 3 months of life, is not related to overfeeding. The deceleration of growth after 3 months is not in itself an indicator to wean. Early weaning is associated with an increased number of respiratory symptoms and has numerous implications for health in later life.

By 6 months, normal physiological development can support the introduction of alternative foods. The baby is able to hold its head erect and can control the movement of its hands to its mouth. The tongue extrusion reflex is waning and can be overcome. Indeed, it is suggested that there is a critical window for introducing solid food, and if it is not done within this window, the baby tends to develop a preference for liquid feeds and may become a child with feeding problems. The kidneys are mature enough to cope with a solute load.

Although the health benefits of breastfeeding are not disputed, opinions and recommendations are divided on the optimal duration of exclusive breastfeeding. Following the WHO recommendations would to exclusively breastfeed for 6 months would have impact on neonatal morbidity and mortality would be significant; it is estimated that the scaling up of breastfeeding would prevent about 823,000 child deaths and 20,000 breast cancer deaths per year (Rollins et al., 2016). Despite this, many authorities argue that there is a lack of clear evidence to either support or refute recommendations for the age of introduction of complementary foods to the breastfed or formula-fed infant to be between 4 and 6 months. Although exclusive breastfeeding for the first 6 months of life can support growth and development in some infants, subgroups have been identified within certain populations who may require complementary feeding prior to this age, particularly larger, and often male, infants. To be confident that exclusive breastfeeding does not increase the risk of undernutrition (growth faltering) in healthy term infants, it may be necessary to make recommendations for infant weight rather than infant age.

Complementary feeding is an important biological and social learning process as well as offering foods of higher nutrient and energy density than milk. Exposing different tastes to children has already begun *in utero* with amniotic fluid and is consolidated by breast milk feeding because compounds ingested by the mother are transported into the milk and create a flavour experience (Birch, 2016). This develops the inherent taste variation of breastfed infants, affecting the development of food preferences; this important learning experience is not received by bottle-fed babies.

KEY POINTS

- The physiological unit of the mammary gland is the alveolus. Prolactin, from the anterior pituitary, stimulates milk production from the alveolar (mammary epithelial) cells. Oxytocin, from the posterior pituitary, stimulates contraction of the myoepithelial cells surrounding the alveoli and the ducts, resulting in milk ejection or 'let-down'.

- Prolactin secretion slowly reaches a peak following stimulation at the nipple. Secretion is pulsatile and circadian and is controlled by the abrogation of tonic inhibition from dopamine produced by the hypothalamus. Prolactin inhibits ovulation thus suppressing fertility.

- Oxytocin release is stimulated by nipple stimulation and by thinking about or hearing the baby. Secretion of oxytocin immediately follows stimulation and can be inhibited by stress.

- The effects of prolactin are thought to be locally controlled by the production of FIL in the milk. Increased concentrations of FIL suppress the response to prolactin thus inhibiting milk production. This is important in mammary gland involution when breastfeeding is curtailed.

- Lactating women appear to have increased efficiency of energy utilization. The nutritional composition of the milk is not affected greatly by maternal diet unless the mother is extremely undernourished; however, concerns have been expressed about effects on maternal calcium balance and the tendency to develop obesity. Breastfeeding is associated with a reduced risk of maternal breast and ovarian cancer.

- Human milk provides optimal nutrition for the human neonate, which has immature renal, hepatic and gastrointestinal functions and a rapidly developing nervous system. Breastfed babies have a lower incidence of infection.

- Colostrum is the early secretion from the breast; it provides important anti-infective properties and promotes favourable microbial colonization of the gut.

- Protein requirements are relatively low as the human neonate has a relatively slow growth rate. Human milk has a high concentration of whey proteins and non-protein nitrogen components, which include growth factors. The amino acid composition of human milk protein compensates for the neonate's limited ability to convert essential amino acids to nonessential amino acids; the net protein utilization of human milk is high.

- Fat is the main energy source in milk and the most variable constituent. The proportion of fat is higher in hindmilk. The fatty acid composition of human milk allows optimum absorption. Human milk fat is rich in polyunsaturated fatty acids required for development of the brain and nervous system.

- Lactose is the major carbohydrate of milk; it provides energy, aids absorption of other nutrients and promotes an environment which is favourable to beneficial microorganisms.

- Human milk has important immunological properties and is associated with a lower incidence of infections and a persistently more responsive immune system in breastfed babies.

APPLICATION TO PRACTICE

It is consistently shown that breastfeeding provides the best start in life for infants and has short- and long-term health benefits. The midwife is uniquely placed to encourage breastfeeding and influence the overall health of the nation. Midwives must ensure that women are aware of what the health benefits of breastfeeding are for both themselves and their babies. Knowledge of lactation and its benefits are important if the midwife is to promote and support breastfeeding in practice.

Many maternity services are now working towards achieving and maintaining the WHO, UNICEF Baby Friendly initiative. This a set of regularly reviewed and revised, evidence-based standards to actively promote and support parents to give their 'babies the love, care and nourishment they need to get the best possible start in life'. Midwives can use the UNICEF standards in their everyday practice, which provide evidence to support practice and guidelines about appropriate advice and interventions. The standards also enable parents to access, balanced evidence-based material to facilitate informed decisions about feeding and caring for their baby.

Following birth, mothers should be encouraged to offer skin-to-skin contact, ideally within the vicinity of the breasts as soon as possible. Placing the naked baby on the abdominal wall of the mother in close proximity to the breasts will enable the baby to spontaneously root, locate, latch or fix and suckle on the nipple. This is important if the baby is cold following delivery and/or required initial resuscitation following birth. Cold-shocked babies are less likely to feed spontaneously and so skin-to-skin contact is not only efficient in warming babies up, it also gives them comfort. Skin-to-skin contact should continue for as long as possible, ideally until, at least an initial feed has been completed. Women who have received pharmacological drugs during labour will need extra help and support as the baby's spontaneous urge to feed may be reduced.

If mother and baby are well and the mother has chosen to breastfeed, then exclusive breastfeeding should be encouraged with adequate, evidence-based and consistent support. If babies are drowsy or seem disinterested in the breast, then the mother should be encouraged to keep offering the breast. The introduction of formula milk or bottles should be avoided as this interferes with the establishment of lactation.

In the exceptional cases where the baby has difficulty latching on, the mother should be encouraged to hand express and the expressed milk (or harvested colostrum) can be offered to the baby via a small cup or spoon to avoid the infant adapting a modified form of sucking to accommodate a teat and bottle feed, which is different to a breastfeeding suckle.

The midwife must ensure that women who have chosen to bottle feed are aware of the need to ensure all equipment used is sterilized and milk made up is appropriately stored to minimize the risk of infection. The milk must be prepared as directed by the manufacturers as diluted or concentrated mixes are potentially harmful to the neonate. Parents must also be informed of the benefits of breastfeeding and against the potential risks associated with artificial feeding.

ANNOTATED FURTHER READING

Anttila-Hughes JK, Fernald LCH, Gertler PJ, et al.: *Mortality from Nestlé's marketing of infant formula in low and middle-income countries*, Cambridge MA, 2018, National Bureau of Economic Research, Working paper 24452.
An interesting calculation of the costs (as infant deaths) of the intensive and controversial marketing (which has not completely stopped) of breast milk substitutes, based on the annual reports of Nestlé, the largest producer of infant formula.
Campbell SH, Lauwers J, Mannel R, Spencer B: *LEAARC: core curriculum for interdisciplinary lactation care*, London, 2018, Jones and Bartlett.
This is essential reading for practitioners who want to extend their knowledge of breastfeeding and lactation and support women in the establishment of breastfeeding.
Eckenrode J: The three B's: bonding, breastfeeding, and baby friendly, *Int J Childbirth Educ* 33:40–42, 2018.
A short article of useful tips and fascinating facts for health professionals encouraging breastfeeding.
Fomon S: Infant feeding in the 20th century: formula and beikost, *J Nutr* 131(2):409S–420S, 2001.
A history of changing infant feeding practices in the 20th century, including the effects of sanitation, dairying practices and milk handling of home and commercially prepared formulas.
Grayson J: *Unlatched: the evolution of breastfeeding and the making of a controversy*, New York, 2016, HarperCollins.
This book gets to the heart of modern misrepresentations about breastfeeding and why humanity has reached such a level of disconnection from natural breastfeeding.
Kaplin M: *Latch: A handbook for breastfeeding with confidence at every stage*, Emeryville, 2018, Rockridge Press.
This book was primarily written for breastfeeding women and is very woman- and baby-focused.
Karakochuk CD, Whitfield KC, Green TJ, Kraemer K: *The biology of the first 1,000 days*, Boca Raton, 2017, CRC Press.
A comprehensive book of all aspects of early nutrition and its importance to human health, which includes the basic and applied biology; each of the 30 chapters is an up-to-date summary of the topic written by an expert in the field.
Palmer G: *Why the politics of breastfeeding Matter*, London, 2016, Pinter & Martin Ltd.
This book explores the influence of artificial feeding on the population from a global perspective. It discusses social, historical and economic factors affecting a woman's decision to breastfeed and the implications of the type of infant feeding method on health, the environment and the global economy with a particular focus on the pressures put on parents to use alternatives to breast milk.
Rollins NC, Bhandari N, Hajeebhoy N, et al.: Why invest, and what it will take to improve breastfeeding practices? *Lancet* 387:491–504, 2016.
The second of two excellent articles about breastfeeding in the global context. This paper investigates the reasons why breastfeeding practices are not optimal and presents an in-depth discussion of the benefits of breastfeeding to the infant, the mother, the national and global economy and the planet.
Sriraman NK: The nuts and bolts of breastfeeding: anatomy and physiology of lactation, *Curr Probl Pediatr Adolesc Health Care* 47:305–310, 2017.
A comprehensive review of how to apply the understanding of the physiology and anatomy of breastfeeding to support the mother–infant dyad.
UNICEF-WHO: *Capture the moment – early initiation of breastfeeding: the best start for every newborn*, New York, 2018, UNICEF.
A joint report from UNICEF and WHO, which succinctly states the advantages of early initiation of breastfeeding and describes worldwide trends over the last 10 years.
Victora CG, Bahl R, Barros AJD, et al.: Breastfeeding in the 21st century: epidemiology, mechanisms, and lifelong effect, *Lancet* 387:475–490, 2016.
The first in the series of two excellent reviews (see Rollins et al., 2016 above), which articulately presents the case for breastfeeding and considers the current trends and historic patterns breastfeeding throughout the world.
Walker M: *Breastfeeding management for the clinician*, ed 4, London, 2016, Jones and Bartlett. revised.
This book focuses on the clinical and practical management of breastfeeding. This latest revision includes latest guidelines and research applied to practice.
Wambach KG, Riordan J: *Breastfeeding and human lactation*, ed 5, London, 2015, Jones and Bartlett.
A comprehensive text on breastfeeding aimed at midwives, breastfeeding consultants, antenatal teachers, dietitians and nutritionists. Covers cultural aspects, anatomy and physiology, breastfeeding education and practical considerations such as breast pumps, donor milk and breastfeeding the ill child.
Whyatt V: A mother-centred approach to breastfeeding support, *J Health Visit* 6:122–124, 2018.
A practical and thorough article in which the author shares her experiences of supporting breastfeeding women.
Wolf JH: 'They lacked the right food': a brief history of breastfeeding and the quest for social justice, *J Hum Lact* 34:226–231, 2018.

A fascinating account of the issues in the 19th century, which led to breastfeeding social justice campaigns and milk crusades.

REFERENCES

Abrahamse E, Minekus M, van Aken GS, et al.: Development of the digestive system – experimental challenges and approaches of infant lipid digestion, *Food Dig* 3:63–77, 2012.

Anderson PO: Drugs in lactation, *Pharm Res* 35:45, 2018.

Andersson Y, Savman K, Blackberg L, Hernell O: Pasteurization of mother's own milk reduces fat absorption and growth in preterm infants, *Acta Paediatr* 96:1445–1449, 2007.

Anttila-Hughes JK, Fernald LCH, Gertler PJ, et al.: *Mortality from Nestlé's marketing of infant formula in low and middle-income countries*, Cambridge MA, 2018, National Bureau of Economic Research, Working paper 24452.

Bazzano AN, Hofer R, Thibeau S, et al.: A review of herbal and pharmaceutical galactagogues for breast-feeding, *Ochsner J* 16:511–524, 2016.

Birch LL: Learning to eat: behavioral and psychological aspects, *Nestlé Nutr Inst Workshop Ser* 85:125–134, 2016.

Bjorksten B: The hygiene hypothesis: do we still believe in it? *Nestlé Nutr Workshop Ser Pediatr Program* 64:11–18, 2009.

Broadhurst CL, Cunnane SC, Crawford MA: Rift Valley lake fish and shellfish provided brain-specific nutrition for early Homo, *Br J Nutr* 79:3–21, 1998.

Burkart JM, van Schaik C, Griesser M: Looking for unity in diversity: human cooperative childcare in comparative perspective, *Proc Biol Sci* 284(1869), 2017.

Crowley WR: Neuroendocrine regulation of lactation and milk production, *Compr Physiol* 5:255–291, 2015.

Dall SR, Boyd IL: Evolution of mammals: lactation helps mothers to cope with unreliable food supplies, *Proc Biol Sci* 271:2049–2057, 2004.

Davies I, Burman-Roy S, Murphy MS: Gastro-oesophageal reflux disease in children: NICE guidance, *BMJ* 350:g7703, 2015.

Dewey KG: Impact of breastfeeding on maternal nutritional status, *Adv Exp Med Biol* 554:91–100, 2004.

Dold S, Zimmermann MB, Jukic T, et al.: Universal salt iodization provides sufficient dietary iodine to achieve adequate iodine nutrition during the first 1000 days: a cross-sectional multicenter study, *J Nutr* 148:587–598, 2018.

Donovan TJ, Buchanan K: Medications for increasing milk supply in mothers expressing breastmilk for their preterm hospitalised infants, *Cochrane Database Syst Rev*, 3: CD005544, 2012.

Echeverría F, Valenzuela R, Hernandez-Rodas MC, Valenzuela A: Docosahexaenoic acid (DHA), a fundamental fatty acid for the brain: new dietary sources, *Prostaglandins Leukot Essent Fatty Acids* 124:1–10, 2017.

Elad D, Kozlovsky P, Blum O, et al.: Biomechanics of milk extraction during breast-feeding, *Proc Natl Acad Sci USA* 111:5230–5235, 2014.

Fu Y, Liu X, Zhou B, et al.: An updated review of worldwide levels of docosahexaenoic and arachidonic acid in human breast milk by region, *Public Health Nutr* 19:2675–2687, 2016.

Gao X, McMahon RJ, Woo JG, et al.: Temporal changes in milk proteomes reveal developing milk functions, *J Proteome Res* 11:3897–3907, 2012.

Gensollen T, Blumberg RS: Correlation between early-life regulation of the immune system by microbiota and allergy development, *J Allergy Clin Immunol* 139:1084–1091, 2017.

Gordon I, Zagoory-Sharon O, Leckman JF, et al.: Oxytocin and the development of parenting in humans, *Biol Psychiatry* 68:377–382, 2010.

Hartmann PE, Sherriff JL, Mitoulas LR: Homeostatic mechanisms that regulate lactation during energetic stress, *J Nutr* 128:394S–399S, 1998.

Hassiotou F, Geddes D: Anatomy of the human mammary gland: current status of knowledge, *Clin Anat* 26:29–48, 2013.

Heise AM, Wiessinger D: Dysphoric milk ejection reflex: a case report, *Int Breastfeed J* 6:6, 2011.

Ho JCS, Nadeem A, Svanborg C: HAMLET – A protein-lipid complex with broad tumoricidal activity, *Biochem Biophys Res Commun* 482:454–458, 2017.

Hunt KM, Foster JA, Forney LJ, et al.: Characterization of the diversity and temporal stability of bacterial communities in human milk, *PLoS One* 6:e21313, 2011.

Innis SM: Palmitic acid in early human development, *Crit Rev Food Sci Nutr* 56:1952–1959, 2016.

Innis SM: Impact of maternal diet on human milk composition and neurological development of infants, *Am J Clin Nutr* 99:734S–741S, 2014.

Julia V, Macia L, Dombrowicz D: The impact of diet on asthma and allergic diseases, *Nat Rev Immunol* 15:308–322, 2015.

Kent JC, Arthur PG, Mitoulas LR, et al.: Why calcium in breastmilk is independent of maternal dietary calcium and vitamin D, *Breastfeed Rev* 17:5–11, 2009.

Kent JC, Gardner H, Geddes DT: Breastmilk production in the first 4 weeks after birth of term infants, *Nutrients* 8:756, 2016.

Koletzko B, Rodriguez-Palmero M, Demmelmair H, et al.: Physiological aspects of human milk lipids, *Early Hum Dev* 65:S3–S18, 2001.

Kovacs CS: Maternal mineral and bone metabolism during pregnancy, lactation, and post-weaning recovery, *Physiol Rev* 96:449–547, 2016.

Kovacs CS: The skeleton is a storehouse of mineral that is plundered during lactation and (fully?) replenished afterwards, *J Bone Miner Res* 32:676–680, 2017.

Kuzawa CW: Adipose tissue in human infancy and childhood: an evolutionary perspective, *Am J Phys Anthropol* 27:177–209, 1998.

Larsson MW, Lind MV, Larnkjaer A, et al.: Excessive weight gain followed by catch-down in exclusively breastfed infants: an exploratory study, *Nutrients* 10, 2018.

Lau Y, Tha PH, Ho-Lim SST, et al.: An analysis of the effects of intrapartum factors, neonatal characteristics, and skin-to-skin contact on early breastfeeding initiation, *Matern Child Nutr* 14:e12492, 2018.

Lawrence RA, Lawrence RM: Maternal nutrition and supplements for mother and infant. In *Breastfeeding: a guide for the medical profession*, ed 8, St Louis, 2015, Elsevier, pp 285–319.

Lee S, Kelleher SL: Biological underpinnings of breastfeeding challenges: the role of genetics, diet, and environment on lactation physiology, *Am J Physiol Endocrinol Metab* 311:E405–E422, 2016.

Lien EL, Richard C, Hoffman DR: DHA and ARA addition to infant formula: current status and future research directions, *Prostaglandins, Leukot Essent Fatty Acids* 128:26–40, 2018.

Lönnerdal B: Trace element transport in the mammary gland, *Annu Rev Nutr* 27:165–177, 2007.

Lönnerdal B: Bioactive proteins in human milk: health, nutrition, and implications for infant formulas, *J Pediatr* 173:S4–S9, 2016.

Lönnerdal B, Erdmann P, Thakkar SK, et al.: Longitudinal evolution of true protein, amino acids and bioactive proteins in breastmilk: a developmental perspective, *J Nutr Biochem* 41:1–11, 2017.

Marshall NE, Lau B, Purnell JQ, Thornburg KL: Impact of maternal obesity and breastfeeding intention on lactation intensity and duration, *Matern Child Nutr* 15:e12732, 2019.

McNeilly AS: Lactational control of reproduction, *Reprod Fertil Dev* 13(7–8):583–590, 2001.

McCreedy A, Bird S, Brown LJ, et al.: Effects of maternal caffeine consumption on the breastfed child: a systematic review, *Swiss Med Wkly* 148:w14665, 2018.

Mennella JA: Ontogeny of taste preferences: basic biology and implications for health, *Am J Clin Nutr* 99:704S–711S, 2014.

Mohd Shukri NH, Wells JCK, Fewtrell M: The effectiveness of interventions using relaxation therapy to improve breastfeeding outcomes: a systematic review, *Matern Child Nutr* 14:e12563, 2018.

Molinari CE, Casadio YS, Hartmann BT, et al.: Proteome mapping of human skim milk proteins in term and preterm milk, *J Proteome Res* 11:1696–1714, 2012.

Moran VH: Nutrient requirements during lactation. In Karakochuk CD, Whitfield KC, Green TJ, Kraemer K, editors: *The biology of the first 1,000 days*, Boca Raton, 2018, CRC Press, pp 53–74.

Mortel M, Mehta SD: Systematic review of the efficacy of herbal galactogogues, *J Hum Lact* 29:154–162, 2013.

Munoz K, Blaszkewicz M, Campos V, et al.: Exposure of infants to ochratoxin A with breast milk, *Arch Toxicol* 88:837–846, 2014.

Napso T, Yong HEJ, Lopez-Tello J, Sferruzzi-Perri AN: The role of placental hormones in mediating maternal adaptations to support pregnancy and lactation, *Front Physiol* 9:1091, 2018.

Neville MC, McFadden TB, Forsyth I: Hormonal regulation of mammary differentiation and milk secretion, *J Mammary Gland Biol Neoplasia* 7:49–66, 2002.

NICE: *Gastro-oesophageal reflux disease in children and young people: diagnosis and management (Clinical Guideline 1)*, London, 2015, National Institute for Health and Care Excellence.

Nommsen-Rivers LA: Does insulin explain the relation between maternal obesity and poor lactation outcomes? An overview of the literature, *Adv Nutr* 7:407–414, 2016.

Nommsen-Rivers LA, Dewey KG: Growth of breastfed infants, *Breastfeed Med* 4(Suppl 1):S45–S49, 2009.

Ojo-Okunola A, Nicol M, du TE: Human breast milk bacteriome in health and disease, *Nutrients* 10, 2018.

Powe CE, Allen M, Puopolo KM, et al.: Recombinant human prolactin for the treatment of lactation insufficiency, *Clin Endocrinol* 73:645–653, 2010a.

Powe CE, Knott CD, Conklin-Brittain N: Infant sex predicts breast milk energy content, *Am J Hum Biol* 22:50–54, 2010b.

Ramsay DT, Kent JC, Hartmann RL, et al.: Anatomy of the lactating human breast redefined with ultrasound imaging, *J Anat* 206:525–534, 2005.

Rodriguez JM: The origin of human milk bacteria: is there a bacterial entero-mammary pathway during late pregnancy and lactation? *Adv Nutr* 5:779–784, 2014.

Rollins NC, Bhandari N, Hajeebhoy N, et al.: Why invest, and what it will take to improve breastfeeding practices? *Lancet* 387:491–504, 2016.

Safari K, Saeed AA, Hasan SS, Moghaddam-Banaem L: The effect of mother and newborn early skin-to-skin contact on initiation of breastfeeding, newborn temperature and duration of third stage of labor, *Int Breastfeed J* 13:32, 2018.

Schaal B: Mammary odor cues and pheromones: mammalian infant-directed communication about maternal state, mammae, and milk, *Vitam Horm* 83:83–136, 2010.

Schack-Nielsen L, Michaelsen KF: Advances in our understanding of the biology of human milk and its effects on the offspring, *J Nutr* 137:503S–510S, 2007.

Seoane LM, Tovar S, Dieguez C: Physiology of the hypothalamus pituitary unit. In Casanueva FF, Ghigo E, editors: *Hypothalamic-pituitary diseases*, New York, 2018, Springer International, pp 1–33.

Sriraman NK: The nuts and bolts of breastfeeding: anatomy and physiology of lactation, *Curr Probl Pediatr Adolesc Health Care* 47:305–310, 2017.

Stinson LF, Payne MS, Keelan JA: Planting the seed: origins, composition, and postnatal health significance of the fetal gastrointestinal microbiota, *Crit Rev Microbiol* 43:352–369, 2017.

Stoutjesdijk E, Schaafsma A, Dijck-Brouwer DAJ, Muskiet FAJ: Fish oil supplemental dose needed to reach 1g% DHA+EPA in mature milk, *Prostaglandins, Leukot Essent Fatty Acids* 128:53–61, 2018.

Strzepa A, Lobo FM, Majewska-Szczepanik M, Szczepanik M: Antibiotics and autoimmune and allergy diseases: causative factor or treatment? *Int Immunopharmacol* 65:328–341, 2018.

Telang S: Lactoferrin: a critical player in neonatal host defense, *Nutrients* 10, 2018.

Triantis V, Bode L, van Neerven RJJ: Immunological effects of human milk oligosaccharides, *Front Pediatr* 6:190, 2018.

Truchet S, Honvo-Houeto E: Physiology of milk secretion, *Best Pract Res Clin Endocrinol Metab* 31:367–384, 2017.

UNICEF-WHO: *Capture the moment – early initiation of breastfeeding: the best start for every newborn*, New York, 2018, UNICEF.

Victora CG, Bahl R, Barros AJD, et al.: Breastfeeding in the 21st century – epidemiology, mechanisms, and lifelong effect, *Lancet* 387:475–490, 2016.

Walsh J, Tunkel D: Diagnosis and treatment of ankyloglossia in newborns and infants: a review, *JAMA Otolaryngol Head Neck Surg* 143:1032–1039, 2017.

Wilde CJ, Prentice A, Peaker M: Breast-feeding: matching supply with demand in human lactation, *Proc Nutr Soc* 54:401–406, 1995.

Witkowska-Zimny M, Kaminska-El-Hassan E: Cells of human breast milk, *Cell Mol Biol Lett* 22:11, 2017.

A

Ablation   Destruction of small amounts of abnormal tissue

Abortifacient   An agent, usually a drug, which induces abortion

Abrogate   To make less

Achondroplasia   Disorder of bone growth that results in dwarfism

Acidosis   Excessive acid in the blood (due to accumulation of acid or depletion of bicarbonate)

Activin   Protein that positively affects production of FSH

Adipocyte   Fat cell or lipocyte

Aerobic metabolism   The production of ATP via oxidative metabolism (requiring oxygen)

Aetiology   The cause of …

Afferent   Afferent neurons (sensory neurons) carry sensory stimuli towards the CNS. Afferent arterioles supply blood to the nephrons in the kidney

Afterpains   Painful uterine contractions experienced after birth of the infant

Agonist   A substance that interacts with a receptor molecule that initiates the same response as the hormone/transmitter usually binding to that site

Aliphatic   An organic compound that contains carbon atoms arranged in a chain rather than a ring formation

Alkalosis   Excessive blood/tissue alkalinity caused by excess bicarbonate or decreased carbon dioxide

Allele   Variant form of a gene

Alloantigens   An antigen present in some individuals which might provoke an immune response in others

Allograft   Transplanted tissue that is of different genetic origin to the donor

Alopecia   The loss of body and scalp hair

Altriciality   The inability of newborns to move around so that nursing is required

Alveolus   Air sac of lung or milk sac of breast

Amenorrhoea   Absence of menstrual cycles

Amniocentesis   Removal of a small volume of amniotic fluid for genetic analysis or infection tests of the fetus

Amoeboid   Appearing and behaving like the large single-celled organism called an amoeba

Amplitude   The difference between the highest and lowest measurement within a regular cycle

Ampulla   A widened region of a duct or tube

Amygdala   A group of neurons in the medial temporal lobe of the brain

Anabolic metabolism   The synthesis of biological compounds involving the expenditure of energy

Anaerobic metabolism   The production of ATP in the absence of oxygen

Analgesic   A drug that relieves pain

Anastomosis   Connection of two tubes, vessels, etc., ensuring that the lumen remains patent between them

Androsperm   A sperm carrying a Y chromosome

Aneuploidy   Presence of an abnormal number of chromosomes

Angiogenesis   The formation of new blood vessels

Anisogamy   Sexual reproduction involving fusion of morphologically dissimilar gametes

Ankyloglossia   Tongue-tie; congenital anomaly that affects mobility of the tongue

Anorexic   Without appetite

Antagonist   A substance that blocks receptor sites and then inhibits any further responses

Anteflexed   Curved inwards

Anteverted   Folded over

Antibody (immunoglobulin)   A large 'Y'-shaped protein that recognises an antigen as part of the immune response; synthesized by B lymphocytes

Antigen   A molecular structure that initiates the immune response

Anti-tocolytic   Drugs that promote labour

Antral   A cavity within the body

Apoptosis   Programmed cell death

Apposition   Positioning close together

Aquatic   Pertaining to an underwater environment

Arborize   To grow in a branch-like formation

Areola   Ring of pigmented skin surrounding the nipple

Aromatase   An enzyme involved in the conversion of an androgen to oestrogen

Arteriosclerosis   Thickening and hardening of arterial walls, age-related

Asphyxia   Deficient oxygen delivery to the body (e.g. from choking) that can cause unconsciousness or death

Asynclitism   To be tilted laterally on either side of the anterior/posterior mid-plane; oblique malpresentation

Atherosclerosis   Narrowing of arteries due to a build-up of plaque

Atony   Loss of muscle strength or tone

Atresia   The abnormal narrowing or closure of the lumen in a tube or vessel

Atretic   Having the characteristics of or pertaining to atresia; without an opening

Atrophy   Decreased function due to cell and tissue loss (hypoplasia) with increasing age

Attenuated   Modified to have less of an effect than normal

Auscultation   Listening to internal body sounds, usually by using a stethoscope

Autocrine   A signalling molecule, which affects the cell that secretes it

Autoimmune   When the immune system attacks a person's own tissues

Autolysis   Destruction of a cell by its own enzymes (self-digestion)

Autophagy   Degradation of cellular components by lysosomes

Autosome   A chromosome that is not a sex chromosome

Azoospermic   Semen that contain no sperm

B

Bactericidal   Containing substances that can kill bacteria

Bacteriostatic   Containing substances that inhibit the reproduction of bacteria

Bariatric   Specializing in the causes, prevention and treatment of obesity

Basal metabolic rate   The amount of energy expenditure required for the maintenance of essential body function only

Behaviour   The study of how organisms interact within the environment

513

Benign A tumour which is not malignant (noncancerous)

Bioavailability (of a nutrient or drug) Proportion of the agent that is absorbed and available to have an effect

Biosynthesis The manufacture of body tissues and substances

Bradycardia Slow heart rate

Breech Pertaining to the fetal rump

Bronchiolitis Infection, usually viral, affecting the bronchioles (small airways)

C

Carotenoid Naturally occurring fat-soluble pigment that colours plants red, yellow, orange or brown

Catabolic metabolism The breakdown of compounds into smaller units usually resulting in the release of energy

Centrioles A pair of minute organelles, which organize the spindle microtubules for chromosome separation in cell division

Centromere Part of the chromosome that attaches to the spindle fibres

Cephalic Pertaining to the head

Cervical dystocia Difficult labour/delivery due to cervix being mechanically obstructed

Chemoattractant A substance that attracts motile cells

Chemosensor A molecule or receptor, which recognizes a particular substance

Chemostasis The maintenance of a chemical balance

Chemotaxis Movement of cells towards a particular chemical signal

Chemotherapy Use of selectively cytotoxic drugs to treat disease, particularly cancer

Chiasmata (singular: chiasma) Where paired chromosomes come into contact and exchange genetic material during meiosis

Cholecalciferol Vitamin D_3, form of vitamin D, which is synthesized in the skin when exposed to ultraviolet light

Chorioamnionitis Infection of the chorion and amnion during pregnancy

Choriocarcinoma Aggressive tumour originating from abnormal placental tissue (e.g. hydatidiform mole)

Cilia Tiny hairlike projections of the plasma membrane in some cell types, which are motile, causing fluid movement

Circadian About 1 day

Climacteric Period of declining fertility leading to menopause

Clonal expansion Rapid production of identical daughter cells from a single cell or lymphocyte as part of the immune response

Cloning Generation of organisms with identical genomes

Co-dominant Expression of both of two differing alleles in the phenotype when present in the genotype

Coitus The act of sexual intercourse

Colloid A protein suspended in a liquid

Colostrum First form of milk produced immediately after birth of the infant, low volume with a high concentration of antibodies and nutrients

Commensal microorganisms Single-celled species, including fungi, archaea, viruses and mainly bacteria, which live in body tissues (particularly the gut) and have many beneficial roles

Complementary feeding Weaning; addition of foods other than milk to an infant's diet

Conceptus The products of conception (embryo, fetus, placenta, etc.) at any stage of development

Congenital (of an abnormality or disease) Present from birth

Conjugation The addition of a chemical moiety, often changing the function and activity of the original substance

Contraception Prevention of pregnancy by intervention

Corpus albicans 'white body' ovarian scar tissue composed of collagen that forms when the corpus luteum degenerates

Corpus luteum 'Yellow body' ovarian structure that secretes hormones; forms from the follicular cells after the ovum has been released

Cortex The outer tissue layer or part of a structure

Cranial Pertaining to the skull

Craniofacial Pertaining to the bones of the skull and face

Cryopreservation Preservation of living cells and tissues using controlled freezing techniques

Cumulus 'Cloud-like' cluster of follicular cells surrounding the ovum when it is released

Cyanosis The bluish appearance of body tissues in situations of hypoxia

Cyclical Repeated on a regular basis

Cytoplasm The intracellular contents contained within the cell membrane. Contents of the cell, excluding the nucleus

Cytotoxic A chemical, drug or other cell type that can kill cells

D

Decidualization The formation of the decidua of pregnancy

Defensins Small antimicrobial polypeptides produced by immune cells and other cell types

Deletion The loss of part of a chromosome

Dermatome Area of skin supplied by a single spinal nerve; derived from segmental development during the embryonic stage

Desaturate Formation of a double bond in a fatty acid

Desquamation The loss of the outer layers of a continuously growing squamous tissue

Detumescence Reduction of swelling or engorgement (e.g. of penis)

Diapedesis The passage of blood cells through the blood vessel wall into the surrounding tissue

Diastasis recti The separation of the two sides of the abdominal muscles

Diastolic The period of relaxation of the ventricles of the heart

Diathermy Medical/surgical procedure using heat or electromagnetic currents

Dichrotic A notch observed on the downstroke of the arterial pressure waveform that indicates the closure of the aortic valve

Dictyate Resting phase of meiosis I of oogenesis occurring from fetal life to just before ovulation

Differentiation Process of specialisation of cells for different functions

Dimorphism The existence of an organism in distinct forms such as male and female

Diploid The normal number of paired chromosomes

Discoid Disc-like

Dispensable (amino acid) Nonessential amino acid, which can be synthesized by the body

Distal Furthest part

Diuresis Production of urine

Diurnal Over a period of 1 day

Dizygotic Embryos and fetuses derived from different ova (fraternal)

Dorsal Pertaining to the back

Downregulation A decrease in secretion of a product or expression of a protein or receptor

Dysbiosis Imbalance in the composition, e.g. of gut microbial species

Dysgenesis Abnormal formation

Dyslipidaemia Abnormal level of lipids (triglycerides, cholesterol and phospholipids) in the blood

Dysmenorrhoea Pain associated with menstruation

Dyspareunia Painful or difficult sexual intercourse

Dysphoria State of profound unease or dissatisfaction

Dyspnoea Difficult or laboured breathing

E

Echogenicity Reflection of an ultrasound wave

Ectopic pregnancy Implantation occurs outside the uterine cavity, usually in a uterine tube

Effacement Softening and thinning of the cervix at parturition

Efferent Efferent neurons (motor neurons) carry stimuli from the CNS to effector tissues (e.g. muscle). Efferent arterioles supply blood to the glomeruli in the kidney

Effusion Accumulation of fluid

Electrolyte Substance that dissociates into ions in solution and can conduct an electrical charge

Elongate (fatty acid) Addition of two carbon atoms

Embolism Materials that cause blockage of blood vessels

Embryogenesis Formation and development of an embryo

Encephalopathy Damage to the brain that affects function and/or structure

Endocrine Pertaining to the secretion of hormones into the blood

Endocytosis The process by which substances are transported into the cell within envelopes formed out of the outer cell membrane

Endogenous Pertaining to the internal physiological environment

Endometriosis Disorder resulting from the abnormal deposition of endometrial tissue at locations outside of the uterus

Endometritis Inflammation of the endometrium

Endometrium Lining of the uterus

Endothermic (animal) Dependant on internal generation of heat (warm-blooded)

Enterocolitis Inflammation of the gut

Entrained Reset by an external factor

Enzyme A protein that is able to speed up a chemical reaction without being structurally altered by the process itself

Epidural Injection of drugs such as anaesthetics into the epidural space around the spinal cord

Epigastric Upper and central region of the abdomen

Epigenetic Changes (which can be inherited) in the expression but not the presence of genes

Episiotomy Surgical incision of the perineum, usually performed to enlarge the vaginal orifice and facilitate delivery of the infant

Epitope An antigenic determinant that evokes an immune response

Ergocalciferol Vitamin D_2, form of vitamin D found in foods of plant origin (and supplements)

Ergometrine A drug derived from alkaloids of ergot that causes a sustained, strong contraction of the myometrium

Erythropoiesis The production of red blood cells (erythrocytes)

Erythropoietin A hormone produced chiefly by the kidneys (in the adult) and by the liver (in the fetus) that initiates red blood cell production

Eugenics The science aimed at producing the perfect individual

Euploidic Contains the normal number of chromosomes

Euthyroid Normal functioning thyroid gland

Evolution The study of genetic variation and change within generations of populations

Exocrine Pertaining to glands that secrete their products into a duct

Exogenous Pertaining to the external environment

Exomphalos Weakness of the abdominal wall in the fetus, which may allow the abdominal organs to protrude

Extended Tilted away

Extracellular matrix The arrangement of extracellular proteins and glycoproteins, which supports cellular integrity

F

Fecundability The probability that a woman will conceive within a certain time period

Fibrinolysis Breakdown of fibrin in blood clots

Fibroblasts Cells that synthesize the collagen and extracellular matrix of connective tissue

Fight-or-flight response The activation of the sympathetic nervous system in response to danger or stress to stimulate body processes to maximize survival

Fimbria/fimbriae The finger-like fringe of tissue at the end of the uterine ducts

Flexed Tilted towards

Follicle Tissue structure that is fluid-filled

Free radical A highly-reactive oxygen-containing molecule which has an unpaired electron

Frenulotomy Surgical procedure to correct ankyloglossia (tongue-tie)

Fundus Part of an organ, e.g. uterus, furthest away from the opening (cervix)

G

Galactopoiesis Maintenance of lactation or milk production once it has been initiated

Gametogenesis The formation of gametes

Gap junctions Junctions between adjacent cells, which allow low molecular weight molecules or ions to pass, to 'orchestrate' cell responses

Gastrulation The formation of the inner layers of the embryo by cell migration in a process of invagination

Gene manipulation The process of modifying gene content or gene sequence to effect a change in a cell or organism

Gene pool The total number of genes within a population

Genome The total number of genes within a single organism

Genotype Set of genes of the organism, responsible for a trait

Glucocorticoids Class of corticosteroids produced by the adrenal gland, which have immunosuppressive and anti-inflammatory activities

Gluconeogenesis The synthesis of glucose from noncarbohydrate sources

Glucosaemia Glucose in blood

Glucosuria Excretion of glucose into urine

GLUT A member of the glucose transporter family

Glycogenolysis Breakdown of glycogen stores in the liver to allow release of glucose into the blood (or in muscle where free glucose produced is used by the myocytes)

Glycolysis The major pathway by which glucose is metabolized

Glycoprotein A protein containing carbohydrate groups, which modify protein structure and function

Gonadotroph Cells of the pituitary gland, which produce gonadotrophins

Gonadotrophin Luteinizing hormone and follicle-stimulating hormone

Graft rejection The rejection of donor tissue by the recipient's immune system

Grey matter of the brain Unmyelinated axons, nuclei and dendrites in the brain

Gynosperm A sperm carrying an X chromosome

H

Haemangioma Collection of small blood vessels under the skin that form a lump (birthmark)

Haematocrit Ratio of red blood cell volume as a proportion of the total blood

Haematospermia The presence of blood in ejaculated semen

Haemochromatosis Genetic disorder of iron transport resulting in iron overload

Haemodilution Increase in plasma volume resulting in a lower concentration of red blood cells, plasma proteins, etc.

Haemoglobinopathy Inherited condition involving the formation of abnormal haemoglobin

Haemolytic Pertaining to the destruction or rupture of red blood cells

Haemopoiesis/Haematopoiesis The production of the different blood cell types

Haemoptysis The presence of blood in sputum

Haemostasis Processes causing bleeding to stop

Half-life The time taken for the reduction by half of the quantity present

Haploid Half of the normal chromosome number (containing only one from each pair of autosomes plus an X or Y)

Hepatitis Inflammation of the liver, often caused by viral infection

Hepcidin Antibacterial protein from liver, which regulates absorption and availability of iron

Herd immunity Protection against the spread of infection when a large enough percentage of the population is immune or vaccinated; the percentage varies with different infections

Hermaphroditism The presence of male and female sex organs within the same individual

Heterozygous Alleles at a particular locus of paired chromosomes each coding for a different phenotype

Hirsutism The presence of excess body hair

Histocompatibility Sufficient similarity between 'self antigens' to allow transplantation of tissue between individuals without immune rejection

Homeobox A conserved DNA sequence present in genes that encode proteins that regulate transcription

Homeostasis Maintenance of a relatively stable internal environment to optimize physiological functions

Homeothermic An organism that maintains a constant body temperature whatever the environmental temperature

Homologous Similar chromosomal or internal structures

Homozygous Having two identical alleles both coding for a particular gene which codes for the same protein function

Humoral immune response The immune mechanisms that are mediated by molecules present or released into blood and other extracellular fluids; these include antibodies

Hydatidiform mole Abnormal growth from a fertilized egg or from the placenta

Hydrolysis Breakdown of a compound in a reaction with water

Hydrophilic Has affinity for water

Hydroxylation The addition of a hydroxyl (-OH) group to a compound

Hygiene hypothesis The hypothesis that the lack of exposure of a child to infectious agents, microorganisms, etc., suppresses the normal development of the immune system and increases susceptibility to allergic diseases

Hyper/hypoglycaemia Abnormally high/low level of glucose within the blood

Hyperaemia An excessive volume of blood

Hyperandrogenism Excess of androgens

Hyperbilirubinaemia Abnormally high level of bilirubin in blood; may result in jaundice

Hypercapnia Raised levels of carbon dioxide in the blood

Hypercholesterolaemia A high level of cholesterol in the blood

Hypercoagulability Predisposition for blood to coagulate, which increases the risk of thrombosis

Hyperemesis gravidarum Severe nausea and vomiting during pregnancy

Hyperlipidaemia Elevated levels of lipids or lipoproteins in blood

Hypernatraemia Abnormally high level of sodium in the blood

Hyperphagia Abnormally increased appetite

Hyperplasia An increase in cell number within a tissue

Hyperprolactinaemia Abnormally raised levels of the hormone prolactin

Hypersensitivity The response of the immune system to harmless molecules such as in allergies or autoimmunity

Hypertrophy An increase in cell size

Hyperventilation Prolonged and rapid breathing resulting in alkalosis

Hypogonadism Decreased function of the gonads, usually due to deceased hormone levels of testosterone (males) or LH/FSH (females)

Hypokalaemia Deficiency of potassium in the blood

Hyponatremia Abnormally low sodium levels in blood

Hypophysectomy Surgical removal of the pituitary gland

Hypotonia Abnormally low muscle tone

Hypovolaemia Loss of body fluids

Hypoxia Deprivation of oxygen

I

Iatrogenic Effects caused by a medication or medical treatment rather than the disease

Immunocompetence The ability of a B or T lymphocyte to recognize a specific antigen

Immunocytochemistry Use of a labelled antibody to localize a component within cells or tissues using microscopy

Immunoglobulins A family of large glycoproteins also termed 'antibodies'

Immunosuppression Suppression of the immune system, e.g. by drugs, to allow tissue transplantation or as a consequence of diseases such as HIV/AIDS

Imprinting (genomic) Phenomenon causing gene expression to be switched on or off

Indispensable Essential

Infarction Inadequate blood supply to a tissue, which causes necrosis or tissue death

Inflammation A normal component of the immune response, and also a cause and consequence of disease

Inhibin Peptide hormone, which inhibits the production of FSH from the anterior pituitary gland

Innate Present from birth, congenital, e.g. a behaviour pattern that is not learnt but is instinctive

Interstitial The fluid-filled spaces within or between tissues

Intrinsic A natural component

Invaginate To fold inwards to form a pouch

Inversion Rearrangement of chromosomal material following a break in which a segment of a chromosome is reversed end to end

Involution Return to normal size (or shrinking) of an organ (e.g. of uterus after childbirth)

Ionophore A lipid soluble chemical, which allows the movement of specific ions across cell membranes

Ischaemia Reduction of blood supply to a tissue or organ which may compromise function

Isoenzyme Form of an enzyme with the same function but different structure to another enzyme, may have different kinetics or regulation

Isoimmunized Production of an immune response against tissue from another person

J

Juxtacrine signalling Signalling between cells that are in close contact

K

Karyotype Set of chromosomes in nucleus of a eukaryotic cell (or organism)

Keratinized Containing the protein keratin

Kernicterus Brain damage due to excess bilirubin accumulating in grey matter of brain and nervous system

Ketonuria Elevated levels of ketone bodies in urine

Ketotic Detectable amounts of ketone bodies present indicating that metabolism of fats is occurring

L

Lactobacilli Bacteria, which converts sugars to lactic acid; important component of the body's microbiota

Lactobezoar Indigestible mass of milk protein and mucus, which gets trapped in the gut (usually of premature infant being fed formula milk)

Lactogenesis Physiological changes, which transform nonsecretory mammary epithelial cells into secretory cells

Lectin Proteins that bind to carbohydrates with a high specificity for particular sugar moieties

Libido Desire for sexual activity

Ligation Surgical procedure of tying a thread around a duct or blood vessel to create a permanent blockage

Lipogenesis Synthesis of triglycerides

Lipolysis The hydrolysis (breakdown) of triglycerides into fatty acids and glycerol

Lipophilic A high affinity for lipids, which facilitates diffusion across cell membranes

Lipoprotein A water soluble protein shell, packed with hydrophobic lipids such as triglycerides and cholesterol

Lipoprotein lipase Enzyme, usually located on the capillary endothelial cells, which breaks down triglycerides

Lochia Vaginal discharge of blood, mucus and endometrial tissue produced after childbirth

Lordosis Inward curve of the spine, which may be pronounced during pregnancy

Luteinization Conversion of the follicular cells after ovulation into the corpus luteum

Luteolysis The degradation and regression of the corpus luteum

M

Macromolecules Large organic compounds

Macronutrients Dietary components (carbohydrate, fat and protein) consumed in large amounts, which can be used as a substrate for energy (ATP) production

Macrosomia Larger than normal body size

Malnutrition Condition due to poor nutrition (nutrient deficiency, excess or imbalance)

Maturation The achievement of full function following a period of growth and/or development

Meconium First faeces of the newborn, which is sometimes also passed, in late pregnancy, into amniotic fluid

Medulla The central part of a tissue or organ

Meiosis Cell division that results in haploid cells (gametes)

Menarche The commencement of the menstrual cycles

Menopause The cessation of the menstrual cycles

Menses The period of shedding of the endometrium during the menstrual cycle

Mentum Pertaining to the fetal chin

Methylation The addition of a methyl group ($-CH_3$) to a molecule

Microbiome The genetic material of the microorganisms (microbiota)

Microbiota The microorganisms (bacteria, fungi, viruses, etc.) of a particular environment

Microcephaly Impaired brain development resulting in a smaller than normal head

Microdeletion Deletion of DNA base-pairs from a chromosome, which may affect several genes and cause genetic disorders

Micronutrients Substances (vitamins and minerals) required in small amounts for normal growth and development; are not oxidized for energy production

Microvilli Projections of the cell membrane present in some cell types, which dramatically increase the surface area

Micturition The voiding of urine

Mitogen A substance that initiates the process of mitosis

Mitogenic Induction of mitosis

Mitosis Cell division resulting in two daughter cells, which have the same diploid chromosome complement as the parent cell

Mittelschmerz 'Middle pain'

Monoclonal antibody An antibody, which recognizes specifically one antigenic determinant or epitope

Monozygotic Siblings (e.g. twins) that develop from one fertilized oocyte (zygote)

Morphogenesis The formation of body structure

Morphology The structure or shape of a tissue

Multigravidae A woman who has been pregnant more than once

Multiparous Having experienced previous childbirth

Mutation Permanent alteration of DNA sequence that comprises a gene

Myometrium Middle smooth muscular layer of the uterine wall

N

Necrosis Cell death, which results from injury and damage

Neocortex A region of the cerebral cortex, which is involved in higher functions

Neoplasia Abnormal cell division or turnover giving rise to benign or cancerous tissue growth

Neurogenic Caused by or associated with the nervous system

Neuroleptic Tranquilizing drug

Neuromuscular Associated with the muscles of the body and the nerves that control them

Neuronal Pertaining to the nervous system

Neurotransmitter A chemical that crosses a synapse to initiate an action potential in the post-synaptic neuron or muscle cell

Neurulation The embryonic formation of the neural tube from the neural plate

Nidation The process of implantation of the blastocyst into the uterine endometrium

Nitric oxide (NO) Compound produced by blood vessel endothelial cells, which has vasodilatory effects and thus increases blood flow

Nocturia The need to void urine frequently at night

Nomenclature Terminology describing systematic naming

Nondisjunction Failure of chromosomes or chromatids to separate correctly during anaphase in mitosis or meiosis

Nonesterified fatty acids Free fatty acids

Non-self Antigens in pathogens or other tissues, which are recognized by the immune system as not our own

Non-trophic hormones Hormones that directly stimulate target cells rather than acting via an intermediate hormone (tropic)

Nuchal thickness Ultrasound measurement of the nuchal fold of skin, which is used to assess the probability of fetal abnormalities such as aneuploidy

Nuchal translucency Ultrasound measurement of the fluid accumulated in the neck of the fetus, which is used to assess the probability of cardiovascular abnormalities and chromosome disorders

O

Obesity State of having excessive body fat, which is likely to compromise health

Occiput A bone at the posterior lower part of the skull

Oedema Excess fluid accumulation in the extracellular compartments or body cavities

Oligosaccharide Carbohydrate polymer composed of 3–10 monosaccharide subunits

Omphalocele A birth defect, which results in the offspring's intestine protruding outside the body near the navel region

Oocyte The female gamete arising from the ovary

Oogenesis Development of an ovum capable of being fertilized

Oophorectomy Surgical removal of one or both ovaries

Operculum Protective plug of mucus that blocks the cervix during pregnancy

Opsonin An antibody or other molecule, which is used to tag an antigen to improve its recognition and destruction by the immune system

Orchitis Inflammation of the testes

Orexia Appetite

Osmosis Passive diffusion of water through a cell membrane towards the higher solute concentration (osmolarity)

Osteoblast Bone cell that produces the matrix that will be mineralized during the synthesis of bone

Osteoclast Large multinucleated bone cell that produces digestive enzymes and breaks down bone

Ovariectomy Surgical removal of one or both ovaries

Oxidation The addition of oxygen to a molecule

Oxidative stress Exposure of cells and tissues to damaging free radicals

P

Palpation Use of the hands and fingers to examine the body by touch and feel

Palpebral Pertaining to the eyelids

Pandemic The spread of disease across multiple countries or continents

Paracrine The effects of hormones and other signals on local tissues via diffusion, rather than via circulation

Parthenogenesis Development of an embryo (parthenote) without the need for fertilization

Partogram A graph showing maternal and fetal measurements recorded during labour

Pathogen A foreign organism that causes harm

Penile Pertaining to the penis

Peptidoglycans Structural polymer comprised of sugars and amino acids, present in bacterial cell walls

Perfusion The flow of blood or other fluids through blood vessels and extracellular fluids

Periconceptual Encompassing the period before conception through early pregnancy

Perineum The area of tissue between the anus and vulva (or scrotum)

Peristalsis Contraction and relaxation of smooth muscle in the intestinal wall that moves luminal contents through the GI tract

Peristaltic Coordinated contraction of smooth muscle around the lumen of a tube or vessel that facilitates the unidirectional movement of the contents within the lumen

Perivitelline space The fluid filled space between the oocyte and the zona pellucida

Phagocytosis The ingestion of foreign material by phagocytes

Phenotype Observed characteristics of an individual due to expression of the genotype and interaction with environmental factors

Phenylketonuria Inborn error of metabolism caused by low expression of phenylalanine hydroxylase, so that phenylalanine is not metabolized normally and builds up, affecting cerebral function and brain development

Pheromone A substance released by an animal into its environment, which has effects on other animals

Philtrum Vertical grove or depression between the upper lip and base of the nose

Phimosis Inability to retract the foreskin past the glans penis

Phosphorylation   The addition of a phosphate group to a molecule which often changes structure and function

Photoperiod   The period of natural daylight exposure

Phytoestrogen   Plant-derived compound, which has oestrogenic properties

Pica   Abnormal appetite or craving for non-nutritious substances (paper, ice, earth, etc.)

Pilonidal   Cyst often containing hair, commonly occurring between the buttocks

Placebo   An inert/harmless substance that has no pharmacological effect, used in double-blind trials in comparison with drugs to assess their clinical effectiveness

Placentation   The formation of the fetal and maternal components of the placenta

Placentome   A lobe of the placenta

Poikilotherm   A cold-blooded animal (which can only regulate its body temperature by changing behaviour)

Polar body   One of two tiny cells that bud off the oocyte during the asymmetrical divisions of meiosis

Polycythaema   An abnormally high number of red blood cells

Polyhydramnios   An excess of amniotic fluid in the amniotic sac

Polyploidy   Cells or organisms containing more than two copies of each chromosome

Polyspermy   Fertilization of an oocyte by more than one sperm

Postprandial   The period following the consumption of a meal

Preantral   Before the antral phase

Preconceptual   Before fertilization

Precursor   A substance that is altered into another substance

Primigravida   A woman who is pregnant for the first time

Primiparous   A woman who has given birth for the first time

Primordial   Existing from the beginning

Progestagen   Synthetic analogues of the hormone progesterone, which has similar effects

Prohormone   A hormone precursor, which is chemically modified to form the active hormone

Proliferative   The ability to increase quickly in numbers

Pronucleus   One of two haploid structures resulting from fertilization, which fuse to form the nucleus of the zygote

Prophylactic   An agent used to prevent disease

Prophylaxis   Treatment aimed at prevention rather than cure

Proprioception   Perception of the position and movement of parts of the body

Prostanoid   A subclass of eicosanoid signalling molecules that includes prostaglandins, prostacyclins and thromboxanes

Prostate-specific antigens (PSA)   A protein produced by the normal and malignant prostate gland, which can be measured in blood as a marker for benign or cancerous prostate enlargement

Proteinuria   Abnormal levels of protein in the urine

Proteolytic   Pertaining to protein breakdown

Proximal   Situated close to

Pruritus   Itching of skin

Pseudopodia   A temporary protrusion in the cell membrane

Psychogenic   The development of the mind

Ptyalism   Real or perceived hypersalivation

Puerperium   Period of about 6 weeks following childbirth when the uterus and other systems return to their nonpregnant state

Pulsatile   Released episodically rather than continuously

Pyrexia   An abnormally high body temperature

Q

Quiescence   A state of inactivity

R

Rate-limiting   A step in the metabolic pathway that regulates or restricts the metabolic flow

Receptor   A molecule that combines with a chemical signal that initiates a response within the cell

Relactation   Induced lactation usually in a woman who did not give birth to the infant she intends to feed

Resection   Surgical removal of tissue of part of an organ

Rete testis   A network of tubules in the testicle, which carries sperm from the seminiferous tubules to the efferent ducts

Reticulocyte   An immature red blood cell

Retrograde   Moving backwards in the opposite way to normal

Rhinitis   Allergic or nonallergic inflammation of the mucous membrane in the nose, causing sneezing and congestion

Rubella   German measles; an infection caused by the rubella virus

S

Sacrum   Triangular shaped bone formed by the fusion of the sacral vertebrae

Sarcomere   Structural unit of a myofibril of skeletal muscle

Sebaceous   Pertaining to a sebaceous gland or its secretion

Second-messenger   Intracellular signals generated by receptor activation on the cell surface to regulate cell function at intracellular sites

Senescence   Age-related deterioration of function

Septum   A structure that divides the body or body area/organ (plural Septa)

Sinciput   Pertaining to the fetal forehead

Single nucleotide polymorphism (SNP)   Common type of DNA sequence variation

Sinus   Cavity in a tissue (or relating to the sinoatrial node of the heart)

Sinusoid   An irregularly shaped vessel carrying blood through tissues (e.g. liver)

Specific gravity   The density of a substance relative to pure water

Spermatogenesis   Male gamete formation

Spermatozoa   The male gamete (plural)

Sphincter   A ring of muscle that can occlude a tube or vessel when contracted

Squamous   Description of cells organized as thin flat plates, giving a scaly appearance

Steroidogenesis   The metabolic production of steroids

Stroma   The structural framework of a cell or organ

Suppository   A medical preparation, which can be inserted into the rectum or vagina where it dissolves to release its active components

Surfactant   Substance that lowers the surface tension between different components of a mixture, such as liquids, solids and gases, to allow these to disperse

Symbiosis   Mutually beneficial relationship between two different organisms

Symphysis pubis   Joint of cartilage between the public bones

Syncytium   A mass of cells, in which the cellular membranes have broken down forming a multi-nucleated cytoplasmic mass

Synergistic   Producing a greater combined effect than expected

Syngamy   The fusion of two gametes, which results from fertilization

Syntocinon   A synthetic analogue of naturally occurring oxytocin, used in obstetrics as a pharmacological method of augmenting uterine contractions via a controlled intravenous infusion

T

Tachycardia   Resting heart rate that is too rapid (e.g. >100 beats/min)

Tachypnoea   Abnormally rapid rate of breathing

Tactile   Pertaining to touch

Talipes   'Clubfoot'; a birth defect in which one or both feet are turned inwards and downwards

Telomere   Repetitive nucleotide sequence at the end of a chromosome, which protects it from loss of genes and fusing with another chromosome; length declines with age

Teratogen   A chemical that interferes with normal embryonic or fetal development and may cause birth defects

Thermogenesis   Production of heat by the body

Thermostasis   The maintenance of a constant body temperature

Thromboembolism   Formation of a blood clot that breaks away from its original site and plugs another blood vessel

Thrombophlebitis   Inflammation, usually in a vein, following the formation of a thrombus

Thrombus   Blood clot formed in a blood vessel, which occludes blood flow

Thyroiditis   Inflammation of the thyroid gland

Thyrotoxicosis   Condition (e.g. hyperthyroidism) due to excessive thyroid hormone production

Tocolytic   An medication, which supresses contractions and premature labour

Tolerogenic   The tolerance mechanisms by which dendritic cells suppress an immune response

Totipotent   A cell from the first few cell divisions of the zygote that has the capability to give rise to all cell types of the embryo, fetus and adult, as well as the extraembryonic tissues (e.g. placenta)

Transcription   The process of synthesizing mRNA from a DNA template

Transgenic   Transfer of genetic material into an organism either naturally or by genetic engineering

Translation   The process of forming an amino acid sequence from the genetic code carried by mRNA

Transudation   Blood plasma that collects within the interstitial space

Triploidy   Having an extra set of chromosomes (total of 69 in humans)

Trisomy   Having an extra copy of a chromosome (e.g. total of 47 in humans causing a developmental abnormality such as Down syndrome in trisomy 21)

Trophic   A hormone that has its effects indirectly by stimulating hormone secretion from another endocrine gland

Tubercle   Small nodule or protuberance

U

Ubiquitin   A small protein present in all eukaryotic cells (ubiquitous), which tags proteins for degradation by the proteosome system

Umbilicus   Navel ('belly button')

Undernutrition   Condition due to inadequate nutrient intake

Unicellular   A single cell organism

Urethritis   Inflammation of the urethra, which carries urine from the bladder for excretion; frequently a result of infection

Uterotonins   Substances that encourage the myometrium to contract

Uterotrophic   Has an effect on the growth of the uterus

V

Vasa efferentia   Ducts that transport sperm from the rete testis to the epididymis

Vascularization   The growth of blood vessels into tissue

Vascularized   Perfused by blood vessels

Vasoactive   Has an effect on vascular smooth muscle

Vasoconstriction   Contraction of smooth muscle of a blood vessel to decrease blood flow

Vasodilation   Relaxation of smooth muscle of a blood vessel to increase blood flow

Ventral   Pertaining to the front

Vestigial   A physical characteristic (structure) in evolutionary decline, i.e. remaining present but no longer necessary for survival

Villi (singular Villus)   Finger-like projections from epithelial sheets to increase surface area

Viraemia   Presence of viruses in the bloodstream allowing widespread access to body tissues

Volatile   Evaporates at ambient temperatures

W

White matter of brain   Bundles of myelinated axons within the brain

X

Xenobiotic   A 'foreign' chemical present in the body that is not naturally produced

Z

Zygote   A totipotent cell formed from the fusion of male and a female gamete

Zymosan   A protein–carbohydrate complex on the surface of fungi, which triggers an immune response

INDEX

Note: Page numbers followed by "f" indicate figures, "t" indicate tables and "b" indicate boxes.